ATLAS OF MINIMALLY INVASIVE SURGICAL OPERATIONS

NOTICE

ATLAS OF MINIMALLY INVASIVE SURGICAL OPERATIONS

Edited By

John G. Hunter, MD, FACS, FRCS Edin (hon)

Executive Vice President and Chief Executive Officer

Oregon Health and Science University (OHSU) Health System

Mackenzie Professor of Surgery, OHSU School of Medicine

Portland, Oregon

Donn H. Spight, MD, FACS, FASMBS

Associate Professor of Surgery

School of Medicine

Oregon Health and Science University

Portland, Oregon, USA

Illustrated By

Corinne Sandone, MA, CMI, FAMI

Certified Medical Illustrator & Associate Professor

Interim Director, Department of Art as Applied to Medicine

Director, Graduate Program in Medical and Biological Illustration

The Johns Hopkins University School of Medicine

Baltimore, Maryland

Jennifer E. Fairman, MA, MPS, CMI, FAMI

Certified Medical Illustrator & Associate Professor

Department of Art as Applied to Medicine

The Johns Hopkins University School of Medicine

Baltimore, Maryland

New York   Chicago   San Francisco   Athens   London   Madrid   Mexico City
Milan   New Delhi   Singapore   Sydney   Toronto

Atlas of Minimally Invasive Surgical Operations

1 2 3 4 5 6 7 8 9 DSS 23 22 21 20 19 18

MHID: 0-07-144905-1
ISBN: 978-0-07-144905-2

This book was set in Minion Pro by Aptara, Inc.
The editors were Andrew Moyer and Regina Y. Brown.
The production supervisor was Rick Ruzycka.
Production management was provided by Indu Jawwad, Aptara, Inc.
The cover designer was Randomatrix.
RR Donnelley was printer and binder.

This book is printed on acid-free paper.

Library of Congress Cataloging-in-Publication Data

Names: Hunter, John G., editor.
Title: Atlas of minimally invasive surgical operations / editors, John
    Hunter, MD, Donn Spight, MD, Corinne Sandone, Jennifer Fairman.
Description: New York : McGraw-Hill, [2018]
Identifiers: LCCN 2018007331 | ISBN 9780071449052 (hardback)
Subjects: LCSH: Endoscopic surgery–Atlases. | BISAC: MEDICAL / Urology.
Classification: LCC RD33.53 .A88 2018 | DDC 617/.057–dc23 LC record available at https://na01.safelinks.protection.outlook.com/
?url=https%3A%2F%2Flccn.loc.gov%2F2018007331&data=01%7C01%7Cleah.carton%40mheducation.com%7Ca173ae00e16e4346049a08d5803adb06%
7Cf919b1efc0c347358fca0928ec39d8d5%7C0&sdata=33FSldJV3ZUGziXIpufk74f%2FLm%2FJ137gmmDsv%2Bcy%2FSI%3D&reserved=0

CONTENTS

PREFACE

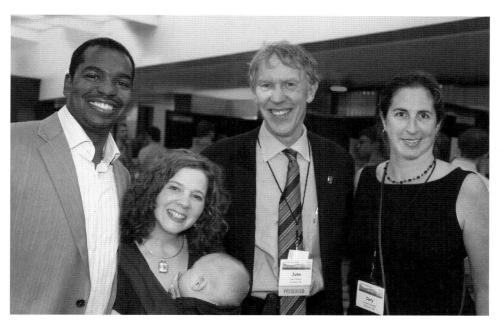

L to R: Donn Spight, MD, Jennifer Fairman, John Hunter, MD and Cory Sandone

INTRODUCTION TO ATLAS OF MINIMALLY INVASIVE SURGICAL OPERATIONS

For the last decade and more, we—the authors of this volume—have been living under the rubric "Rome was not built in a day!"—and indeed, this *Atlas of Minimally Invasive Surgical Operations* has taken nearly as long as Rome to build. If my memory allows, I would like to take you back 15 years to where the story starts. . . .

In 2003, before the birth of Facebook, Twitter, and many other institutions of the 21st century, I was approached by McGraw-Hill to create an atlas of minimally invasive surgery (MIS) to accompany their best-selling *Atlas of Surgical Operations*, also known as "Zollinger" by many generations of surgical residents. It was becoming clear that MIS was fast on its way to replacing many common (and uncommon) operations. I responded that I would be interested—if, and only if, I could pick the best medical artist in the country, Cory Sandone, to illustrate this work. As well, I asked McGraw-Hill to allow us 800 figures, or 200 plates, to richly illustrate these procedures, similar to the Zollinger atlas. They agreed, *if* I could find a corporate partner to help support so much artwork. Chuck Kennedy of U.S. Surgical, then Covidien, then Medtronic, agreed. (I think you are now getting a perspective of the length of time it took to create this atlas!) The next element we needed was expertise in areas where we clearly weren't experts. The authors contributing to this work, including Wexner, Schauer, Soper, Young-Fadok, and others, are household names to most GI surgeons, widely acclaimed international experts in their respective fields. For other topics, a stellar array of interested and accomplished surgeons from Oregon Health & Science University (OHSU) jumped in to help, each of them now accumulating recognition and reputation in their own fields. With all the elements in place, we were off to the races. Cory and I met by phone weekly, often interrupted by other duties at Hopkins or in Oregon . . . and the years ticked by. Finally, about 5 years in to this project, Cory realized that she needed help if we were ever to get this done, and I took another year or so to stumble to the same conclusion. We can't begin to thank Jennifer Fairman and Donn Spight for agreeing to take on this "labor of love." Without their efforts, there is little doubt in my mind that we would have a pile of half-finished drawings and rough drafts of procedure descriptions lying around. With them, we have a new atlas that we are all extremely proud of. We'd also like to recognize and thank Andrew Moyer, Brian Belval, Regina Brown, Marsha Gelber, Indu Jawwad, and Marc Strauss at McGraw-Hill, as well as April Hill, Timoree Leggett, and Pamela Sidis at OHSU, for their assistance on this project.

The *Atlas of Minimally Invasive Surgical Operations* represents the best thoughts and voluminous experience of the pioneers in laparoscopic surgery in the United States who have taken common open operations and adapted them to an MIS environment, bringing things they learned from each other and from masters in Europe, Asia, South America, and Australia into focus at the end of a rod lens telescope. These procedures have evolved over a quarter of a century—they have even evolved since we drew our first figure, forcing us to revise the atlas as we created it. Since our first "draft" table of contents, we have added such things as single-port laparoscopic surgery, natural orifice transluminal surgery (NOTES), and robotic surgery. As soon as the presses start to roll on this first edition, we know that we will need to be back to work, as new technology and new ideas drive procedure evolution.

This is the video generation, and some would suggest that line drawings are out of date, replaced by the surgical video, rendering an atlas such as this anachronistic. While we have been creating educational videos since the beginning of laparoscopic surgery, we realize that line drawings can do something that video struggles to accomplish. The creation of key figures by great illustrators unlocks the difficult steps of laparoscopic surgery, such as the takedown of the splenic flexure of the colon, the "shoeshine" maneuver during laparoscopic Nissen, or obtaining the "critical view of safety" during laparoscopic cholecystectomy. To demonstrate this, I'd like the surgeons reading this introduction to do an exercise: Close your eyes and picture laparoscopic inguinal hernia anatomy. Do you see a video in your mind, or do you see a line drawing or a color figure illustrating this perspective? I will bet that for most of you it is the artist's figure that you visualize as you step to the operating table, running the operation start-to-finish in your mind, as a slalom racer runs the gates in his or her mind before leaving the starting gate. Hard to believe that a static illustration can be so powerful in something as dynamic as video surgery, isn't it?

Every good scientific manuscript ever written contains a paragraph on limitations, so let me suggest the limitations of this atlas. Fundamentally, we illustrate *one* way of accomplishing each operation. Where there are two equally compelling techniques, we have tried to illustrate the alternative method, but we fully recognize that for each procedure we show you, there are 10 (at least) other ways to accomplish the goal with equal, maybe greater, efficiency and expertise. Some of these methods, as we learn them, will appear in the next edition of the atlas. Some may stay rooted in a single surgeon or single institution. As well, we do not yet have companion videos for each of these procedures. Many companion videos can be found online, on Access Surgery or YouTube. With the next edition, we hope to create to links from the atlas to a video demonstrating each step of the technique, but we didn't want to delay another fortnight in getting this atlas into your hands. I hope, on behalf of Cory, Jeni, Donn, and myself, that you enjoy this work.

John G. Hunter, MD, FACS, FRCS Edin (Hon)
Portland, Oregon, March 5, 2018

INTRODUCTION FROM THE ILLUSTRATORS

The opportunity to work on a major surgical atlas is the dream of many medical illustrators. When John Hunter proposed the idea to create a companion to *Zollinger's Atlas of Surgical Operations* describing minimally invasive procedures, we were very familiar with the 5th edition of *Zollinger's* in our department library. We often referred to it for operative information and artistic inspiration.

This was a great opportunity: to learn and understand procedures at the forefront of surgical advancement, to collaborate with a surgeon who valued illustrations enough to support an ambitious art budget for this *Atlas of Minimally Invasive Surgical Operations*, and to communicate surgical content in black-and-white illustrations when the emerging mode for depicting minimally invasive surgery was full-color videos that captured what the camera could—and no more. A medical illustrator can communicate far more in well-designed images, often "zooming out" to provide more anatomic context; using transparency to indicate the position of underlying structures; and incorporating cross sections, diagrams, and cutaway views to illustrate concepts not easily observed through the limited view of the scope. We accepted the challenge of this bicoastal collaboration to depict a comprehensive series of minimally invasive surgical operations.

It didn't take long to realize this project would go much faster and be more fun if we brought on an additional illustrator and author. Jennifer Fairman and Donn Spight joined the team. Donn's tireless, careful review was essential to the accuracy of the figures; his unwavering enthusiasm for the process made this project a joy. The *Atlas* was greatly enhanced by the outstanding illustration and design talents of Jennifer Fairman. Both artists trained at Johns Hopkins and currently teach in the graduate program in the Department of Art as Applied to Medicine. To maintain a consistent illustration style, we shared techniques in graphite and Adobe Photoshop to develop an efficient, smooth workflow.

Most appealing about this project was Dr. Hunter's positive response to the dynamic, robust quality of our sketches. Often, the authors would provide text and a video or photo and say, "What you can't see here is that. . . ." We'd work up a quick sketch to be sure we understood the concept. In earlier stages, Dr. Hunter would often respond more positively to the sketch than to the final illustration. These sketches had the energy and immediacy that can sometimes get "polished off" in refining them. He'd suggest we use the first sketch—it captured the concept! We made sure the images were clear and accurate while retaining a vigorous drawing style.

We had Friday phone calls for over a decade to create this massive body of work—nearly a thousand illustrations. We would review iterations of the figures, ask questions, and clarify content. The authors would teach us surgery, one hour a week, calling in at 11:00 a.m. Baltimore time and 8:00 a.m. Portland time. As procedures changed, we'd revise earlier illustrations and add or replace figures. As we worked together illustrating chapters, we continued to hone our skills as effective communicators of surgical technique. Our individual approaches blended into one unique style that is signature to this *Atlas*.

Minimally invasive surgery continued to evolve throughout the development of this comprehensive work. Technical innovation in these procedures will persist, making it challenging to bring a project of this scope to completion. With the support of McGraw-Hill and the entire team, it is our pleasure to bring this *Atlas of Minimally Invasive Surgical Operations* to print.

Corinne Sandone and Jennifer E. Fairman
Baltimore, Maryland

ASSOCIATE EDITORS

James I. Cohen, MD, PhD, FACS
Head and Neck Surgery
Professor of Otolaryngology-ENT
OHSU School of Medicine
Otolaryngology, Portland VAMC
Portland, Oregon

Michael J. Conlin, MD, FACS
Urologic Surgery
Professor of Urology
OHSU School of Medicine
Assistant Chief of Surgery, Portland VAMC
Portland, Oregon

Clifford W. Deveney, MD, FACS
Bariatric Surgery
Professor of Surgery
Division of Bariatric Surgery
OHSU School of Medicine
Portland, Oregon

James Fleshman Jr., MD, FACS, FASCRS
Colorectal Surgery
Chief of Surgery
Chairman of the Department of Surgery
Baylor University Medical Center
Dallas, Texas

Daniel O. Herzig, MD, FACS, FASCRS
Colorectal Surgery
Associate Professor of Surgery
Division of Gastrointestinal and General Surgery
OHSU School of Medicine
Director of Surgical Informatics, OHSU
Portland, Oregon

John D. Horton, MD, FACS
Pediatric Surgery
Chief, Pediatric Surgery, Department of Surgery
Madigan Army Medical Center
Adjunct Instructor, Pediatric Surgery
OHSU School of Medicine
Tacoma, Washington

Blair A. Jobe, MD, FACS
Foregut Surgery
Director, Esophageal and Lung Institute
Clinical Professor, Surgery
University of Pittsburgh School of Medicine
Pittsburgh, Pennsylvania

Christopher Komanapalli, MD, FACS, FACC
Thoracic Surgery
Adult Cardiothoracic Surgeon
Medical Director
Division of Cardiovascular and Thoracic Surgery
Des Moines, Iowa

Sanjay Krishnaswami, MD, FACS, FAAP
Pediatric Surgery
Associate Professor of Surgery and Pediatrics
Program Director, Pediatric Surgery Fellowship
OHSU School of Medicine
Portland, Oregon

David M. Le, MD, FACS
Gastrointestinal Surgery
Advanced Minimally Invasive Gastrointestinal Surgery
Clinical Lead, Gastric Cancer Surgery
Northern California Kaiser Permanente
San Francisco, California

Kim C. Lu, MD, FACS, FASCRS
Colorectal Surgery
Associate Professor of Surgery
Division of Gastrointestinal and General Surgery
OHSU School of Medicine
Portland, Oregon

David L. Maccabee, MD, FACS, FASMBS
Gastrointestinal Surgery
Director, Weight Loss Surgery Institute of the Central Coast
Minimally Invasive and Bariatric Surgery
MBSAQIP Accredited Comprehensive Center
Dignity Health—Marian Regional Medical Center
Santa Maria, California

John C. Mayberry, MD, FACS
General Surgery
Clinical Professor of Surgery
University of Washington
Ketchum, Idaho

Adrian Park, MD, FRCSC, FACS, FCS (ECSA)
Gastrointestinal Surgery
Chair of the Department of Surgery
Professor or Surgery
Anne Arundel Medical Center
Annapolis, Maryland

Stephen C. Rayhill, MD, FACS
Transplant and Liver Surgery
Professor of Surgery
Director, Transplant Clinical Services
Co-Director, Kidney and Pancreas Transplantation
Division of Transplant Surgery
University of Washington Medical Center
Seattle, Washington

Robert W. O'Rourke, MD, FACS
Bariatric Surgery
Professor, Department of Surgery
Michigan Medicine
University of Michigan Medical School and
   Ann Arbor VA Hospital
Ann Arbor, Michigan

Philip R. Schauer, MD, FACS
Bariatric Surgery
Professor of Surgery
Cleveland Clinic Lerner College of Medicine
Director of the Cleveland Clinic Bariatric and Metabolic Institute
President of the American Society for Bariatric Surgery
Cleveland, Ohio

Paul H. Schipper, MD, FACS, FACCP
Thoracic Surgery
Professor of Surgery
Program Director, Cardiothoracic Residency Section of
   General Thoracic Surgery
OHSU School of Medicine
Portland, Oregon

Brett C. Sheppard, MD, FACS
Pancreas Surgery
Professor and Vice-Chair of Surgery
Division of GI and General Surgery
Oregon Health and Science University
Portland, Oregon

Section I
GENERAL CONSIDERATIONS AND PRINCIPLES OF ACCESS

PRINCIPLES OF ROOM SETUP AND PORT PLACEMENT FOR MINIMALLY INVASIVE SURGERY

More than two decades after the replacement of much traditional open abdominal and chest surgery by minimally invasive surgery (MIS), certain observations have become accepted truths. For the minimally invasive surgeon, little is more important than understanding that poor port position not only impairs operative performance, it leads to career shortening injuries, particularly carpal tunnel syndrome, rotator cuff and other shoulder injuries. In addition, sore necks, sore backs, sore hands, and sore feet can impair performance, especially at times when patience is required. In this chapter we address patient positioning, monitor placement, and trocar positioning to optimize ergonomics for the busy minimally invasive surgeon.

ROOM SETUP In each chapter of this atlas, we demonstrate the room setup for that particular operation. The general principles of room setup are focused on the "delivery" of the target organ to the surgeon with optimal ergonomics. The first principle in room setup is to align the primary monitor, the operative target, the laparoscope, and the surgeon in a single straight line. This is possible for most, but not all, MIS procedures. For right upper quadrant procedures (e.g., cholecystectomy), the surgeon's primary monitor is placed above the patient's right shoulder, the laparoscope is placed in the umbilicus, and the surgeon stands off the patient's left hip, facing the monitor over the patient's right shoulder (**FIGURE 1A**). For surgery around the esophageal hiatus (e.g., hiatal hernia repair), the monitor is placed over the head of the patient, the laparoscope is positioned near the midline, usually above the umbilicus, and the surgeon stands between the abducted legs (**FIGURE 1B**). For right lower quadrant procedures (e.g., appendectomy), the monitor is placed over the patient's right hip, the laparoscope is placed in the umbilicus, and the surgeon stands adjacent to the patient's left costal margin (**FIGURE 1C**). Although this principle works for almost all procedures, such an alignment cannot be applied to pelvic surgery, as the surgeon would have to straddle the patient's head. It is for this reason, among others, that robotic surgery is particularly popular for pelvic procedures, as it is difficult to optimize ergonomics for procedures in this region.

PATIENT POSITIONING In open surgery, exposure is gained by proper retraction of the abdominal wall, chest wall, and structures blocking access to the organ of interest. In MIS, abdominal and chest wall retraction is unnecessary. Structures blocking access are moved with retractors, such as the right lobe of the liver for right adrenalectomy. The small and large bowel is displaced from the field of interest with gravity rather than retraction. For upper abdominal MIS, the patient is placed in steep reverse Trendelenburg position, and for pelvic surgery, Trendelenburg is used to displace the small bowel toward the diaphragm. For right upper quadrant surgery, the patient is rolled to the left and placed in reverse Trendelenburg to elevate the right upper quadrant. As well as displacing the small bowel from the field, such positioning shortens the distance between the surgeon and the target organ. For retroperitoneal organs, such as the kidneys and adrenal glands, the patient is placed in a lateral decubitus position, and the operating table

is "broken" in the middle to open up the space between the ribs and the pelvic brim, improving access to the retroperitoneal organs (**FIGURE 2**).

Correct arm positioning is critical. If mobile video carts are used and the patient is supine, it is best to tuck both arms, as table position changes during the operation may result in the arm boards, or the patient's hands or fingers, bumping into the video carts. With overhead-mounted monitors, it may be possible to leave the arms out on arm boards, but this position may restrict the surgeon's ability to stand at the patient's shoulder, and it may be hard to keep the arm on the arm board without pressure points, especially when the patient is in steep or reverse Trendelenburg position. As a rule, we tuck both arms for procedures about the diaphragmatic hiatus (e.g., laparoscopic hiatal hernia repair), leave the right arm extended for cholecystectomy (so the C-arm can be brought in from the left without an arm in the way), and leave the right arm extended for appendectomy, as the surgeon and assistant are on the patient's left. For pelvic procedures and hernia repair, tucking both arms is best, as it allows the surgeon and assistant to stand adjacent to the axillae without bumping into the arms. For bariatric procedures, the size of the patient frequently precludes tucking either arm at the patient's side.

For thoracic procedures, the most frequent positioning is a pure decubitus position, as it would be for posterolateral thoracotomy (**FIGURE 3**). The head of the table is elevated to work at the apex of the thorax (reverse Trendelenburg) and dropped to work on the peridiaphragmatic tissues (Trendelenburg). Single-lung ventilation allows the lung to be deflated during the operation. Some surgeons prefer to place the patient in the prone position for access to the esophagus and posterior thoracic cavity. In this position, gravity retracts the lung(s) anteriorly, making single-lung ventilation unnecessary if a low-pressure pneumothorax (5–8 mm Hg) is maintained.

SURGEON AND ASSISTANT POSITION Whenever possible, the surgeon stands on the opposite side of the table from the organ of interest, moving to a position between the patient's legs for upper abdominal surgery, as stated earlier. For pelvic surgery, the surgeon usually stands on the patient's right side. It is often necessary for the surgeon to move around the table for more extensive colon resections. Operating ports should be placed to allow the surgeon a comfortable arm position, with elbows at the side and the monitor dropped to a 10-degree position below a horizontal sight line (**FIGURE 4**). Reaching an arm across the table or abducting the shoulder is a fatiguing position and impairs performance of delicate tasks, such as suturing and knot tying.

The first assistant is usually placed across the table from the surgeon, but when the first assistant must also hold the camera, it makes sense to stand on the same side of the table as the surgeon for certain procedures. Laparoscopic appendectomy is an example of this principle. Although some surgeons will place their assistant across the table for this operation, the assistant may become extraordinarily fatigued if they are required to reach across the operating table to hold the laparoscope for long periods of time.

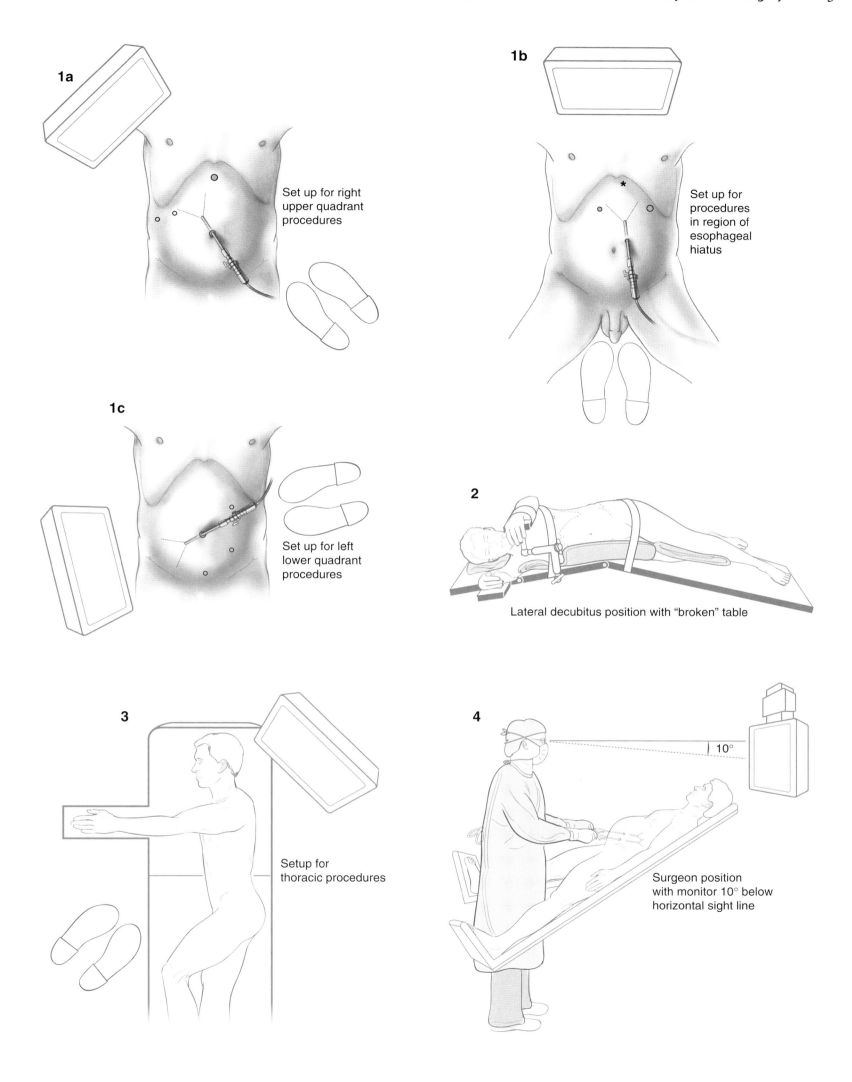

1a

Set up for right upper quadrant procedures

1b

Set up for procedures in region of esophageal hiatus

1c

Set up for left lower quadrant procedures

2

Lateral decubitus position with "broken" table

3

Setup for thoracic procedures

4

10°

Surgeon position with monitor 10° below horizontal sight line

PORT PLACEMENT There is nothing more important in facilitating laparoscopic surgery than choosing the optimal trocar positions. Understanding that surgeons should operate with both hands (and not hold the video laparoscope with the nondominant hand), we first focus on organization of the primary (laparoscope) port and the surgeon's right- and left-hand ports. Secondarily, we focus on the appropriate placement of the assistant's ports.

The standard laparoscope is 30 cm from tip to the right-angle entry point for the optical bundle. A straight tip scope can be used but generally a forward oblique viewing angle (30 or 45 degrees) gives more options for intracavitary viewing (**FIGURE 5**). Longer scopes, 45 cm in length, have been developed for bariatric surgery, but for this description, we focus on the appropriate use of the 30-cm laparoscope. The first principle is that it is easiest to use a laparoscope if half of the shaft is inside the patient and half is out. In other words, the primary trocar site should be 15 cm away from the target tissue, so that half the scope is in and half the scope is out. Not only does this allow the greatest flexibility for moving closer to or farther from the target, but a one-to-one relationship of tip movement to outside motion of the scope is established. For example, a 1-cm leftward movement of the laparoscope results in a 1-cm rightward movement of the tip of the laparoscope when the laparoscope is working at its fulcrum, in which half the shaft is in and half the shaft is out (**FIGURE 6**).

When the laparoscope port is too far from the target, a small movement of the camera on the outside will cause a much greater movement on the inside, accentuating the inherent tremor of the laparoscope operator. In addition, if the primary port is too far away, the laparoscope may be maximally inserted (into its hub) without getting close enough to the target to provide the surgeon adequate operative detail. Conversely, when the laparoscope is too close to the operative target, it is necessary to swing the laparoscope through long arcs to effect relatively small movements on the inside of the patient. Also, the length of the port projecting into the abdominal cavity (usually 3–10 cm) will impair the ability to get a broad view without retracting the laparoscope into the port. The surgeon's reaction to this problem is to withdraw the port, which frequently leads to the end of the port being pulled back into the abdominal wall. Losing abdominal access will make reentry of the scope or other instrument difficult if not impossible. Suffice it to say, it is important to get the primary trocar site correct.

The standard length of the laparoscope was chosen to be able to reach most points in the abdominal cavity easily from the umbilicus. Placement of the primary port just above, just below, or through the umbilicus is the most common primary port site. It turns out—in an average-sized adult—that the distance between the umbilicus and many intraabdominal targets (e.g., gallbladder, appendix, ovary) is almost exactly 15 cm, offering the ideal operating conditions for the laparoscope. However, in many circumstances, especially when working deep in the pelvis or at the diaphragmatic hiatus, the umbilicus is too far from the operative target, and a primary trocar position must be chosen that is closer to the target. In this circumstance we generally draw an imaginary line between the surgeon and the target organ (as mentioned earlier), then mark a point on the patient's abdominal wall that is 15 cm from the surface projection of the target. This principle is also important for performing standard laparoscopic procedures on large patients, where the primary port for a standard operation, such as laparoscopic cholecystectomy, might need to be closer to the costal margin than the umbilicus allows. (**FIGURE 7A,B**). Although the use of a bariatric-length scope is helpful when the primary port is too far away, picking a longer scope is not an adequate substitute for choosing the correct primary port position at the start.

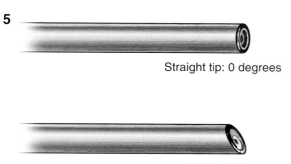

5

Straight tip: 0 degrees

Angled tip: 30 degrees

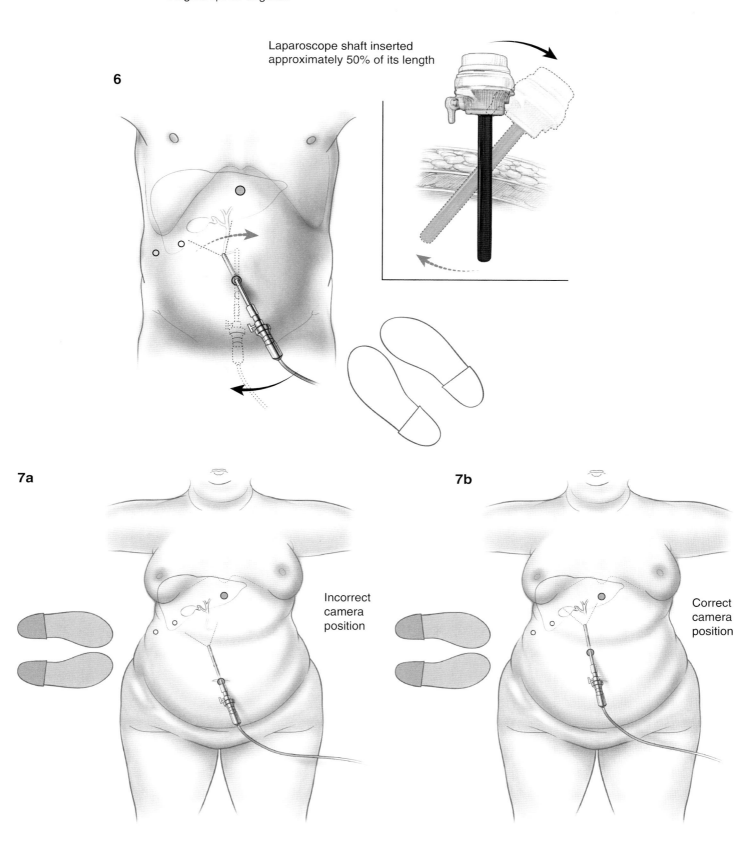

6

Laparoscope shaft inserted approximately 50% of its length

7a   Incorrect camera position

7b   Correct camera position

PORT PLACEMENT The surgeon's right- and left-hand operating ports are placed to the left and the right of the line between the target tissue and the port for the laparoscope. When complete, the operative target, the primary port, and the two operative ports create a "baseball diamond," or a square rotated 45 degrees. The instruments arriving at the target from the left and right operating port will arrive 90 degrees from each other, giving the maximum flexibility for tissue, suture, and needle manipulation (**FIGURE 8**). As a general rule, it is a good idea to separate all port sites by at least 10 cm, to avoid "sword fighting" inside the abdomen or chest. When the right- and left-hand ports are placed too close together, the ability to manipulate tissue is limited to the single axis of the instruments. As well, the surgeon feels that he or she is always looking down the shaft of the instrument, better able to see its shaft than discern what is happening at its tip (**FIGURE 9**). A less frequent problem is excessive separation of instruments, which will force the surgeon to lift his or her arms and shoulders into ergonomically uncomfortable positions ("wing out" in surgical jargon) under which operative acuity is severely impaired (**FIGURE 10A–C**).

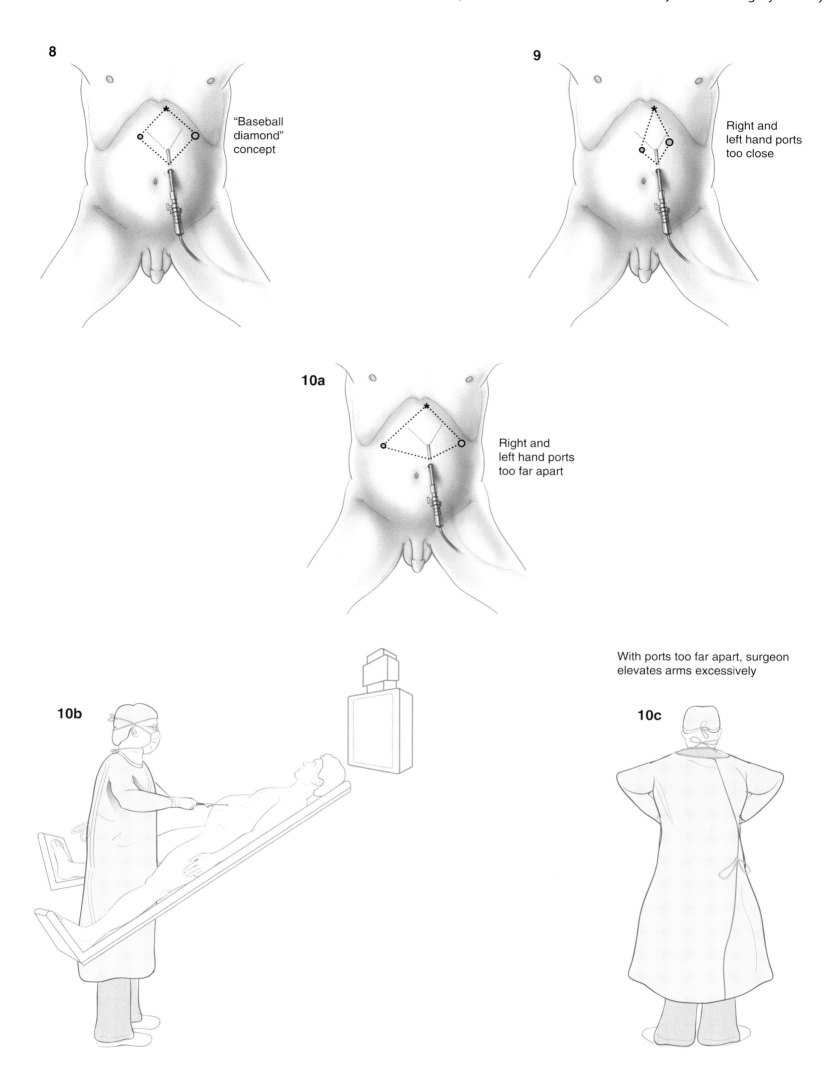

8

"Baseball diamond" concept

9

Right and left hand ports too close

10a

Right and left hand ports too far apart

10b

With ports too far apart, surgeon elevates arms excessively

10c

PORT PLACEMENT The assistant's trocar positions are a little less critical, but are—at a minimum—placed outside the "diamond" created earlier. Which side of the diamond the assistant works from is variable from operation to operation, depending on the requirements of the procedure. In laparoscopic cholecystectomy, where the assistant's job is to elevate the gallbladder fundus, it works best to have the assistant standing on the patient's right side (**FIGURE 11A**). For a laparoscopic Nissen fundoplication, the need to divide the short gastric arteries with an ultrasonic scissors in the surgeon's right-hand trocar would dictate that the assistant enter from the patient's left side (**FIGURE 11B**).

The principle of working at the fulcrum of the instrument is as valuable for the assistant as it is for the surgeon. Again, this would suggest that the assistant's port(s) should be 15 cm from the point at which they will be retracting, often several centimeters from the site at which the surgeon is working. When the assistant's port is too far from the operative field, it may be necessary to resort to longer instruments (initially made for bariatric surgery, but now widely available) or to move the assisting port closer to the target tissue. Additional assisting ports and liver-retracting ports are addressed in each chapter where they are necessary.

CAMERA AND RETRACTOR MANAGEMENT When the surgeon is operating with two hands, laparoscope management falls to the first assistant. Because a still laparoscope is paramount to efficiency, we prefer to use a passive robotic "camera holder" for longer and delicate procedures (**FIGURE 12**). There are many of these on the market. When the operation is short or the operative field is constantly changing, a steady-handed camera operator will suffice.

Table-mounted retractors are common in open surgery. Many of these systems have been modified to add arms that will grasp a laparoscopic retractor (often a liver retractor) and maintain position until released (**FIGURE 13A,B**). Operative performance is enhanced by elimination of the human variables caused by handheld cameras and handheld liver retractors. The ultimate step of removing all humans from the operative field—robotic surgery—is addressed in the subsequent chapters. ■

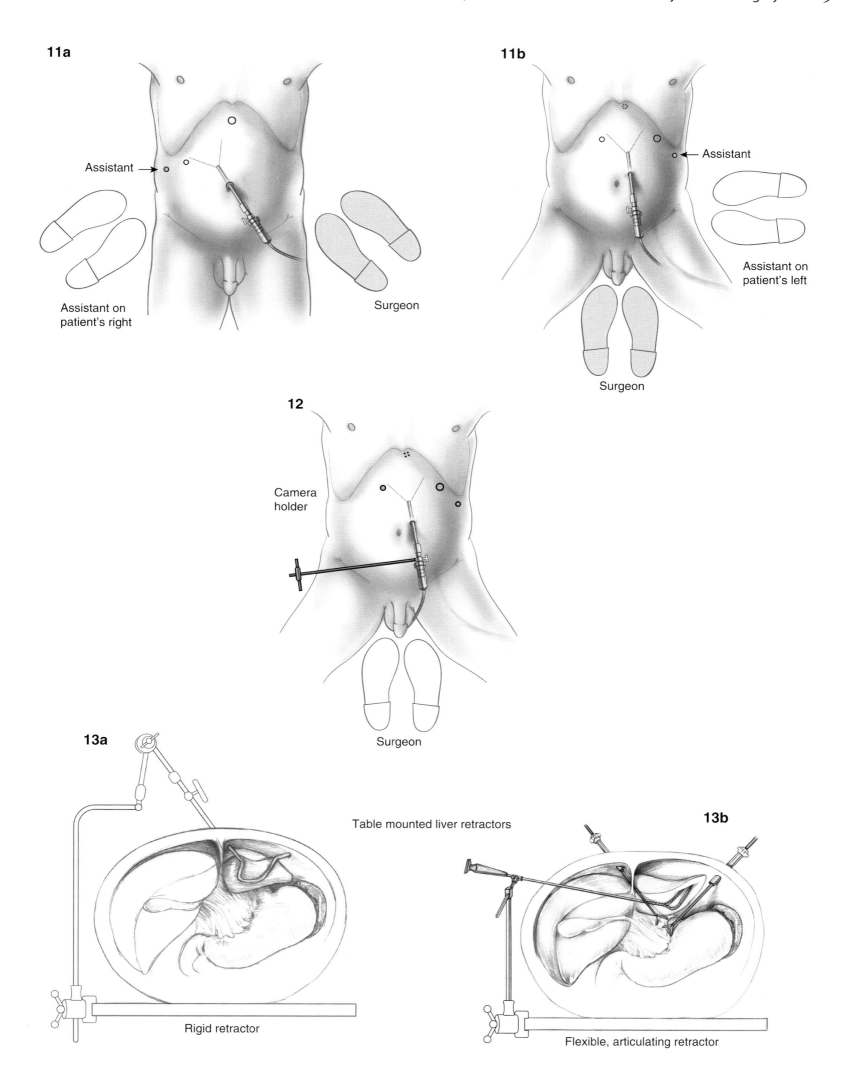

11a

Assistant →

Assistant on patient's right

Surgeon

11b

→ Assistant

Assistant on patient's left

Surgeon

12

Camera holder

Surgeon

13a

Table mounted liver retractors

13b

Rigid retractor

Flexible, articulating retractor

CHAPTER 2

GENERAL PRINCIPLES OF LAPAROSCOPIC ACCESS

Paramount to proper visualization of intraabdominal structures is the ability to safely introduce gas into the peritoneal cavity (pneumoperitoneum). Techniques available to accomplish this objective can generally be divided into closed and open categories. Specific choice depends on surgeon experience and preference as well as careful patient selection. The primary tools used to create pneumoperitoneum by the closed technique are the Veress needle and optical viewing trocar. The alternative "open" technique uses the Hasson trocar or hand port to provide initial access.

The Veress needle allows for rapid access into the peritoneal cavity through an incision the diameter of the needle. Its two-stage mechanism features an outer barrel with a beveled point designed to penetrate tissue (**FIGURE 1A**). The inner cannula is a spring-loaded obturator that retracts during the passage through tissue, exposing the cutting outer barrel. Once the inner cannula passes into the peritoneal cavity, the sudden decrease in resistance allows the inner cannula to spring forward, shielding the outer barrel (**FIGURE 1B**). At this point insufflation gas can be passed through the needle into the peritoneal cavity.

An optical viewing trocar is a second, less frequently used tool for creation of pneumoperitoneum by closed technique. In this technique a camera is positioned inside of a pyramidal or bladed trocar, allowing visualization of the layers of the abdominal wall as they are traversed by direct force (**FIGURE 2**). A thorough understanding of the anatomy of the abdominal wall is critical for safe application of this technique.

Significant risk of damage to underlying structures is inherent with the closed techniques. In patients who have had multiple or extensive abdominal operations, the Veress needle or optical trocar should be used with extreme caution. In these circumstances, trocar insertion through a surgically created defect in the abdominal wall is often the best technique. The "open" technique for the attainment of pneumoperitoneum will not prevent the aforementioned injuries but will, it is hoped, allow early recognition.

The Hasson trocar is a blunt instrument that can be passed directly through a 10-mm fascial defect and held in position by sutures anchored to the fascia (**FIGURE 3**). Alternatively, a skin incision and fascial defect approximately the size of the surgeon's hand can be created to allow the insertion of a mechanical valve type apparatus creating a "hand port" (**FIGURE 4**). Position and use of the hand port are largely dependent on the surgical procedure, surgeon facility with totally laparoscopic dissection, and size of the specimen to be removed.

Patient selection is a critical element for safe application of these techniques. Ideal candidates for the closed techniques are those without prior history of open abdominal surgery. Open abdominal surgery can result in dense adhesion formation between the greater omentum, small bowel, or colon and the anterior abdominal wall. This is often especially dense in the area of the previous incision. Placement of a Veress needle or optical trocar through a scar can be hazardous and lead to bowel injury or bleeding from omental vessels. An alternative site away from the scar should be chosen.

Morbid obesity can create challenges for both closed and open techniques. Dense subcutaneous fat between the skin and anterior abdominal fascia makes it difficult to elevate the abdominal wall away from the underlying viscera. This prevents the creation of a space between the posterior abdominal wall and the viscera below, increasing risk of bowel injury with the closed technique. The alternative "open approach" often requires a generous incision to identify the underlying fascia and is sometimes no less difficult.

Adherence to technical detail can allow safe access for establishment of pneumoperitoneum using either closed or open techniques, even in the morbidly obese.

PREOPERATIVE PREPARATION The patient should be evaluated for suitability to undergo a laparoscopic procedure. Significant comorbidities should be thoroughly evaluated (e.g., cardiac insufficiency, pulmonary dysfunction, or increased intracranial pressure). A complete understanding of the patient's previous surgical history will help determine the most appropriate method of access and site of entry to optimize safety and success.

ANESTHESIA General anesthesia with endotracheal intubation is necessary for this operation. Neuromuscular blockade is required. Intravenous antibiotics are administered as indicated for the specific operation. Local anesthetic should be administered at the skin and fascial level for each trocar placed.

POSITION Operative procedure will dictate the patient's position. Surgeon and assistant should stand on either side of the patient for initial trocar insertion. In general, the supine or lateral decubitus position provides optimal access to the abdominal wall.

OPERATIVE PREPARATION A Foley catheter and an orogastric tube are placed after the induction of anesthesia, as indicated. The abdomen of the patient is shaved with clippers after induction of anesthesia and is sterilely prepped in the routine manner.

INCISION AND EXPOSURE The most frequent access point for "open" or closed techniques is near the umbilicus, where the abdominal fascia is thinnest. The abdominal fascia is fused along the midline where the anterior and posterior rectus sheaths come together to form the *linea alba*. This location is ideal for placement of the Veress needle, optical trocar, Hasson trocar, or hand port because there are fewer layers to pass through before penetration into the peritoneal cavity. The umbilical stalk provides an excellent point of countertraction against the pressure needed to advance the Veress needle through the fascia and peritoneum.

Patients who have undergone prior open abdominal surgery resulting in large midline scars require a different strategy. Adhesion formation is likely to occur below the scar but is less common along the lateral aspect of the abdomen and flank region. Trocar insertion at these lateral points, however, is challenging and may result in injury to visceral structures such as the colon. An "open" technique such as the Hasson trocar enables safe identification of underlying structures in circumstances in which there is a question about proximity of underlying structures. Alternatively, placement of a Veress needle in the right or left upper quadrants below the costal margin can be performed safely. The costal margins are often a virgin region of the abdomen that provides excellent countertraction to the puncture of the Veress needle. Caution must be maintained to avoid injury to the liver below the right subcostal border and to the stomach, colon, or spleen below the left. Because puncture of the liver is hard to feel, and insufflation of CO_2 may lead to gas embolus, most laparoscopic surgeons favor the left subcostal position. If the left subcostal border is chosen as an access point, it is important that the patient have tube decompression of the stomach via orogastric or nasogastric routes. Often the stomach is hyperinflated during intubation, increasing the risk of inadvertent needle insertion into the stomach if access is attempted.

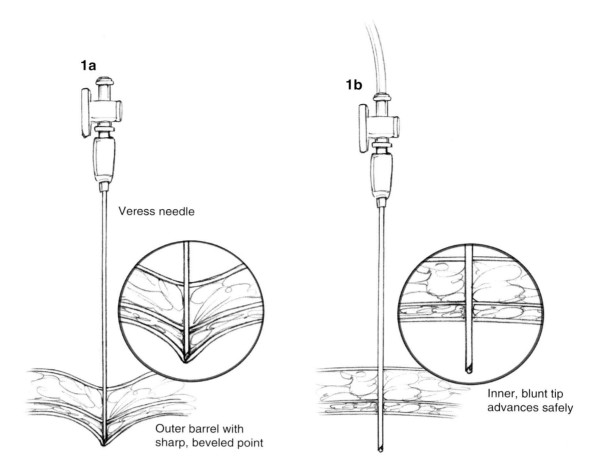

1a

Veress needle

Outer barrel with
sharp, beveled point

1b

Inner, blunt tip
advances safely

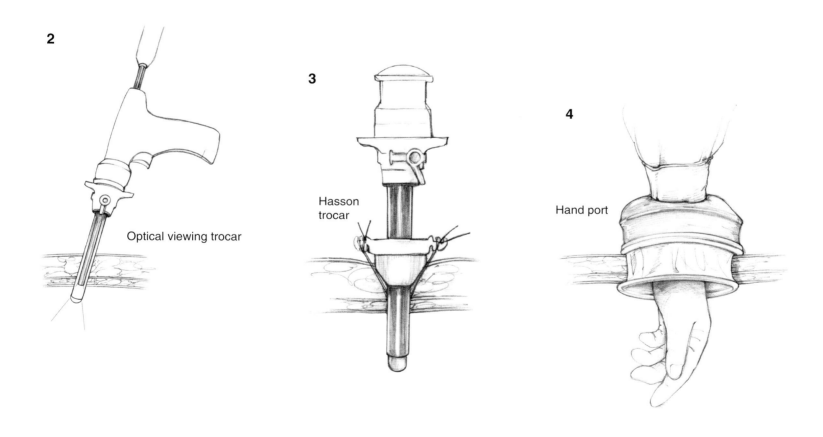

2

Optical viewing trocar

3

Hasson
trocar

4

Hand port

DETAILS OF PROCEDURE

Veress Needle Technique Local anesthetic is injected in the umbilical region prior to skin incision. The length of the skin incision depends on whether the location is to be used solely for establishment of pneumoperitoneum or for eventual trocar placement. If the site is to be used solely for establishing pneumoperitoneum, a 1-mm supraumbilical incision can be made with a #11 blade scalpel. If a trocar is to be placed through the site, an umbilical incision equal to the width of the trocar should be made. A transverse or vertical incision can be made within the umbilicus or in a supraumbilical or infraumbilical position, depending on the surgeon's preference. Transverse incisions can be cosmetically more appealing if placed in the natural umbilical fold. However, if there is a high probability of conversion to an open operation, a vertical trocar incision can be incorporated into a midline vertical incision with greater success.

The abdominal wall is elevated to create countertraction. This can be performed with penetrating towel clamps or a tracheal ring hook. The Veress needle is then inserted into the abdomen perpendicular to the abdominal fascia (**FIGURE 5**). Two abdominal wall layers are often felt as the needle is inserted (fused midline fascia and peritoneum). Once through the peritoneum, the outer cannula springs forward and a "popping" sensation may be appreciated as the tip enters the low-resistance intraabdominal space. A saline-filled syringe is attached to the end of the Veress needle, and the plunger is removed. Free flow of saline into the abdomen helps confirm intraabdominal placement (**FIGURE 6**). If the saline does not flow freely, it is likely that the Veress needle is resting in the preperitoneal space, in the greater omentum, or within loops of bowel and therefore needs to be repositioned. This is best done by removal of the needle and reinsertion. Once proper positioning has been confirmed, the insufflator is attached to the end of the Veress needle (**FIGURE 7**). It is important at this time to visualize the pressure readings on the insufflator. Typical maximum pneumoperitoneum pressure is set at 15 mm Hg. If the Veress needle is located in the intraabdominal space, pressures should be in a range of normal intraabdominal pressure (3–8 mm Hg). A high gas flow (3 L/min via Veress) should be able to be sustained (**FIGURE 8**). High pressure readings or poor gas flow indicate improper placement of the Veress needle and require readjustment.

After pneumoperitoneum is attained, the Veress needle is removed and the initial trocar can be placed cautiously into the abdomen using a step system or pyramidal trocar. In the VersaStep system, the sheath and Veress needle are reinserted into the abdomen together (**FIGURE 9**). The Veress needle is removed, leaving the sheath in place (**FIGURE 10**). The trocar is passed through the radially expanding sheath using a forceful twisting motion (**FIGURE 11**). The camera is then inserted. Initial inspection should include the region directly beneath the trocar and in the trajectory of the Veress needle. After confirmation of safe entry, the gas flow can be turned up to 20 L/min through this larger-diameter conduit. The abdomen is insufflated to 15 mm Hg and maintained at this level throughout the case.

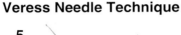

Veress Needle Technique

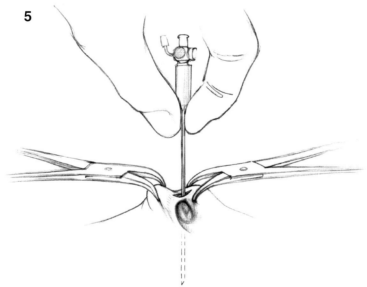

5

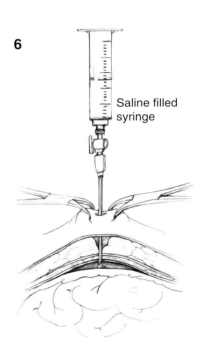

6

Saline filled syringe

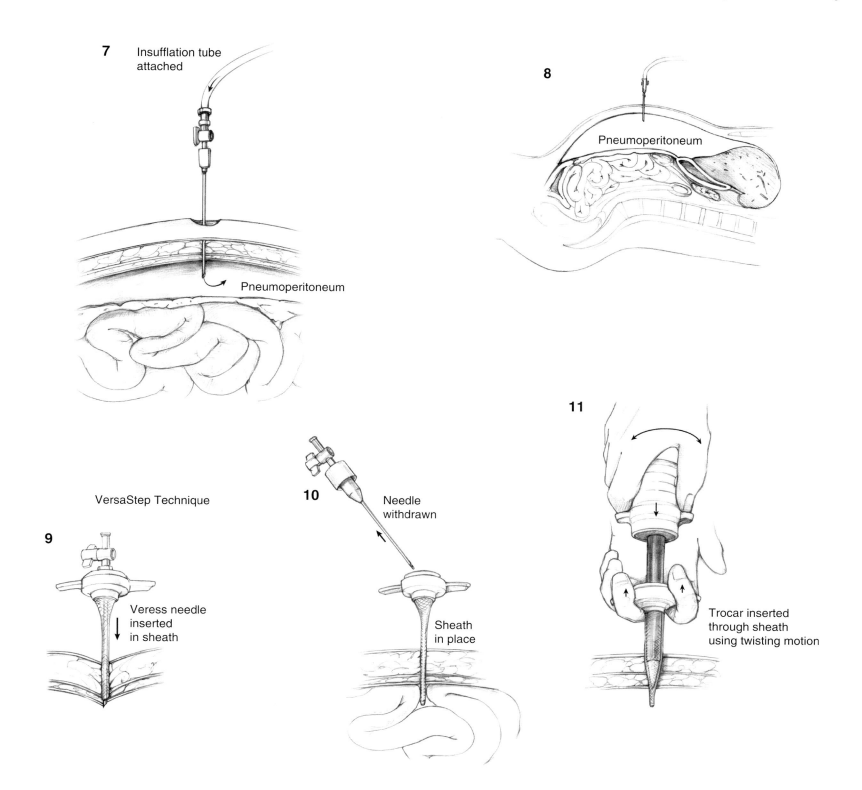

7 Insufflation tube attached

Pneumoperitoneum

8 Pneumoperitoneum

VersaStep Technique

9 Veress needle inserted in sheath

10 Needle withdrawn

Sheath in place

11 Trocar inserted through sheath using twisting motion

Optical Trocar Technique Local anesthetic is injected in the umbilical region prior to skin incision. An umbilical incision is made with a #11 blade scalpel equal to the width of the optical trocar. A transverse or vertical incision can be made within the umbilicus or in a supraumbilical, or infraumbilical position depending on the surgeon's preference. Transverse incisions can be cosmetically more appealing if placed in the natural umbilical fold. However, if there is a high probability of conversion to an open operation, a vertical trocar incision can be incorporated into a midline vertical incision with greater success. A laparoscope is placed within the trocar obturator, and the entire complex is carefully directed into the wound via a twisting motion or blade application (**FIGURE 12A**). To enable controlled entry into the abdomen, many surgeons insufflate the abdomen with a Veress needle prior to trocar insertion. Alternatively, the abdominal wall can be grasped en masse with the nondominant hand to provide countertension as the trocar is advanced. Subcutaneous fat, fascia, preperitoneal fat, peritoneum, and omentum are visualized in succession (**FIGURE 12B**). Caution must be exercised to ensure controlled guidance and immediate recognition of abdominal wall structures. Overshooting the trocar placement into the omentum or mesentery can quickly result in bowel or major vascular injury (portal vein, aorta, inferior vena cava). After proper positioning, the obturator is removed and the trocar is attached to the insufflation apparatus. The camera is then reinserted into the abdomen. The initial inspection should include the region directly beneath the trocar and in the trajectory of the initial entry. The abdomen is insufflated to 15 mm Hg and maintained at this level throughout the case.

Open Hasson Technique Local anesthetic is injected in the umbilical region prior to skin incision. An umbilical incision is made with a #11 blade scalpel equal to the size of the trocar. A transverse or vertical incision can be made in the supraumbilical or infraumbilical position, depending on the surgeon's preference. Transverse incisions can be cosmetically more appealing if placed in the natural umbilical fold. However, if there is a high probability of conversion to an open operation, a vertical trocar incision can be incorporated into a midline vertical incision with greater success. Blunt dissection is carried down to the level of the abdominal fascia with a standard dissection clamp. Using handheld retractors to optimize visualization, small Kocher clamps are used to grasp the fascia at the medial and lateral aspects of the incision elevating it from the underlying structures. A #11 blade scalpel is used to incise the fascia vertically (**FIGURE 13**). The Kocher clamps are removed. Hemostats are used to grasp the peritoneum and elevate it into the field (**FIGURE 14**). The peritoneum is incised sharply to open the abdominal cavity. A finger is inserted into the abdomen to ensure a clear path for blunt Hasson trocar insertion. Anchoring sutures are placed at the lateral aspects of the wound through the peritoneum and fascia (**FIGURE 15**). The Hasson trocar is inserted and secured by wrapping the anchoring sutures onto the trocar posts (**FIGURE 16**). The abdomen is insufflated to 15 mm Hg.

After camera insertion, initial inspection should include the region directly beneath the trocar.

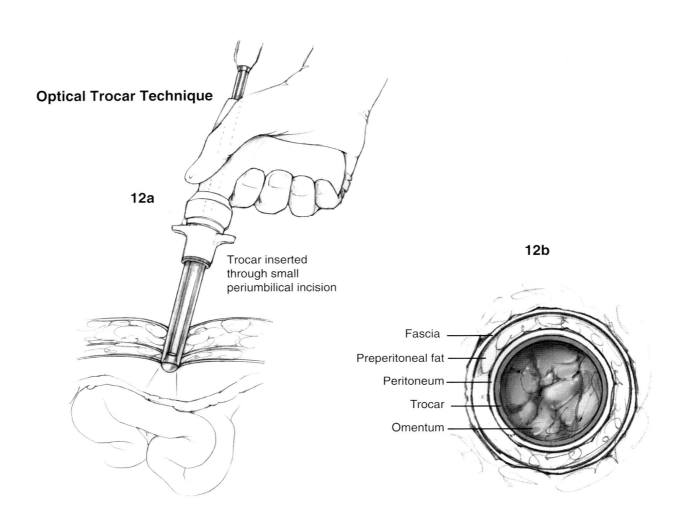

Optical Trocar Technique

12a

Trocar inserted through small periumbilical incision

12b

Fascia
Preperitoneal fat
Peritoneum
Trocar
Omentum

Open Hasson Technique

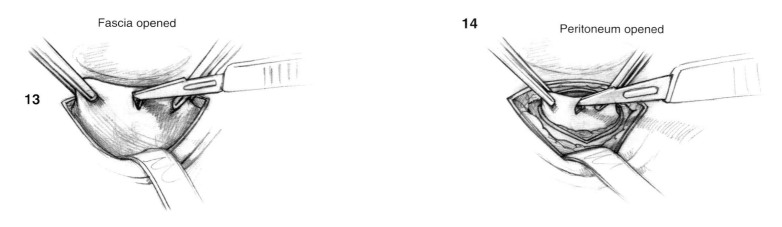

Fascia opened

13

14   Peritoneum opened

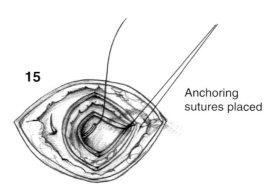

15

Anchoring
sutures placed

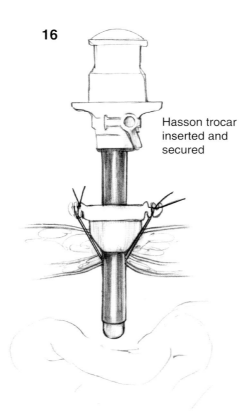

16

Hasson trocar
inserted and
secured

Hand Port Technique Position of the hand port is chosen based on the procedure to be performed. Local anesthetic is administered along skin and subcutaneous tissues. The diameter of the hand port incision should be equivalent to the diameter of the surgeon's closed fist (**FIGURE 17**). The incision is carried down to the fascia using cautery. The fascia and peritoneum are incised sharply. The inner lip of the hand port device is inserted into the peritoneal cavity, sandwiching the abdominal wall between its inner and outer aspects (**FIGURE 18**). The gel cap is then attached to the transabdominal portion (**FIGURE 19**). A trocar can be inserted into the assembled hand port to facilitate insufflation and initial abdominal inspection using the camera, followed by insertion of a hand (**FIGURES 20 AND 21**).

CLOSURE Radially expanding trocars rarely need closure, but all trocar sites 10 mm or greater at the umbilicus or lower should be closed with interrupted sutures placed via a transfascial suture passing device or open technique. The skin is reapproximated with a subcuticular suture and Steri-Strips or reapproximated with tissue glue. ∎

Hand Port Technique

17

Width of fist = width of incision

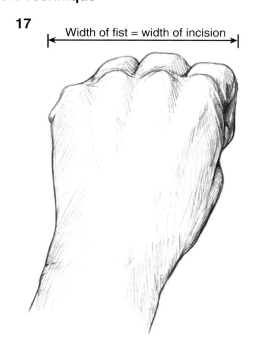

18

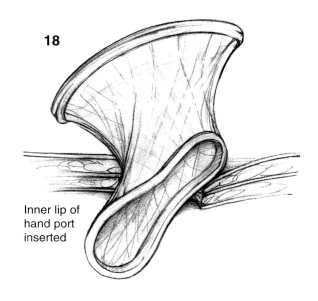

Inner lip of
hand port
inserted

19

Gel port

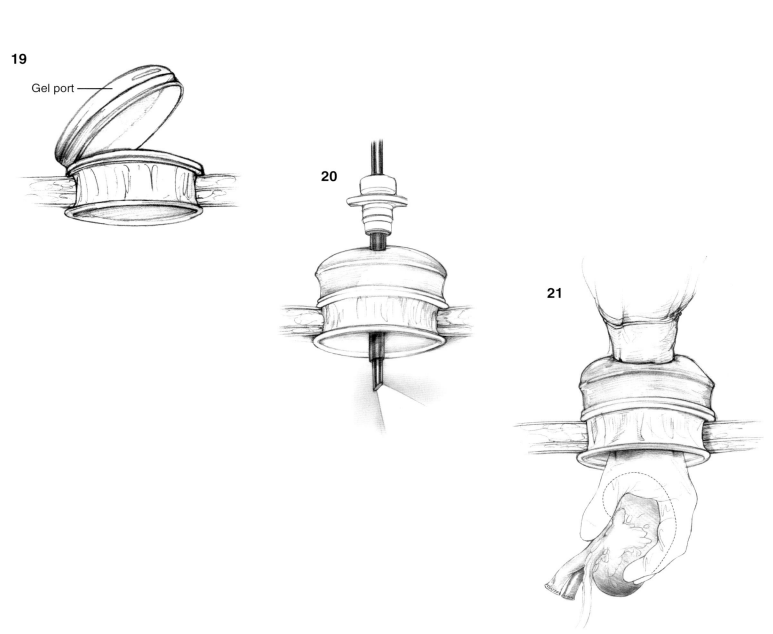

20

21

PRINCIPLES OF THORACIC ACCESS

INDICATIONS Video-assisted thoracic surgery (VATS) is a general term used to describe operations on the thorax accomplished with the use of a video camera, monitor, and long instruments. This approach using only a thoracoscope was originally described in 1910, but had limited application due to poor visibility. With the advent of high resolution cameras and monitors it has been increasingly applied over the last 10 to 20 years to operations traditionally performed through a thoracotomy. VATS is now commonly used to treat diseases of the lung, pleura and mediastinum.

PREOPERATIVE PREPARATION The preparation required depends largely on the procedure to be accomplished. Although VATS may be accomplished with the patient prone, using a low-pressure pneumothorax (<8 mm Hg) and a standard endotracheal tube, most patients undergoing VATS surgery require single-lung ventilation, as the standard is not to use positive-pressure pneumothorax. In most circumstances this mandates pulmonary function testing. A forced expiratory volume of greater than 1 liter in 1 second (FEV$_1$ >1 L) generally represents adequate lung function. Functional testing is also useful, with patients able to tolerate climbing at least one flight of stairs without stopping to catch their breath representing adequate function. As with other thoracic operations, VATS procedures are commonly carried out on relatively sick patients, and an electrocardiogram and laboratory evaluation including complete blood count, electrolytes, glucose, blood urea nitrogen, creatinine, and prothrombin and partial thromboplastin times are generally recommended. All patients undergoing VATS procedures should have a current type and screen.

Chest radiograph, computed tomography (CT) scan, and positron emission tomography (PET) scan are done as part of the investigation of the primary problem for which thoracoscopy is being performed.

ANESTHESIA General endotracheal anesthesia with single-lung ventilation either via a double-lumen endotracheal tube or a bronchial blocker is generally necessary. The other option is CO_2 insufflation of the thoracic cavity. This provides a working space without single-lung ventilation, but limits the ports and instruments that can be used, because an airtight seal must be present and mini-thoracotomy is not possible.

The double-lumen endotracheal tube should be placed with the distal balloon in the left main-stem bronchus to avoid occlusion of the right upper-lobe bronchus. Flexible bronchoscopy down the proximal lumen should reveal the carina, right upper-lobe bronchus, and bronchus intermedius. The blue balloon will be visible in the left main-stem bronchus (**FIGURE 1**). Care should be taken to identify the right upper-lobe bronchus, as its absence may indicate that the distal balloon is in the right bronchus intermedius, and the bifurcating airway that you see is the take-off of the right upper-lobe bronchus rather than the carina.

A bronchial blocker offers a reasonable alternative to achieve single-lung ventilation. Blocking the left main-stem bronchus with confirmation via bronchoscopy is generally straightforward (**FIGURE 2**). Blocking the right main-stem bronchus is often difficult because the short main-stem bronchus predisposes the balloon to herniation into the trachea or migration distally, incompletely occluding ventilation of the right upper lobe. In either case, effective single-lung ventilation is important in establishing and maintaining a clear surgical field.

In addition to single-lung ventilation, two large-bore intravenous lines are needed, and an arterial line is helpful for most procedures. A central line should be placed if needed for postoperative monitoring. Depending on the procedure, either a thoracic epidural catheter should be placed preoperatively, or an intercostal nerve block should be performed during the procedure (**FIGURE 3**). A Foley catheter should be placed.

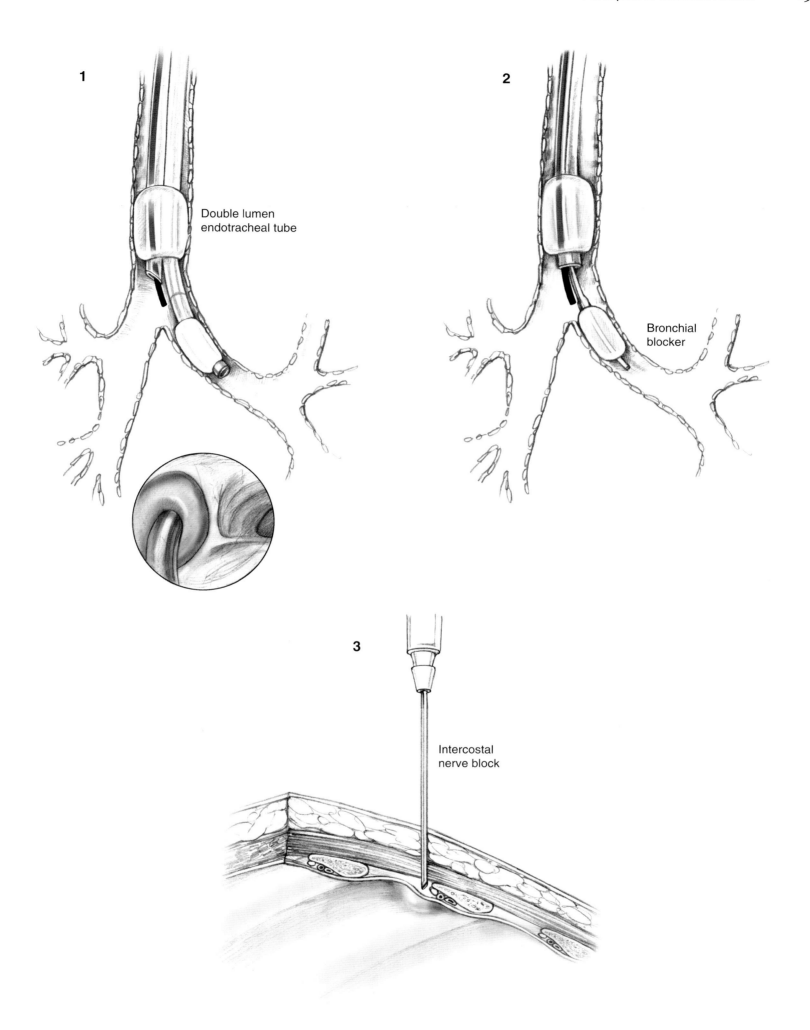

1

Double lumen
endotracheal tube

2

Bronchial
blocker

3

Intercostal
nerve block

POSITION After induction, the patient is placed in the lateral decubitus position with the operative side up. The table is flexed to open the intercostal spaces, which allows for easier access through the working incision (**FIGURE 4**). The whole bed is placed in reverse Trendelenburg position to avoid having the patient's head down for the procedure. Whether the patient should be leaning slightly anteriorly or posteriorly depends on the procedure. When the hilum is to be dissected, the patient should be leaning posteriorly; if the posterior mediastinum is to be dissected, the patient should be leaning anteriorly. Patients are supported in this position with a beanbag and an axillary roll with the arm on a padded support. The patient is further stabilized on the operating table by taping from anterior to posterior over the hip (**FIGURE 5**). A lower body warming blanket is applied from the waist down. The lower extremities are padded with pillows.

The surgeon stands in front of the patient with the assistant standing to the surgeon's left or behind the patient. The anesthesiologist stands at the head of the patient. The surgical nurse stands opposite the side of the surgical assistant. Monitors are positioned at the head of the bed and on either side of the patient (**FIGURE 6**).

OPERATIVE PREPARATION A preoperative dose of cefuroxime or piperacillin-tazobactam is administered half an hour before the skin incision is made. The skin of the chest is sterilized from the shoulder to the iliac crest with either an iodine preparation or chlorhexidine. Care is taken to extend the surgical field to the sternum anteriorly and to the spinous processes posteriorly. Drapes should be placed in such a way that a thoracotomy can be performed if needed. Instrumentation needed for VATS includes a 10-mm diameter, 30-cm long, 30-degree thoracoscope and thoracoscopic ring clamps, tonsil sponges, thoracoscopic scissors, thoracoscopic vascular clamp, curved Yankauer sucker, and electrosurgical and ultrasonic energy devices.

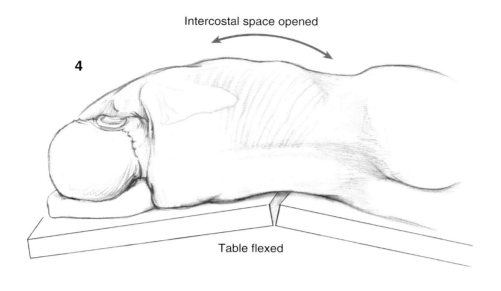

4

Intercostal space opened

Table flexed

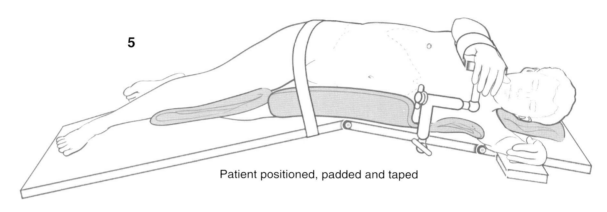

5

Patient positioned, padded and taped

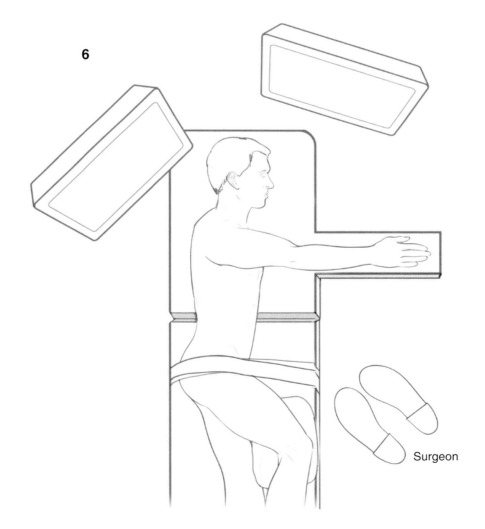

6

Surgeon

DETAILS OF THE PROCEDURE In general, the ports are placed with the camera port in the seventh intercostal space in line with, or anterior to, the anterior iliac spine. This port may need to be more posterior on the left to avoid the heart. The working incision is placed through the fourth or fifth intercostal space between the anterior and midaxillary line (**FIGURE 7**). A non–rib-spreading minithoracotomy (5 cm) may be used for the anterior working incision (no port) with a Weitlaner retractor to spread the soft tissues. The intercostal incision (indicated by dashed line) is made longer than the skin incision, as this allows the easy insertion of a wider variety of instruments as well as the ability to place two or three instruments at once through this incision (**FIGURE 8**). This technique may avoid the need for a fourth port.

Alternatively, a "baseball diamond" configuration of three ports can be used. The camera is situated at home plate, first and third bases are working ports, and the pathology of interest is triangulated at second base (**FIGURE 9**). An important principle is to keep the ports placed as widely spaced as possible to avoid instruments clashing with each other during the operation.

Once the camera port has been placed, it is often helpful to visualize the target area within the chest with the thoracoscope before deciding on the placement of the working incision or the two ports.

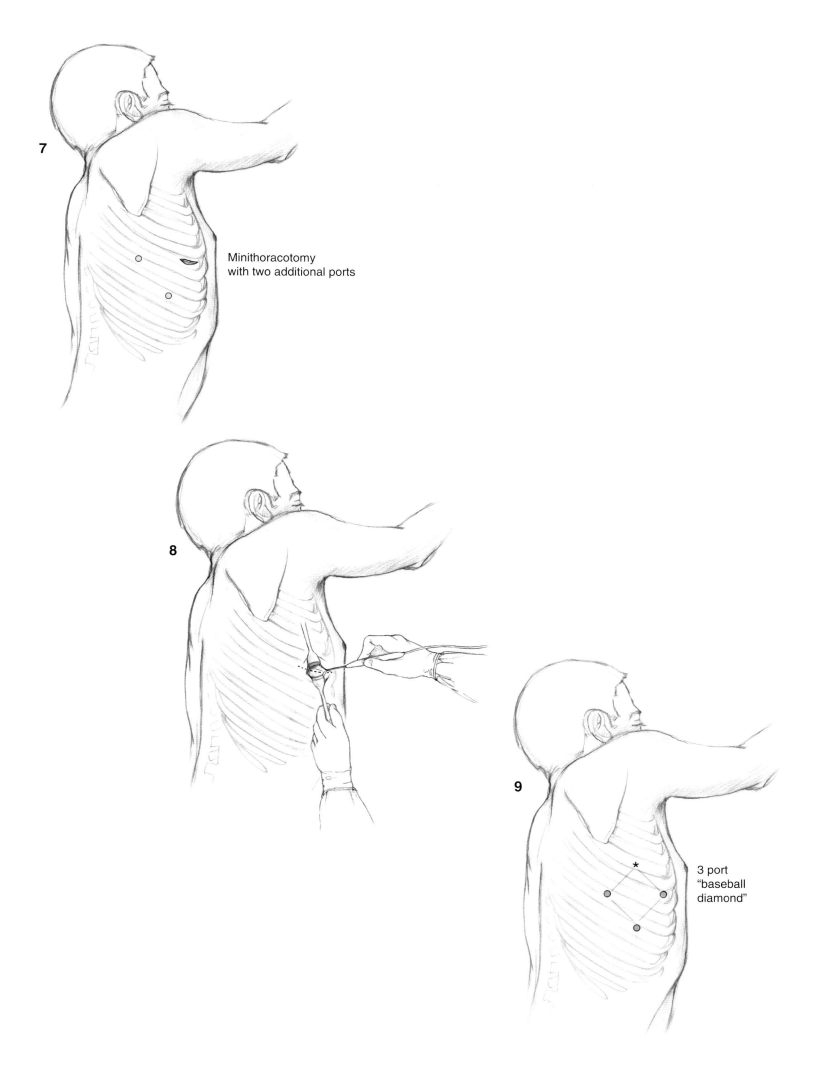

7

Minithoracotomy
with two additional ports

8

9

3 port
"baseball
diamond"

DETAILS OF THE PROCEDURE Another important consideration for port placement is elevation of the diaphragm. If the diaphragm is elevated and/or fused to the chest wall, there is a risk of diaphragmatic injury and entry into the abdomen during port placement. Even if this does not occur, if the ports are too low, the diaphragm may obstruct the view and prevent free movement of instruments throughout the procedure. Therefore, moving the ports superiorly in patients with an elevated diaphragm is strongly recommended. If, after port placement, the superior excursion of the diaphragm is problematic, a figure-of-eight stitch may be used to retract the diaphragm inferiorly to facilitate the operation. Aspiration of the stomach, reverse Trendelenburg position, and downward pressure on the diaphragm with a sponge stick through the working incision are also helpful to move the diaphragm out of the operative field (**FIGURE 10**).

Initial entry into the chest is accomplished through the 2.5-cm incision in the seventh intercostal space. Dissection can be performed with cautery or sharply in the intercostal space down to the pleura. Retraction with two army-navy retractors is helpful. The pleura is entered bluntly with a finger or incised using cautery or sharply with a scissors while ventilation is held. A 10-mm port is placed after probing the pleural space with a finger. The 30-degree scope is introduced to examine the chest and select the site of the working incision (minithoracotomy).

The working incision is next made after injecting 0.25% bupivacaine into the appropriate intercostal space (fourth or fifth). Under thoracoscopic vision, local anesthetic is injected into the intercostal space to elevate the parietal pleura. Dissection is performed using cautery just above the lower rib of the intercostal space, and entry into the pleural cavity is thoracoscopically visualized. A Weitlaner retractor is used to hold the soft tissues open; this allows suction to be used with in the chest without the lung reexpanding, as there is free passage of air into and out of the chest.

A third, more posterior port can be inserted if needed (see Figure 8). Thoracoscopic instruments can be introduced via the working incision. The thoracoscope can be placed through the working incision when an instrument needs to be placed through the camera port, because it provides a better working angle within the chest.

When the procedure is completed, hemostasis is secured with cautery and the chest irrigated. This is best done by pouring the irrigant through a bulb syringe with the bulb removed, positioned through the working incision. The irrigant is usually saline. Water is used if cancer is found in the chest. The fluid is sucked out of the chest, and one or two 28 French chest tubes are placed. The first tube is placed through the camera incision (posterior), and if a second tube is needed, it is placed through a separate incision anterior to the camera port (**FIGURE 11**). The chest tube position is confirmed by thoracoscopic visualization, and the tube is secured to the chest wall with a figure-of-eight 2-0 nylon stitch. Intercostal nerve blocks are performed above, below, and within the space of all incisions. The lung is reexpanded, and this is also confirmed thoracoscopically before ending the procedure. The camera is removed from the chest, and the working incision is closed with running 2-0 Vicryl for the muscle layer and the subcutaneous tissue. The skin is closed with subcuticular 4-0 Vicryl. The patient is extubated in the operating room.

POSTOPERATIVE CARE Most patients are extubated in the operating room and then taken to either an intensive care unit or step-down unit by way of the postanesthesia care unit. Every patient should receive a postoperative chest radiograph to ensure good expansion of the lung and effective chest tube placement. Except as noted below, chest tubes are generally left to water seal and removed when output is less than 250 mL/24 hr and there is no air leak. Special attention should be paid to pulmonary hygiene and pain control throughout the postoperative period, with the use of incentive spirometry and, in many cases, an epidural catheter (placed preoperatively). Most patients walk by postoperative day 1 and are discharged within 3 to 5 days. ∎

10

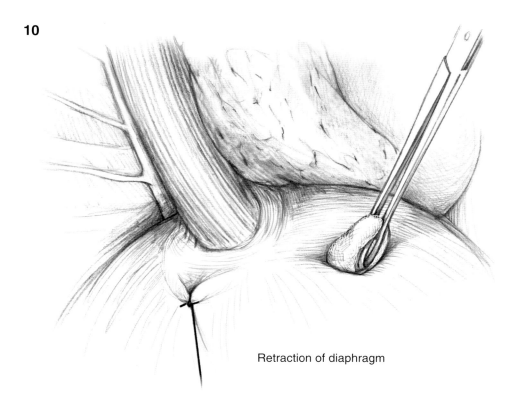

Retraction of diaphragm

11

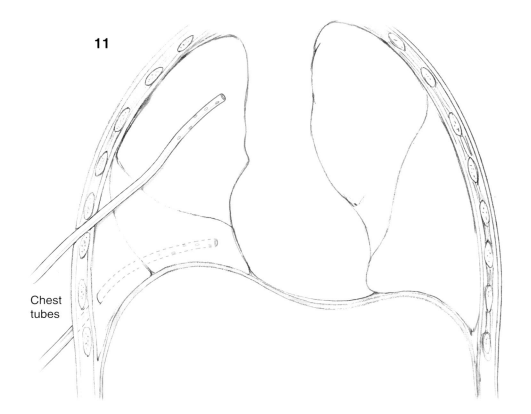

Chest
tubes

MINIMALLY INVASIVE SUTURING AND KNOT TYING

In laparoscopic and thoracoscopic surgery, suturing and knot tying are considered difficult skills, leading to billions of dollars of technology development to make suturing easier for the surgeon. The primary problem begging solution is the loss of the wrist in laparoscopic instruments. The only technology to have adequately solved this engineering problem is the surgical robot, but this multimillion-dollar solution is unnecessary for the bulk of suturing tasks encountered in minimally invasive surgery. Simple suturing and knot tying without robots, articulated needle holders, or "instant" knots can be learned in a simulator with the investment of a few hours. Mastery of these techniques may take more time, so practice in a simulator or box trainer is advised. It is preferable to ascend the suturing and knotting learning curve in a simulator, rather than wasting valuable time in the operating room. No professional athlete, pilot, or concert musician learns their skill without hours of practice "off stage." As surgeons, our obligation to our patient requires similar practice outside of the operating room. By convention, descriptions in this section are written for the right-hand-dominant surgeon.

INTRODUCING AND REMOVING THE NEEDLE   For laparoscopic suturing, the needle cannot be introduced on the needle holder, as the trocar is not wide enough. The suture is grasped with the needle holder adjacent to the needle and passed through the trocar (**FIGURE 1**). Clearly quick release (pop-off) needles cannot be used. A 10-mm trocar is needed, at a minimum, to introduce the needle.

NEEDLE POSITIONING   Positioning the needle in the needle holder is one of the more difficult tasks for the beginner. This becomes a one-handed task for the expert, but for the beginner, the simplest way to do this is to pick up the suture 1 or 2 centimeters above the needle, allowing the tip of the needle to dangle (**FIGURE 2A**). The needle is then lowered so the tip touches the tissue. Moving the left hand around causes the needle to pivot on its tip, allowing almost any position desired by the surgeon. Generally a position that will allow a 90-degree angle between needle holder and needle is desirable (**FIGURE 2B**). Once this position is achieved, the right hand is brought into view, and the needle grasped in the middle of its arc or several degrees toward the tail with a specialized laparoscopic needle holder (**FIGURE 2C**). The convex surface of the needle holder is aligned with the tip of the needle, to allow angulation of the needle (if desired) and to keep the

tip of the needle holder from digging into tissue as it is rotated. With certain suturing tasks, the needle may need to be angled 100 to 120 degrees away from the needle holder (e.g., for suturing the left crus of the diaphragm). In other circumstances the needle will need to be loaded up backhanded, and occasionally, even for "righties," a left-handed approach is necessary to accomplish the suturing task at hand. After many years of design, two types of needle holders remain popular, the Castro-Viejo type and the simple ringed handle, both analogous to similar open surgical needle holders.

SUTURING   Most laparoscopic suturing is done as a series of interrupted stitches. At the beginning, specially designed straight and ski needles were created for laparoscopic surgery, but—as skill was attained—most surgeons returned to the round needles used for open surgery. Suturing can be performed with any suture material, but suture with too little memory ("wilted" silk) or too much memory (polypropylene) makes knot tying more difficult. The suture should be cut to a length of 15 to 20 cm for most simple suturing. Passing the needle through tissue is one of the easier steps. As in open surgery, a tissue entry and exit site are planned in the surgeon's mind. The needle tip is placed on the entry point, and the instrument is rotated in a shallow arc (small bite of tissue) or a deep arc (large bite of tissue) (**FIGURE 3A**). When the tip of the needle emerges, it may be adequate to disengage the needle holder without grasping the tip of the needle, as the needle will sit without moving. In some situations it is best to grasp the tip of the needle as it emerges from tissue with the left hand to avoid it slipping back, or the tip rotating out of sight. If possible, it is always best to let the tissue hold the needle, then regrasp the needle for the next pass before pulling it out of the tissue (**FIGURE 3B**). This step is repeated until all the tissue to be approximated is gathered together.

A running suture is popular in laparoscopic surgery for creating purse strings, closing enterotomies, and oversewing staple lines. The suture length may be extended to 25 to 30 cm for this exercise, but a full-length suture should not be used, as it is difficult to effectively manage such a long suture in the MIS field. The needle is passed into the abdomen and through tissue as described earlier. Maintaining tension on the running suture is accomplished by the surgeon or first assistant grasping the tail of the suture, (also known as "following" in surgical jargon) as the surgeon prepares for the next bite through tissue (**FIGURE 4**). Methods of beginning and ending running suture lines are discussed in the next section.

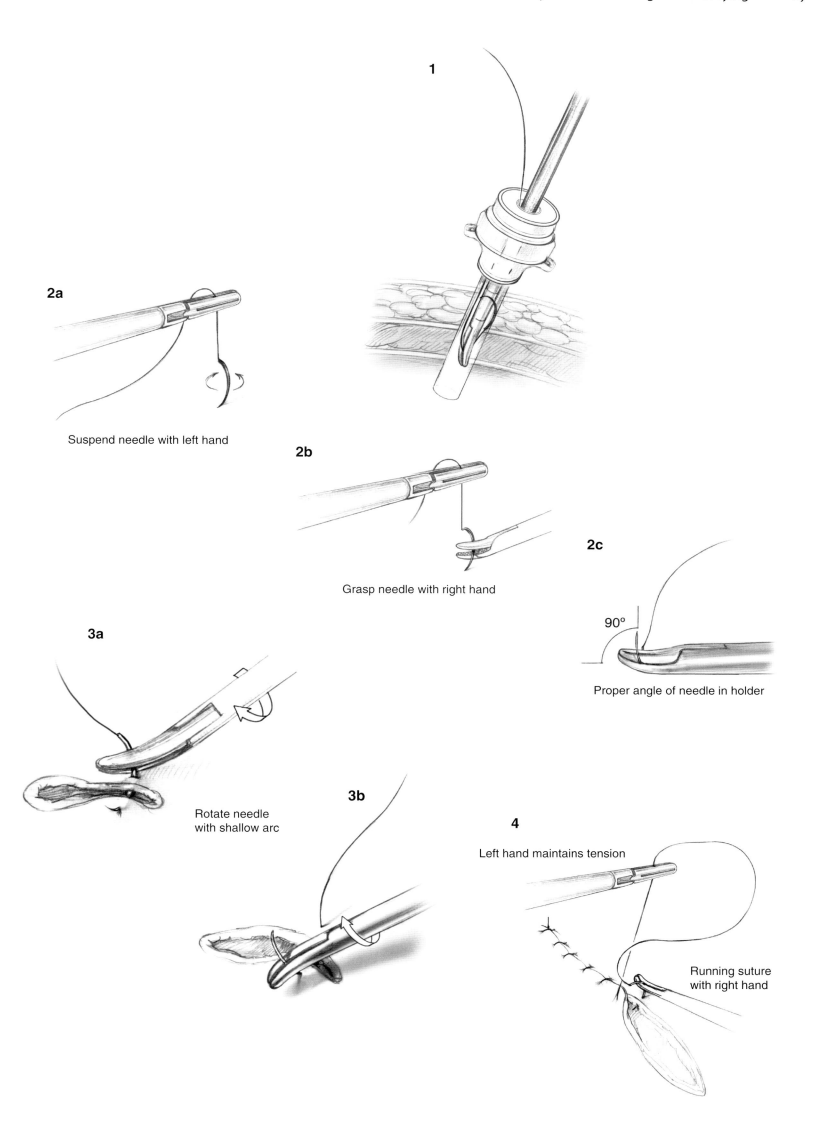

1

2a

Suspend needle with left hand

2b

Grasp needle with right hand

2c

90°

Proper angle of needle in holder

3a

Rotate needle
with shallow arc

3b

4

Left hand maintains tension

Running suture
with right hand

INTRACORPOREAL KNOTTING The simplest knot, applicable to most situations, is the square knot. Placed as a "sliding slip knot," the square knot is extremely flexible. The desired tension of tissue apposition is achieved with the knot in one configuration (two half hitches) where it will slide freely. The knot is locked in position by conversion of the two half hitches to a more stable configuration (the square knot). The sliding slip knot is created by throwing two overhand knots; the second is the mirror image of the first.

To start, the surgeon grasps the suture body adjacent to the needle with the right hand. A C loop is created between the tissue exit point of the suture and the needle (**FIGURE 5A**). The left hand is passed over the back of the C loop, then dropped as the right hand passes the C loop around the tip of the left hand instrument (**FIGURE 5B**). The left hand is advanced through the loop to grasp the suture tail (**FIGURE 5C**). The tail is pulled back through the loop to create an overhand knot (**FIGURE 5D**). The knot is not snugged down if the surgeon plans to convert to a slip knot. The body of the suture is then passed to the left hand and grasped next to the needle (**FIGURE 5E**).

A reverse C is created, and the surgeon passes their right hand behind the C, dropping through the loop and advancing through the loop to pick up the suture tail (**FIGURE 5F**) and pull it back through the loop (**FIGURE 5G**). This creates a square knot.

The knot is converted to two half hitches by pulling on one leg (usually the left leg, on the screen) and the corresponding suture tail (**FIGURE 6A**). This will convert the square knot, which will not slide, to two half hitches, which can be slid (**FIGURE 6B**). Holding the body of the suture in the right hand, the knot is slid down (**FIGURE 6C**) to achieve desired tightness (**FIGURE 6D**). Pulling on the body and tail in opposite directions (**FIGURE 6E**) will reconvert the two half hitches into a square knot (**FIGURE 6F**). Two more overhand knots, thrown on top of the square knot, in alternating directions will create a secure knot using all but the slipperiest suture. If there is any concern about suture slippage, additional overhand knots can be thrown. The suture is cut immediately above the knot and the excess suture material is removed.

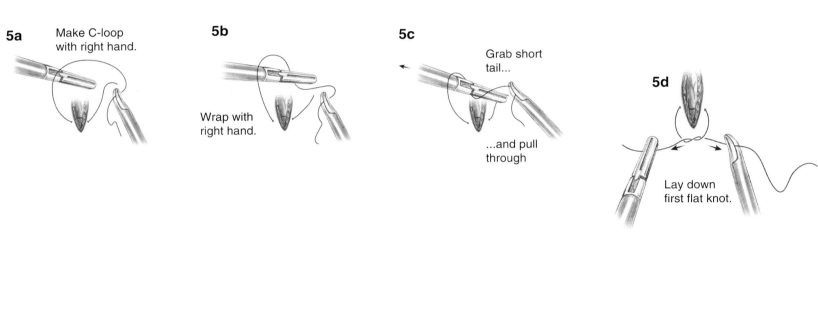

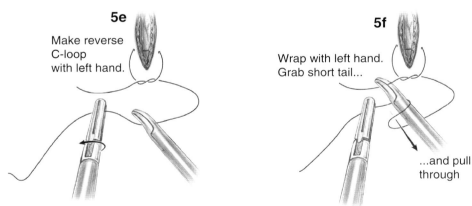

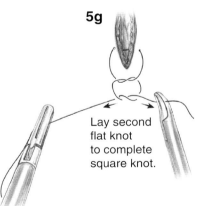

Conversion of square knot to slip knot

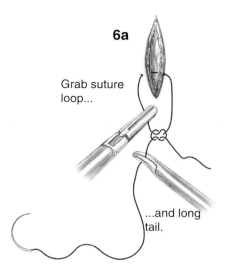

6a

Grab suture loop...

...and long tail.

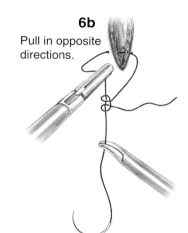

6b

Pull in opposite directions.

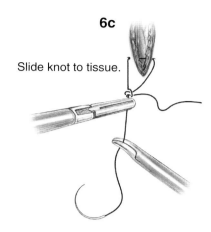

6c

Slide knot to tissue.

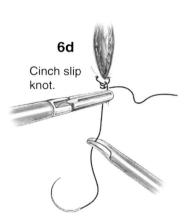

6d

Cinch slip knot.

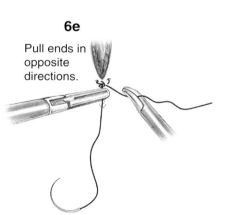

6e

Pull ends in opposite directions.

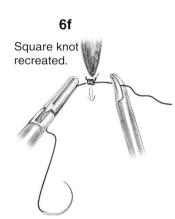

6f

Square knot recreated.

INTRACORPOREAL KNOTTING Two variations on this technique deserve mention. The first is the reef knot. This is a form of sliding square knot, but does not require the surgeon to transition the suture back and forth between their left and right hands. Instead, the square (two mirror-image overhand knots) is formed by looping behind the C for the first overhand knot and in front of the C for the second overhand knot (**FIGURE 7A–D**). On the creation of the second knot (**FIGURE 7E–G**) it is necessary for the surgeon to cross the instrument tips to pull the body and tail of the suture in opposite directions to create the square knot (**FIGURE 7H**).

The second variation is used when the suture will not slide through the tissue as the knot is tightened. Examples of this situation are the end of a running suture, or after a "Z" stitch is placed across a bleeding vessel. Under these circumstances, a "surgeon's knot" (a doubly looped overhand knot) is used as the first throw and cinched down tightly. A tight surgeon's knot will usually keep the suture locked well enough that a mirror-image overhand knot can be placed before the knot slips.

The first knot in a running suture is usually a sliding slip knot as described earlier. At the end of a running suture, the knot created will have a doubled tail (the last pass through the tissue) and a single body (**FIGURE 8A**). The needle is removed. A sliding slip knot is impossible at the end of a running suture, so the first knot thrown should be a surgeon's knot (**FIGURE 8B**) followed by a series (three to five, depending on suture material) of alternating overhand knots to secure the suture line effectively (**FIGURE 8C**).

EXTRACORPOREAL KNOTTING Although most knot tying can be done with intracorporeal techniques, as shown previously, there are situations in which extracorporeal knotting may be preferable—for example, when the working space does not allow sufficient instrument freedom for intracorporeal knotting. During transabdominal extraperitoneal (TEP) hernia repair, it is difficult to ligate a large indirect hernia sac with intracorporeal techniques. Some individuals also like to close the diaphragmatic hiatus with extracorporeal knotting.

The first step in extracorporeal knotting is choosing the correct suture material. Braided or monofilament suture material may be used, but suture that frays easily, such as silk, may be damaged during knot sliding. A 45- or 60-cm-long suture is passed down a 10-mm or larger trocar, looped behind the structure(s) to be ligated, then pulled back out through the trocar. A simple overhand knot is created near the mouth of the trocar, and the suture ends are held under tension with a hemostat. A specialized knot pusher is placed on top of the knot, and the knot is pushed down the trocar until it is snug around the structure to be ligated (**FIGURE 9**). The knot pusher is removed as tension is kept on the suture ends. A second overhand knot, oriented in the opposite direction from the first knot, is created at the mouth of the trocar, and the process is repeated until the desired number of overhand knots have been placed. The suture is cut immediately above the knot, and the excess suture material is removed.

OTHER TECHNIQUES Suturing techniques using specialized devices, and knotting techniques used by laparoscopic surgeons in some environments, including Roeder's knots and jamming knots, are beyond the scope of this atlas. The techniques described in this chapter will serve the surgeon for almost all basic and advanced minimally invasive surgery. ■

Reef knot (alternating direction of wrap)

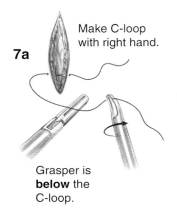

7a Make C-loop with right hand. Grasper is **below** the C-loop.

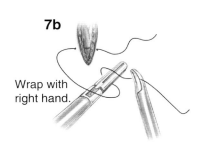

7b Wrap with right hand.

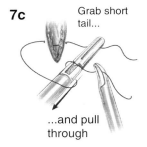

7c Grab short tail... ...and pull through

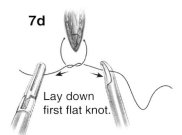

7d Lay down first flat knot.

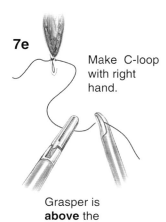

7e Make C-loop with right hand. Grasper is **above** the C-loop.

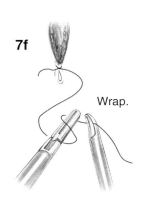

7f Wrap.

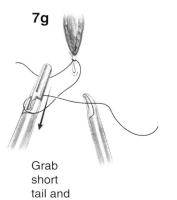

7g Grab short tail and pull through.

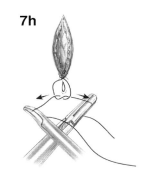

7h Cross hands to lay second knot flat.

Surgeon's knot (doubly looped overhand knot)

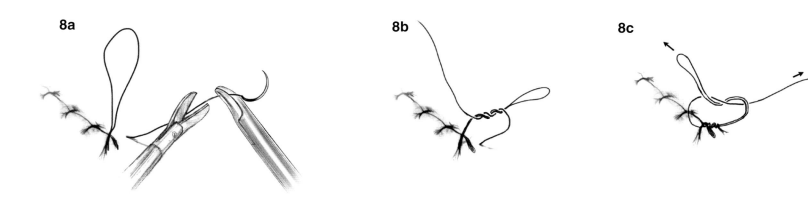

8a   8b   8c

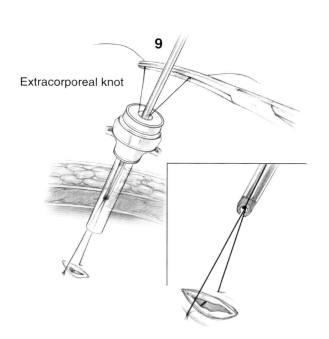

9

Extracorporeal knot

CHAPTER 5

ADVANCED MINIMALLY INVASIVE SURGICAL TECHNIQUES: SINGLE-INCISION LAPAROSCOPIC SURGERY, ROBOTICS, AND NATURAL-ORIFICE TRANSLUMINAL ENDOSCOPIC SURGERY

In recent years advances in optics, instrumentation, and technical skill coupled with a desire to further minimize operative wounds has led to the proliferation of new highly sophisticated techniques. These newer modalities often challenge the traditional tenets of modern laparoscopy. Single-incision laparoscopic surgery (SILS) uses specialized access devices or multiple tightly spaced fascial incisions at the umbilicus to accomplish what has been traditionally done through multiple port sites. To accomplish an operation in such a limited space requires the laparoscopic surgeon to work in a cross-handed manner and employ specialized curved instruments. Robotic surgery removes the operating surgeon from the bedside and places him or her at a console where hand motions are translated electronically into actions. Natural-orifice transluminal endoscopic surgery (NOTES) uses advanced endoscopic techniques to traverse the upper or lower GI tract or vagina to reach the targeted surgical area. To date, a wide array of surgical procedures have been attempted using these advanced minimally invasive surgery techniques with varying degrees of success. Outcomes data to justify increased costs and OR times has lagged behind market demand in all three of these areas.

SINGLE-INCISION LAPAROSCOPIC SURGERY SILS techniques have now been applied to a number of different procedures, but the most established application for this technique has been for cholecystectomy. SILS cholecystectomy is described in Chapter 33. The major advantage of this technique is improved appearances, resulting from a single scar that can often be hidden in the umbilicus (**FIGURE 1**).

The main disadvantage of the SILS approach lies in its technical challenges, which require some time to master. Whether performed through specialized trocars or multiple tightly spaced facial openings, traditional ergonomics is significantly compromised (**FIGURES 2, 3**). Operative times—initially quite long with SILS—decrease significantly after the first 10 cases

are completed. Another disadvantage of SILS is the requirement for customized articulating instruments that allow the operating surgeon a sufficient degree of angulation from the target to complete the procedure. Postoperative pain following SILS cholecystectomy may be more of the same as standard laparoscopic surgery. Studies suggest that complication rates and outcomes are comparable to those for laparoscopic cholecystectomy, but the rate of incisional hernia appears to be greater after SILS access.

Choosing patients with modest body mass index and without extensive past surgical history is critical during initial SILS learning curve. Operative indications for specific procedures are the same for the traditional laparoscopic procedure. Expertise in traditional advanced laparoscopy and a low threshold for placement of additional trocars when patient safety requires it are prerequisites for safe SILS.

SILS access is obtained through a vertical skin incision through the umbilicus. Three 5-mm laparoscopic ports are introduced into the SILS port, and carbon dioxide (CO_2) insufflation is initiated through the insufflation cuff until a pneumoperitoneum of 12 to 14 mm Hg pressure is achieved. The decision to proceed along conventional laparoscopic lines should be liberally applied, particularly early on in a surgeon's learning curve, if there is evidence of severe inflammatory disease. Transabdominal sutures many be used in place of trocars to aid in retraction, as seen for laparoscopic cholecystectomy (**FIGURE 4**).

With the SILS approach, the dissection is frustrated by the close grouping of the trocars at the umbilicus, the need to cross operating instruments inside the abdomen (**FIGURE 5**), the lack of commonly accepted sturdiness of the current-generation SILS instruments, and the inability to completely retract the tip of the gallbladder in a cephalad fashion or manipulate the organ to assist with visualization or dissection. Frustration or difficulty in these areas generally decreases as surgeon experience increases.

1

**Single-Incision
Laparoscopic
Surgery (SILS)**

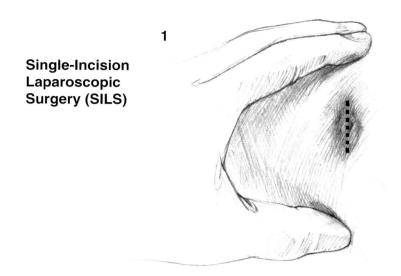

2

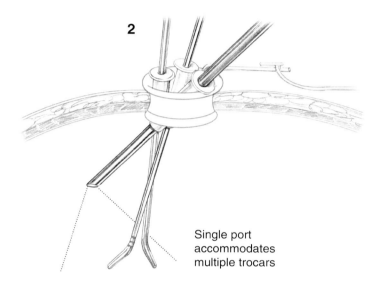

Single port
accommodates
multiple trocars

3

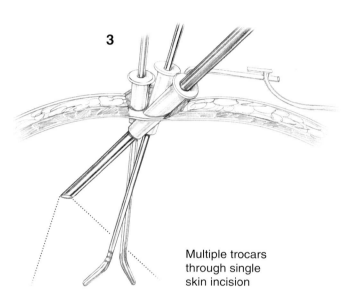

Multiple trocars
through single
skin incision

4

Transabdominal
suture for
retraction

SILS
port

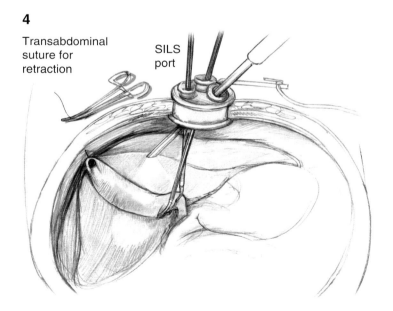

5

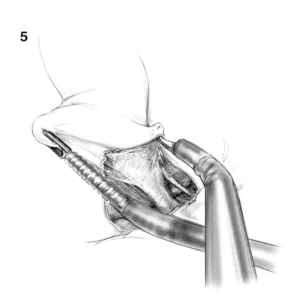

ROBOTIC SURGERY The da Vinci robotic surgical system consists of a surgeon console, a multiple-armed robotic cart, and a high-definition stereoscopic 3D camera (**FIGURE 6**). Efficient implementation of the technology requires a dedicated team familiar with setup and intraoperative management. In fields such as urology and gynecology, use of robots has grown rapidly, resulting from surgeons' reduced learning curve, ergonomic advantage, and specific suitability for pelvic operations. The robotic platform requires that the patient be stationary once docked. The inability to change patient position intraoperatively makes proper positioning and trocar placement critical to operative success (**FIGURE 7**). Improper spacing of trocars and robot arms can create clashes as the robot attempts to move through its full range of motion. Limitations in tools for the robot such as suction/irrigation and advanced energy sources mean that a trained bedside surgical assistant is needed to assist with most procedures. This assistant is also necessary to make robotic instrument exchanges as required (**FIGURE 8**).

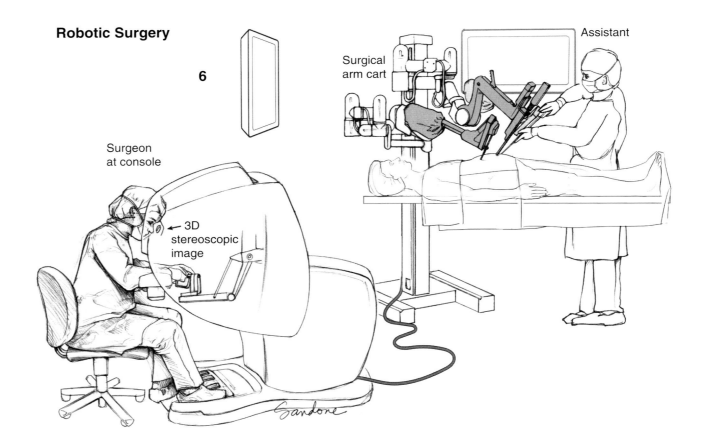

Robotic Surgery

6

Surgical arm cart

Assistant

Surgeon at console

← 3D stereoscopic image

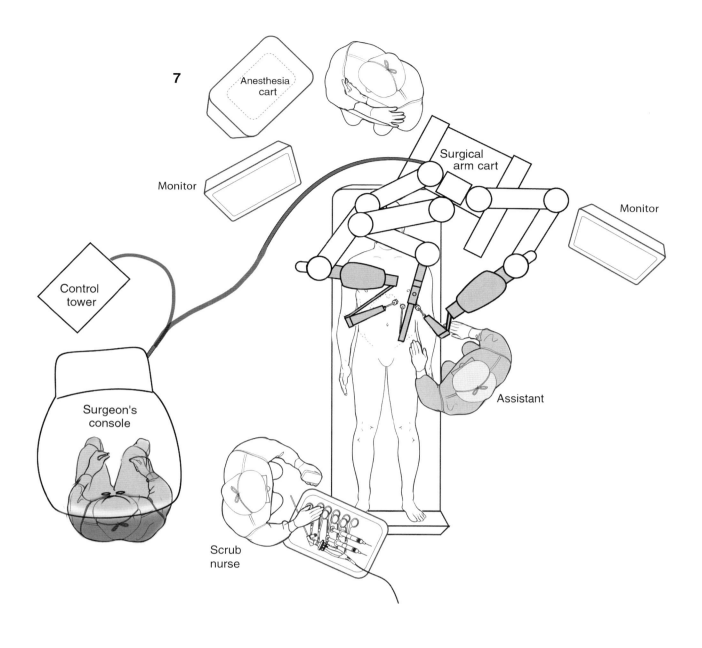

7

Anesthesia cart

Surgical arm cart

Monitor

Monitor

Control tower

Surgeon's console

Assistant

Scrub nurse

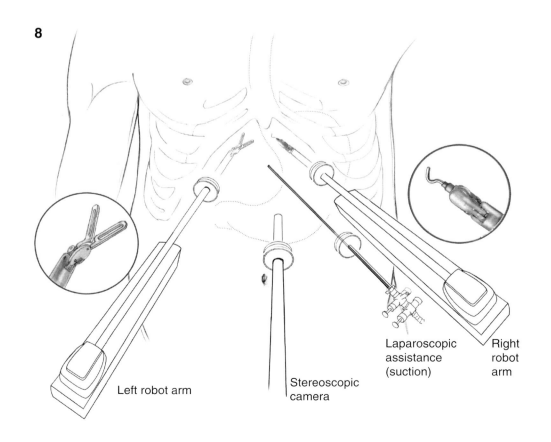

8

Left robot arm

Stereoscopic camera

Laparoscopic assistance (suction)

Right robot arm

ROBOTIC SURGERY The wrist action of the robotic instruments provides additional freedom of motion over traditional laparoscopic instruments. This is particularly useful in procedures such as the robotic Heller myotomy, in which upward wrist action allows safe dissection of circular muscle fibers off of the underlying mucosa (**FIGURE 9**). Although the current robotic platform lacks tactile feedback, the high-definition 3D visualization enables highly complex dissection capability.

Robotic surgery has proven efficacy for complex dissections in the foregut and pelvis. The lymph node dissection of a D2 gastrectomy, total mesorectal excision in colorectal procedures, and radical prostatectomy are all procedures in which the increased dexterity afforded by the robot has shown superiority over traditional laparoscopic instrumentation.

Current robotic technology facilitates the application of SILS concepts through the reassignment of arms at the console to restore normal surgeon motion despite the arms working in a "crossed hands" position at the bedside (**FIGURE 10**).

9

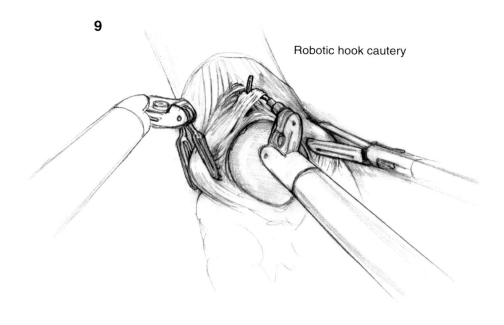

Robotic hook cautery

Robotic SILS

Left
robotic arm

Stereoscopic
camera

Right
robotic arm

10

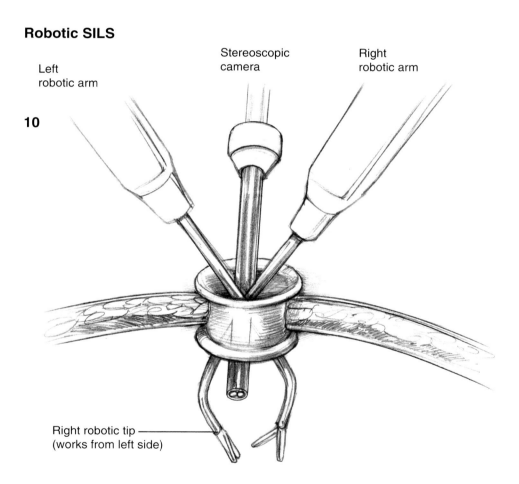

Right robotic tip
(works from left side)

NATURAL-ORIFICE TRANSLUMINAL ENDOSCOPIC SURGERY NOTES has been applied to a variety of surgical procedures around the world. Portals of access to the peritoneal cavity include transgastric, transvaginal, and transrectal puncture (**FIGURES 11, 12**).

Although the first NOTES procedures to receive acclaim were the NOTES appendectomy (transvaginal or transgastric) and cholecystectomy (transvaginal or transgastric), these procedures are performed in only a few centers. The most widely used new NOTES procedure is peroral endoscopic myotomy (POEM) for achalasia (see Chapter 15). Patients found to have severe dysphagia related to the absence of esophageal body peristalsis and incomplete relaxation of the lower esophageal sphincter tone are candidates for this approach.

The greatest advantage of POEM is the ability to perform an esophageal myotomy without any incision on the abdominal wall. A surgeon and OR team with expertise in advanced therapeutic techniques and specialized instrumentation is a requirement. The procedure, in brief, goes as follows: A transparent endoscopic cap is placed on the end of a standard endoscope to allow greater viewing perspective and prevent smudging of the optical surface. An electrosurgical needle knife is then used to make a mucosal incision in the esophagus approximately 10 cm above the GE junction. A biliary sphincterotomy balloon is inserted into the incision and inflated to facilitate creation of a submucosal tunnel (**FIGURE 13**). The scope is advanced into the tunnel with the assistance of the balloon, then advanced distal to the lower esophageal sphincter (LES) (**FIGURE 14**). A triangular-tip electrosurgical knife is used to create a myotomy in the circular muscle fibers of the esophagus in a proximal to distal direction (**FIGURE 15**). The endpoint of myotomy is at least 2 to 3 cm distal to the gastroesophageal junction. Closure of the mucosotomy is performed with a series of endoscopically placed hemostatic clips.

POEM is one of the first widely accepted NOTES procedures, but there is little doubt that other similar procedures will be developed. ■

11

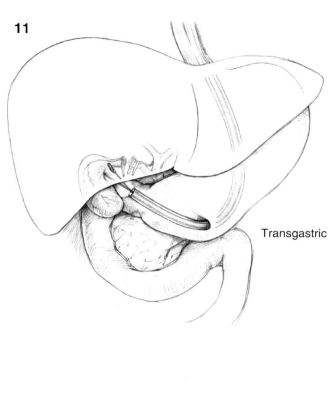

Transgastric

12

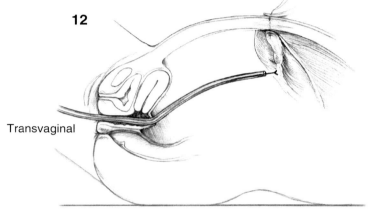

Transvaginal

POEM

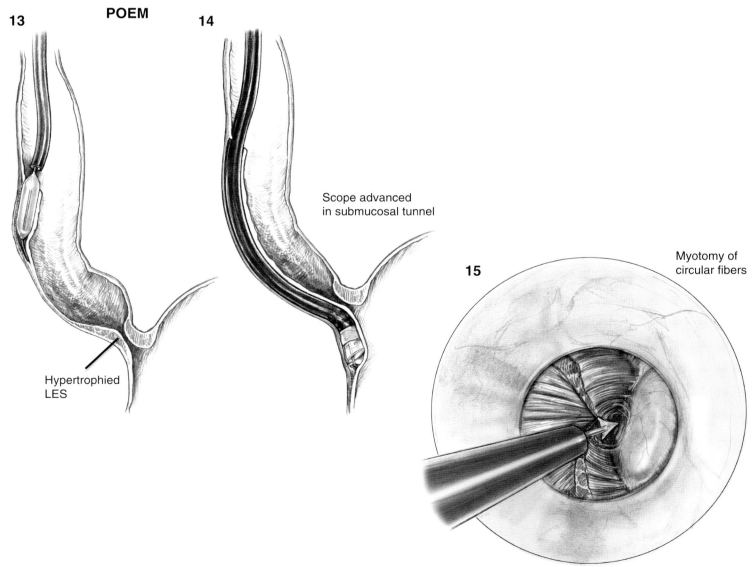

13

Hypertrophied
LES

14

Scope advanced
in submucosal tunnel

15

Myotomy of
circular fibers

SECTION II
MINIMALLY INVASIVE THORACIC SURGERY

MEDIASTINOSCOPY

INDICATIONS Mediastinoscopy is indicated for the staging of the mediastinal lymph nodes in cases of suspected or confirmed non–small cell lung cancer or to obtain diagnostic tissue in other cases of mediastinal lymphadenopathy. Level 2, 4, and 7 paratracheal lymph nodes are generally accessible to the mediastinoscope (**FIGURE 1**). Relative contraindications include prior thoracic radiation, previous mediastinoscopy, aortic arch aneurysm, tracheal resection, or functioning tracheostomy.

PREOPERATIVE PREPARATION Computed tomography scanning of the chest as well as a whole-body positron emission tomography (PET) scan are helpful both in evaluating other areas of disease and in identifying areas within mediastinum that are of particular interest. Many of these patients have extensive comorbidities, and an electrocardiogram and laboratory evaluation including complete blood count, electrolytes, blood urea nitrogen, creatinine, glucose, and prothrombin and partial thromboplastin times are generally recommended.

ANESTHESIA General anesthesia with endotracheal intubation should be used. An arterial line and two large-bore intravenous lines should be placed, and the anesthesiologist should be prepared for an emergent sternotomy in case excessive bleeding is encountered.

POSITION The patient is placed supine on a flat table with a shoulder roll placed to extend the neck. The surgeon stands at the head of the patient, and the assistant stands to the surgeon's right side. The surgical nurse stands on the right side toward the foot of the patient. The anesthesiologist stands to the patient's left side (**FIGURE 2**).

1

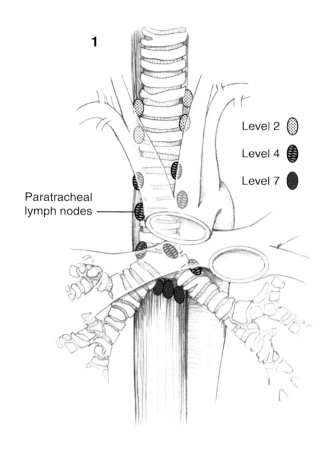

Level 2
Level 4
Level 7

Paratracheal
lymph nodes

2   Surgeon

Assistant

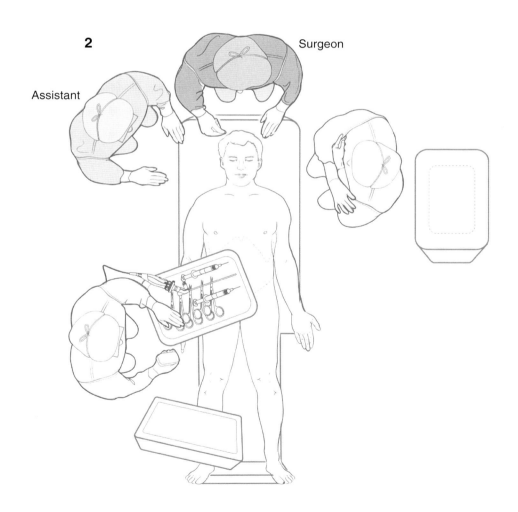

OPERATIVE PREPARATION The skin of the neck and entire chest should be prepared in the usual manner. Care should be taken that the operative field and drapes are placed such that emergent sternotomy is possible if bleeding is encountered.

DETAILS OF THE PROCEDURE A 2.5-cm transverse incision is made two fingerbreadths above the sternal notch. The platysma is divided transversely, and the strap muscles are divided vertically through the median raphe. Dissection is carried down to the trachea. Once the trachea is exposed, blunt dissection with a finger allows development of the pretracheal space (**FIGURE 3**). If dense adhesions are encountered, the procedure should be aborted. Throughout the procedure, it is important to stay immediately on the trachea to ensure that the surgeon is posterior to the great vessels crossing anteriorly.

At this point, the video-mediastinoscope is inserted (**FIGURE 4**). Attention is paid to staying immediately on the trachea as it is advanced inferiorly. The right level 2 nodes are accessible immediately after entry into the paratracheal soft tissue space and just inferior to the innominate artery after opening the mediastinal pleura with the suction/cautery (**FIGURE 5**).

3

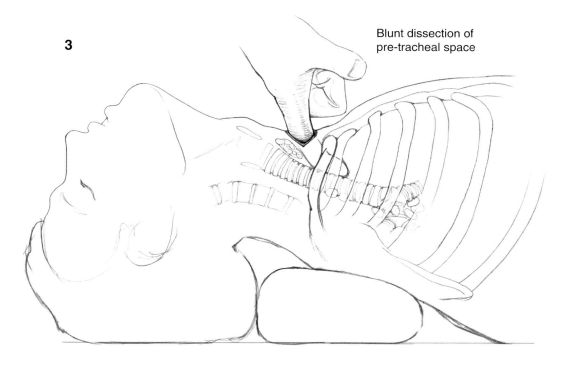

Blunt dissection of
pre-tracheal space

4

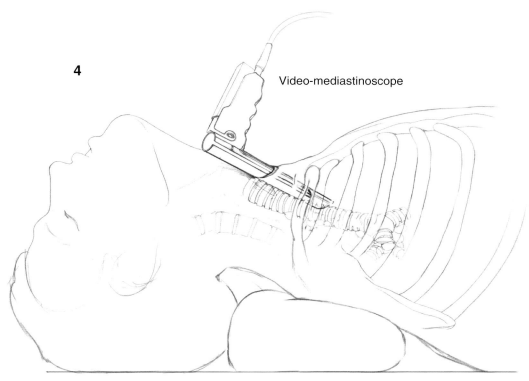

Video-mediastinoscope

5

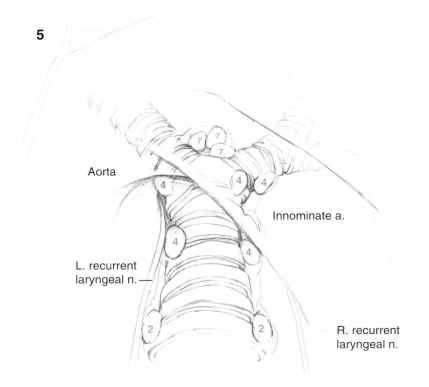

Aorta

Innominate a.

L. recurrent
laryngeal n.

R. recurrent
laryngeal n.

DETAILS OF THE PROCEDURE The nodes can be identified as blue-gray structures on either side of the trachea. Before biopsy, care should be taken to identify the innominate artery. At this and every level, each structure should be aspirated prior to biopsy to ensure that it is not a vessel, as the appearance can be very similar (**FIGURE 6A,B**).

Using cautery or blunt dissection, the pleura is opened, continuing inferiorly along the trachea to identify the right level 4 nodes. Inferior dissection is halted when the right main-stem bronchus is encountered. The pleura is gently dissected anterior to the carina, and the subcarinal area is identified. Bluntly dissecting to the left will help identify the left main-stem bronchus and the aortic arch. Cautery should not be used in this portion of the dissection to avoid injury to the recurrent laryngeal nerve. Once both mainstem bronchi are identified, level 7 nodes can be biopsied, taking care to not injure the pulmonary artery inferiorly and anteriorly or the esophagus posteriorly (**FIGURE 7**). Continuing back up the left side, the left level 4 nodes are biopsied, followed by the withdrawal of the mediastinoscope to the superior aspect of the aortic arch, where the left level 2 nodes are identified and biopsied (**FIGURE 8**).

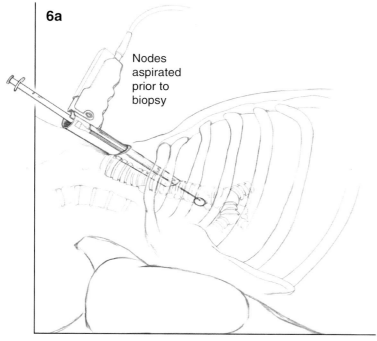

6a

Nodes aspirated prior to biopsy

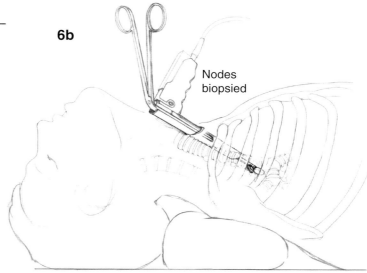

6b

Nodes biopsied

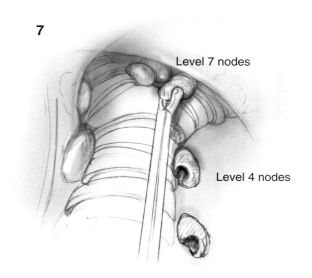

7

Level 7 nodes

Level 4 nodes

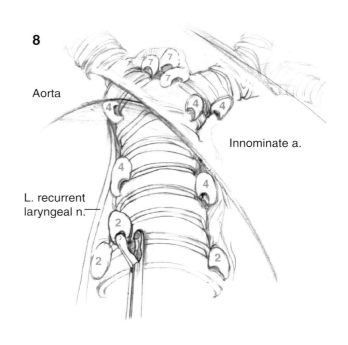

8

Aorta

Innominate a.

L. recurrent laryngeal n.

DETAILS OF THE PROCEDURE After any biopsy, the area should be inspected for bleeding. Some oozing is common and controlled by packing the mediastinum with a gauze for 2 to 5 minutes or by the limited use of electrocautery (**FIGURE 9**). Bleeding not controlled by packing or that rapidly fills the wound is serious and will require sternotomy or right thoracotomy for control.

Once all biopsies have been obtained, the mediastinoscope is removed and the mediastinum is packed with a gauze pad and left for at least 3 minutes (**FIGURE 10**). The packing is then removed and the mediastinoscope reinserted. The mediastinum is inspected to ensure good hemostasis. Once hemostasis has been achieved, the mediastinoscope is removed and the strap muscles of the neck are closed with an interrupted 2-0 absorbable suture. The platysma is closed with a running 3-0 absorbable suture, and the skin is closed with a subcuticular 4-0 absorbable suture.

POSTOPERATIVE CARE After mediastinoscopy, patients should be observed in the postanesthesia care unit for a couple of hours. During that time, a chest radiograph is obtained to ensure that there is no pneumothorax. The patient can then be safely discharged home. ■

9

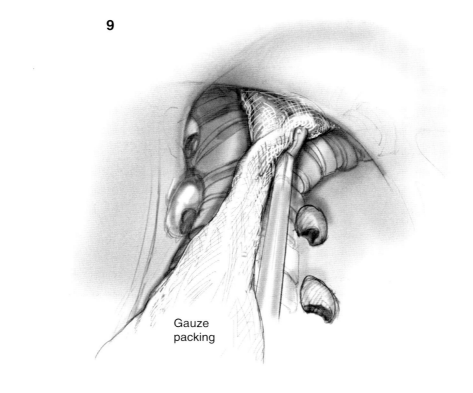

Gauze
packing

10

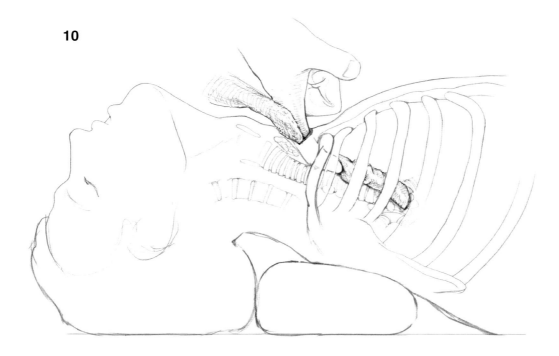

BLEBECTOMY AND PLEURECTOMY

INDICATIONS Blebectomy and pleurectomy is recommended for the second episode of ipsilateral spontaneous pneumothorax, or the first episode of spontaneous pneumothorax with an apical bleb on CT scan. Patients who are severely symptomatic during the first spontaneous pneumothorax, or who may not be able to obtain rapid treatment for a second spontaneous pneumothorax by virtue of poor access to specialized care, may benefit from pleurectomy after a single spontaneous pneumothorax.

PREOPERATIVE PLANNING A CT scan of the chest identifies the target areas, usually in the apices of the lung (**FIGURE 1**). A bleb may also be seen in the superior segment of the lower lobe. Women should be questioned about their menstrual history to rule in (or out) catamenial pneumothorax. Underlying emphysema is not a contraindication to surgery but substantially increases its complexity and postoperative morbidity. With underlying emphysema, the area of potential air leak is less predictable, occurring anywhere along the surface of the lung, and is therefore more difficult to localize. The delicate nature of emphysematous lung and the often-associated pleural adhesions require expertise in lung handling. Routine use of gentle lung handling, buttressed staple lines, and mechanical pleurodesis or pleurectomy are required.

ANESTHESIA General anesthesia is performed with single-lung ventilation. A double-lumen tube allows the anesthesiologist to assist in localizing blebs with gentle hand ventilations on the ipsilateral side, while still fully ventilating the contralateral side.

POSITION The patient is placed in the appropriate lateral decubitus position, slightly rolled forward in case of the need for posterolateral thoracotomy. The surgeon stands in front of the patient with the assistant standing to the surgeon's left or behind the patient. The anesthesiologist stands at the head of the patient. The surgical nurse stands on the same side as the surgical assistant. Monitors are positioned at the head of the bed and on either side of the patient (**FIGURE 2**).

OPERATIVE PREP The skin may be prepared using any suitable prep, but the prep should anticipate the possibility of a thoracotomy. The skin prep should be from the nipples medially, to the spine laterally; and from above the shoulder superiorly, to below the level of the costal margin inferiorly.

INCISION AND EXPOSURE The incision for the thoracoscope is placed in the 7th intercostal space (ICS) in the midaxillary line. A 5-mm port in the 5th ICS posteriorly can be used for retraction and may provide the best angle for stapling of the bleb. A second 2- to 3-cm incision is made in the 4th intercostal space between the midaxillary line and the anterior axillary line (**FIGURE 3**).

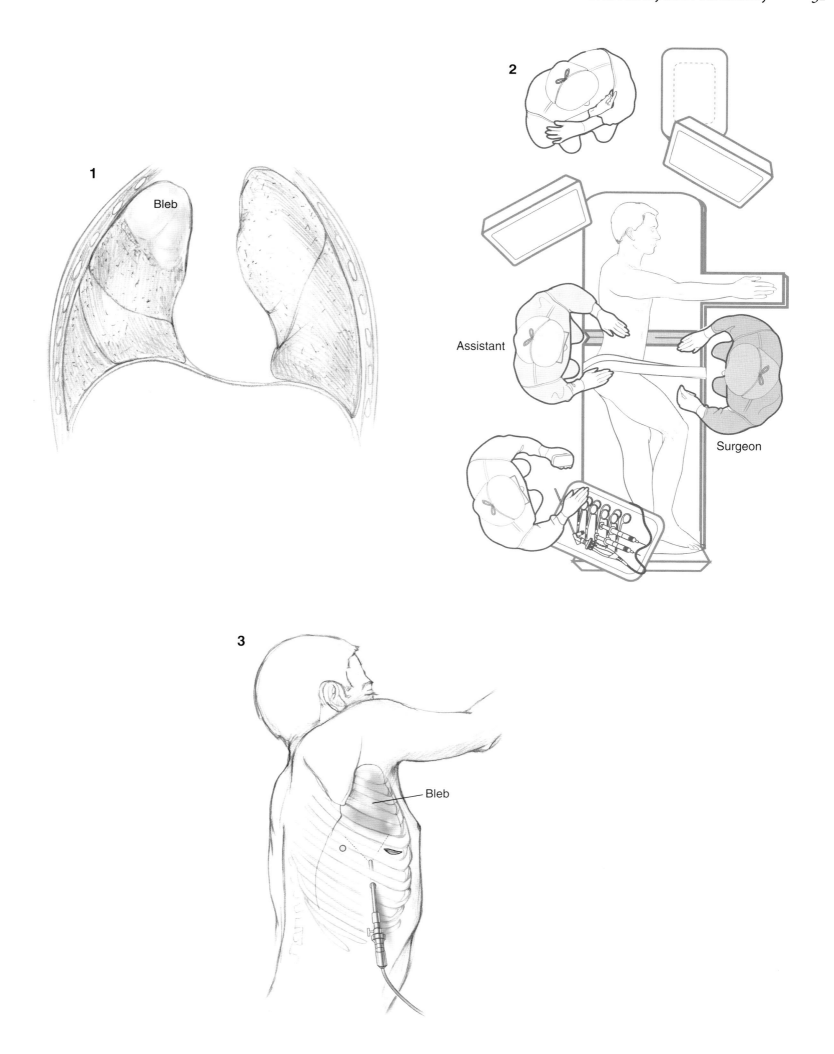

Bleb

2

Assistant

Surgeon

3

Bleb

DETAILS OF THE PROCEDURE The lung is collapsed and any adhesions divided sharply or with electrosurgery. If a pleural tent is to be performed, as may be done for treatment of a pneumothorax secondary to emphysema, a decision is made as to what lung will need to be resected and what parietal pleura used for the pleural tent. Care is taken not to injure lung left in situ or parietal pleura used for a tent. Once the lung is free, a ring clamp is used to grasp the apex of the lung and bring it into view. The bleb is identified and held within a ring clamp. Blebs that cannot be located can often be visualized by gentle ventilation of the ipsilateral lung. The highly compliant bleb will ventilate and fill before the less compliant surrounding lung.

A linear stapler with an intermediate-length staple load (45-mm length, purple tristapler, or 3.5-mm staple height) is introduced into the chest, passing under the ring clamp, and applied to the lung parenchyma caudad to the ring clamp to include normal lung parenchyma. This part of the lung is then resected by firing the stapler (**FIGURE 4**). The superior segment of the lower lobe is inspected for any other blebs, as is the rest of the lung. In the case of catamenial pneumothorax, the diaphragm is inspected for fenestrations and the pleural surfaces for endometriosis. Fenestrations should be suture closed and endometriosis removed as much as possible. If no further blebs are identified, a pleurectomy is performed.

The parietal pleura is divided with electrosurgery starting posteriorly and progressing anteriorly in the line of the working incision (4th space) (**FIGURE 5**). While the anterior edge of the upper pleura is held in a ring clamp, a Kittner dissector is used to develop an extrapleural plane (**FIGURE 6**). Once this plane is well established, the pleura is stripped from the chest wall posteriorly, anteriorly, and laterally using a sponge stick. The dissection proceeds to the apex of the chest (**FIGURE 7**). For a pleural tent, the pleura is allowed to fall over the area of lung suspected to be the source of the pneumothorax. Two 28 French chest tubes are placed, one anteriorly outside of the tent and the other posteriorly to drain the chest and reexpand the lung (**FIGURE 8**).

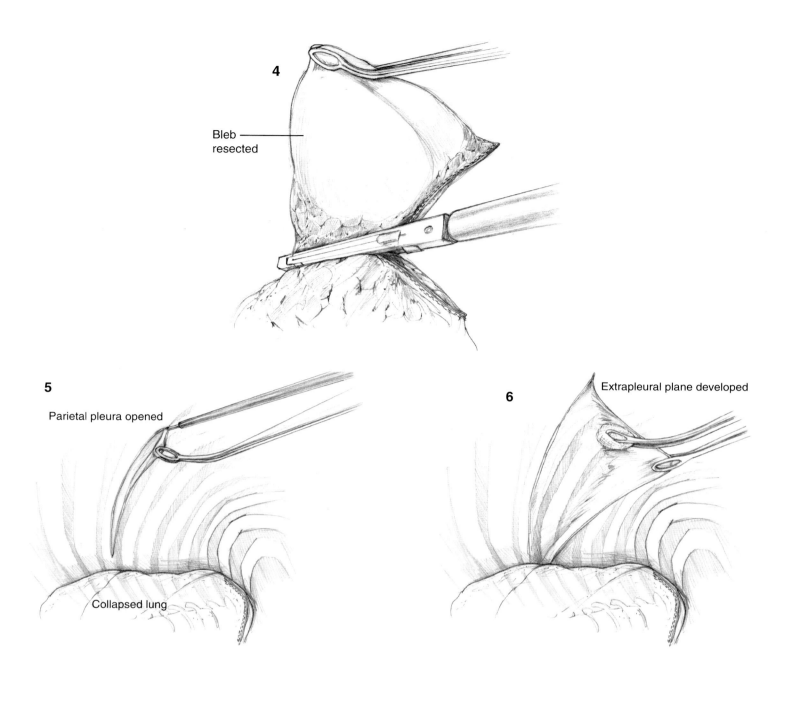

4

Bleb resected

5

Parietal pleura opened

Collapsed lung

6

Extrapleural plane developed

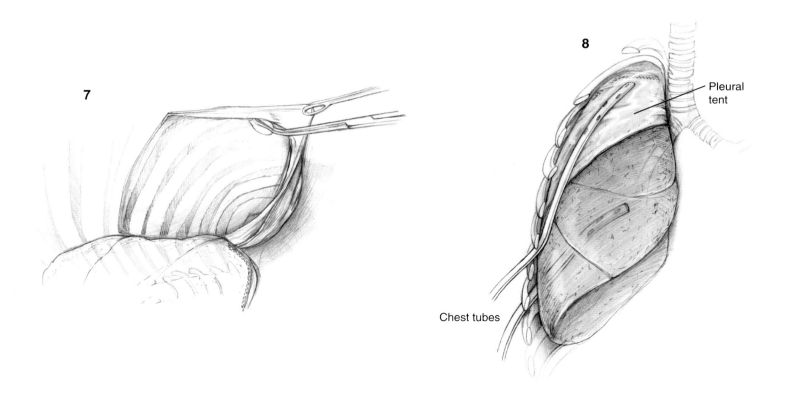

7

8

Pleural tent

Chest tubes

DETAILS OF THE PROCEDURE   Alternatively, for a pleurectomy, the pleura is transected at its reflection with the mediastinal pleura anteriorly and posteriorly (**FIGURE 9**). The mediastinal and diaphragmatic pleura can be abraded to roughen these surfaces using an electrocautery scratch pad held with a ring clamp. Care must be taken not to damage the phrenic nerve if diaphragmatic pleurodesis is performed. Hemostasis must be meticulous after pleurectomy, and this is accomplished by cauterizing any bleeding areas on the chest wall and/or placing a laparotomy pad into the chest against the pleural surface (**FIGURE 10**). The ipsilateral lung is inflated for 5 to 10 minutes to provide mechanical pressure on the laparotomy pad and thus the sites of bleeding. The pad is then removed and hemostasis confirmed. Two 28 French chest tubes are placed, one anteriorly and the other posteriorly, to drain the chest and reexpand the lung.

POSTOPERATIVE MANAGEMENT   The chest tubes are maintained on suction for the first day after the operation and then placed to waterseal. Chest tube drainage can be high for the first 48 hours, after which a marked decrease is seen. The chest tubes are removed when drainage is less than 150 mL/day. If an air leak persists for more than 3 days, one of the tubes is left in the chest and the patient discharged with a pneumostat device (Heimlich valve) or a mini pleur-evac. Often a small apical pneumothorax is seen, which is usually of no significance and resolves over the next 2 to 4 weeks. ■

9

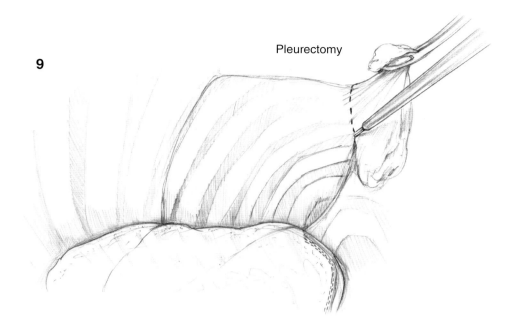

Pleurectomy

10

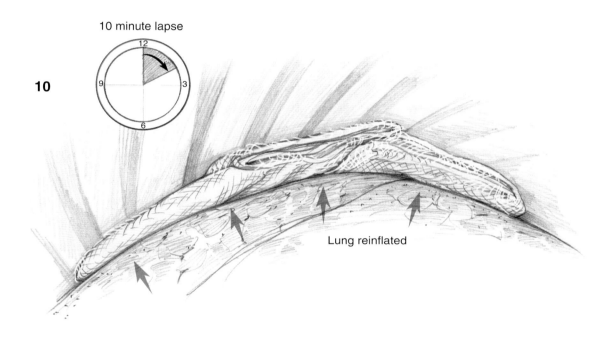

10 minute lapse

Lung reinflated

PLEURODESIS

INDICATIONS VATS pleurodesis is done to cause pleural symphysis. It is most commonly done to prevent the reaccumulation of symptomatic pleural effusions, malignant or benign, in a patient with otherwise good performance status (**FIGURE 1**). In addition, it can be used to treat spontaneous or secondary pneumothoraces and manage thoracic duct leak, in conjunction with ligation of the thoracic duct.

PREOPERATIVE PREPARATION A CT scan of the chest is performed to evaluate the anatomy of the pleural space. Loculations and adhesions are noted. Chest CTs or chest radiographs performed after thoracentesis are reviewed to evaluate the ability of the lung to expand and touch the chest wall—visceral to parietal pleural apposition. Without visceral to parietal pleural apposition, pleurodesis *will not* be effective.

ANESTHESIA General anesthesia with single-lung ventilation is required. Epidural analgesia is avoided, as it may cause profound hypotension following talc pleurodesis. Intercostal nerve blocks are performed at the end of the procedure. Prior to positioning, bronchoscopy is performed to rule out obstructive lesions in the airway that could prevent reexpansion of the lung. Obstructing lesions that can be removed, reestablishing distal aeration, do not prevent an effective pleurodesis. If an obstructing lesion cannot be removed and would prevent reexpansion of the lung on the involved side, pleurodesis is not performed and a long- or intermediate-term tunneled indwelling pleural catheter is placed to manage the effusion.

POSITION The patient is placed in the appropriate lateral decubitus position slightly rolled forward (**FIGURE 2**). The surgeon stands in front of the patient, with the assistant standing to the surgeon's left or behind the patient. The anesthesiologist stands at the head of the patient. The surgical nurse stands opposite the side of the surgical assistant. Monitors are positioned at the head of the bed and on either side of the patient.

INCISION AND EXPOSURE A single 1.5-cm incision is made in the 8th intercostal space along the midaxillary line and thoracic access is obtained as in Chapter 3. The ipsilateral lung is then dropped by isolating ventilation to the contralateral lung.

PROCEDURE A Yankauer suction catheter is used to drain the effusion through this access point, and the 10-mm thoracoscope introduced. If the lung is trapped and cannot expand to touch the chest wall, a 19-French Blake drain or tunneled indwelling catheter can be placed and the incision closed, as pleurodesis will be ineffective. If the lung is able to completely expand to meet the chest wall after draining the effusion, pleurodesis can be performed.

TALC PLEURODESIS Talc is insufflated into the pleural cavity using an atomizer with a long nozzle through the original incision. The parietal and visceral pleura are coated with talc by directing the nozzle appropriately. If the nozzle is floppy and difficult to direct, it can be lightly held and directed with a ring clamp (**FIGURE 3**). A total of 6 to 8 g of talc is used. The talc can be kept from escaping the chest cavity into the operating room by wrapping a wet towel or laparotomy pad around the port and infusion catheter. Before infusing the talc, to ensure uniform and complete distribution of the talc, the surgeon forms a mental image of the chest cavity and a pattern of how the talc will be directed. Talc cannot be placed under direct vision, because once infusion starts, the thoracoscope, if left in the chest cavity, experiences a "whiteout." If the talc is insufflated using an atomizer, the atomizer must be held upright. Otherwise, the propellant is expelled and the talc left in the atomizer.

MECHANICAL PLEURODESIS A mechanical pleurodesis is accomplished using a Bovie scratch pad folded and held in a ring clamp. The ring clamp with folded pad is introduced through a separate 1.5-cm incision in the anterior axillary line, 7th interspace (**FIGURE 4**). The pad is used to abrade the pleura until the faint and diffuse speckling of capillary bleeding is achieved (**FIGURE 5**). It is not necessary to completely remove the pleura—this is better accomplished by pleurectomy, detailed in another chapter. To avoid injury to the phrenic nerve, the diaphragm and mediastinal pleura are not abraded. To avoid lung injury, the visceral pleura is also not abraded. If good single-lung ventilation is achieved, and in thinner patients, a thorough mechanical pleurodesis can be accomplished by palpating and directing the abrasion process externally with the nondominant hand. Chest tubes (28 French) are placed through both access points, and the lung is reexpanded.

POSTOPERATIVE CARE The patient is observed in an ICU or stepdown unit. Fever, hypotension, or tachycardia may be seen because of the inflammatory response caused by talc. These can be treated with fluid and pressors. The chest tube(s) is kept on suction for the first 24 hours and then to waterseal until the output is less 150 mL 24 hours. Allergic pneumonitis and respiratory failure can be seen in 5% of patients and is related to the amount of talc insufflated. More than 10 g is associated with a higher incidence of this complication. ■

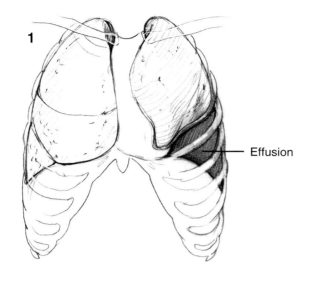

Effusion

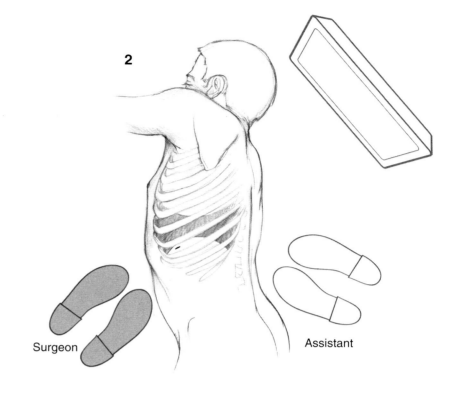

Surgeon

Assistant

Talc pleurodesis

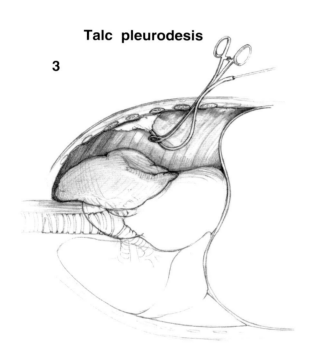

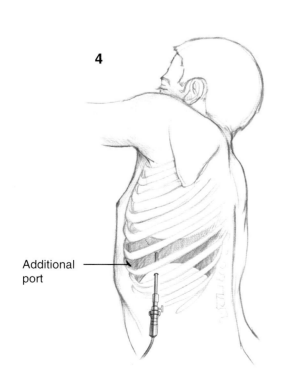

Additional
port

Mechanical pleurodesis

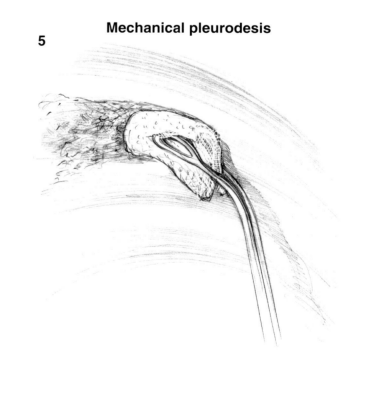

SYMPATHECTOMY

INDICATIONS VATS sympathectomy is indicated for patients with socially disabling axillary or palmar hyperhidrosis refractory to all conservative measures.

PREOPERATIVE PREPARATION Prior to surgery, a chest x-ray is performed to rule out unsuspected pathology in the chest. A preoperative type and screen is also obtained. The patient is informed about possible aftereffects of sympathectomy, including chest wall paresthesias and compensatory truncal sweating (present in 30%–70% of patients).

ANESTHESIA General anesthesia with single-lung ventilation via a double-lumen endotracheal tube or single-lumen tube with bronchial blocker is usually performed. Intraoperative monitoring includes a Foley catheter and pulse oximetry.

POSITION The patient is placed supine with a beanbag under the back with their arms out. The chest and axillae are prepped. The surgeon stands on the operative side with the assistant. The surgical scrub nurse stands on the opposite side. The anesthesiologist stands at the head of the bed. Monitors are positioned at the head of the bed and on either side of the patient (**FIGURE 1**).

INCISION AND EXPOSURE Bilateral sympathectomies are performed during the same operation. For the right thorax, 0.5% bupivacaine is infiltrated into the right 3rd intercostal space (ICS) in the anterior axillary line. Because of the position of the heart, the primary incision is made more laterally (midaxillary line) on the left. A stab incision is made with a #15 blade, and using a tonsil clamp the subcutaneous tissue is dissected up to the intercostal (IC) muscle. A 5-mm port is introduced into the chest as described in Chapter 3. The ipsilateral lung is deflated, and CO_2 is insufflated into the chest to a pressure limit of 8 mm Hg. A 5-mm-angled laparoscope is placed through this port. A second incision is made in the 5th ICS in the midclavicular line on the right, and the anterior axillary line on the left. A second 5-mm trocar is placed under thoracoscopic visualization.

DETAILS OF THE PROCEDURE A Kittner sponge stick is introduced into the chest, the lung is retracted inferiorly, and the Kittner is removed. Should it be necessary to keep the Kittner in place, another 5-mm port may be placed farther laterally. On the left side, extra care is taken to direct the trocars away from the heart. The 5-mm thoracoscope is introduced via the 3rd IC port and a hook cautery through the 5th IC port. The electrosurgical unit is set at 20 W for coagulation and cutting currents. The sympathetic chain is identified running over the neck of the ribs posteriorly (**FIGURE 2**). The ribs are counted from superior to inferior, making note of the 2nd to 4th ribs. Next, the parietal pleura over the sympathetic ganglia is opened with the L hook from the top of the 2nd rib and inferiorly to the 4th rib (**FIGURE 3**). Care is taken to avoid the intercostal veins and the stellate ganglion, overlying the first rib. Once the chain is isolated, T_2–T_4 ganglia and nerve fibers in between are removed by clipping the chain superiorly and inferiorly with the 5-mm endoclip applier and then dividing it using endoscopic shears (**FIGURE 4**). The chain is then removed with a grasper (**FIGURE 5**) and sent for frozen section to confirm removal of nerve tissue. The sympathectomy is completed by coagulating laterally from the neck of T_2–T_4 ribs for approximately 5 cm (**FIGURE 6**). This destroys any accessory sympathetic pathways (nerves of Kuntz). A #12 red rubber catheter is then introduced via the 5th IC port and the tail end placed in in a bowl of saline, creating a waterseal. The lung is reexpanded under thoracoscopic vision, then a Valsalva maneuver is performed and the red rubber catheter is withdrawn with the ports. The skin incisions are closed with subcuticular 4-0 Vicryl after injecting 0.5% bupivacaine.

POSTOPERATIVE CARE A chest x-ray is taken with the patient intubated to make sure no large pneumothorax is present. The patient is then extubated and transferred to the recovery room. The patient is monitored for 4 to 6 hours. If stable and pain free, the patient may be discharged to home on the day of surgery. ∎

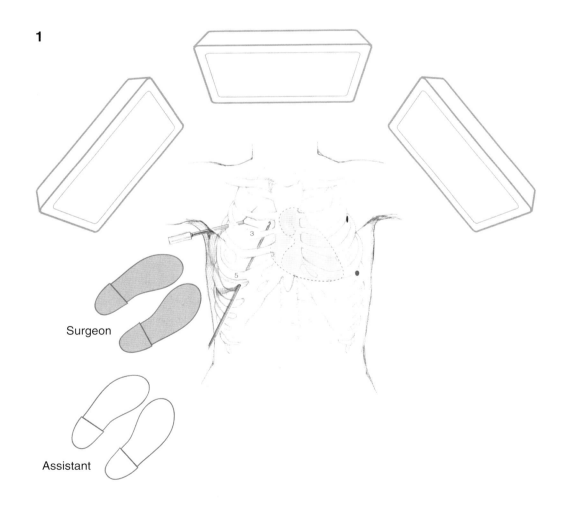

1

Surgeon

Assistant

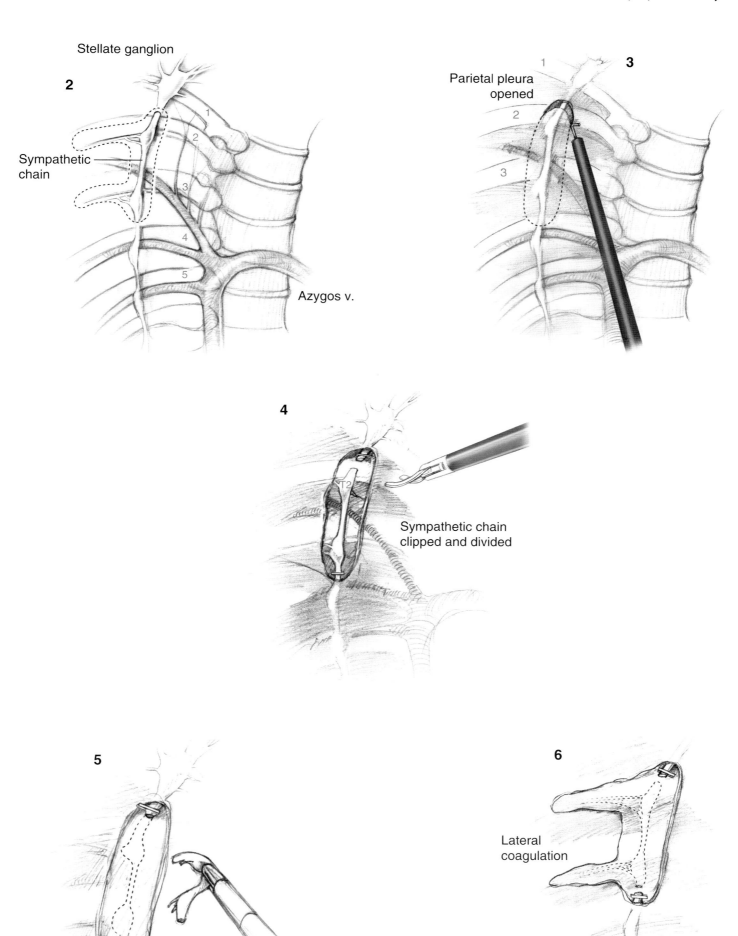

2

Stellate ganglion

Sympathetic chain

1
2
3
4
5

Azygos v.

3

Parietal pleura opened

1
2
3

4

T2

Sympathetic chain clipped and divided

5

6

Lateral coagulation

CHAPTER 10

WEDGE RESECTION OF THE LUNG

INDICATIONS Video-assisted thoracoscopic wedge resection is most commonly used to obtain tissue diagnosis in patients with either suspected interstitial lung disease or lung nodules. It is also indicated for the treatment of known lung cancers less than 3 cm in diameter in patients whose comorbidities or lung function suggest they will not tolerate an anatomic lung resection.

PREOPERATIVE PREPARATION A current computerized tomography scan of the chest is essential as a roadmap to identify the area to be resected. For nodules, the location, depth, and size of the nodule are noted, as well as position relative to the pulmonary arteries, pulmonary veins, and airway. Nodules that are too small or located too deep to be found by visual inspection of the surface of the lung or by palpation can be needle localized prior to surgery. For interstitial disease, the lobes or segments affected are noted. As with other thoracic procedures, a type-and-screen should be available. Routine laboratory examination including blood counts, prothrombin time (PT), partial thromboplastin time (PTT), electrolytes, electrocardiogram, and pulmonary function testing are recommended.

ANESTHESIA General anesthesia with single-lung ventilation is standard. A large-bore intravenous line and pulse oximetry are required. Arterial-line blood pressure monitoring and Foley catheter placement may be necessary, based on the individual patient and the anticipated length of the procedure.

POSITION The patient is placed in the lateral decubitus position, as for thoracotomy. A slight lean toward the back may facilitate instrument placement and manipulation anteriorly. The surgeon stands in front of the patient with the assistant standing to the surgeon's left or behind the patient. The anesthesiologist stands at the head of the patient. The surgical nurse stands opposite the side of the surgical assistant. Monitors are positioned at the head of the bed and on either side of the patient (**FIGURE 1**).

OPERATIVE PREPARATION The skin of the chest is sterilized from the shoulder to the iliac crest with either an iodine or chlorhexidine preparation. Care is taken to prep to the sternum anteriorly, to the spinous processes posteriorly, superiorly to above the shoulder, and inferiorly to below the costal margin. Drapes should be placed in such a way that conversion to thoracotomy is possible if necessary.

DETAILS OF THE PROCEDURE The incision for the thoracoscope is made in the 7th intercostal space in the anterior axillary line or anterior to the anterior superior iliac spine. The lung is deflated and the 30-degree thoracoscope introduced. If the nodule was wire localized, the wire is brought into the chest cavity before full deflation of the lung is attempted. This prevents the wire from pulling out of the lung as the lung falls away from the chest wall. The working incision, 3 to 4 cm in length, is placed between the mid and anterior axillary line in the 4th or 5th intercostal space, depending on the lobe to be biopsied (**FIGURE 2**).

If a lung biopsy is being performed for diagnosis of interstitial disease, all lobes on the surgical side are biopsied. If a nodule is being removed, the target lobe is first inspected and then grasped with a ring clamp and brought to the working incision. A finger can be introduced next to the ring clamp and the nodule palpated (**FIGURE 3**). Small (<1 cm) or deep nodules occasionally require palpation of the entire lobe. This can be accomplished by mobilizing the mediastinal pleura with cautery or scissors and, for the inferior lobes, dividing the inferior pulmonary ligament (**FIGURE 4**). Until all suspect nodules are located, the lung should be grasped and handled as little as possible. Iatrogenic trauma to the lung can make palpation, visualization, and ultimately localization of nodules difficult or impossible. Nodules identified by palpation are found by the relative difference in density between the nodule and the surrounding lung. Lung that has become edematous or hemorrhagic will approach the same density as the nodules and obscure them. Care should be taken not to grasp the nodule directly to minimize disrupting a nodule and causing intraparenchymal spread of its contents.

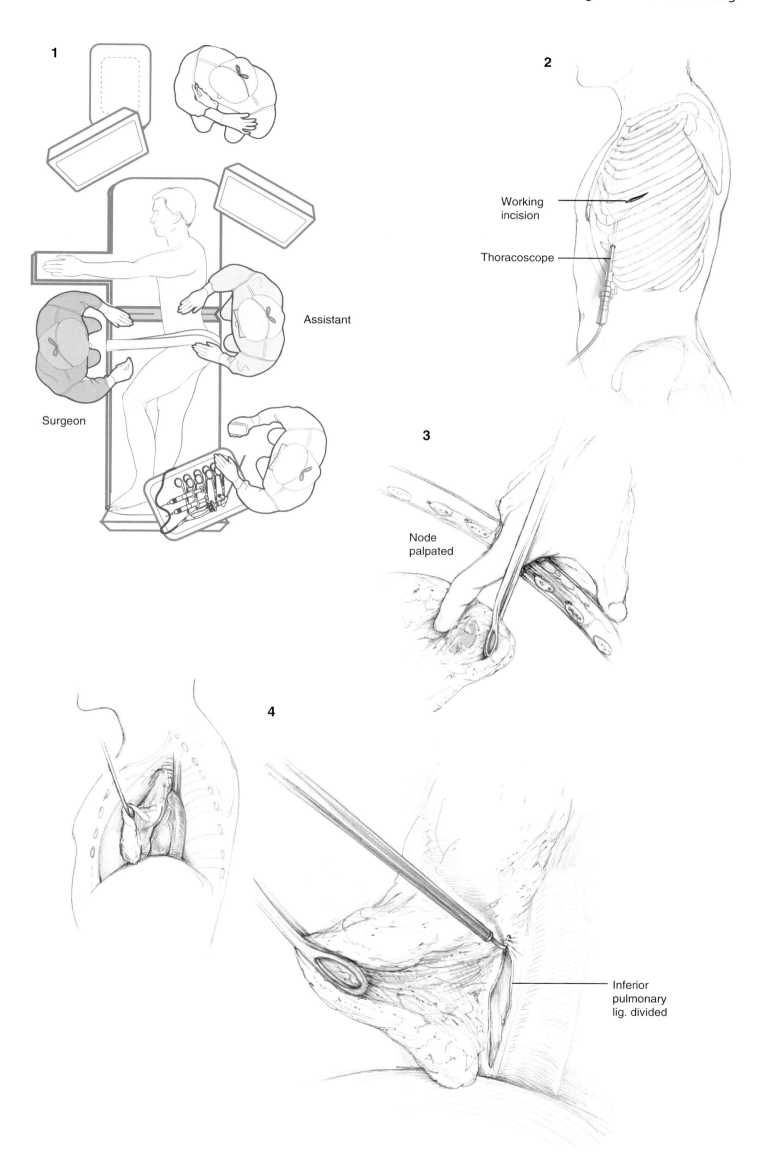

1

Assistant

Surgeon

2

Working
incision

Thoracoscope

3

Node
palpated

4

Inferior
pulmonary
lig. divided

DETAILS OF THE PROCEDURE Once the target area is identified, the lung is grasped with a ring clamp and retracted toward the lateral chest wall. An endoscopic stapler cutter with a 4.5-mm staple height and 45- or 60-mm length is introduced into the chest (**FIGURE 5**). Once open, the stapler is manipulated around the lung to be resected. The stapler is closed, its top and bottom distal end visualized, and then fired. Multiple firings may be necessary to complete the resection. Regrasping the lung closer to the distal end of the staple line after each firing allows a wedge to be constructed (**FIGURE 6**) and avoids needlessly resecting a long horizontal strip of lung (**FIGURE 7**). If there is suspicion of malignancy, the specimen is placed in an endoscopic retrieval bag (**FIGURE 8**) and the specimen is removed through the working incision.

The muscle layers of the 7th intercostal incision are closed and a 28 French chest tube is placed through same skin incision but passed through one rib space above the intercostal port site (**FIGURE 9**). This is done to minimize the chance of iatrogenic pneumothorax with chest tube removal. The tube is directed to the apex of the chest under thoracoscopic vision. The lung is reinflated and complete expansion confirmed. The working incision is closed in layers with absorbable suture.

POSTOPERATIVE CARE The patient is extubated in the operating room, and the chest tube is placed to waterseal. As with other thoracic procedures, incentive spirometry, early ambulation, and pain control are important. The chest tube is removed when there is no air leak and drainage is less than 200 mL/24 hr. ■

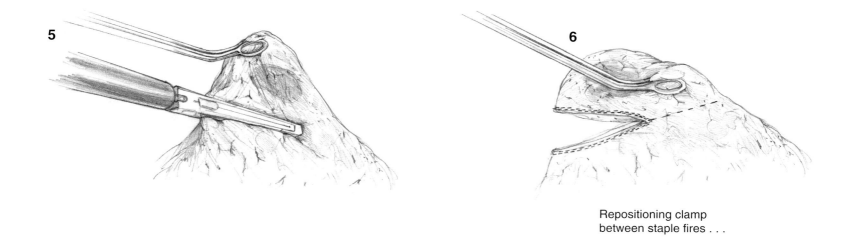

5

6

Repositioning clamp
between staple fires . . .

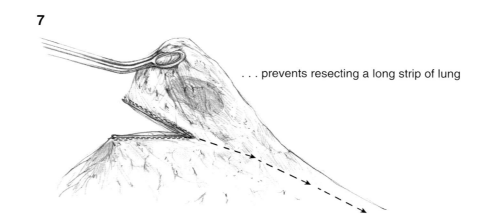

7

. . . prevents resecting a long strip of lung

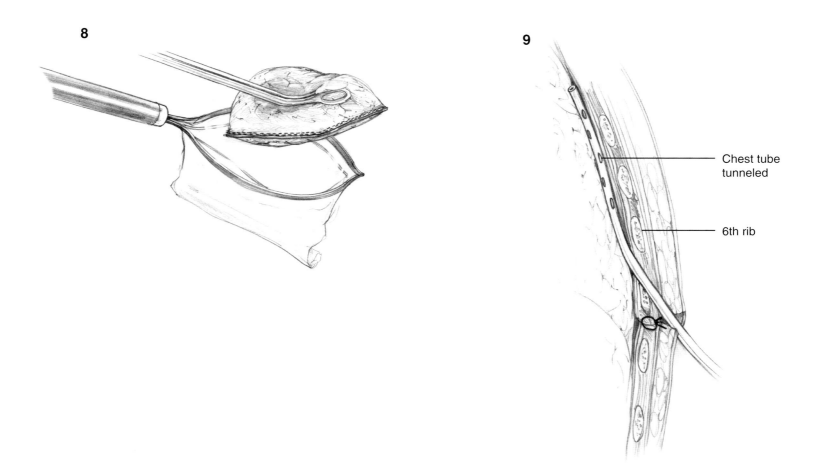

8

9

Chest tube
tunneled

6th rib

PULMONARY LOBECTOMY

INDICATIONS Video-assisted thoracic surgery (VATS) is indicated for resection of early-stage lung cancer (stages I and II). In experienced centers, VATS lobectomy can also be performed for more advanced-stage disease (stage IIIA).

PREOPERATIVE PREPARATION Preparation focuses on accurate staging of the malignancy, including computed tomography scanning of the chest and whole-body positron emission scanning. Mediastinal staging with endobronchial ultrasound or mediastinoscopy should be performed before resection and can be incorporated into the same operation, as long as frozen-section pathology is available before resection is attempted. Pulmonary function tests should be completed, including diffusion capacity of the lungs for carbon monoxide (DLCO). In general, patients with a postoperative predictive forced expiratory volume in 1 second (FEV_1) and a DLCO greater than 50% can tolerate a lobectomy via either thoracotomy or thoracoscopy. Patients with lung function below this must be considered on a case-by-case basis. Before operation, patients should also be counseled to quit smoking, and two units of packed red blood cells should be cross-matched and available.

ANESTHESIA General endotracheal anesthesia with single-lung ventilation via either a double-lumen endotracheal tube or a bronchial blocker is essential. An arterial line and two large-bore intravenous lines are needed. A central line should be placed if needed for postoperative monitoring. A thoracic epidural catheter can be considered for postoperative pain relief;

however, in most cases pain can be controlled with intercostal nerve blocks and oral narcotics. A Foley catheter should be placed.

POSITION The patient should be placed in the lateral thoracotomy position. The patient should be leaning slightly posterior to allow instrument placement and increased exposure of the anterior hilum of the lung. The surgeon stands in front of the patient with the assistant standing to the surgeon's left or behind the patient. The anesthesiologist stands at the head of the patient. The surgical nurse stands opposite the side of the surgical assistant. Monitors are positioned at the head of the bed and on either side of the patient (**FIGURE 1**).

OPERATIVE PREPARATION The skin of the chest is sterilized from the shoulder to the iliac crest with either an iodine preparation or chlorhexidine. Care is taken to extend the surgical field to the sternum anteriorly and to the spinous processes posteriorly. Drapes should be placed in such a way that emergent thoracotomy is possible.

DETAILS OF THE PROCEDURE: LEFT UPPER LOBECTOMY The working port is a 3- to 5-cm incision in the 5th or 6th intercostal space between the mid and anterior axillary lines. The camera port is in the 7th or 8th intercostal space in line with the midaxillary line for the two-incision technique (**FIGURE 2**). To allow for additional retraction or stapling, a third port can be placed posteriorly below the tip of the scapula for the first assistant (**FIGURE 3**). When using this three-incision technique, the camera port is placed more anteriorly, in line with the anterior iliac spine.

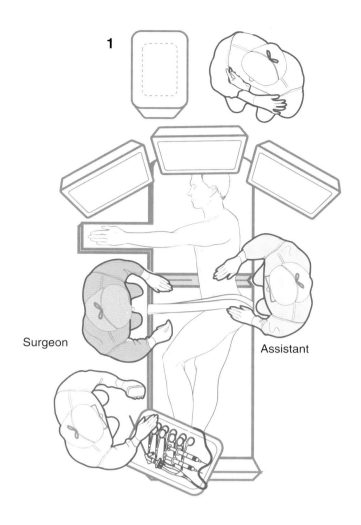

Surgeon

Assistant

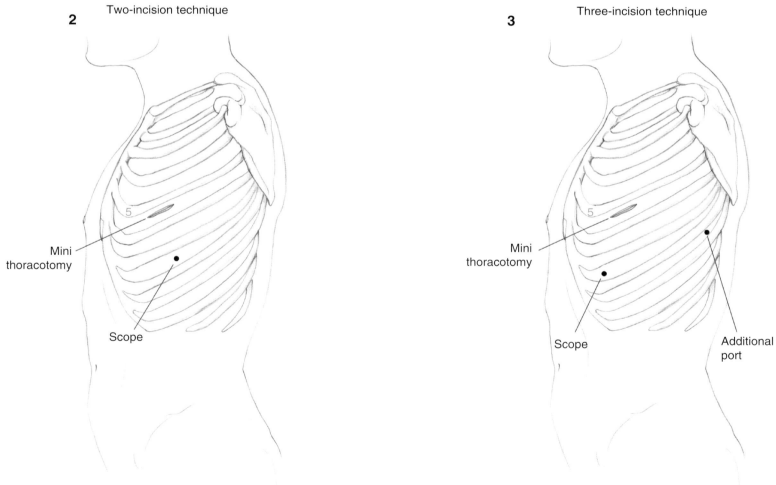

2 Two-incision technique

Mini thoracotomy

Scope

3 Three-incision technique

Mini thoracotomy

Scope

Additional port

DETAILS OF THE PROCEDURE: LEFT UPPER LOBECTOMY Once the camera is in place, a curved thoracoscopic ring clamp is introduced via the working incision and used to grasp the lobe being resected. This lobe is retracted superiorly and posteriorly to expose the hilum anteriorly and to place mild tension on the hilar structures, including the superior pulmonary vein (SPV), inferior pulmonary vein (IPV), pulmonary artery (PA), and bronchus (Br) (**FIGURE 4**). The hilum is dissected anteriorly with Metzenbaum scissors, opening the pleura around the hilum (**FIGURE 5**). The pulmonary vein is the first structure to be dissected using a combination of sharp and blunt dissection (**FIGURE 6**). The vein is isolated and a C clamp or renal pedicle clamp is used to obtain circumferential control (**FIGURE 7**).

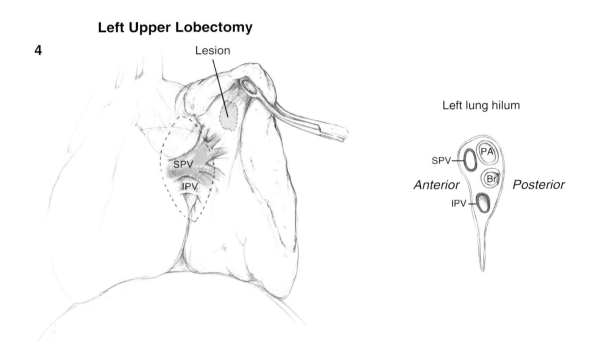

Left Upper Lobectomy

4

Lesion

SPV

IPV

Left lung hilum

SPV

PA

Br

IPV

Anterior   *Posterior*

5

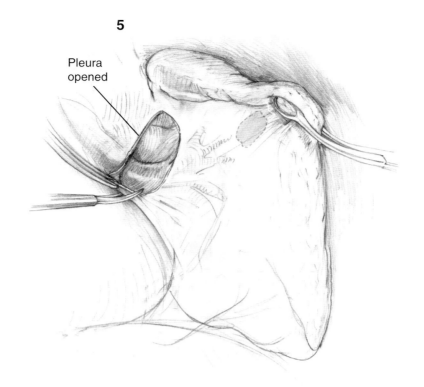

Pleura opened

6

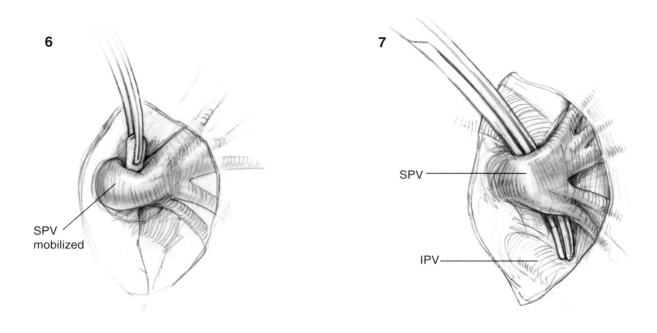

SPV mobilized

7

SPV

IPV

DETAILS OF THE PROCEDURE: LEFT UPPER LOBECTOMY The camera is then moved to the working incision and an endoscopic vascular stapler (30 mm) is introduced through the camera port (**FIGURE 8**). Alternatively, the stapler can be introduced through the posterior port, if using a three-port technique. The stapler jaws are negotiated around the vein and closed. The stapler jaws are checked to make sure they completely enclose the vein before firing. A sponge stick (a tonsil sponge in a ring clamp) is always kept readily available to compress bleeding if it occurs (**FIGURE 9**).

8

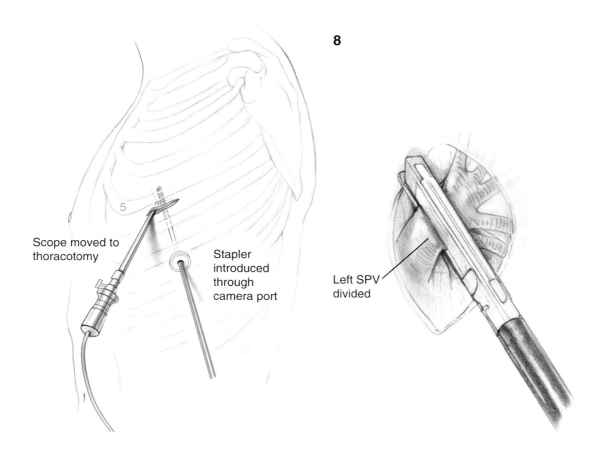

Scope moved to
thoracotomy

Stapler
introduced
through
camera port

Left SPV
divided

9

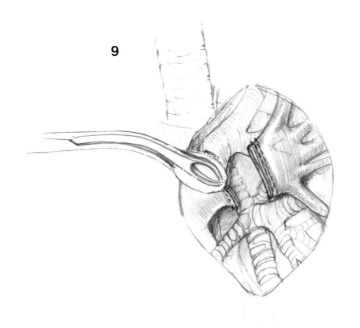

DETAILS OF THE PROCEDURE: LEFT UPPER LOBECTOMY After division of the vein, the camera is switched back to the inferior port. Next the pulmonary arterial branches are dissected by a combination of sharp and blunt dissection and divided by a vascular stapler. Then the bronchus is dissected and clamped while the lung is briefly ventilated to ensure good expansion of the lower lobe. The patient is returned to single-lung ventilation, and the bronchus is divided with a 45 mm × 3.5 mm endoscopic stapler passed through the inferior port while the camera is temporarily moved to the working incision (**FIGURE 10**). The lobar bronchus is then divided with a 45-mm medium-thickness stapler (**FIGURE 11**). Finally, the interlobar fissure division is completed with a medium-thickness stapler (**FIGURE 12**).

Once the lobe has been resected, an endobag is introduced through the mini-thoracotomy and used to bag the specimen before removal. The bag is extracted with a gentle rocking motion (**FIGURE 13**). At this time a mediastinal lymph node dissection is performed. On the left side, the dissection includes levels 5, 6, 7, 8, and 9 lymph nodes (**FIGURES 14 AND 15**).

The chest cavity is filled with sterile water and the bronchial stump tested to 30 cm water pressure. Once hemostasis has been achieved, a 28 French chest tube is placed through the camera port. The lung is inflated and the working incision closed in layers with absorbable suture and a sterile dressing placed.

10

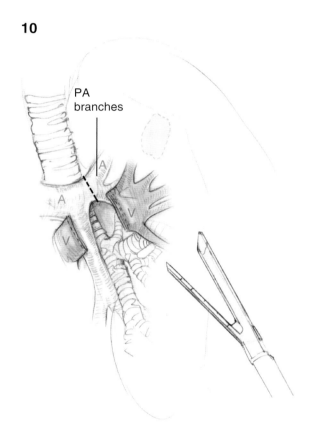

PA
branches

11

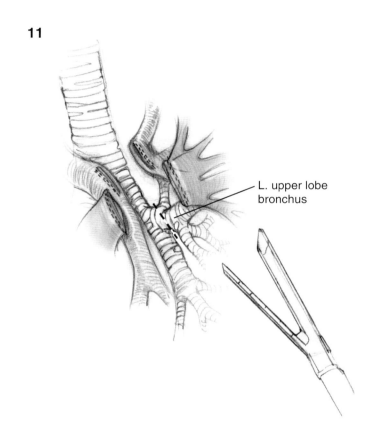

L. upper lobe
bronchus

12

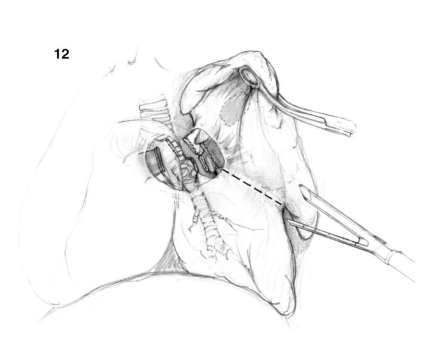

13

Lung in endobag

Thoracotomy

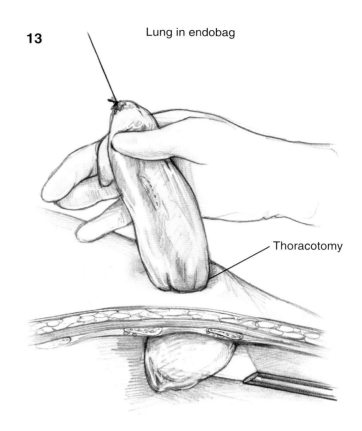

14

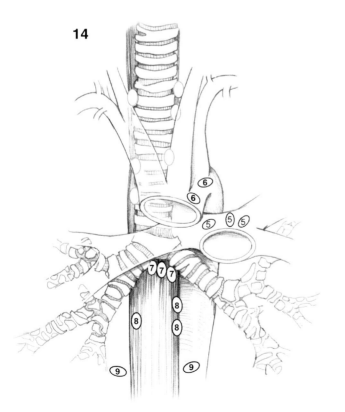

**Mediastinal
lymph nodes**

15

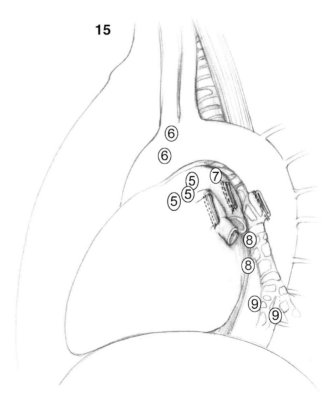

ALTERNATE APPROACH: RIGHT LOWER LOBECTOMY When a lower lobectomy is to be performed, the operative steps differ. The inferior pulmonary ligament is first divided with an electrosurgical hook (**FIGURE 16**). The anterior and posterior pleural reflection is divided sharply and the inferior pulmonary vein is identified. The vein is bluntly dissected out with a Kittner or curved suction tip (**FIGURE 17**). Next, the pulmonary artery is dissected in the fissure and branches to the lower lobe divided using a vascular stapler. The stapler can be placed through the working incision, as this allows adequate access to the hilar structures of the lower lobe (**FIGURE 18**). The vein is divided with a vascular stapler (**FIGURE 19**). The bronchus to the lower lobe is dissected and divided with a medium-thickness stapler (**FIGURE 20**). The fissure dissection is completed with a medium-thickness stapler (**FIGURE 21**). On the right side, lymph nodes at levels 2, 4, 7, 8, and 9 are removed (**FIGURES 22 AND 23**).

POSTOPERATIVE CARE The patient is extubated in the operating room. Patients with significant comorbidities should be monitored overnight in the intensive care unit, but lower risk patients can be sent to the regular surgical ward. Excellent pain control, the use of incentive spirometry, and early ambulation are very important. The patient can generally be returned to a full diet as soon as awake and should be ambulating by postoperative day 1. The chest tubes can be removed when there is no air leak and output is less than 200 mL/24 hr. ∎

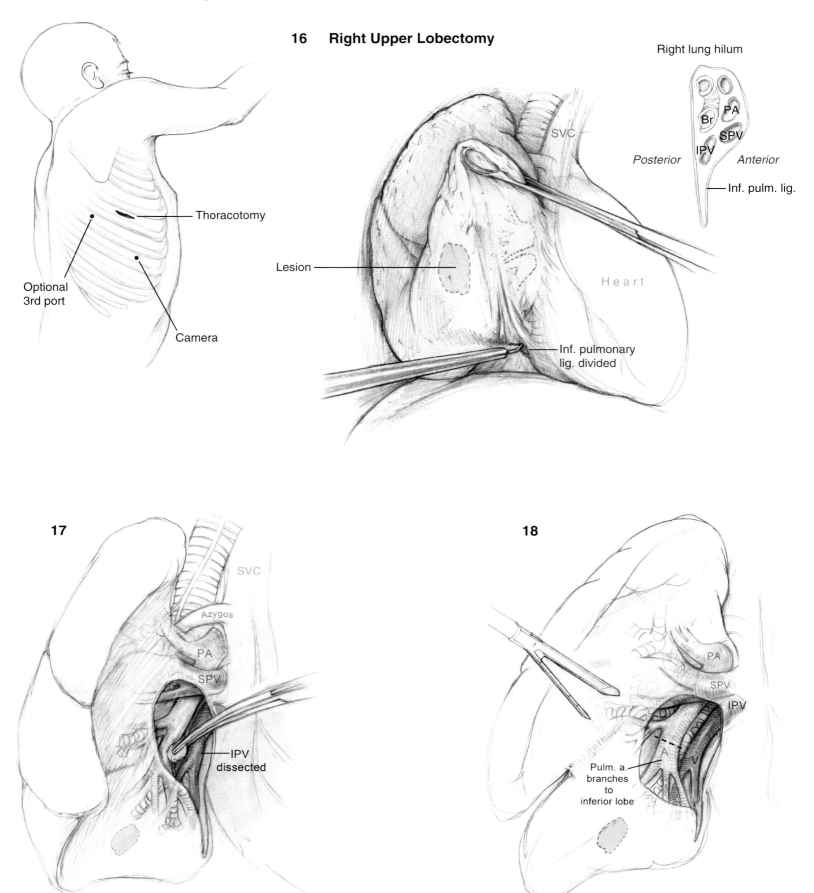

16   Right Upper Lobectomy

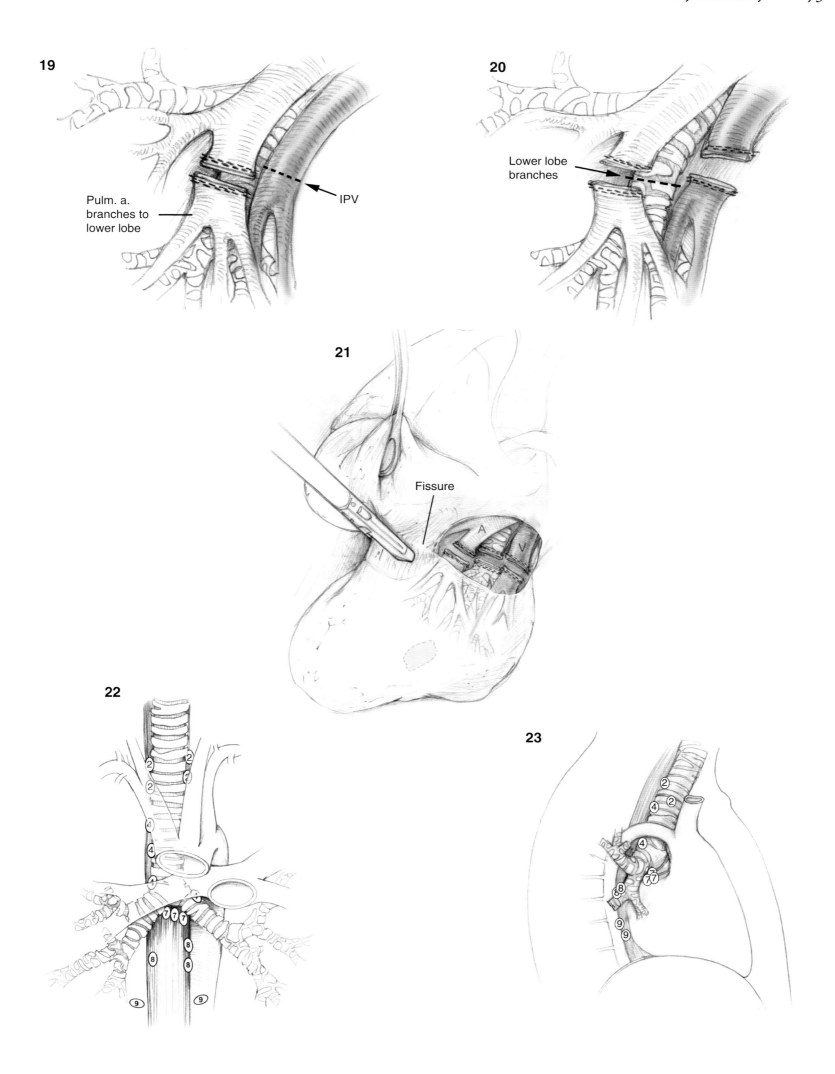

19

Pulm. a.
branches to
lower lobe

IPV

20

Lower lobe
branches

21

Fissure

A

V

22

23

RESECTION OF A MID-ESOPHAGEAL DIVERTICULUM WITH MYOTOMY

INDICATIONS Esophageal diverticula are rare entities. They are commonly categorized by anatomic location and etiology. Epiphrenic diverticula occur in the distal third of the esophagus and develop by increased intraesophageal pressure secondary to a motility disorder. They are considered pulsion diverticula. Midesophageal diverticula have traditionally been considered traction diverticula and are associated with mediastinal inflammation. Recent work would suggest that most midesophageal diverticula are in fact pulsion diverticula and are associated with motility disorders. Patients with minimal symptoms or small diverticula should not be repaired because of postoperative anastomotic leak rates ranging from 6% to 18% and a perioperative morbidity rate of 33% to 45%. Diverticulectomy and myotomy can be recommended in patients who are symptomatic. The repair of large asymptomatic diverticula may warrant repair as well. Symptoms typically include dysphagia, regurgitation, or weight loss. Less often, chest pain, heartburn, aspiration pneumonia, or vomiting have been noted. It is sometimes difficult to determine the contribution of a diverticula versus a primary motility disorder as the cause of a patient's symptoms.

The traditional approach to an epiphrenic or midesophageal pulsion diverticulum would be a left thoracotomy, diverticulectomy, and myotomy. Depending on the extent of the myotomy, a Belsey Mark IV or other antireflux procedure would be considered. MIS diverticulectomy and myotomy should be tailored to the location of the diverticulum, its etiology, and the surgeon's experience. Diverticula close to the esophageal hiatus can be approached with laparoscopy. A diverticulectomy, myotomy, and antireflux procedure can be performed through the laparoscope as described in Chapter 17. Care should be taken in the preoperative evaluation to ensure the diverticulum is within reach of the laparoscope. The esophageal hiatus is located at the 10th or 11th thoracic vertebra. The dome of the diaphragm can rise up to the level of the 4th thoracic vertebra, and a diverticulum, while appearing below the dome of the diaphragm, may be at the level of the carina and in the midesophagus. Thoracoscopy and diverticulectomy is indicated if laparoscopy fails to safely identify the diverticulum or finds the diverticulum too high in the chest to resect. In this situation, the lower extent of the myotomy and any required antireflux procedure would be performed through the laparoscope. The procedure would then be converted to right thoracoscopy for completion of the myotomy and resection of the diverticulum. Planned thoracoscopy and myotomy is indicated for midesophageal diverticula. The entire extent of the thoracic esophagus is most easily approached through the right chest. Procedures on the gastroesophageal junction, however, are very difficult from the right chest. If an antireflux procedure is needed, this should be performed through laparoscopy. Laparoscopy should be done first in order to prevent losing pneumoperitoneum through the thoracoscopy field. A long esophageal myotomy can be started 1 cm below the gastroesophageal junction thorough the laparoscope and completed later in the procedure through the thoracoscope. Left thoracoscopy, diverticulectomy, myotomy, and Belsey Mark IV fundoplication has been performed but was associated with a 5% perioperative mortality, 10% anastomotic leak rate, and 26% rate of recurrence of the diverticulum. This procedure cannot be recommended at this time, and a midesophageal diverticulum requiring a left-sided approach is better performed open.

Previous ipsilateral thoracic procedure is a relative contraindication to thoracoscopy, but not absolute.

PREOPERATIVE PREPARATION Before an esophageal diverticulectomy is performed, the location and etiology of the diverticulum need to be determined. At a minimum, an esophagram, esophagogastroduodenoscopy (EGD), and esophageal manometry should be performed. The Gastrografin swallow can locate the diverticulum as well as evaluate for underlying esophageal pathology (achalasia, distal stricture, mass lesions, corkscrew esophagus, etc.). EGD can confirm the location of the diverticulum and rule out endoluminal masses, Barrett esophagus, dysplasia, or strictures. Because the manometry catheter enters the diverticulum as opposed to passing distally into the esophagus, it may be difficult to place. The catheter can be positioned endoscopically. The information received from a well-positioned manometry catheter is invaluable in determining the need for an esophageal myotomy. The presence of normal distal esophageal function would make a myotomy unnecessary. This situation is rare. Diverticulectomy without myotomy is associated with increased recurrence and suture line leak. 24-hour pH testing is not necessary unless reflux disease is suspected.

Because thoracoscopic esophageal procedures require single-lung ventilation, lung function should be accessed. In addition, patients with large diverticula or esophageal dysmotility can have silent aspiration and develop insidious deterioration of lung function. A patient able to climb two flights of stairs without stopping or walk two blocks on the level without stopping will likely tolerate single-lung ventilation. Questionable candidates should undergo spirometry. A patient with an $FEV_1 > 1$ L or greater than 50% of predicted will likely tolerate single-lung ventilation.

Patients are generally continued on all preoperative medications prior to surgery. Anticoagulants should be discontinued at an appropriate interval prior to surgery to allow metabolism and restoration of normal coagulation. Antiplatelet agents (e.g., aspirin) are discontinued 1 week preoperatively, when feasible. Diabetes should be controlled and cardiac status thoroughly evaluated with appropriate testing and consultation prior to surgery. Colon prep is unnecessary; however, patients with large diverticula may have food material contained in the sac. Endoscopy with "washout" of the diverticulum the day before surgery, followed by a liquid diet, is prudent for all but the smallest diverticula.

ANESTHESIA General endotracheal anesthesia with the capability for single-lung ventilation is necessary for this procedure. A double-lumen tube is ideal for both left- and right-sided procedures. If thoracoscopy is planned, an epidural catheter is placed preoperatively, used during the case as an adjunct to the general anesthetic, and used postoperatively for pain control. Alternatively, intercostal blocks can be placed as described elsewhere in this text. A urinary catheter is placed. Arterial and central lines are generally not necessary, but may be used if the patient's medical condition otherwise warrants. Before positioning the patient for thoracoscopy, an endoscope is passed into the esophagus and the diverticulum located. The endoscope is then left in position for use later in the procedure (**FIGURE 1**).

POSITION The position for right thoracoscopy is full left lateral decubitus (left side down). Arms are positioned straight in front of the patient, with the ipsilateral arm depressed as much as possible without putting strain on joints or pressure points to allow instruments to be directed toward the diaphragm without interference from the arm. The operative table is flexed to open up the interspaces. The patient should be secured to the table at the hips and legs using belts or tape. Care should be taken to not place a tight band across the thigh and injure the lateral femoral cutaneous nerve. Once ports are placed, the table is tilted to the left such that the lung falls anteriorly. The surgeon stands in front of the patient with the assistant standing to the surgeon's left or behind the patient. The anesthesiologist stands at the head of the patient. The surgical nurse stands opposite the side of the surgical assistant. Monitors are positioned at the head of the bed and on either side of the patient. If laparoscopy is planned as part of the procedure, this is done first and positioning is supine. Once the laparoscopic portion is completed, drapes are removed and the patient repositioned for the thoracoscopic portion. The operative surgeon stands in front of the patient (**FIGURE 2**).

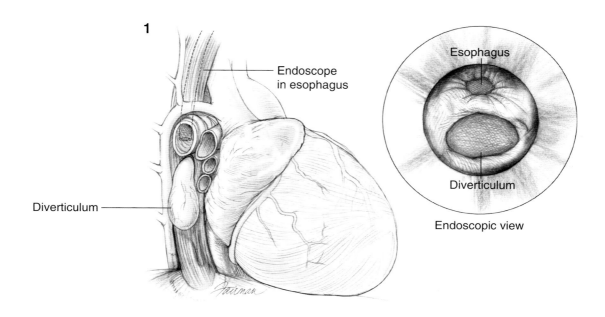

Endoscope
in esophagus

Diverticulum

Esophagus

Diverticulum

Endoscopic view

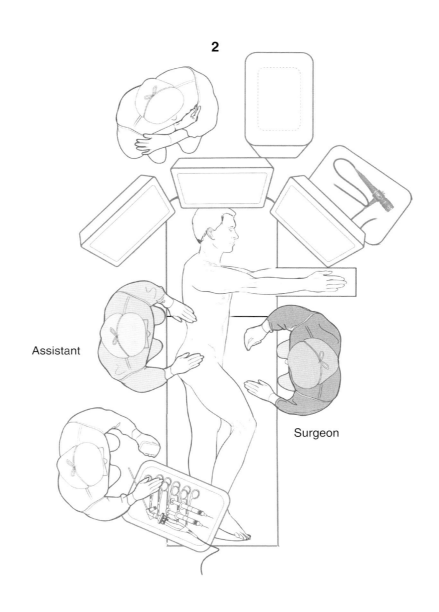

Assistant

Surgeon

DETAILS OF THE PROCEDURE

Place Ports and Locate Diverticulum A 1.5-cm incision is made at the anterior axillary line, approximately the 7th interspace. This incision is carried down to the chest wall and the pleural cavity entered directly on top of the rib. To avoid damage to the underlying lung, the pleura is incised with a Metzenbaum scissors. Once the lung has fallen away from the chest wall, the intercostal incision is widened to 1.5 cm. This gives adequate room for the camera and prevents port-site bleeding. A 12-mm metal trocar is used for the camera port. Before placing additional ports, the chest is inspected, including the position of the diaphragm and the esophagus. A long ring forceps with a curve at the end can be placed through the same thoracoscopy port as the camera, outside the trocar, to provide retraction of the lung for better visualization. The diverticulum is sought immediately, as manipulation near the esophagus can sometimes cause protruding mucosa to return inside the esophageal wall, and the site of pathology disappears. If the diverticulum is not localized at this stage, mobilization of the esophagus ensues. In general, two additional access sites are used. One is a mini-thoracotomy placed anteriorly at the 5th interspace. It is 3 to 4 cm in length and allows access by several instruments simultaneously (**FIGURE 3**). An additional port is occasionally placed posteriorly, at the axillary line approximately the 6th or 7th interspace to provide countertraction for dissection of the esophagus and triangulation for intracorporeal suturing.

The table is tilted anteriorly so the lung falls onto the middle mediastinum. The right lower lobe of the lung is grasped and brought into the upper chest, exposing the inferior pulmonary ligament. This ligament is taken with hook electrocautery. The top of this dissection is the inferior pulmonary vein. This vein is recognized as a pericardial invagination into the right lower lobe. There is often a lymph node at the top of the inferior pulmonary ligament, guarding the pulmonary vein. The pulmonary ligament is taken close to lung parenchyma in order to avoid inadvertent injury to the esophagus or thoracic duct. Care must be taken in retracting the ligament, such that both the anterior and posterior sides are visualized. The ligament can be pulled against the middle mediastinum, which risks thermal injury to the phrenic nerve (**FIGURE 4**).

Mobilize Esophagus The esophagus is located posterior to the pericardium behind the left atrium and anterior to the azygos vein. The pleura over the esophagus and slightly anterior is grasped and incised, opening this pleura from the level of the diaphragm to the arch of the azygos vein. For midesophageal diverticula, the underside of the azygos vein is bluntly exposed, separating it from the trachea/right main-stem bronchus and esophagus. The pleura above the azygos vein is then incised. A 30-mm endoscopic stapler with a vascular load is used to divide the arch of the azygos vein in its midportion (**FIGURE 5**).

An Endoloop can be passed over the divided posterior portion of the azygos vein, tightened, and the suture brought out through the posterior port. This can provide additional exposure of the underlying esophagus. Mobilization of the esophagus continues by defining the anterior wall. To avoid injury to the vagus nerve, the vagus is kept attached to the esophagus. Difficult dissections are aided by using the inferior pulmonary vein to identify the pericardium over the left atrium. This will often lead into the plane between the left atrium and esophagus. Mobilization is continued in this fashion up to the level of the azygos vein. As the dissection proceeds superiorly, the bronchus intermedius and right main-stem bronchus will gradually approach the esophagus and eventually come to lie next to each other as the tracheoesophageal groove forms. The posterior wall of the esophagus is mobilized, grasping the posterior pleural edge and peeling it off the esophagus. Again, care is taken to keep the vagus nerve attached to the esophagus. A spoon clamp or right angle clamp is passed around the esophagus in its midportion. A 4-inch-long Penrose drain is placed around the esophagus and secured with an Endoloop (**FIGURE 6**).

If a large diverticulum is present, this will need to be mobilized from whatever structures it adheres to. Placement of the Penrose drain, superior or inferior to the diverticulum where planes can be identified, can aid in identifying the dissection planes in the vicinity of the diverticulum. The esophagus does not need to be mobilized completely from its bed, only enough to find the diverticulum and expose 1 to 2 cm of normal esophagus superior to the diverticulum and esophagus down to the level of the diaphragm. If the diverticulum cannot be located, the esophagoscope can be used to assist. The light from the esophagoscope can be seen through the esophageal wall in the chest. In addition, gentle insufflation from the esophagus can inflate and reveal a previously hiding diverticulum.

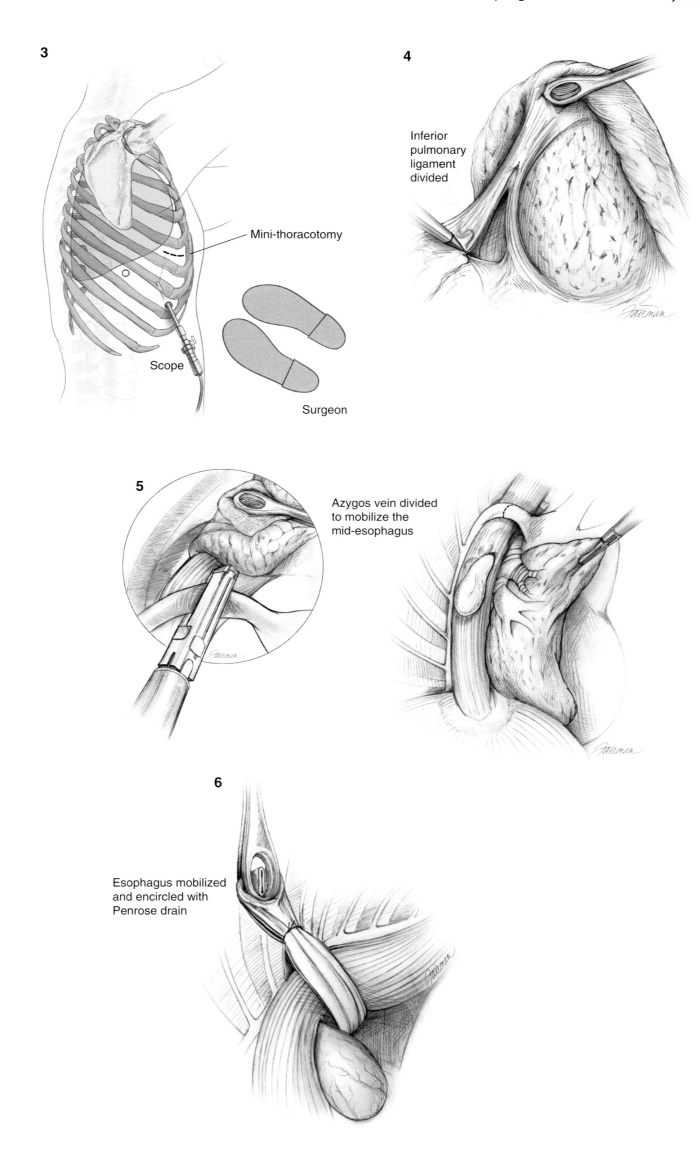

3

Mini-thoracotomy

Scope

Surgeon

4

Inferior
pulmonary
ligament
divided

5

Azygos vein divided
to mobilize the
mid-esophagus

6

Esophagus mobilized
and encircled with
Penrose drain

Diverticulectomy For a traction diverticulum, a diverticulectomy is performed as well as a mediastinal lymph node dissection. The level 7 (subcarinal) and 4R (right paratracheal) lymph nodes are removed to prevent formation of further diverticula. All other diverticula are considered pulsion diverticula, even if situated in the midesophagus, and mandate an esophageal myotomy, but not lymphadenectomy.

The diverticulum is composed of mucosa, occasionally with thinned-out strands of esophageal muscle. As the edge of the diverticulum is found, these thinned-out strands thicken until the esophageal wall is identified. This is often a gradual process. The muscle wall of the esophagus should be dissected and identified on all sides of the diverticulum. Enough substance needs to be found to allow suture closure of the muscle over the diverticulectomy. Once the diverticulum is free, a 40 French bougie is passed through the mouth into the esophagus and into the stomach. The bougie will help ensure preservation of enough esophageal mucosa to maintain esophageal patency. The superior and inferior poles or the anterior and posterior poles of the diverticulum are grasped. A 60-mm endoscopic stapler with a medium-tissue load is placed across the base of the diverticulum against the bougie. Occasionally a very thick-walled diverticulum will require use of a thick-tissue (4.8 mm) staple load. If multiple firings are required, care should be taken to exactly line up the staple lines to prevent a sawtooth appearance. A stapler placed transversely across the diverticulum has a theoretical advantage of not causing a stricture. This orientation is generally easier via thoracoscopy. If the stapler lines up better longitudinally, it is fired in this orientation (**FIGURE 7**). The staple line is tested with air insufflation under water, looking for bubbles. Any leaks are repaired with interrupted 3-0 silk sutures. The esophageal wall is then closed over the top of the diverticulectomy with simple interrupted non absorbable sutures (**FIGURE 8**).

Mediastinal Lymph Node Dissection: Subcarinal Lymph Nodes A traction diverticulum requires a mediastinal lymph node dissection. This can be done thoracoscopically. The subcarinal nodes are defined by locating the bronchus intermedius and using electrocautery and blunt dissection to mobilize the nodal packet to the level of the carina. At the carina, a large bronchial artery is often encountered and should be clipped with a 5-mm endoclip. The dissection continues from the carina, down the left mainstem bronchus until the lymph node packet is free.

Mediastinal Lymph Node Dissection: Right Paratracheal Lymph Nodes The pleura just posterior to the superior vena cava is incised vertically to just below the brachiocephalic artery. Electrocautery too close to the right brachiocephalic artery risks injury to the right recurrent laryngeal nerve. The plane between the lymph node packet and the superior vena cava is developed bluntly with a Yankauer sucker. Any dense adhesions are divided with electrocautery. The packet is then grasped with a ring forceps and brought anteriorly. The plane between the lymph nodes and the right anterior wall of the trachea is developed. The packet is then divided inferiorly from its attachments to the right main pulmonary artery. Last, the

packet is divided superiorly at a point approximately 1 cm below the brachiocephalic artery. This chain of lymph nodes will extend into the neck, so lymphatic material is often crossed at this point. The packet should now be free and is removed from the chest through the working port.

Myotomy An esophageal myotomy is not continued from the same defect in the esophageal wall as the diverticulum. Because of the increased incidence of leaks, the wall of the esophagus is always closed over the diverticulectomy. The esophagus is then rotated 180 degrees and a myotomy performed. Myotomy techniques are similar to those for a laparoscopic Heller myotomy. The 40 French bougie may be left in the esophagus and serves to define the mucosa. The muscle wall is superficially scored with electrocautery. Two atraumatic graspers are used to grab muscle on either side of this score and bluntly pull the outer longitudinal muscle apart. Blunt dissection continues until the mucosa is visualized. A fine network of vessels on top of the mucosa indicates that the proper depth has been found. The dissection then continues superiorly to 1 cm above the level of the diverticulum (**FIGURE 9**). If manometry indicated esophageal dysfunction in the upper esophagus, this myotomy can be continued above the azygos arch. The myotomy should be continued distally to meet with the previously performed laparoscopic myotomy. Without the aid of laparoscopy, an esophageal myotomy from the right chest can be performed to within 1 cm of, but not across, the gastroesophageal junction. Leaving distal esophagus without a myotomy can potentiate suture-line leaks and recurrent diverticula.

Closure The pleura may be closed over the esophagus if it comes together easily. It may also be left open. A single 28 French chest tube is placed through the skin incision of the camera port, but directed through the intercostal space superior. This is done to create a subcutaneous tunnel so, when the chest tube is removed, there is not a straight line into the chest, and a chest tube pulling pneumothorax is prevented. The chest is copiously irrigated with warm normal saline. The bougie is removed under direct vision through the thoracoscope. Once the bougie is removed, no further tubes are placed into the esophagus to avoid accidental disruption of the repair. Muscle layers of the port sites are closed with interrupted figure-of-eight 2-0 Vicryl sutures. Skin is closed with a 4-0 running subcutaneous suture of absorbable monofilament.

Postoperative Care A nasogastric tube is *not* used. Postoperative nausea is preempted with a dose of ondansetron prior to emergence from anesthesia. Postoperative pain control is with epidural anesthesia or nonsteroidals. Narcotics are used judiciously. Careful attention is paid to pulmonary hygiene, and patients are ambulated beginning POD 1. Patients are kept NPO for 3 days, and then an Omnipaque esophagram is performed. If there is no evidence of suture-line leak or stenosis on the swallow, patients are advanced to a clear liquid diet followed by full liquids. Most patients go home on POD 3 or 4. A full liquid diet is continued for 2 weeks at home, and then patients allowed to gradually advance their diet on their own. ∎

7

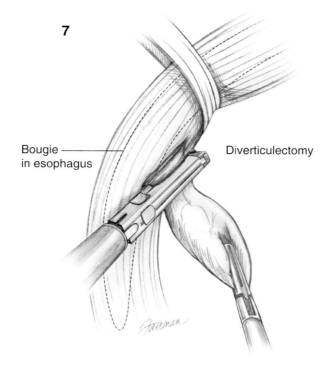

Bougie
in esophagus

Diverticulectomy

8

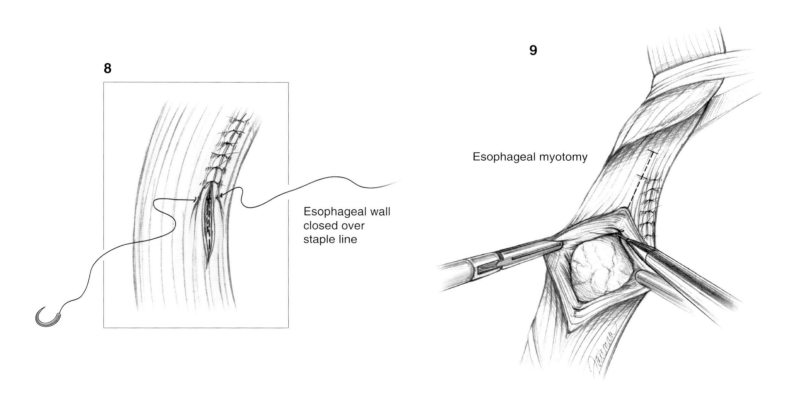

Esophageal wall
closed over
staple line

9

Esophageal myotomy

Two- and Three-Field Esophagectomy

INDICATIONS The technique of minimally invasive esophagectomy (MIE) can be applied to almost any condition for which resection is indicated. Current indications include neoplasms, end-stage achalasia, esophageal perforation, Barrett esophagus with high-grade dysplasia, and complications of severe gastroesophageal reflux disease (GERD), especially undilatable strictures. Although initial experience with MIE primarily involved patients with Barrett esophagus and high-grade dysplasia, it has evolved to include most patients with resectable malignant lesions, including those with nodal involvement and patients who have undergone prior neoadjuvant chemoradiation therapy. Although there are no absolute contraindications for MIE, resection of large bulky tumors, reoperative upper abdominal or thoracic operations, and the need for colon interposition would commonly necessitate an open approach. Occasionally, a patient may be a candidate for a "hybrid" procedure: a patient with previous mediastinitis may need a thoracotomy and laparoscopy, or a patient with multiple previous abdominal operations may need a laparotomy but has no contraindication to thoracoscopy. There are many variations of MIE, but three approaches predominate: (1) thoracoscopic and laparoscopic dissections with cervical anastomosis (three-field esophagectomy), (2) laparoscopic and thoracoscopic dissections with intrathoracic anastomosis (Ivor-Lewis technique), and (3) laparoscopic transhiatal technique with cervical anastomosis (inversion esophagectomy) (**FIGURE 1**). In this chapter we describe the first two operations; laparoscopic transhiatal esophagectomy is described in Chapter 22.

PREOPERATIVE PREPARATION Patients undergoing MIE must be carefully evaluated prior to surgery. The evaluation of a suspected malignancy includes a thorough staging workup. This should include computed tomography (CT) of the chest, abdomen, and pelvis; an esophagogastroduodenoscopy (EGD); a bronchoscopy for mid to upper esophageal tumors; an endoscopic ultrasound; and a combined CT and positron emission tomography (PET) scan to provide clinical staging for all locally advanced tumors. Occasionally laparoscopic and/or thoracoscopic staging is needed to confirm or rule out extraesophageal metastases, but this is not routinely necessary. Cardiopulmonary risk stratification and optimization is pursued for all patients. Functional testing includes stair climbing and/or a 6-minute walk. Physiologic evaluation includes pulmonary function tests, an echocardiogram, and a stress test. Patients are placed on an exercise program, and smoking cessation is mandatory. In addition, all patients meet with a dietician preoperatively to promote nutritional optimization. In patients who are diabetic, tight control of serum blood glucose is achieved several weeks prior to surgery. Screening colonoscopy and visceral angiography is obtained in selected cases where there is a concern that the stomach will not be an adequate conduit for reconstruction. If there is any concern about other comorbidities, appropriate consultation is obtained preoperatively. Patients at high risk for arrhythmia or myocardial ischemia are placed on perioperative beta blockers. Anticoagulants, nonsteroidal anti-inflammatory agents, and antiplatelet agents are discontinued approximately 7 days prior to surgery if possible. Other preoperative medications are continued until the morning of surgery.

ANESTHESIA AND POSITION Prophylactic antibiotics are administered and antiembolism pneumatic stockings are placed before the induction of general anesthesia. Preoperatively, cervical range of motion should be evaluated to gauge the patient's ability to tolerate varying degrees of extension necessary for completion of a cervical anastomosis. A double-lumen endotracheal tube is inserted and proper positioning confirmed with bronchoscopy. Two large-bore intravenous lines or a central venous catheter is placed. If a central venous catheter is required, a right-sided subclavian or internal jugular approach should be used to maintain access to the left neck for the anastomosis. A radial artery line and Foley catheter are placed. On-table upper endoscopy is routinely performed to assess the location and extent of the tumor, the length of Barrett involvement, and the suitability and extent of the gastric conduit. This information solidifies preoperative planning for the surgical technique to be used. A nasogastric tube is passed into the stomach and placed on low continuous suction. A body warmer is applied after the final positioning, padding the pressure points, and securing the patient to the operating table.

DETAILS OF THE PROCEDURE If a three-field technique is indicated, dissection is begun in the thorax and then followed by a combined laparoscopic and cervical approach. The two-field (Ivor-Lewis) technique requires the reverse order of dissection. Despite variability in the order and combination of the different phases of the operation, positioning and compartment-specific conduct remain consistent. The thoracoscopic, abdominal, and cervical phases of the three-field approach are described in detail. This is followed by illustrating key differences in thoracic access and anastomotic technique for the two-field (Ivor-Lewis) esophagectomy.

THORACOSCOPIC PHASE

Position The patient is positioned on a beanbag in a left lateral decubitus position with the right side up. An axillary roll is used and the left arm is positioned on an arm board. The right arm is suspended and the table is flexed. The surgeon stands posterior and the assistant anterior to the patient (**FIGURE 2**). The operating table is flexed and placed in slight reverse Trendelenburg position to expand the intercostal spaces and depress the diaphragm. All ports are placed under direct visualization, and the operative monitor is placed close to the patient's head.

Port Insertion The thoracoscopic phase of MIE most commonly requires a four-trocar technique. The camera port (10 mm) is placed at the 8th intercostal space anteriorly. Upon entry to the chest, the lung is "dropped" by the anesthesiologist ceasing ventilation on the right lung of the double-lumen tube. A 5-mm port is placed at the 8th or 9th intercostal space 2 cm posterior to the posterior axillary line, for the ultrasonic coagulating shears and other dissecting instruments (**FIGURE 3**). Care is taken to avoid placing this port lower, which would make access to the upper chest difficult. Two additional ports are placed: one 5-mm port is placed posterior to the tip of the scapula, and one 10-mm port is placed at the fourth intercostal space at the anterior axillary line for lung retraction and countertraction during the esophageal dissection. These two additional trocars are frequently omitted in favor of a 4- to 6-cm mini-thoracotomy in the midaxillary line, in the 4th or 5th interspace. To optimize visualization at the diaphragmatic hiatus, a single retracting suture may be placed in the central tendon of the diaphragm and brought out of the inferior, anterior chest wall through a 1-mm skin incision. This suture allows downward traction on the diaphragm and excellent exposure of the distal esophagus, thus eliminating the need for an additional retractor.

Thoracoscopic Mobilization of the Esophagus After a thorough inspection of the chest, the inferior pulmonary ligament is divided to the level of the right inferior pulmonary vein (**FIGURE 4**). The mediastinal pleura overlying the esophagus is opened from the diaphragm to the level of the azygos vein, staying close to the pericardium and hilar structures. Great care is used in dissecting near the membranous trachea and bronchi to avoid injury.

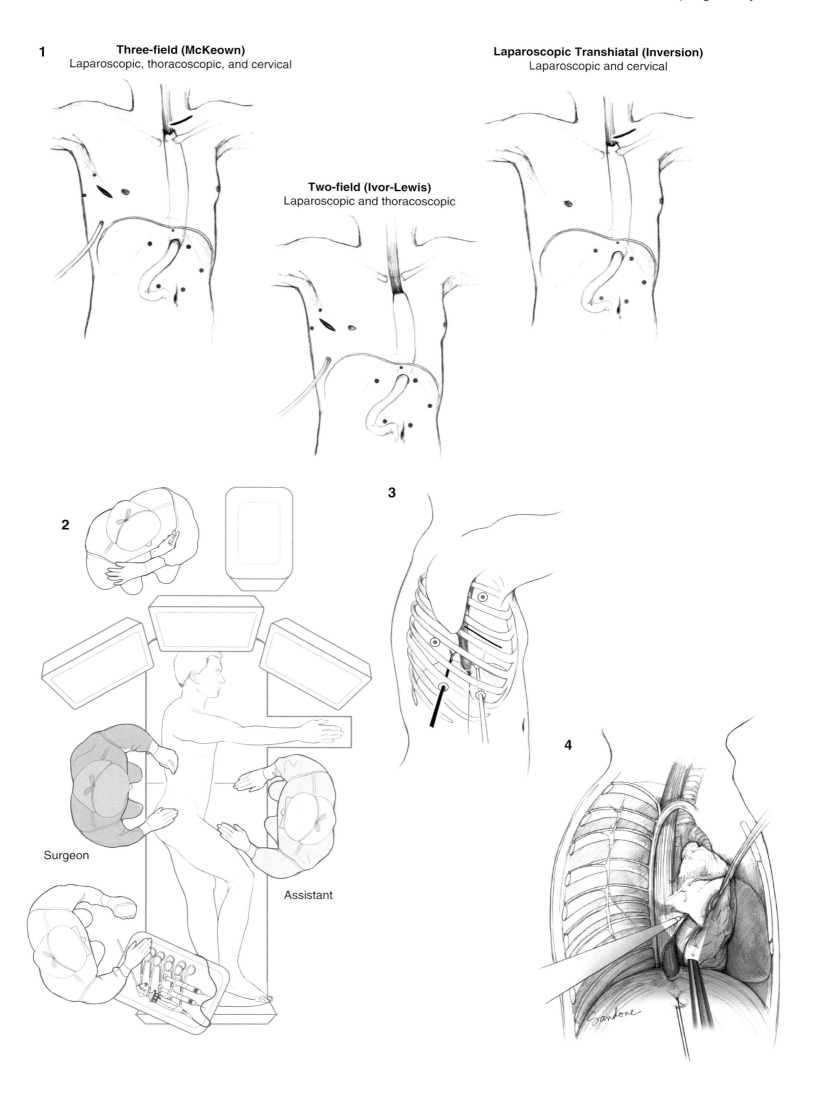

1

Three-field (McKeown)
Laparoscopic, thoracoscopic, and cervical

Laparoscopic Transhiatal (Inversion)
Laparoscopic and cervical

Two-field (Ivor-Lewis)
Laparoscopic and thoracoscopic

2

Surgeon

Assistant

3

4

Thoracoscopic Mobilization of the Esophagus The azygos vein is divided using an endoscopic stapler with a vascular load (**FIGURE 5**). Care is taken to preserve the mediastinal pleura above the azygos vein. The integrity of the pleura helps to maintain the gastric tube in a mediastinal location, and may also be useful to seal the plane around the gastric tube near the thoracic inlet, thereby minimizing the downward extension of a cervical leak.

A Penrose drain is placed around the esophagus to facilitate traction and exposure. The esophagus is retracted medially, and the parietal pleura is divided just anterior and medial to the line of the azygos vein and thoracic duct. Tributaries from the thoracic duct and azygos vein are carefully clipped to minimize the potential for chylous leak. Circumferential mobilization of the esophagus is performed up to the level of 1 to 2 cm above the carina, including all surrounding lymph nodes, periesophageal tissues and fat, and the plane along the pericardium, aorta, and contralateral mediastinal pleura, up to but not including the thoracic duct and azygos vein laterally (**FIGURE 6**).

The entire subcarinal node packet is removed with the specimen; lymph nodes from the upper esophagus, trachea, and adjacent to the recurrent nerve are only sampled for gastroesophageal (GE) junction cancers, but midesophageal cancers require more complete upper mediastinal lymph node clearance.

Care is taken to achieve hemostasis of the bronchial vessels supplying the lymph nodes. As the dissection proceeds toward the thoracic inlet, care is taken to stay near the esophagus, so as to avoid injury to the membranous trachea and the recurrent laryngeal nerves. The vagus nerves are typically divided at the level of the carina, and all periesophageal tissue is gently preserved above this level to avoid injury to the recurrent nerves, which are generally not visualized. Large clips are used during the dissection of the mid- and lower esophagus to avoid lymphatic bleeding from aortoesophageal vessels posteriorly. The distal dissection continues until visualization of the crura is obtained. This will facilitate connecting the dissection planes during the laparoscopic portion of the operation. After complete mobilization of the esophagus has been achieved, the Penrose drain is tucked high into the thoracic inlet or removed (**FIGURE 7**).

Regional anesthesia for up to 12 hours is achieved by injecting each intercostal space with 1 to 2 mL of 0.5% bupivacaine with epinephrine if an epidural catheter has not been placed preoperatively. The lung is gently inflated to search for air leaks from the trachea and proximal bronchus. A single 28 French chest tube is inserted through the camera port and positioned in the posterior mediastinum. All other port sites are closed with absorbable sutures.

5

Azygos v.
divided

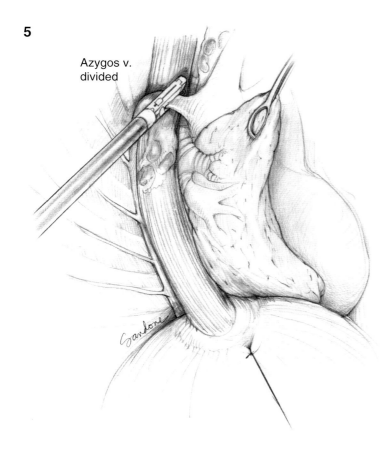

6

Esophagus
mobilized

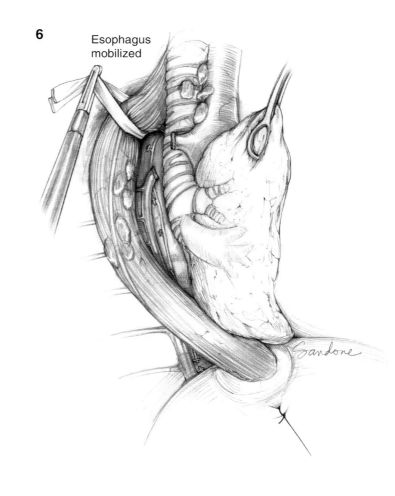

7

Vagus n.
divided

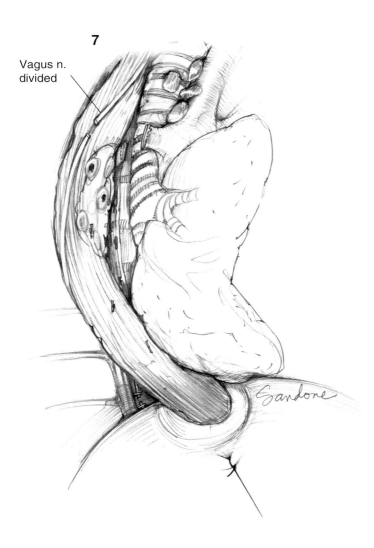

ABDOMINAL PHASE

Position The surgeon and assistant remain in the room to help with repositioning. With an organized team approach, the entire breakdown, repositioning, and repreparation can be accomplished in a timely fashion. The patient is placed in a supine split-legged position with padded leg straps and foot rests. A left chest tube should be placed before starting the abdominal phase, to prevent the development of left tension pneumothorax when the abdominal and chest dissection fields are joined. This positioning allows for the patient to be placed into steep reverse Trendelenburg position, which improves exposure of upper abdominal anatomy. A large gel roll is placed behind the patient's neck between the scapulae to facilitate slight extension of the neck. The bag is inflated before performance of the cervical mobilization and anastomosis. All pressure points are properly protected and padded. The surgeon stands between the patient's legs with the first assistant located at the patient's left, and the second assistant or scrub nurse stands at the patient's right (**FIGURE 8**).

Port Placement The laparoscopic portion of the esophagectomy procedure is performed with a 6 port technique. Three 5-mm ports, two 11- or 12-mm ports, and one 15-mm port are used (**FIGURE 9**). Precise localization of the laparoscopic ports is made according to the patient's body habitus. Although in patients with previous abdominal surgery the port placement may require a creative approach, the definitive port distribution generally approximates that for the Nissen fundoplication, but is 1 to 3 cm lower to allow access to the greater curvature of the stomach. Paradoxically, dropping the trocar positions lower is more important in thin individuals, as the diaphragms tend to be lower and flatter, moving the stomach a bit more inferiorly.

A CO_2 pneumoperitoneum is created using the Veress or Hasson technique as described in Chapter 2. The upper limit of insufflation pressure is set at 15 mm Hg. The primary port is placed approximately 17 cm below the xiphoid to the left of the umbilicus. This placement facilitates alignment with the esophageal hiatus and its oblique entry into the abdominal cavity. The primary port serves as the location for the camera. The entire abdomen is closely examined for evidence of metastatic cancer, which may have not been detected with CT scan. Subsequent upper abdominal ports should be placed high enough to be able to reach the upper abdomen with the surgical instruments, but low enough to reasonably work along the greater curvature of the stomach, the gastroepiploic arcade, and the pylorus. A 12-mm port is placed under direct vision approximately 12 cm lateral to the tip of the sternum, and 3 cm inferior to the left costal margin. This port provides access for the surgeon's right hand. A third trocar is placed 8 cm lateral to the port previously described along the same subcostal line. This 5-mm trocar serves as the primary port site for the first assistant. The fourth site of access is created immediately to the left of the xiphoid process for placement of the liver retractor. A 5-mm cutting trocar is used to create a passageway for the Nathanson liver retractor, which is placed through the track of the trocar (percutaneously) once the trocar is removed. The left lobe of the liver is elevated and the Nathanson liver retractor is then attached to a table-mounted holder (**FIGURE 10**). The fifth port is placed inferior to the right costal margin to the right of the falciform ligament. This 12-mm port provides access for the surgeon's left hand and for the endoscopic stapling device at the time of the creation of the gastric conduit. This port site should be placed as far lateral as possible, without compromising access to the esophageal hiatus and posterior mediastinum. The sixth port site is placed in the patient's right midabdomen and is tailored based on internal anatomy. This 5-mm port provides access for the second assistant's instrument. It is through this port that the assistant elevates the gastric antrum during mobilization of the greater curvature.

8

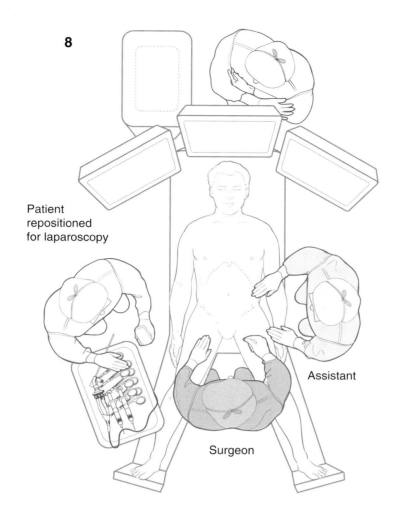

Patient repositioned for laparoscopy

Surgeon

Assistant

9

6 port technique

10

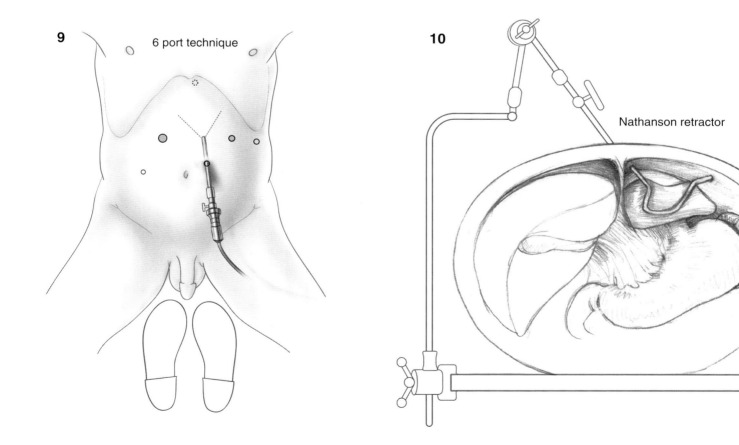

Nathanson retractor

Esophageal and Gastric Mobilization The laparoscopic dissection starts by dividing the gastrohepatic ligament toward the right crus of the diaphragm with the ultrasonic dissector. The hepatic branch of the vagus nerve is divided. The first assistant grasps the epiphrenic fat pad and places the phrenoesophageal membrane on tension. The right crus is exposed and dissected from the top of the hiatus to the decussation with the left crus. This plane is then developed cephalad along the left crus to develop a retroesophageal window (**FIGURE 11**). Care is taken during the early steps of the dissection to avoid complete division of the phrenoesophageal ligament, to avoid entry into the thoracic cavity with subsequent loss of pneumoperitoneum and the exposure difficulties that result from loss of the pneumoperitoneum. If early entry into either thoracic cavities occurs, the chest tubes should be placed to suction to make sure both lungs are allowed to fully expand, and all CO_2 is removed as it enters. We have also found that lowering the insufflating pressure in the abdomen minimizes the transdiaphragmatic air leak. In many cases, an adequate laparoscopic view can be maintained with insufflating pressures in the range of 8 to 12 mm Hg.

Dissection is then taken to the superior portion of the esophageal hiatus toward the upper portion of the left crus. In this area, division of the upper phrenogastric attachments toward the highest short gastric vessels will help with mobilization of the spleen and cardia area away from the diaphragm. This generally makes division of the upper short gastric vessels easier.

At this point, attention is directed toward the greater curvature of the stomach just opposite the inferior pole of the spleen. This anatomic landmark approximates the end of the left gastroepiploic arcade and the beginning of the short gastric vessels.

The assistant grasps the greater omentum adjacent to the greater curvature of the stomach and elevates it anteriorly and laterally. With the surgeon's left hand, the anterior wall of the stomach is retracted medially and posteriorly, toward the spine. The Harmonic scalpel is used to divide the gastrosplenic ligament and the intervening splenic vessels, entering the lesser sac in the progress (**FIGURE 12**). As the highest short gastric is approached, both surgeon and first assistant retract the stomach. The surgeon grasps the fundus of the stomach on the anterior surface, and the first assistant grasps the fundus of the stomach on the posterior surface. The surgeon retracts anteriorly and to the patient's right. The first assistant retracts posteriorly and to the patient's right. This opens up the field at the superior pole of the spleen (**FIGURE 13**).

The retroesophageal plane is cleared more thoroughly as the greater curvature of the stomach is rolled toward the right crus. All tissue posterior to the esophagus is cleared from the diaphragm (at the union of crura and over the preaortic fascia) and maintained en bloc with the esophagogastric junction (**FIGURE 14**). As the GE junction is lifted and rolled to the right, the superior border of the pancreas and the splenic artery are visualized. As one proceeds along the left crus posteriorly, continuity will be established with the right-sided dissection at the base of the right crus, and thus the posterior esophageal window is created.

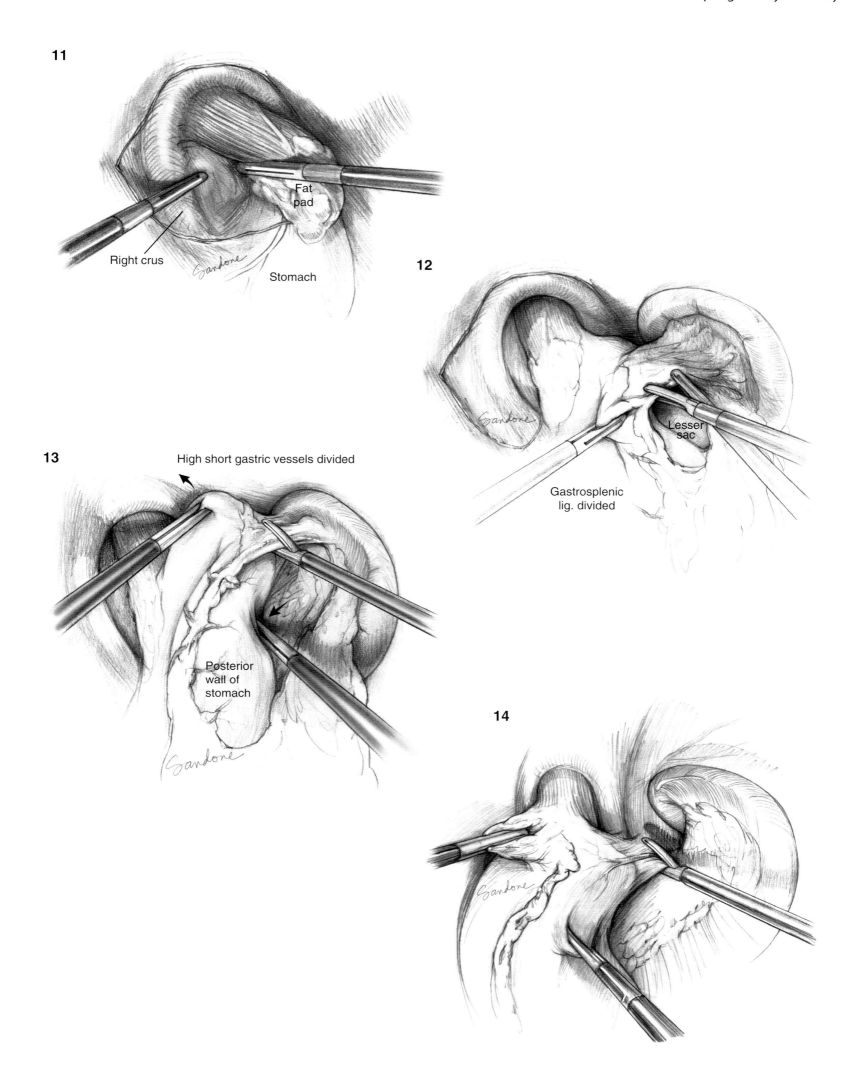

11

Right crus

Fat pad

Stomach

12

Lesser sac

Gastrosplenic lig. divided

13

High short gastric vessels divided

Posterior wall of stomach

14

Esophageal and Gastric Mobilization Next, the central lymph node compartment is cleared, including lymph node (LN) stations 7, 8, 9, and 11, along the hepatic artery and the splenic artery at the superior pancreatic border, then across to the base of the crura (**FIGURE 15**). To expose this region for dissection, the first assistant slides an atraumatic grasper beneath the stomach to the left of the left gastric artery and elevates the stomach anteriorly. This places tension on the left gastric vessels and allows visualization in the retrogastric region. The second assistant may need to retract inferiorly (and gently) on the superior border of the pancreas to expose the LN basins along the hepatic and splenic arteries (**FIGURE 16**). In the course of this dissection, the left gastric vein is identified and divided with clips. The left gastric artery is divided at the level of the celiac trifurcation after clipping or with a vascular load of the linear stapler. This device can be placed through either upper abdominal port, whichever gives the best view of the closed stapler (**FIGURE 17**).

The plane along the greater curvature of the stomach is developed and continued distally, care being taken to avoid injury to the right gastroepiploic arcade. This arcade must be identified and preserved, as it constitutes the major source of blood flow to the gastric tube. In addition, the transverse mesocolon may be fused posteriorly to the gastrocolic ligament, putting the middle colic vessels at risk of injury by the unsuspecting surgeon. The first and second assistants grasp the body and antrum of the stomach, respectively, and retract in a superior and anterior direction. This movement serves to place the gastrocolic ligament on tension, displaying the gastroepiploic vessels. Once the gastroepiploic vessels are clearly in view, the gastrocolic ligament is divided (**FIGURE 18**).

It is important to insure that the entire gastrocolic ligament is divided all the way to the hepatic flexure, as the proximal transverse colon can serve as a point of tension that will prohibit a tension-free pull-up of the neoesophagus. At this point it becomes necessary for both assistants to grasp the posterior aspect of the stomach to facilitate mobilization of the posterior gastric wall away from the anterior surface of the pancreas (**FIGURE 19**). There are four potential pitfalls in this dissection: (1) injury to the transverse colon, especially in cases where diverticulosis is present; (2) injury to the transverse colon blood supply, especially when there is fusion of the greater omentum and transverse mesocolon; (3) gastric perforation secondary to overly aggressive retraction; and perhaps most importantly, (4) injury to the right gastroepiploic vessels along the greater curvature of the stomach, or to the gastroduodenal artery as it passes posterior to the duodenal bulb. The posterior gastric and duodenal dissection is completed at the point when the pulsations of the gastroduodenal artery are visualized. Care should be taken to preserve enough tissue to keep a healthy arcade without leaving too much tissue, which will result in excessive bulk on the gastric tube. Excess fat along the greater curvature can also lead to tension on the arcade or make it difficult for the gastric tube to ascend through the hiatus along the left crus.

The dissection along the greater curvature continues toward the hepatoduodenal attachments. These are divided along the lateral duodenum and gallbladder area to complete the Kocher maneuver. This portion of the dissection is ergonomically easier if the surgeon moves their left-handed grasper to the lowest right-sided trocar, allowing an assistant on the right side of the table to place countertraction on the lateral peritoneal reflection while the assistant on the left side of the table retracts the pylorus and proximal duodenum to the left (**FIGURE 20**). The Kocher maneuver is complete when the third portion of the duodenum is visualized as it curves medially and the pylorus is easily elevated to the diaphragmatic hiatus. If gentle lifting of the pylorus does not allow an easy, tension-free reach to the right crus, further duodenal and infrapyloric mobilization should be performed.

15

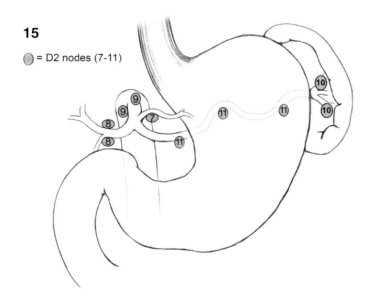

= D2 nodes (7-11)

16

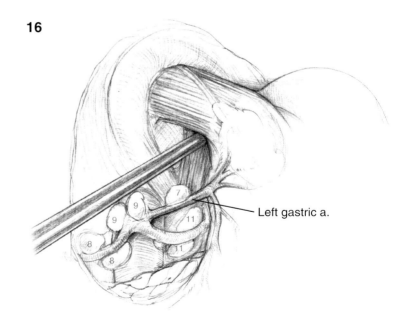

Left gastric a.

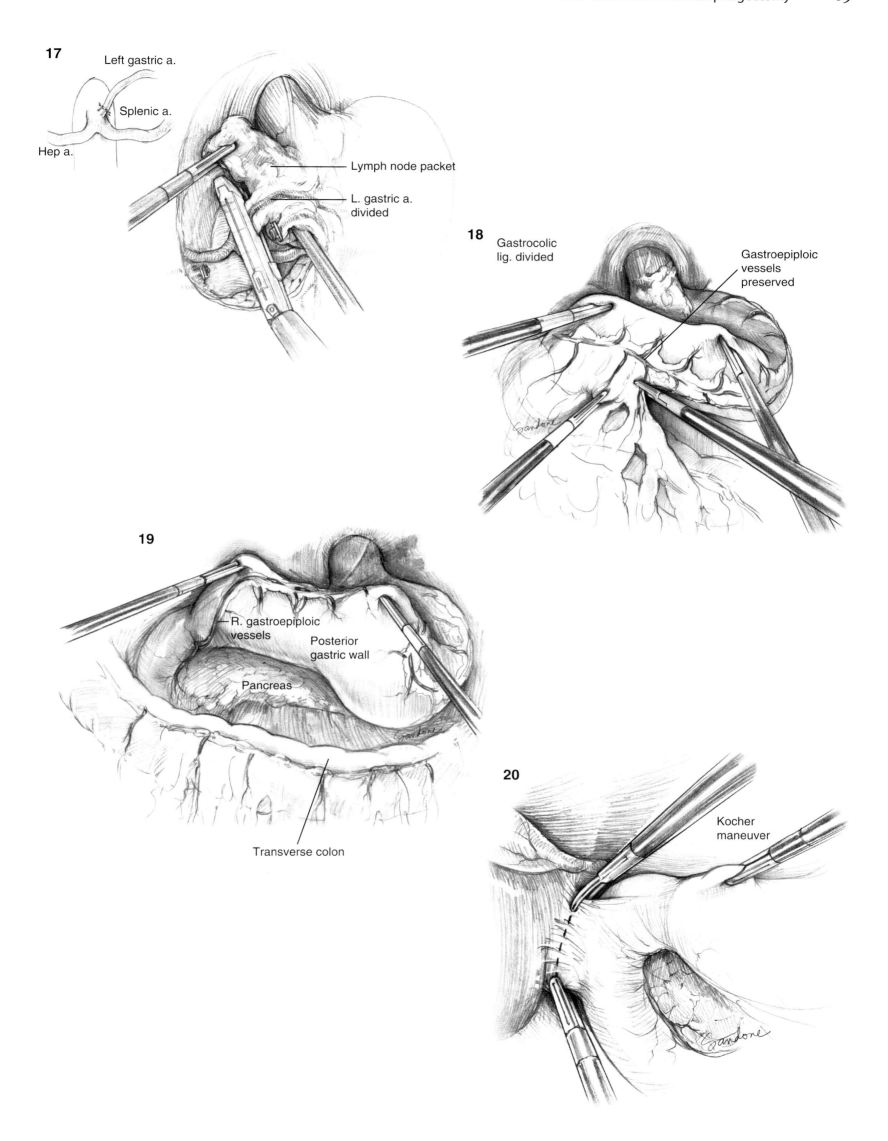

17

Left gastric a.

Splenic a.

Hep a.

Lymph node packet

L. gastric a. divided

18 Gastrocolic lig. divided

Gastroepiploic vessels preserved

19

R. gastroepiploic vessels

Posterior gastric wall

Pancreas

Transverse colon

20

Kocher maneuver

Creation of the Gastric Tube The nasogastric tube is pulled back to a position within the thoracic esophagus, no more than 40 cm in from the nasal ala. A site, 2 to 4 cm proximal to the pylorus, is identified on the gastric lesser curvature, sparing two or three branches of the right gastric artery. At the point selected, the lesser omentum is divided down to the substance of the stomach with the ultrasonic dissector in preparation for stapling. The surgeon, standing between the patient's legs and working through the left upper and right lower trocars, orients the lesser curvature for the second assistant, who creates the gastric tube through the right upper quadrant port. The first assistant places another atraumatic grasper along the greater curvature and gently stretches and flattens the stomach as the site for each stapler firing is chosen. The endoscopic tri-stapling device with a purple cartridge (or other equivalent stapler) is introduced through the 12-mm port site located in the patient's right upper abdomen. The first load is fired in a perpendicular orientation to the lesser curve and parallel to the greater curvature (**FIGURE 21**). Serial stapling is performed by the second assistant standing on the patient's right side to create a conduit approximately 3 to 4 cm wide. As the gastric tube stapling progresses cephalad, the first assistant's traction point is moved up the greater curvature to keep the tube "on stretch," lengthening it. Meanwhile, the surgeon is providing countertraction by pulling the staple lines toward the right lower quadrant and into the jaws of the stapler, with atraumatic graspers in both hands. The goal is to make the stomach appear like a tabletop before each firing of the stapler (**FIGURE 22**).

For patients with cancer of the mid or distal esophagus, the neoesophagus is completed at the tip of the gastric fundus. In patients who have malignancy of the GE junction, it may be necessary to include a larger portion of the proximal stomach in the resection.

Once the neoesophagus is constructed, the distal margin on the specimen side is sent for frozen section examination. This tissue is obtained with an endoscopic stapler to avoid opening the proximal stomach, usually at the far end of the staple line, nearest to the GE junction.

Attention is turned to the distal esophageal mobilization. With the first assistant grasping the gastric remnant of the specimen, the esophagus and stomach are retracted inferiorly and slightly to the patient's left. The distal esophagus is circumferentially mobilized with its accompanying lymphatic tissue. The posterior mediastinum is cleared of all tissue to visualize the pericardium anteriorly, the right and left pleura laterally, and the surface of the aorta posterolaterally (**FIGURE 23**). Lymph nodes and periesophageal fat are generally left with the specimen, but may be individually removed if they separate from the specimen during dissection. Upon completion of the mediastinal resection, the GE junction and the angle of His are pushed through the esophageal hiatus, leaving only a small tip of the distal lesser curve of the specimen visible (**FIGURE 24**). The tip of the gastric tube is sewn to this tip of the specimen, minimizing the overall profile for advancement of the neoesophagus to the neck (**FIGURE 25**).

21

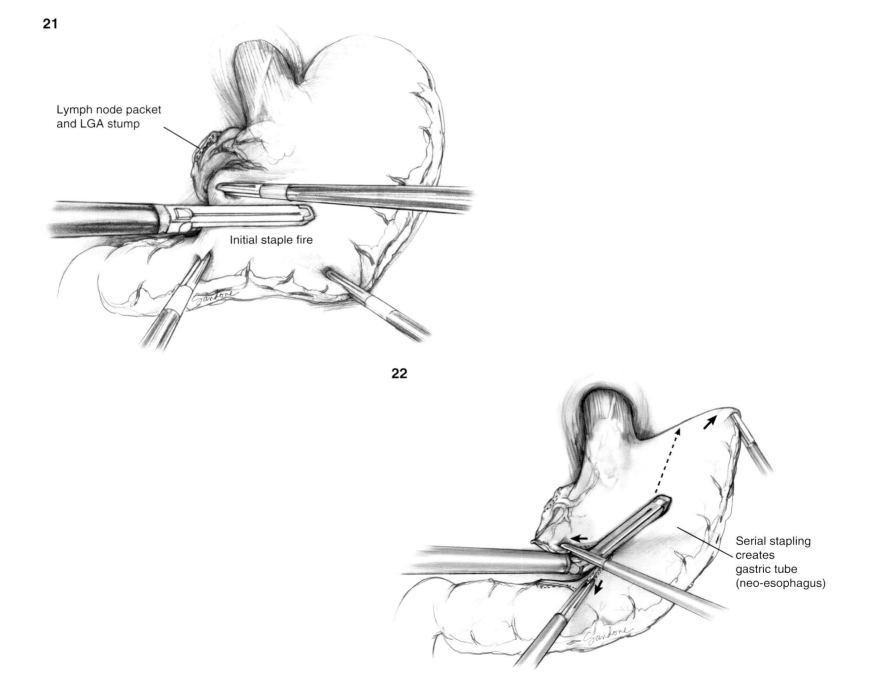

Lymph node packet
and LGA stump

Initial staple fire

22

Serial stapling
creates
gastric tube
(neo-esophagus)

23

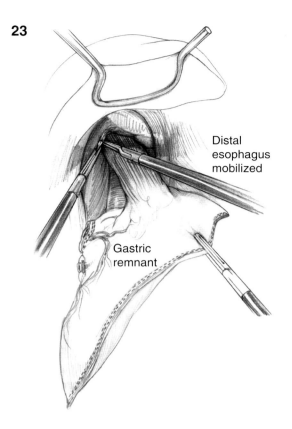

Distal
esophagus
mobilized

Gastric
remnant

24

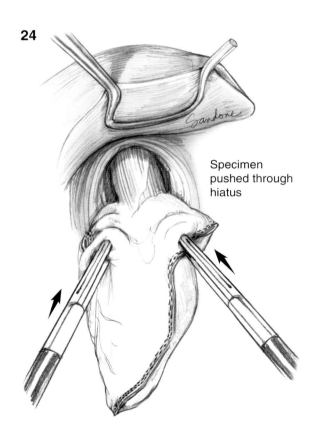

Specimen
pushed through
hiatus

25

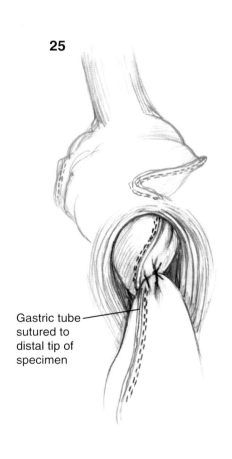

Gastric tube
sutured to
distal tip of
specimen

Pyloromyotomy and Pyloroplasty At this point, a pyloroplasty or pyloromyotomy is performed; we prefer pyloromyotomy. A suture is placed across the pyloric muscle superiorly, and elevated by the second assistant through the RUQ port. With the heel of an "L" hook, the serosa overlying the pylorus is scored for approximately 3 to 5 cm (**FIGURE 26**). The hook is then slid along the gastric mucosa, beneath the pyloric muscle, which is elevated and divided with the hook (**FIGURE 27**). The pyloromyotomy is spread open with an atraumatic grasper, which allows visualization of the base of the gastric and duodenal mucosa, ensuring that all muscle fibers have been divided (**FIGURE 28**). If the mucosa is perforated, the pyloromyotomy is converted to a pyloroplasty (**FIGURES 29 AND 30**). For details of laparoscopic pyloroplasty, refer to Chapter 24.

Feeding Jejunostomy If two teams are employed, laparoscopic placement of a feeding jejunostomy can be performed concurrently with the neck dissection (**FIGURE 31**). Alternatively, it can be performed at the completion of the case. For details of laparoscopic feeding jejunostomy tube placement, refer to Chapter 28.

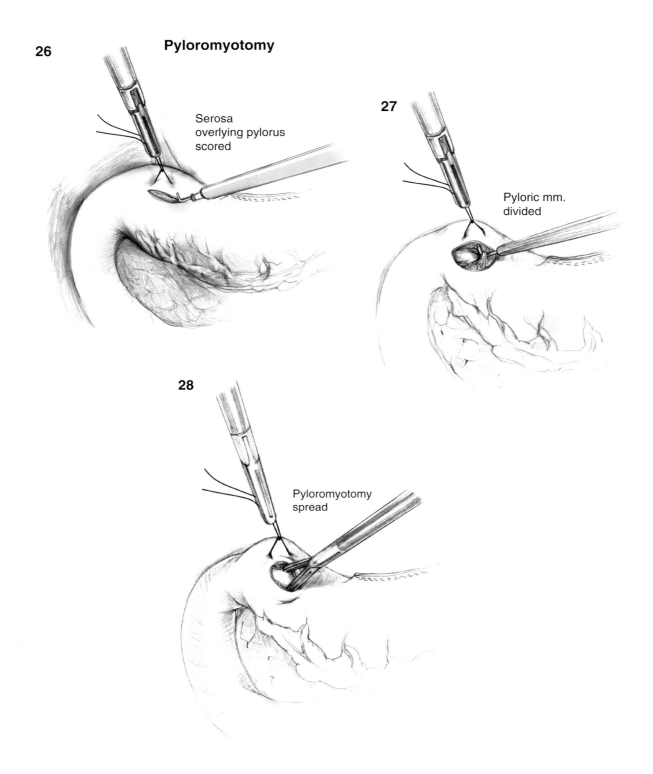

26

Pyloromyotomy

Serosa overlying pylorus scored

27

Pyloric mm. divided

28

Pyloromyotomy spread

Pyloroplasty

29

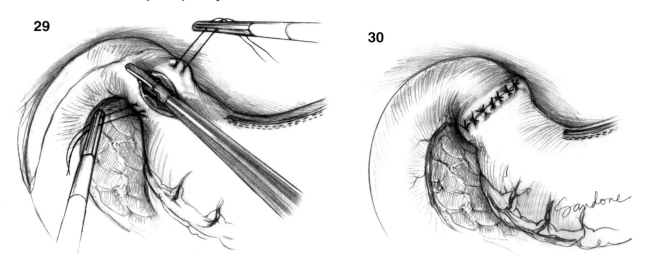

30

31

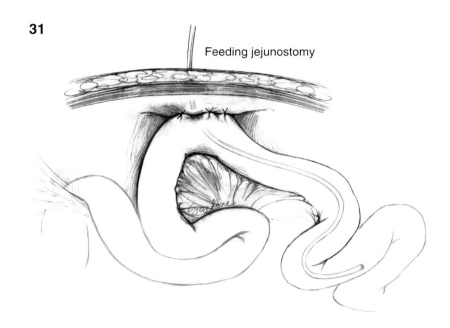

Feeding jejunostomy

CERVICAL PHASE

Position For the cervical esophageal mobilization, the surgeon stands on the patient's left side with the neck extended by a gel roll beneath the shoulders (**FIGURE 32**).

Exposure of the Cervical Esophagus A 5-cm transverse incision is made in the left neck approximately one fingerbreadth above the clavicle (**FIGURE 33**). The subcutaneous tissue and platysma muscle are divided using electrocautery, thereby exposing the anterior border of the sternocleidomastoid muscle. A blunt, self-retaining retractor is applied to the skin edges medially and the sternocleidomastoid muscle laterally. The omohyoid muscle is identified running in a transverse plane across the wound. This muscle is divided, thereby opening the fascia, which leads to the deep neck structures. At this point, the contents of the carotid sheath will be retracted laterally, and the fascia lateral to the strap muscles is opened with electrosurgery. The lateral borders of the sternothyroid and the sternohyoid muscles are grasped with Allis clamps, sequentially, and a Kittner is used to free the muscle bellies, posteriorly. Both muscles are divided over a right-angle clamp below the inferior pole of the thyroid, to maximize exposure of the esophagus. During this portion of the procedure, the surgeon's and assistants' fingers are used for retraction. We avoid using any retractors deep in the neck, to avoid traction injury on the recurrent laryngeal nerve or vagus nerve. The left lobe of the thyroid gland is carefully grasped with two Babcock clamps and retracted medially (**FIGURE 34**). Should the middle thyroid vein or inferior thyroid artery obscure the deeper neck structures, they are divided between clamps and ligated.

At this point, the superior mediastinum should be easily accessed by placing a finger along the anterior spine and using blunt dissection to open this space. With the assistant's index finger rotating and retracting the larynx and trachea medially, and the surgeon retracting the sternocleidomastoid and carotid sheath laterally, the esophagus and recurrent laryngeal nerve become apparent (**FIGURE 35**). After sharply incising the tissue posterolateral to the tracheoesophageal groove, the anterior wall of the esophagus can be mobilized away from the membranous trachea, using blunt dissection. This is continued in superior and inferior directions, so as to increase esophageal mobility. The lateral and posterior aspects of the esophagus are mobilized with blunt dissection using a Kittner and a finger. Once the esophagus is circumferentially mobilized, an umbilical tape is passed around the esophagus (**FIGURE 36**).

32

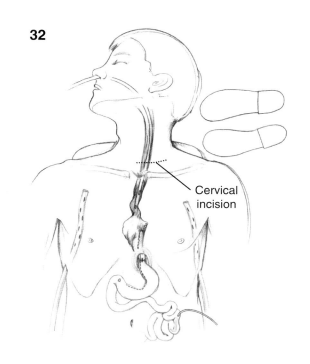

Cervical
incision

33

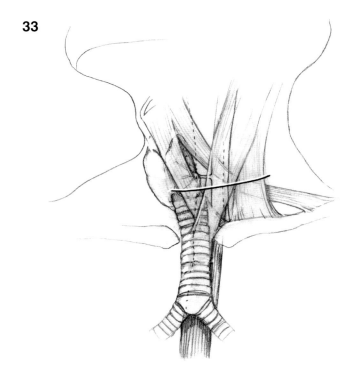

34

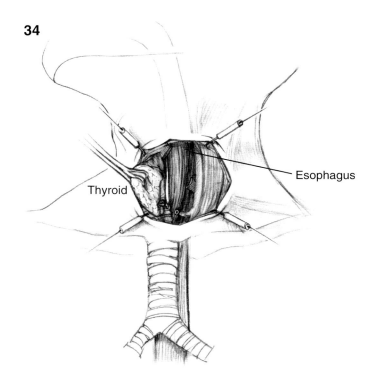

Thyroid

Esophagus

35

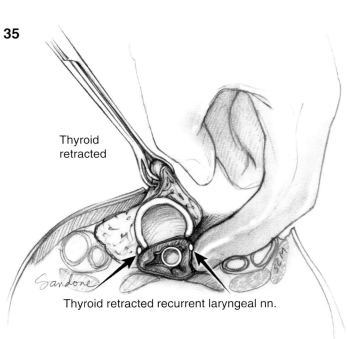

Thyroid
retracted

Thyroid retracted recurrent laryngeal nn.

36

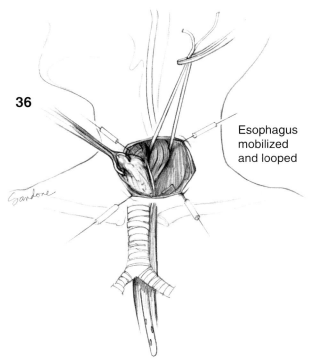

Esophagus
mobilized
and looped

Exposure of the Cervical Esophagus At this point, the surgeon stays at the neck to pull up the gastric tube as the abdomen is insufflated and the laparoscopic view is reestablished, allowing direct visualization as the gastric tube ascends through the hiatus. The resected esophagogastric specimen is removed through the cervical incision, and the gastric tube is pulled up to the neck (**FIGURE 37**). Care is taken to maintain visualization of the conduit from above and below to ensure proper orientation of the gastroepiploic arcade toward the left crus and the staple line toward the right crus. This avoids spiraling of the gastric tube. Care should be taken to avoid tension on the gastroepiploic arcade as the conduit traverses the hiatal opening. The gastric tube is assessed for viability and adequate tension-free length. The esophagus is then divided at an oblique angle using heavy scissors (**FIGURE 38**).

Cervical Anastomosis The method of anastomosis can be hand sewn, side-to-side stapled, or end-to-side stapled. We perform a stapled, end-to-side cervical anastomosis as described by Orringer. The staple line of the lesser curvature resection site is maintained toward the right. If the tip of the conduit is redundant or ischemic, it is removed with an endoscopic stapling device. The resulting staple line may be oversewn with interrupted sutures.

A traction suture is placed on the neoesophagus at the inferior aspect of the cervical incision to elevate it to the skin level. A second stay stitch is placed in the anterior wall of the remaining esophagus to keep it oriented correctly. By lowering the cut end of the remaining esophagus to the conduit, the site of anastomosis is defined. A 1.5-cm gastrotomy is created on the anterior wall of the stomach, adjacent to the greater curvature, and just above the gastric stay stitch. Two lateral sutures are placed and tied, to line up posterior wall of the divided esophagus to the edge of the gastrotomy. A 45-mm-long endoscopic stapling device (purple cartridge or equivalent) is introduced into the esophagus and gastrotomy. We put the thinner, anvil portion of the stapler through the gastrotomy, and the cartridge side within the esophagus. The traction sutures are drawn inferiorly as the stapler is advanced (**FIGURES 39A, B**). It is critical that the posterior wall of the esophagus and anterior wall of the stomach be appropriately aligned and that the gastric conduit staple line not be included in the esophagogastrostomy. The stapler is fired, and the anastomosis is inspected for hemostasis. The nasogastric tube is carefully passed through the anastomosis and positioned distally in the gastric conduit, bridging the diaphragm (**FIGURE 40**). This is done under laparoscopic visualization. The gastrotomy and esophagotomy are closed in two layers, with 3-0 monofilament absorbable suture in a running fashion, followed by interrupted Lembert sutures (**FIGURE 41**).

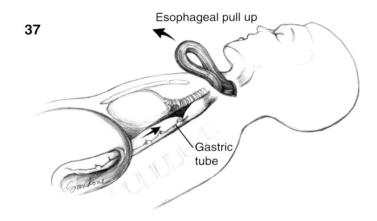

37   Esophageal pull up

Gastric tube

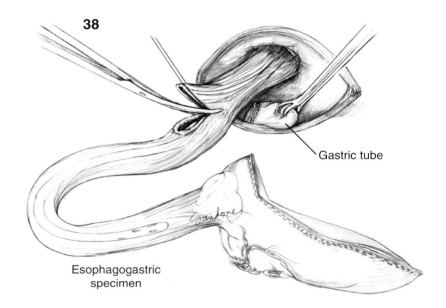

38

Gastric tube

Esophagogastric specimen

Cervical anastomosis

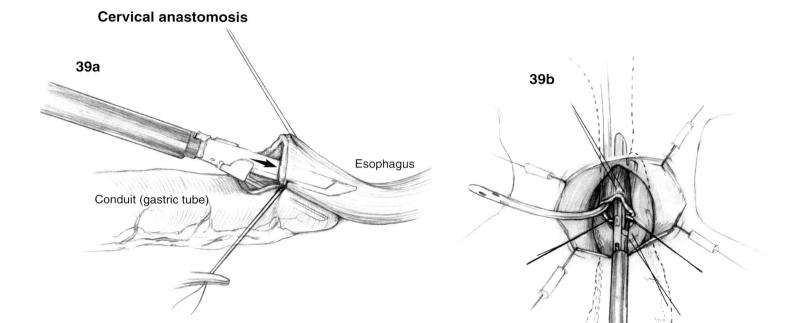

39a

Esophagus

Conduit (gastric tube)

39b

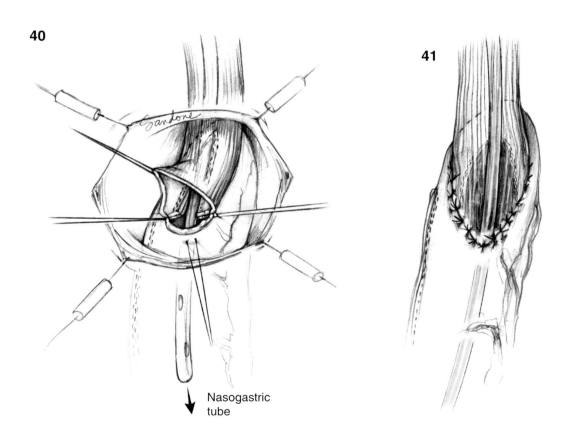

40

41

Nasogastric
tube

Cervical Anastomosis Alternatively an end-to-side anastomosis can be performed using a circular stapler. As the specimen is pulled out of the neck, slight tension is placed on the remaining cervical esophageal attachments. Once the cervical esophagus is adequately mobilized, it is placed on slight tension and a 45-mm auto-purse-string device is fired across the esophagus 2 to 3 cm distal to the cricopharyngeus. The esophagus is divided distal to the purse-string device. The purse string device is removed and the esophagus is lubricated, and gently dilated. A 25-mm anvil to the stapler is inserted into the cervical esophageal stump and the purse string is tied. The distal end of the conduit staple line is carefully opened and the gastric tube is suctioned clean (**FIGURE 42, INSET**). A 25-mm stapler is inserted into this opening. The exit point of the stapler is out of the posterior gastric tube 4-6 cm distal to the tip, avoiding the area of the short gastrics laterally and the lesser curve staple line medially. The stapling device is docked with the anvil and fired (**FIGURE 42**). A nasogastric tube is manually guided across the anastomosis and the tip positioned in the gastric tube above the diaphragm. The opening in the tip of the gastric tube is amputated with a linear stapling instrument.

The proximal esophagus and anastomosis are replaced in the superior mediastinum, posterior to the trachea. The neck is irrigated and hemostasis is ensured. A 10-mm closed suction drain is placed in the superior mediastinum, lateral to the anastomosis. The platysma muscle is reapproximated with an interrupted 3-0 Vicryl suture. The skin is closed with 4-0 monofilament suture or surgical staples.

Gastropexy and Colopexy The last two steps close the diaphragm around the gastric tube and fix the colon in the abdomen to avoid colonic herniation. The gastric tube is gently grasped near the pylorus, and downward traction is applied until all redundancy is reduced back into the abdomen. The gastric tube is tacked to the diaphragmatic hiatus with 4 to 6 interrupted sutures to prevent herniation of other abdominal viscera and rotation of the gastric conduit (**FIGURE 43**). Despite this fixation, colonic herniation is a risk unless the colon is secured in the abdomen. To avoid this, the splenic flexure may be sutured to the left abdominal wall, and the mid–transverse colon may be sutured, like a clothesline, to the round ligament in the midline.

The liver retractor and all trocars are removed under direct vision. The abdomen is de-insufflated. All trocar sites 10 mm or greater are closed and the skin is approximated with subcuticular absorbable sutures. If the patient is to remain intubated, the double-lumen tube is exchanged to a single lumen prior to transfer to the ICU.

Postoperative Care Patients are routinely transferred to ICU. The nasogastric tube is typically removed between POD 3 and 5. Routine esophagography is performed on POD 7. The patient remains NPO until after the esophagram. A clear liquid diet is started after a negative radiographic and speech pathology evaluation (optional). Jejunostomy tube feeding is initiated at trophic levels on POD 1 and is gradually advanced to goal as tolerated. We convert to cyclic feeds (5 PM to 9 AM) before discharge. The chest tubes are removed when outputs are below 200 mL/day of drainage. Average hospital discharge is on POD 8 or 9 for the MIS three-field esophagectomy.

42

**Alternate:
Circular stapled
anastomosis**

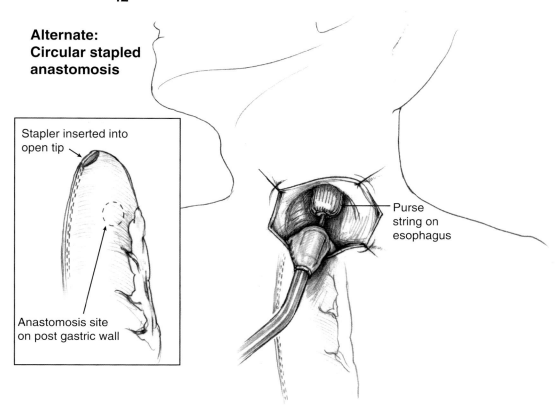

Stapler inserted into
open tip

Anastomosis site
on post gastric wall

Purse
string on
esophagus

43

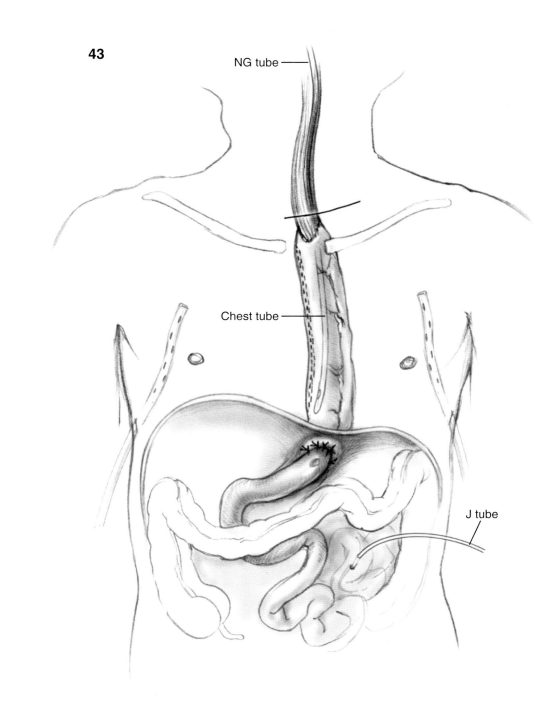

NG tube

Chest tube

J tube

TWO-FIELD ESOPHAGECTOMY Although the order is reversed, mobilization of the specimen and creation of the gastric conduit is the same as above. After completion of the laparoscopic steps, the conduit is affixed to the proximal stomach (**FIGURE 44**). The patient is repositioned in the left lateral decubitus position, and thoracic access with a mini-thoracotomy is attained (**FIGURE 45**). The esophagus is circumferentially mobilized above the level of the divided azygos arch. It is transected using endoscopic scissors (without cautery) (**FIGURE 46**).

44

**Alternate:
Two field esophagectomy**

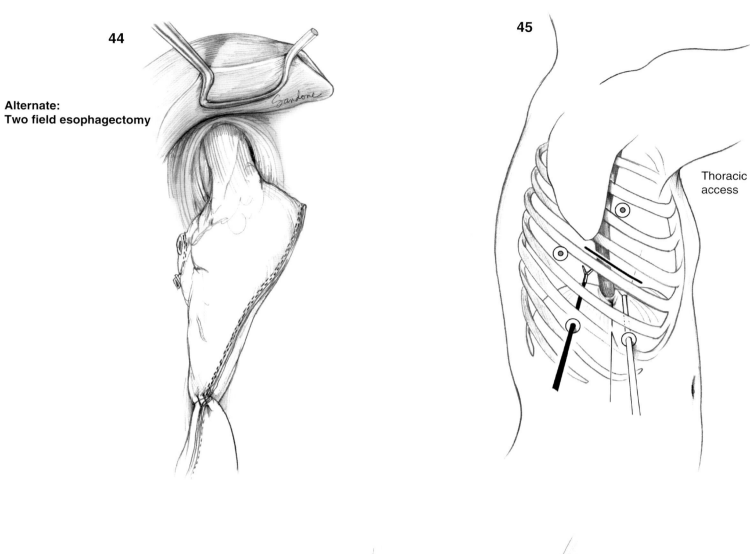

45

Thoracic
access

46

Esophagus mobilized
and transected

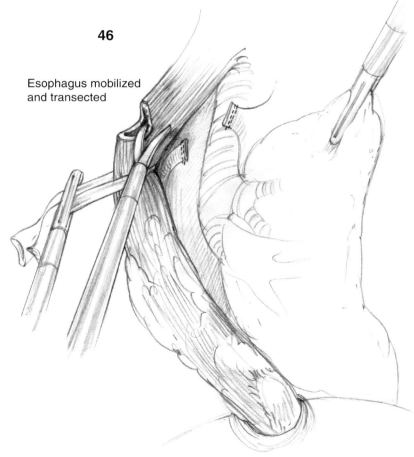

TWO-FIELD ESOPHAGECTOMY The posterior 9th interspace port is enlarged to 4 cm and a wound protector is placed through the incision. A 25- or 28-mm circular stapler anvil is introduced and placed in the proximal esophageal lumen. It is secured with a purse-string suture. The distal esophagus and gastric conduit are then pulled through the hiatus and brought out of the thoracic cavity (**FIGURE 47**).

The gastric conduit tip is opened and the stapler handle is introduced (**FIGURE 48**). The point of the stapler should exit the greater curve 4 to 6 cm distal to the tip, avoiding close proximity to the lesser curve staple line.

The stapling device and conduit are docked with the anvil, and the stapler is fired (**FIGURE 49**). A nasogastric tube is inserted across the anastomosis with the tip positioned in the gastric tube above the pylorus. The enterotomy in the tip of the gastric tube is amputated with a linear stapling instrument (**FIGURE 50**). As a final step, the gastric tube is gently retracted downward to minimize its intrathoracic redundancy and sutured to the crus to avoid rotation of the conduit (**FIGURE 51**). A 28 French thoracostomy tube is introduced via the camera access site (**FIGURE 52**). The trocar sites are closed with absorbable suture.

Postoperative Care Bronchoscopy is performed and the patient is extubated in the OR or left intubated in the ICU overnight. Our current practice for Ivor-Lewis MIE patients is to remove the NG tube on POD 3 to 5 (when the ileus resolves) and get an esophagram on POD 7. We start oral liquids if the study is negative. J-tube feeding is as described above. The chest tube is maintained until after starting a liquid diet and confirmation of no leak. Epidural or paravertebral blocks are initially used for pain control, with conversion to narcotic elixir when tolerating oral intake. ■

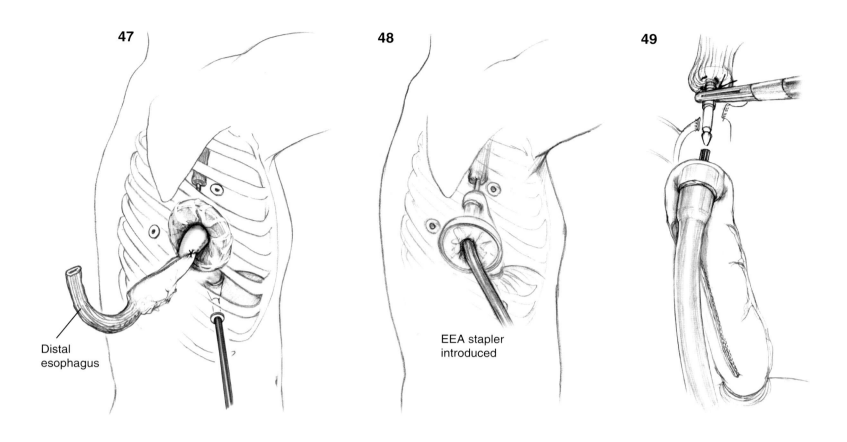

47

Distal
esophagus

48

EEA stapler
introduced

49

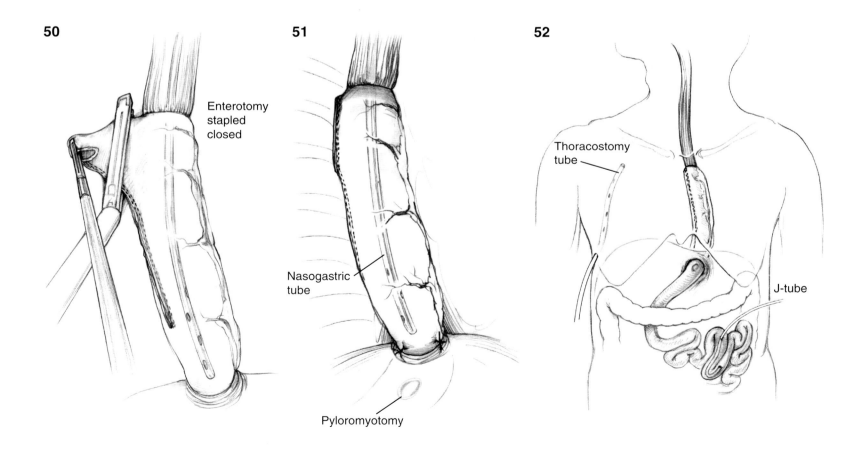

50

Enterotomy
stapled
closed

51

Nasogastric
tube

Pyloromyotomy

52

Thoracostomy
tube

J-tube

MINIMALLY INVASIVE UPPER GI TRACT SURGERY

Transoral Cricopharyngeal Myotomy and Zenker Diverticulectomy

A Zenker diverticulum is a pulsion diverticulum that occurs between the cricopharyngeus muscle inferiorly and the inferior constrictor superiorly as a result of relative obstruction to swallowing at the esophageal introitus by a "tight" cricopharyngeus muscle (**FIGURE 1A**). As the diverticulum develops and extends inferiorly and posteriorly, the cricopharyngeus muscle is enveloped by mucosa from the posterior wall of the esophageal introitus and the anterior wall of the diverticulum (**FIGURE 1B**). This relationship allows transoral division of the common wall between the esophagus and diverticulum, and cricopharyngeal myotomy with a single firing of a linear stapler inserted into the diverticulum (one jaw) and across the upper esophageal sphincter (cricopharyngeus muscle) (**FIGURE 1C**). An important anatomic fact that supports the safe performance of the cricopharyngeal myotomy is that the hypopharynx, diverticulum, and cervical esophageal complex are surrounded by the middle layer of the deep cervical fascia, which protects against leakage into the mediastinum.

INDICATIONS Surgical management of Zenker diverticulum is indicated in individuals who have hypopharyngeal, laryngeal, or swallowing symptoms that can be correlated with the presence of the diverticulum and its associated cricopharyngeal spasm. Typical symptoms include: (1) pharyngeal regurgitation of food often in association with coughing, sometimes with a long latency after eating; (2) difficulty swallowing, particularly solid boluses; (3) cough from the microaspiration that occurs when food and liquid matter in the diverticulum refluxes into the hypopharynx. (4) As symptoms worsen, weight loss may become a major issue.

Because of the low morbidity of the endoscopic approach to Zenker diverticulum and cricopharyngeal myotomy as compared to the external approach, many patients are now eligible for surgical management who, in the past, would have been felt to be at high risk for general anesthesia. Many of these patients are old and cachectic with significant pulmonary comorbidities. Endoscopic management of this condition can generally be performed on an outpatient basis with less than 60 minutes of general anesthesia. It is contraindicated in relatively few patients.

PREOPERATIVE PREPARATION A modified barium swallow performed by a qualified team of speech and language pathologists and radiologists is a prerequisite to surgical management of this disease process. The purpose of the swallowing evaluation is not only to determine the size and location of the diverticulum but also to look at associated problems with swallowing in the oral, pharyngeal, and esophageal phases. Many patients with a Zenker diverticulum have associated esophageal dysmotility that may ultimately influence their swallowing result. Although these patients can still undergo surgical management, preoperative counseling as to the likelihood of resumption of normal swallowing will be tempered by these findings. Generally, a modified barium swallow examination will look at all aspects of swallowing with particular focus on the oropharyngeal, hypopharyngeal, and esophageal phases, whereas a regular barium swallow done by radiology alone tends to focus only on the esophageal phase. There must be a correlation between the patient's symptoms and the presence of a diverticulum before surgery should be considered. Patients with significant esophageal dysmotility that is responsible for their dysphagia, who are found to have an associated asymptomatic Zenker diverticulum, should not be operated on.

At the time of modified barium swallow, the Zenker diverticulum should be visualized in the anterior and lateral planes to determine the length and the thickness of the common wall between the diverticulum and the esophagus. Often placing a marker of known size, such as a penny, on the patient during examination will help with calibration. In general, the diverticulum should be more than 2.5 to 3 cm in length for the patient to be a good candidate for endoscopic management. This length will provide adequate exposure of the cricopharyngeus muscle for complete sectioning, which is the key to success of the operation. A thick common wall between the diverticulum and the esophagus makes it more difficult to engage the stapler and adequately section the cricopharyngeus muscle simultaneously. The ideal diverticulum is more than 2.5 to 3 cm in length but does not reach below the clavicle and has a well-defined, relatively thin partition between itself and the esophagus.

In addition to radiographic imaging of the diverticulum, the patient should be assessed for their degree of mouth opening and neck mobility. Patient positioning for appropriate placement of the diverticuloscope requires significant mouth opening, neck flexion at the shoulders, and head extension similar to operative laryngoscopy. Significant neck arthritis or temporomandibular joint (TMJ) problems may make exposure difficult. The size of the diverticuloscope, its configuration, and the requirement that it rest on the upper incisors make chipping of the upper front incisors a real possibility despite the use of a tooth protector.

ANESTHESIA This operation is performed under general anesthesia. The patient should be intubated with a relatively small endotracheal tube to maximize the space in the oropharynx and hypopharynx for the diverticuloscope. A wire-reinforced tube may be helpful in preventing kinking during the performance of the procedure (not depicted). Preoperative antibiotics with good coverage for upper aerodigestive tract aerobes and anaerobes are generally given in case a perforation should occur. Perioperative steroids given as a single dose preoperatively may used to minimize postoperative tongue swelling.

POSITIONING The patient is positioned supine on the operative table with the bed turned 90 degrees from the anesthesiologist. The monitor is placed at the patient's feet, which will allow an unobstructed view during the procedure itself. A Mayo stand is placed over the patient's chest for support of the suspension arm that is attached to the diverticuloscope. The light source is positioned off to the surgeon's left so that the cords do not interfere with instrumentation (**FIGURE 2**).

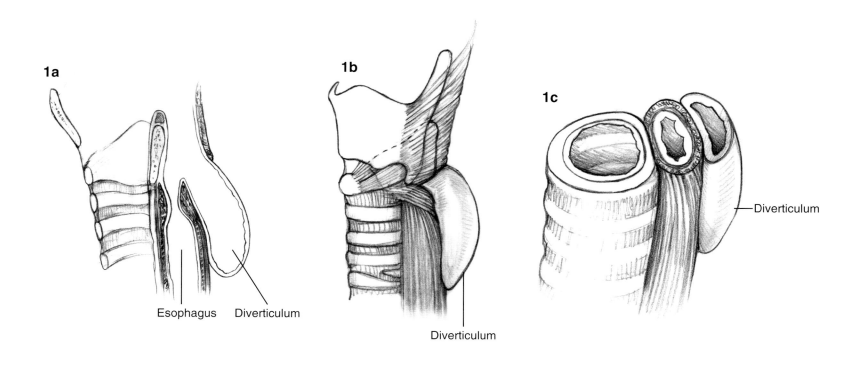

Esophagus   Diverticulum

Diverticulum

Diverticulum

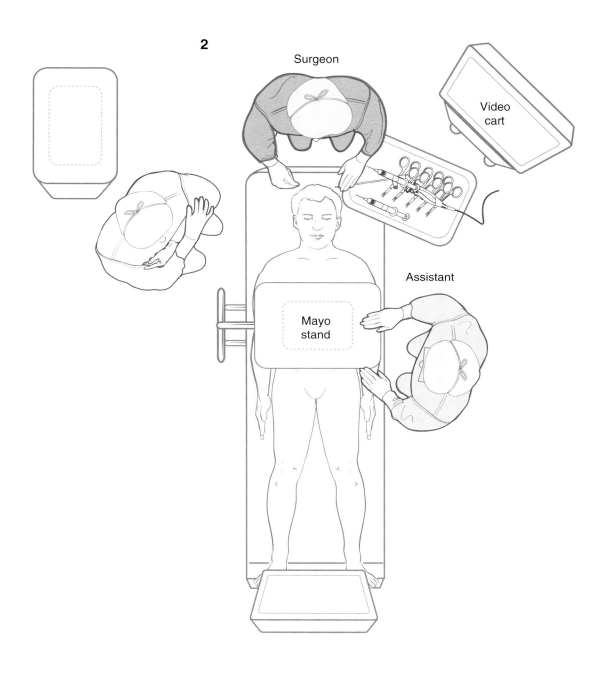

OPERATIVE PROCEDURE With the patient in position and fully relaxed, the diverticuloscope is introduced transorally. The diverticuloscope can be opened in two dimensions—distally, which increases the room for operative manipulation and instrumentation at the operative site; and proximally, which allows access for the scope from the side for visualization of what is happening in the hypopharynx without interfering with the placement of the stapling device (**FIGURE 3**). With the scope closed proximally and opened only minimally distally, it is introduced orally and gradually advanced into the hypopharynx. In general, the diverticulum will be seen first (usually with debris or residual barium from the preoperative examination within it), as it is in the most direct line with the hypopharynx. Once the diverticulum has been visualized, the scope is withdrawn slightly and suspended anteriorly, which will bring the esophageal introitus into view at the most anterior aspect of the visual field.

The tip of the upper blade of the diverticuloscope is advanced minimally into the esophageal introitus so that it engages the cricopharyngeus muscle and stabilizes the tracheoesophageal complex on the diverticuloscope. Care must be taken to advance the scope slowly, only as far as the mucosa will allow. This will prevent perforation of the often inflamed mucosa. The scope is then suspended in position with the suspension arm on the Mayo table (**FIGURE 4**). The distal blades are then gradually opened. The posterior blade will engage the inferior aspect of the inferior constrictor muscle that is seen as a fold across the inferior half of the field and push it out of the way, thereby maximizing exposure of the diverticulum. The proximal part of the scope is then opened carefully and slowly, being sure that the amount of pressure on the upper teeth that have been protected with a tooth guard is monitored. A 0- or 30-degree scope is then introduced down the side of the diverticuloscope so that the operative field can be visualized, and this is held in position by the first assistant.

Debris is suctioned out of the Zenker diverticulum, and exposure is gradually adjusted so that the esophageal introitus and Zenker opening can be well seen in the field. The common wall will be displayed horizontally between them. When the surgeon is satisfied with the exposure, a 16 French nasogastric tube is introduced into the esophageal introitus and advanced down it to confirm that it indeed does represent the esophagus (**FIGURE 4**). Once this has been confirmed, it is withdrawn.

An endoscopic linear stapler, with 45 cm of working length with 3.5-mm GI staples, is introduced into the operative field. Generally, because the proximal end of the diverticuloscope is smaller relative to its open distal end, it must be introduced closed and opened once it reaches the hypopharynx. The staple cartridge, which is the longer end of the working stapler, is placed anteriorly so as to maximize the amount of the common wall that can be engaged by the stapler. The shorter end of the stapler, the anvil, is placed in the sac. Stapler insertion is limited by the point at which the jaws come to rest against the distal end of the sac (**FIGURE 5**).

One of the more difficult aspects of the procedure is caused by the fact that the esophageal introitus and common wall are often quite anterior within the operative field. Although they can be well visualized (particularly with a 30-degree scope), the stapler itself will not angle sufficiently anteriorly to allow introduction of the anvil into the esophageal introitus. Usually, manipulation with suction to pull the common wall posteriorly will allow it to be engaged, and then the stapler can be gradually advanced.

Occasionally, one or two silk stay sutures may be placed through the common wall between esophagus and diverticulum to maintain upward traction during stapler firing, thereby maximizing the length of the stapled cricopharyngeal myotomy.

Once the stapler has been advanced as far as possible into the sac, it is closed and rotated to visualize that the common wall is properly and fully engaged. At times, an edematous common wall that seems to limit full advancement of the stapler can be dealt with by first closing the stapler over it for 30 to 45 seconds to compress the tissue into a thinner configuration. Caution must be exercised while advancing the stapler to avoid pushing too hard against the distal sac with the posterior blade of the stapler, as this is the most common cause of sac perforation.

When the surgeon is satisfied with the exposure and engagement of the common wall, the stapler is fired, opened, and withdrawn. The cricopharyngeus muscle pulls the two cut edges laterally so that a common lumen between the sac and the esophageal introitus is well seen (**FIGURE 6**). If there is significant length of common wall and Zenker diverticulum still remaining, a second load of the stapler can be introduced. In general, if at least 2.5 to 3 cm of the common wall has been divided, the cricopharyngeus muscle will have been fully sectioned and the level of the common wall sufficiently lowered that it will empty into the esophagus rather than the hypopharynx, thereby relieving symptoms. Attempts to engage and section small distal remnants of the common wall only serve to increase the risk of sac perforation. Because the stapling device generally does not cut as far distally as it staples, an endoscopic scissors can be used to gain more length complete the myotomy and further marsupialize the diverticulum. The diverticuloscope is withdrawn and the procedure is terminated.

If, on exposure of the diverticulum, it becomes apparent that significant engagement of the common wall will not be possible (because either the diverticulum is too short or the common wall is too edematous), we prefer to abort the procedure from a transoral standpoint and convert to an external approach. Endoscopic attempts in this situation seldom result in long-term relief of symptoms and generally will complicate the subsequent open approach by creating scarring between the mucosa of the sac, cricopharyngeus muscle, and esophagus.

If perforation of the sac occurs during the endoscopic attempt, ideally the cricopharyngeal myotomy should be completed as planned so as to minimize distal obstruction to swallowing, and then the perforation should be stitched shut. The patient is kept NPO for 48 hours, and if a barium swallow shows no leakage, oral intake can be started. In contrast, minor mucosal lacerations without violation of the muscular or fascial layer do not require special management.

POSTOPERATIVE MANAGEMENT The patient is allowed to start a diet as tolerated postoperatively and is discharged home on the same day. Counseling is given for the signs of perforation, such as back pain, fever, or tachycardia. Patients are seen in the office generally 7 to 10 days after the procedure. In the absence of symptoms, repeat modified barium swallow is not performed, as residual diverticulum is routinely seen. If symptoms remain persistent or recur, a repeat barium swallow can help distinguish between residual diverticulum or an associated oropharyngeal, hypopharyngeal, or dysmotility problem. ■

3

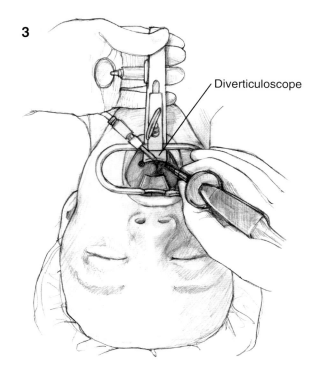

Diverticuloscope

NG tube
confirms
identification
of esophagus

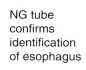

4

Diverticulum

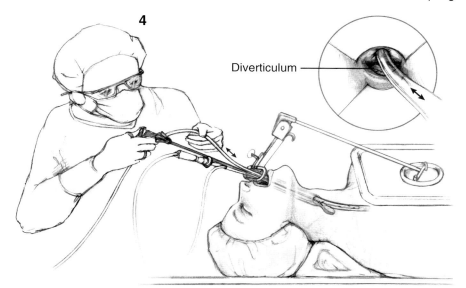

5

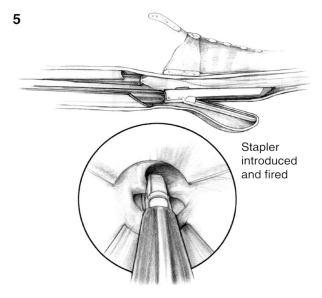

Stapler
introduced
and fired

6

Common wall
divided

Tr.

Eso.

Div.

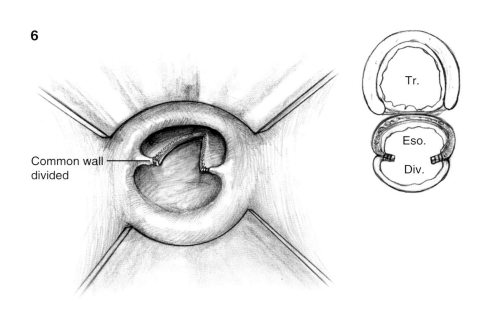

PERORAL ENDOSCOPIC MYOTOMY (POEM)

INDICATIONS Patients found to have achalasia are candidates for peroral endoscopic myotomy (POEM). Workup should include endoscopy, upper GI series, and high-resolution esophageal manometry to confirm the diagnosis of achalasia and rule out paraesophageal hernia or other pathology that might confound the creation of a submucosal tunnel. Although the presence of a hiatal hernia is not a strict contraindication to POEM, the patient should be counseled about the likelihood of reflux that will occur, because an antireflux procedure is not associated with this approach as with a traditional laparoscopic Heller myotomy. Patients should also be consented for laparoscopic surgery so that the threshold to convert to a laparoscopic or hybrid approach is low in the event of safety concerns.

PATIENT POSITIONING The procedure should be performed in a traditional operating room capable of conversion to laparoscopic or open procedures if the need should arise. The bed is turned from the anesthesia console to allow maximal access to the head and neck region.

ANESTHESIA General anesthesia should be performed to allow for maximal relaxation and safe manipulation of complex endoscopic equipment.

An esophageal overtube should be placed to allow frequent exchanges of the scope when necessary.

OPERATIVE PROCEDURE A transparent endoscopic cap attachment is placed on the end of a standard endoscope to allow greater viewing perspective and prevent smudging of the optical surface. A needle knife and triangular-tip knife are used for creation of the submucosal tunnel and myotomy (**FIGURE 1A, B**). Endoscopic insufflation should be performed with CO_2 rather than air as a pneumomediastinum is not unusual. A formal endoscopy is performed to identify the gastroesophageal (GE) junction and decompress the stomach. A dilute mixture of methylene blue and epinephrine is injected to tattoo the lesser curvature 2 to 3 cm distal to the GE junction.

The procedure begins by raising a submucosal wheal approximately 10 cm above the GE junction with a sclerotherapy needle and a dilute mixture of epinephrine and methylene blue. A needle knife is used to start the initial mucosal incision of the esophagus (**FIGURE 2**). A biliary dilation balloon is inserted into the incision and inflated to facilitate creation of a submucosal tunnel (**FIGURES 3 AND 4**).

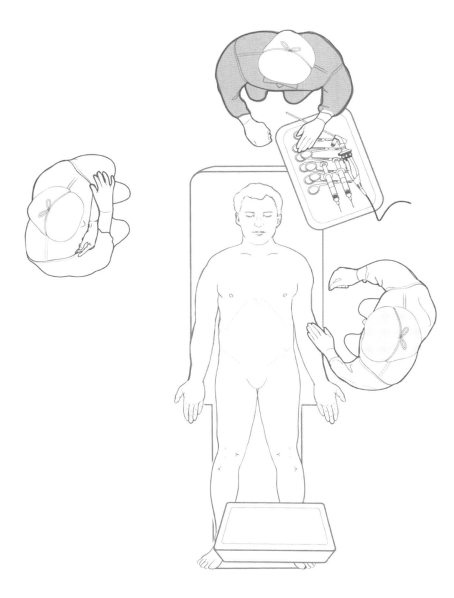

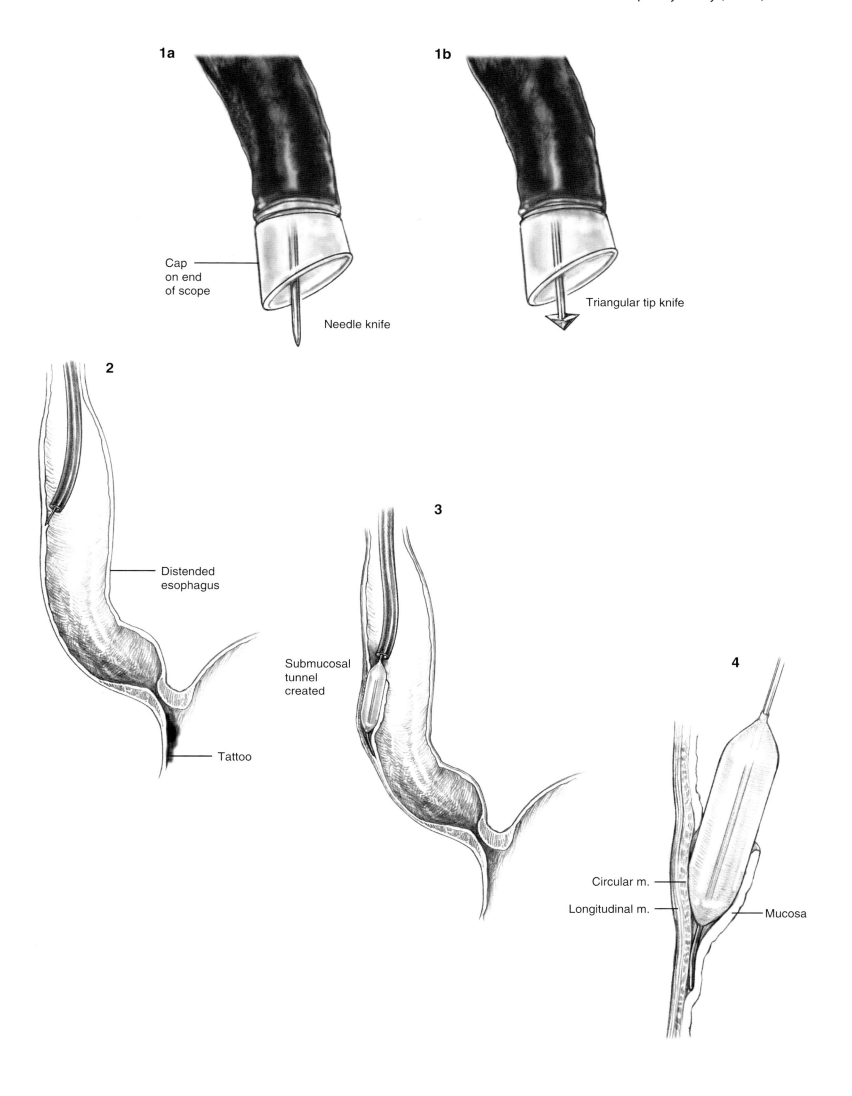

1a

Cap on end of scope

Needle knife

1b

Triangular tip knife

2

Distended esophagus

Tattoo

3

Submucosal tunnel created

4

Circular m.

Longitudinal m.

Mucosa

OPERATIVE PROCEDURE The scope is advanced into the tunnel with the assistance of the needle knife to open the mucosotomy further if necessary. A triangular-tip cautery knife with a spray setting of 20 W is used in a proximal-to-distal direction to complete the submucosal tunnel approximately 2 to 3 cm on to the stomach (**FIGURE 5**). Care must be taken to avoid injury to the mucosal surface of the tunnel while dissecting.

After completion of the submucosal tunnel, attention is turned to creation of the myotomy in the circular muscle fibers of the esophagus. The scope is returned to the top of the mucosotomy. Decompression of the stomach and assessment of the mucosotomy is performed from the lumenal side. The submucosal tunnel is then reentered for creation of the myotomy. Cautery energy is increased to a spray setting of 40. The triangular-tip knife is used to divide the circular muscle fibers in a proximal-to-distal direction (**FIGURES 6 AND 7**).

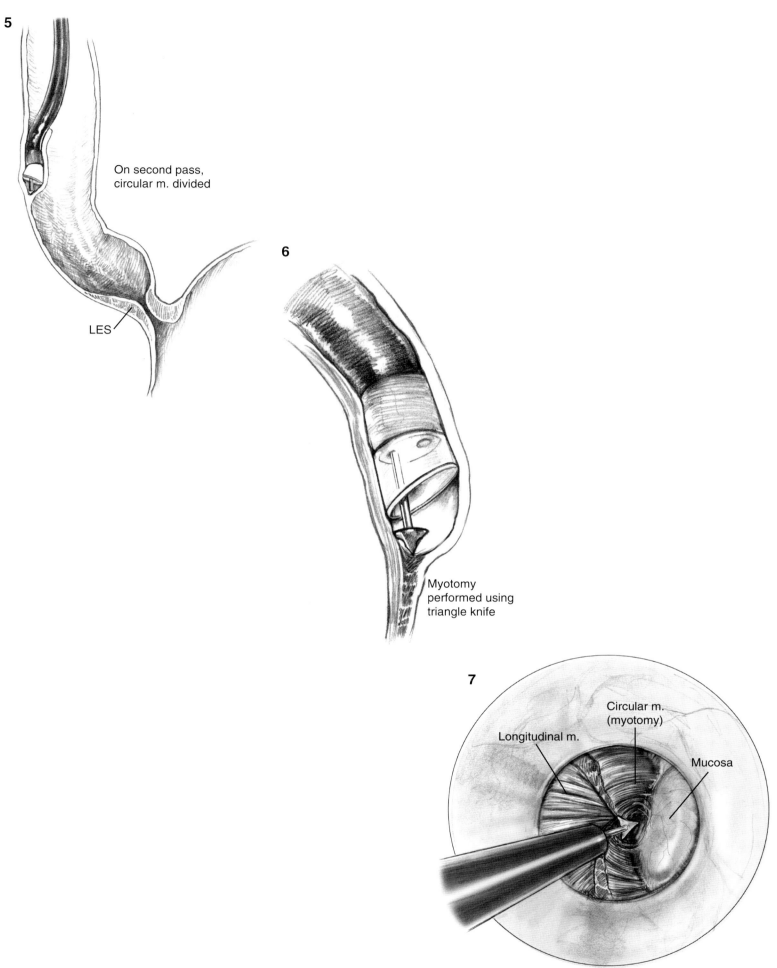

5

On second pass,
circular m. divided

LES

6

Myotomy
performed using
triangle knife

7

Circular m.
(myotomy)

Longitudinal m.

Mucosa

Endoscopic view of myotomy

OPERATIVE PROCEDURE The endpoint of the myotomy is a minimum of 2 to 3 cm distal to the GE junction (**FIGURE 8**). After completion of the myotomy, the endoscope is returned to the esophageal lumen and advanced into the stomach to assess completeness of the dissection. The appearance of the previously injected methylene blue is helpful to assist in visualization that muscle fiber division is complete. Total myotomy length should be approximately 10 cm at completion (**FIGURE 9**). Closure of the mucosotomy is performed with a series of endoscopically placed hemostatic clips (**FIGURE 10**).

POSTOPERATIVE CARE Patients experience minimal pain or discomfort after the procedure. Relief of dysphagia is often immediate. Narcotic pain medications are provided as necessary. Patients are often discharged the same day, although they should be carefully counseled regarding the signs and symptoms concerning for esophageal perforation, including fever, accelerated heart rate, and persistent chest pain. A liquid diet may be started shortly after completion of the procedure. A week of liquids will minimize the risk that the esophageal clips will be prematurely dislodged. ∎

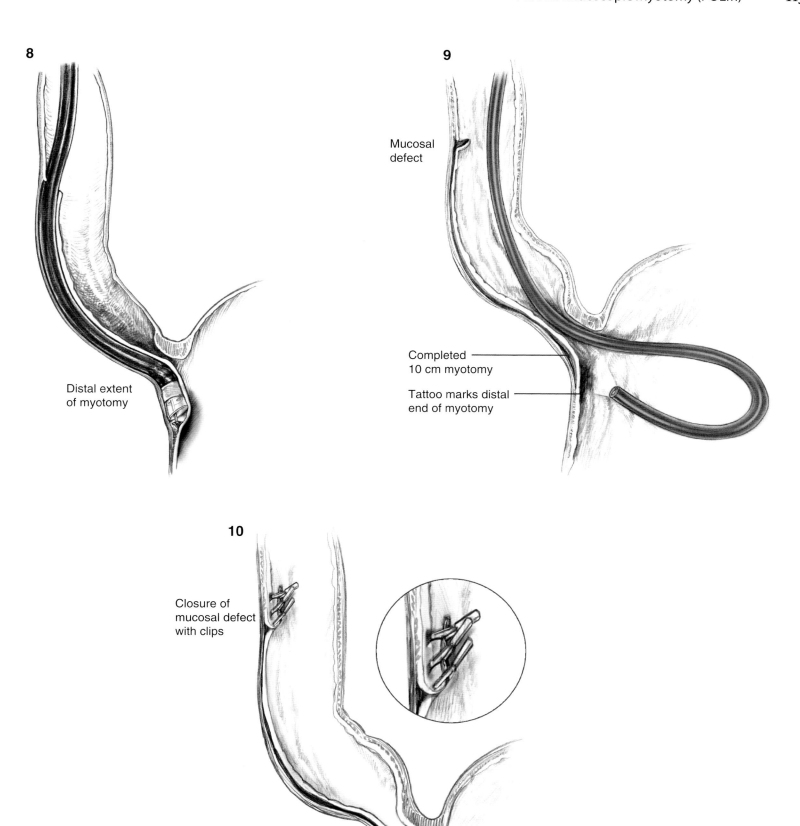

8

Distal extent
of myotomy

9

Mucosal
defect

Completed
10 cm myotomy

Tattoo marks distal
end of myotomy

10

Closure of
mucosal defect
with clips

Tattoo marks
distal end of myotomy

HELLER MYOTOMY WITH PARTIAL FUNDOPLICATION

INDICATIONS AND EVALUATION Laparoscopic Heller myotomy is indicated for individuals with well-documented achalasia. This procedure may also be used in association with diverticulectomy for patients with epiphrenic diverticula, and for hypertensive lower esophageal sphincter (LES). The preoperative evaluation of the patient with achalasia includes a barium swallow, esophageal motility study, and upper endoscopy. For atypical presentations, a CT scan is often added to rule out extrinsic compression of the distal esophagus by tumor, aortic aneurysm, or pancreatic pseudocyst. These entities may mimic the endoscopic and radiologic findings of achalasia and are therefore called *pseudoachalasia*. A Nissen fundoplication that is too tight can create pseudoachalasia as well.

Although Heller myotomy is established as the optimal primary therapy for individuals with achalasia, forceful pneumatic dilatation with balloons measuring 30 to 40 mm in diameter is an acceptable option for those averse to surgical intervention. These patients must be aware that esophageal perforation may result from balloon dilatation, requiring emergency operation. Botulinum toxin injection into the LES may be indicated in patients who are an extraordinarily high risk for Heller myotomy. In addition, in patients when the diagnosis of achalasia is unclear, clinical responsiveness to injection of botulinum toxin usually predicts a good response to Heller myotomy. Peroral endoscopic myotomy (POEM), as described in chapter 18, is also an option, particularly valuable in individuals who have had open upper abdominal surgery, previously, and those patients with type 3 (spastic) achalasia.

PREOPERATIVE PREPARATION Before performing Heller myotomy, the diagnosis must be confirmed. In addition, it is important to try to empty the esophagus of solid food. In patients with a normal esophageal diameter, this may only mean overnight fasting. In individuals with a very large, tortuous esophagus, this may require a liquid diet for 4 to 5 days preoperatively, and even this may not be successful. Additionally, in patients undergoing diverticulectomy we have found it wise to endoscope the patient the day before surgery to make sure the diverticulum is emptied of food. If it is full of food, it can generally be lavaged with vigorous irrigation and suction. Failure to take this extra precaution may give the surgeon the uneasy sensation of stapling across lettuce or other foodstuff at the time of diverticulectomy. Clearly this is not desirable.

ANESTHESIA General anesthesia with endotracheal intubation is necessary for this operation. Complete neuromuscular blockade is required. A first-generation cephalosporin is administered, although entry into the GI tract is rare. A Foley catheter and an orogastric tube are placed after the induction of anesthesia. The upper abdomen is shaved with clippers, and the abdomen is sterilely prepped and draped. Before the patient emerges from anesthesia, it is important that they be aggressively treated for postoperative nausea with ondansetron and phenergan or its equivalent. Some anesthesiologists also add low doses of steroids for their antiemetic effects. Last, if there has been little bleeding during the dissection, we administer ketorolac to our patients to diminish postoperative pain.

POSITION Laparoscopic Heller myotomy is generally performed with the patient in the supine position with the legs extended and abducted 30 to 60 degrees on leg boards so the surgeon may stand between the legs to perform the operation. Once the trocars are placed, steep reverse Trendelenburg position brings the operating trocars to the surgeon and allows gravity to retract the intestine from the operative field. Although many surgeons use the low lithotomy position to perform this operation, this position is less desirable, as peroneal nerve injury, deep vein thrombosis (DVT), and patient movement while in reverse Trendelenburg position may occur. Additionally, some surgeons prefer to perform this operation with the patient in the supine position, either operating from the left or from the right side of the patient. Although trocar positions have been adapted to

perform myotomy ergonomically from the side of the patient, the surgeon is always addressing the hiatus obliquely from this position. Clearly, optimal positioning is a split-leg position with the surgeon standing between the legs. Under this scenario, the assistant may stand on the left or the right side of the patient. If the assistant stands on the left side of the patient, they are able to hold the laparoscopic camera with their left hand and operate an assisting trocar (see below) with their right hand. Alternatively, a mechanical (or robotic) arm may be attached to the operating table to hold the videolaparoscope. Optimally, the operative monitor is placed over the patient's head, fixed on a ceiling-mounted boom (**FIGURE 1**).

INCISION AND EXPOSURE Laparoscopic Heller myotomy is performed with a five-port technique: Except in the pediatric population, we have obtained the maximum flexibility by using two 10-mm ports and three 5-mm ports (**FIGURE 2**).

The operation begins with insufflation of the abdomen using the Veress needle technique placed through the umbilicus. Alternatively, some surgeons prefer to obtain primary access with the open laparoscopy (Hasson technique) at the site of the operating laparoscope (see Chapter 2).

After obtaining a pneumoperitoneum, the primary puncture is placed 15 cm below the costosternal junction slightly to the left of the midline. By placing the primary puncture to the left of midline, and obliquely entering the abdomen—aiming toward the esophageal hiatus—the surgeon avoids the risk of postoperative port-site hernia, stays out of a fatty ligamentum teres, stays farther from the left lobe of the liver, and more accurately aligns the laparoscope with the trajectory of the esophagus (right to left) as it traverses the diaphragm.

After placement of the primary port, an angled (30 or 45 degree) laparoscope is introduced through this trocar and a brief abdominal survey is performed. All secondary trocars are placed under direct vision, and all trocar sites are infiltrated with one-half percent bupivacaine before the incision is made. The second trocar is introduced along the left costal margin 11 to 12 cm from the base of the sternum. This trocar is generally a 10-mm trocar, but a 5-mm trocar may be used, especially in children. The 10-mm trocar facilitates the passage of suture and suturing devices and is useful for the placement of endoscopic clips when necessary. The third trocar placed is a 5-mm trocar, generally placed 8 to 10 cm farther down the left costal margin than the second trocar. This trocar should not be placed farther lateral than the anterior axillary line and may be limited by the reflection of the left colon.

The left lobe of the liver is elevated with a Nathanson liver retractor. This retractor is placed through the track of a cutting 5-mm port that has been introduced and removed just inferior and left of the xiphoid process, high in the epigastrium (**FIGURE 3**). After being placed into position, the retractor is secured using a mechanical arm fixed to the left side of the operating table. Alternatively, a 5-mm trocar can be placed near the right costal margin 12 to 15 cm from the sternal base. After this trocar is placed, an articulated liver retractor is inserted, formed into position, and used to elevate the left lobe of the liver maximally. The optimal placement of a liver retractor allows access to the anterior arch of the hiatus as well as thoroughly defining the right crus of the diaphragm. With extremely "floppy" livers it may be necessary to fold over the left lobe of the liver with the liver retractor, and in extremely fatty livers, it may be necessary to introduce a second liver retractor to achieve adequate visualization.

The fifth, and final, trocar is used for the surgeon's left-hand instrument and is placed along the right costal margin just inferior to the edge of the retracted left lobe of the liver. The point at which this trocar is placed is determined by external rather than internal anatomy, and therefore may be somewhat variable in its superficial projection. It is generally desirable to have this trocar as high and as wide as is possible without going into the left lobe of the liver or achieving placement to the right side of a fatty umbilical ligaments.

1

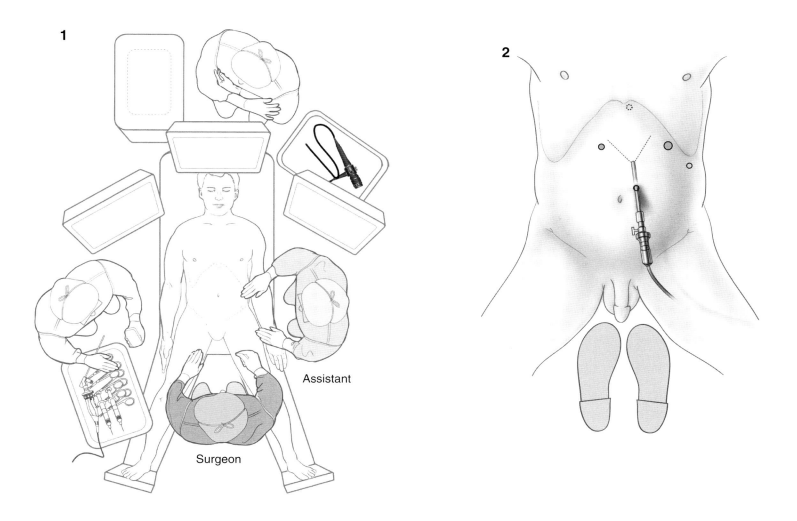

Assistant

Surgeon

2

3

Nathanson
liver retractor

Liver

Stomach

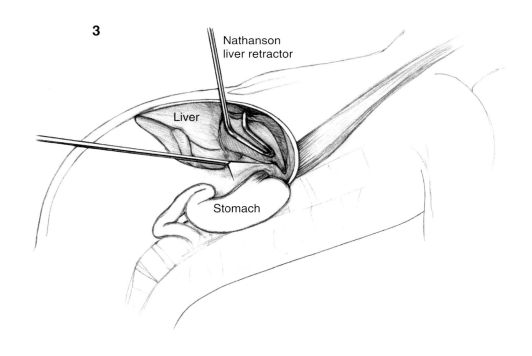

DETAILS OF THE PROCEDURE Dissection commences by placing an atraumatic grasper (Hunter type) through the assistant's port, grasping the epiphrenic fat pad, and retracting inferiorly, slightly toward the patient's left. This puts the phrenoesophageal ligament on stretch and demonstrates the hepatic branch of the vagus. The gastrohepatic omentum is opened above and below the hepatic branch of the vagus. Although some surgeons divide the hepatic branch routinely, it is generally not necessary to do so. After division of the gastrohepatic omentum above and below the hepatic branch of the vagus, the phrenoesophageal ligament (visceral peritoneum) is opened with electrosurgery or Harmonic scalpel along the right crus of the diaphragm and across the crural arch, anteriorly (**FIGURE 4**). Next, the surgeon places two blunt atraumatic graspers through the newly created gap in the peritoneum spreading horizontally to open the plane between the esophagus and right diaphragmatic crus (**FIGURE 5**).

The dissection proceeds around the arch of the hiatus and down the left pillar of the diaphragm as low as easily visualized. Access to the mediastinum is obtained by placing two blunt graspers (closed) between the esophagus and the left crus of the diaphragm, then spreading horizontally and vertically as was done on the right of the esophagus (**FIGURE 6**). The anterior vagus nerve is generally directly attached to the esophagus, and

the posterior vagal nerve is not visible at this time. The anterior crural arch is separated from the esophagus, leaving the vagus against the esophagus. This completes the preliminary phase of crural dissection.

There are two approaches toward the remainder of distal esophageal dissection for Heller myotomy. Some surgeons will not disrupt the posterior gastric attachments to the retroperitoneum, as they feel this helps anchor the gastroesophageal (GE) junction in the abdomen. Other surgeons, including ourselves, perform a circumferential esophageal dissection as we do for laparoscopic Nissen fundoplication in order to place a drain behind the esophagus and provide inferior traction that allows a greater cephalad extension of the Heller myotomy. If a full dissection of the GE junction is to be performed, the right crus is dissected down to its junction with the left crus which is visible from the right side of the esophagus.

In addition, some surgeons do not mobilize the greater curvature of the stomach or take down the short gastric vessels with the performance of a Dor or Toupet fundoplication. However, we believe that this dissection is imperative to perform fundoplication without tension or fundic distortion. The detailed technique of short gastric mobilization (**FIGURE 7**) is described in Chapter 18. Once the posterior window has been made behind the esophagus, a Penrose drain is passed behind the esophagus (**FIGURE 8**) and secured with an Endoloop.

4

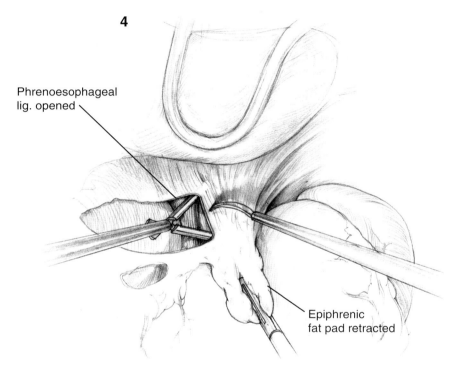

Phrenoesophageal lig. opened

Epiphrenic fat pad retracted

5

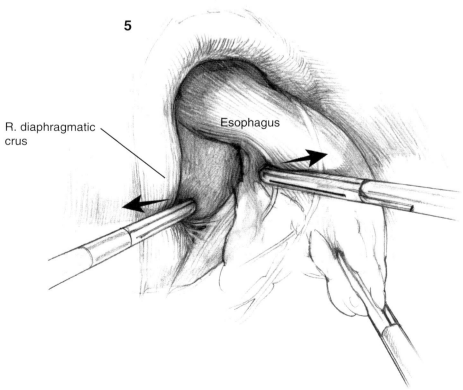

R. diaphragmatic crus

Esophagus

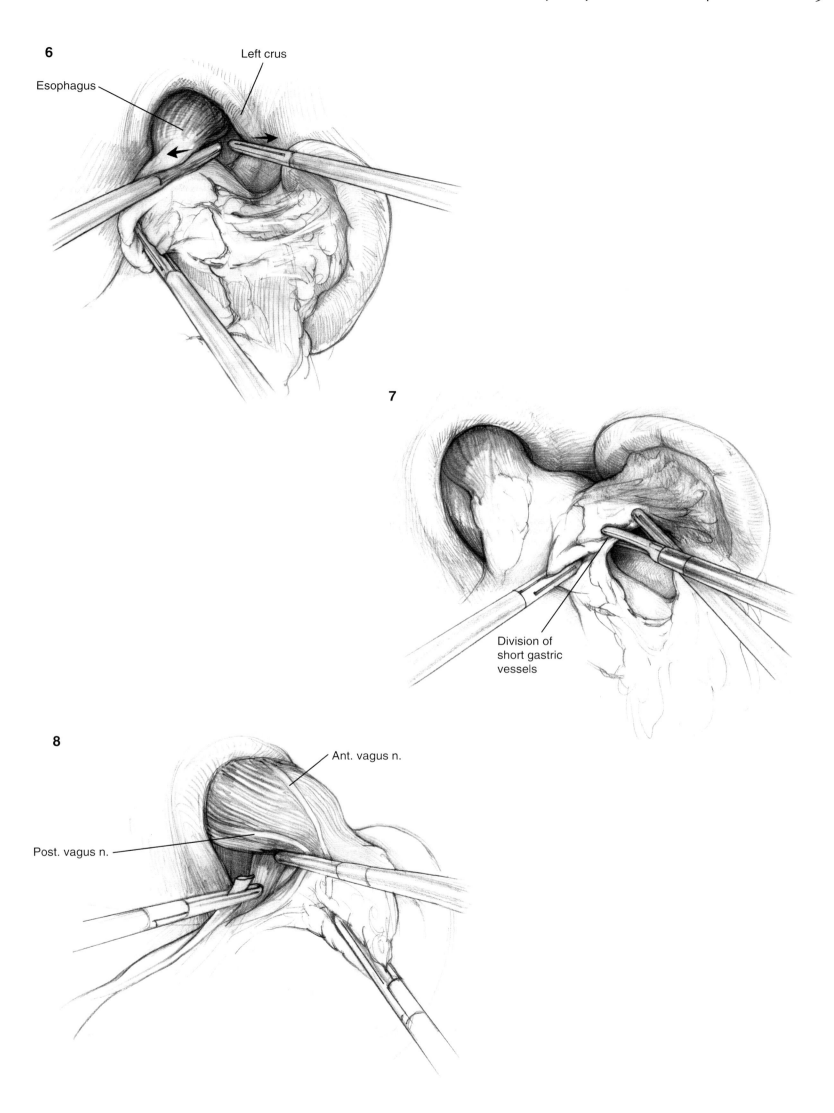

6

Esophagus

Left crus

7

Division of
short gastric
vessels

8

Ant. vagus n.

Post. vagus n.

DETAILS OF THE PROCEDURE Following Penrose drain placement, the Heller myotomy procedure diverges from the Nissen fundoplication rather radically. Instead of performing extensive mediastinal dissection to achieve esophageal length, the Heller myotomy proceeds by dividing the epiphrenic fat pad on the anterior surface of the esophagus just to the left of the anterior vagus nerve. This is accomplished by retracting the fat pad to the right with the surgeon's left hand and to the left with the first assistant's grasper (**FIGURE 9**).

Although the esophagus does not have any serosa, there is a layer of periesophageal tissue overlying the longitudinal muscle of the esophagus that is rich in blood supply. The Heller myotomy can be performed with little bleeding if this layer is divided with the Harmonic scalpel before the myotomy is started (**FIGURE 10**). Great care must be taken to identify and preserve the anterior vagus nerve. If the anterior vagus nerve crosses the anterior esophagus close to the GE junction, it may be necessary for the surgeon to elevate the vagus nerve and create a "tunnel" beneath it as they clean the adventitia superiorly. Alternatively, if the anterior vagus truly lies on the anterior esophagus, the entire myotomy may be performed to the left of the anterior vagus without displacing it.

9

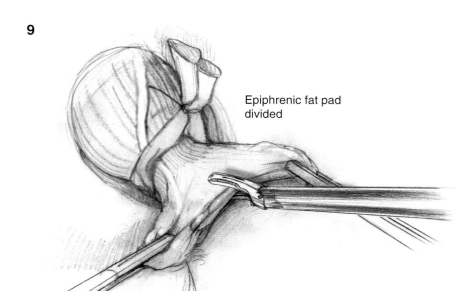

Epiphrenic fat pad
divided

10

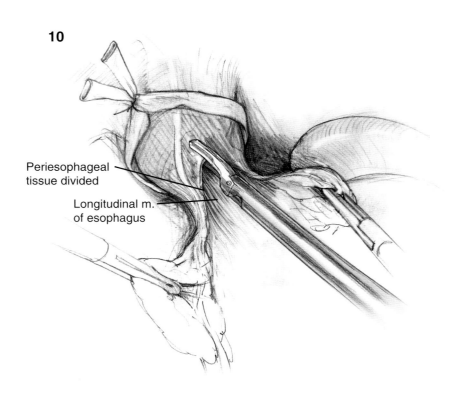

Periesophageal
tissue divided

Longitudinal m.
of esophagus

DETAILS OF THE PROCEDURE To start the myotomy, the GE junction is retracted to the patient's left with the assistant's grasper on the divided fat pad retracting toward the left side of the abdomen and the first assistant's grasper on the right portion of the divided epiphrenic fat pad pulling to the right of the patient. Using a pair of scissors, the longitudinal muscle is divided, and the circular muscle then comes into view (**FIGURE 11**). The closed scissor tip is slid beneath the circular muscle to elevate it away from the submucosa (**FIGURE 12**). No electrocautery is used here, as thermal injury to the esophageal mucosa is to be avoided at all cost. An opened

sponge in the abdomen is helpful at this point to tamponade the small amount of bleeding that may occur using sharp dissection. This sponge technique can be augmented by soaking it with epinephrine prior to introduction into the abdomen.

Once in the submucosal plane, the circular muscle is divided sharply with scissors (**FIGURE 13**). At this point, it is relatively easy to bluntly dissect in the submucosal plane superiorly using a blunt grasper. To best do this, the surgeon and first assistant retract the cut edge of the myotomy with two atraumatic graspers (**FIGURE 14**).

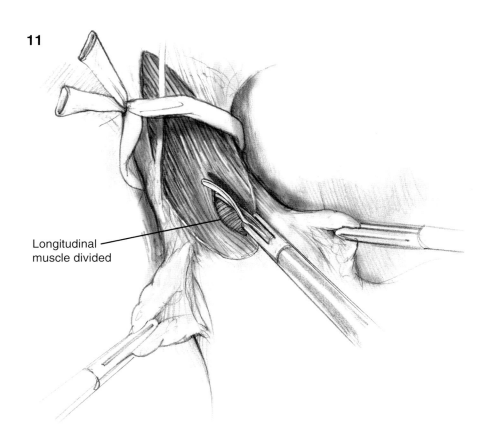

11

Longitudinal muscle divided

12

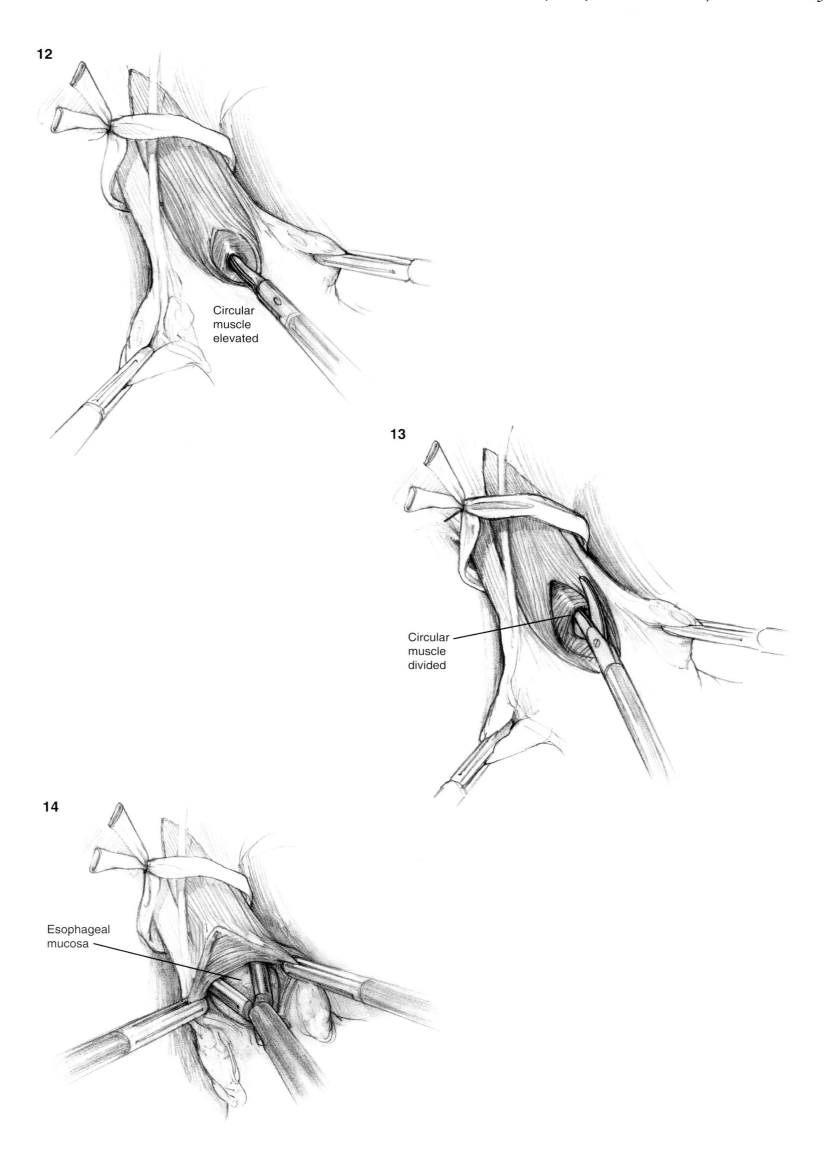

Circular
muscle
elevated

13

Circular
muscle
divided

14

Esophageal
mucosa

DETAILS OF THE PROCEDURE   If botulinum toxin has been injected into the submucosa, one may find some obliteration of this submucosal plane. If this blunt dissection encounters resistance, application of excessive force may end up perforating the esophageal mucosa. This is a gentle, delicate dissection and little resistance should be encountered. Once in the appropriate plane, the division of the esophageal muscle superiorly is quite easy and can be done with one of three techniques. Sharp division with the Metzenbaum scissors is our preference (**FIGURE 15**).

Two alternative techniques are effective in dividing the circular muscle. The first technique is to rupture the muscle by traction of the circular muscle between two graspers (**FIGURE 16**). The second technique involves the use of a monopolar hook cautery, which can be slid beneath the circular muscle and with small bursts of cutting current the muscle is divided (**FIGURE 17**). The primary risk of this technique is that the heel of the hook is often quite close to the mucosa, and great care must be used to avoid thermal injury to the mucosa or delayed perforation may occur. For the same reason, the Harmonic scalpel should not be used to perform this dissection, as the active blade will very rapidly penetrate or thermally injure the mucosa, leading to immediate or delayed perforation.

The superior terminus of the dissection is judged by one of two parameters: either until the dissection is carried 6 cm above the GE junction (measured), or until the dilated portion of the esophagus has been reached. The superior terminus of the myotomy can be confirmed to be a dilated esophagus by use of endoscopic assistance (see later discussion).

15

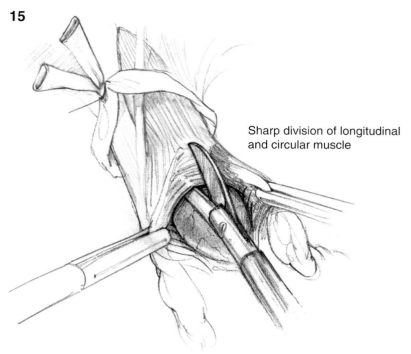

Sharp division of longitudinal
and circular muscle

16

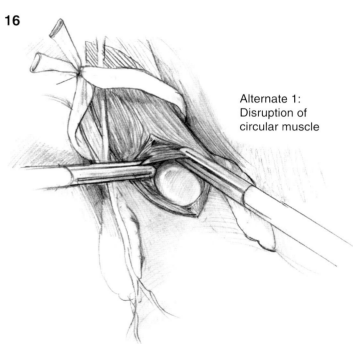

Alternate 1:
Disruption of
circular muscle

Alternate 2:
Hook cautery
division of
circular muscle

17

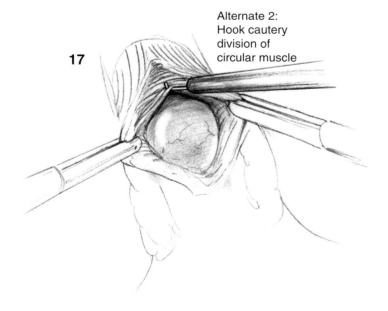

DETAILS OF THE PROCEDURE The gastric portion of the Heller myotomy should extend 2 to 3 cm onto the stomach to ensure that the gastric portion of the LES is entirely divided. This portion of the myotomy may in fact be the most difficult, and most likely to produce a perforation of the mucosa, as the collar and sling musculature of the gastric portion of the sphincter is quite adherent to the mucosa. Two strategies are most effective for dividing this muscle without perforating the mucosa. Generally, we work down from the GE junction with two blunt graspers, teasing the muscle fibers apart bluntly with firm and opposite traction (**FIGURE 18**). Submucosal vessels may be torn in this process, but bleeding can be easily tamponaded with an open gauze sponge for a minute or two until the field is dry.

Alternatively, one can begin 3 cm down from the GE junction with the closed scissor tip hooking beneath the muscularis opening, then dividing the gastric muscle (**FIGURE 19**). We find this technique slightly more risky, as it is relatively easy to tent a piece of mucosa over the scissor tip and incise the gastric lumen. Again, the L hook can be helpful in teasing these fibers apart, but fiber rupture is preferable to using electrosurgery in this region. Although it is tempting to coagulate the small bleeding submucosal vessels, these will usually stop with direct compression, which minimizes the risk of mucosal injury. This completes the myotomy. The cephalad portion of the myotomy usually extends 4 to 7 cm above the GE junction. The caudad portion of the myotomy extends 2.5 to 3 cm below the GE junction (**FIGURE 20**).

When the myotomy is complete, the integrity of the mucosa should be tested by one of two methods. In the first method, 250 mL of dilute methylene blue may be placed in the stomach and esophagus via a nasogastric tube. Areas of mucosal leak will become immediately apparent. Areas where the mucosa has become thinned by thermal injury or mechanical abrasion will stain blue. These areas should be treated like frank perforations and oversewn with a fine (4-0) Vicryl suture, then retested with additional methylene blue.

A second method, which we prefer, is the performance of intraoperative endoscopy. A video endoscope is introduced through the mouth and advanced under direct vision into the distal esophagus. The area of myotomy is made readily apparent by the strong transillumination of the laparoscopic light into the esophagus. The upper end of transillumination should appear in the dilated portion of the esophagus. The endoscope should pass through the region of the myotomized LES and enter the stomach without resistance. In addition, the distal end of transillumination, in the stomach, should be visible below the narrow point of endoscopy. As one retracts the endoscope into the esophagus, it should be easy to view directly into the stomach without any closure of the GE junction. Endoscopic leak testing may be accomplished by filling the upper abdomen with saline through the irrigation system and ensuring that no bubbling from the distended esophagus and stomach is visualized. Before removing the endoscope, all air is removed from the stomach and esophagus.

At this point we pass a 56 French Maloney dilator into the stomach. This serves two functions. First, it allows the surgeon to see any intact muscle fibers that will be on tension around the dilator. Second, it reinforces the completeness of the myotomy by observation of the slack mucosa around the dilator in the myotomized portions of the esophagus and stomach. The mucosa is still quite tight to the dilator under most circumstances in the area of the LES. Last, the presence of the dilator in the esophagus allows formation of the fundoplication over a "mold" that will prevent any anatomic distortion. If the dilator still appears snug within the myotomized segment of the esophagus, and especially if muscle fibers are viewed bridging the gap between the myotomy and mucosa, the submucosal plane can be further mobilized by bluntly undermining the muscularis on the lateral edges of the myotomy (**FIGURE 21**). In general, the cut edges of the muscularis should be adequately retracted in the region of the LES such that the bare mucosa contributes about 50% of the circumference of the esophagus. A well-done Heller myotomy allows the circumference of the LES region to double. The left edge of the cut muscle is generally not visible, as it is retracted around the esophagus posteriorly.

18

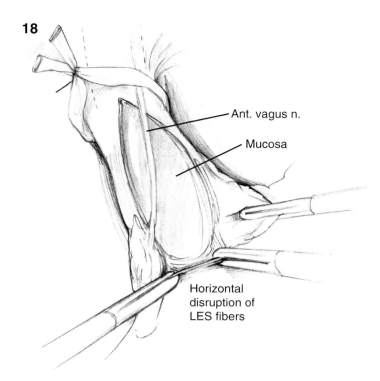

Ant. vagus n.

Mucosa

Horizontal
disruption of
LES fibers

19

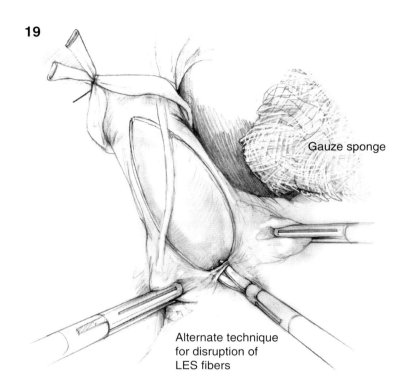

Gauze sponge

Alternate technique
for disruption of
LES fibers

20

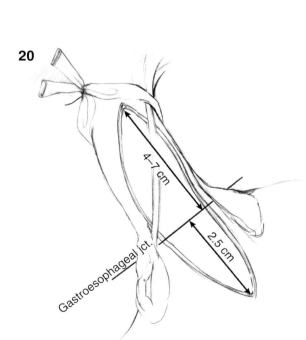

4–7 cm

2.5 cm

Gastroesophageal jct.

21

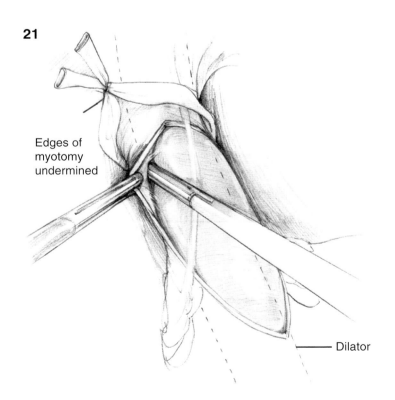

Edges of
myotomy
undermined

Dilator

PARTIAL FUNDOPLICATIONS (DOR AND TOUPET) With the dilator in place, the anterior partial fundoplication (Dor fundoplication) creates a flap valve using the greater curvature of the stomach folded anterior to the intraabdominal portion of the distal esophagus. The first step in this fundoplication is to roll the fundus of the stomach around to the anterior surface of the distal esophagus. This is done with two blunt atraumatic graspers, which place the greater curvature vessels into the 12 to 1 o'clock position (viewing the esophagus as a clock face from the foot of the patient). The fundus should sit very comfortably in this position without any lines of tension.

Once the dilator has been situated, anterior partial fundoplication is performed with 5 to 7 sutures. The first suture is placed between the cut edge of the myotomy on the left, usually at the high end of the myotomy, as the muscle in the region of the LES is retracted too far posteriorly to be found. The point on the stomach chosen is on the posterior wall of the stomach immediately posterior to the cardiophrenic angle **(FIGURE 22)**. 2-0 silk or braided nonabsorbable suture should be used for the fundoplication. The second stitch approximates the superior portion of the fundus—just posterior to the line of short gastric vessels—to the left side of the crural arch **(FIGURE 23)**. As with the Nissen fundoplication, we prefer intracorporeal suturing. Two additional sutures are placed across the crural arch. completing the "hanging" of the fundus from the arch **(FIGURE 24)**. The last one or two sutures of the fundoplication incorporate the fundus of the stomach with the right cut edge of the myotomy or the right crus of the diaphragm. When the fundoplication is complete, the myotomy has been completely covered by the fundoplication **(FIGURE 25)**. The dilator is then removed. Alternately the partial fundoplication can be performed in the Toupet fashion **(FIGURE 26)**. More details on partial fundoplications can be found in Chapter 19.

POSTOPERATIVE CARE Essential elements to postoperative care include aggressive treatment of nausea intraoperatively and postoperatively with ondansetron and other agents. Pain relief is usually obtained with intravenous ketorolac and judicious use of narcotics. The Foley catheter is removed in the recovery room, and the patient transferred to an inpatient room. The vast majority of surgeons and patients prefer at least an overnight stay to ensure pain control and resumption of a diet. The patient is kept without oral intake until the morning after operation. At this point a water-soluble contrast radiograph of the esophagus is performed to make sure there is no mucosal leak. Although this is an extremely rare event, the adverse consequences of discharging a patient with a leaky esophagus are formidable. If a leak is seen, the patient is immediately returned to the OR and the esophagotomy is repaired with interrupted sutures. Postoperative edema about the GE junction creates a "tight" appearance on the radiograph, but this should not concern the surgeon, as the patient will usually note that their swallowing is much improved from preoperatively, despite the edema. A liquid diet is started, and the patient is discharged that evening or the next morning. Because of distal esophageal edema, we have used a conservative dietary approach which includes 5 days of full liquids, followed by 3 weeks of a modified esophageal diet, which avoids breads, meats, and raw vegetables. With strict adherence to this dietary protocol, few patients complain of postoperative dysphagia. Without such aggressive management, food impaction, nausea, retching, and wrap disruption have been reported.

As well, we urge the patients to resume the activities of daily living immediately, but avoid events involving intraabdominal straining (particularly heavy lifting) for 6 to 8 weeks to allow the fundoplication to heal and to minimize the likelihood of acute paraesophageal herniation of the fundoplication. This latter complication is the most immediately life-threatening complication that may occur to these patients, especially if unrecognized. Last, the most fundamental caveat of postoperative care is that any patient who fares poorly for any reason (increasing pain, tachycardia, tachypnea, pleural effusion, fever, retching, or confusion) should be immediately studied with a barium swallow to rule out esophageal perforation or herniation of the fundoplication. Most catastrophes following laparoscopic Heller myotomy are treatable without great patient morbidity if they are recognized and treated early. ■

Dor Fundoplication

22

First suture

23

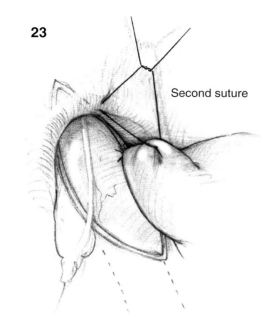

Second suture

24

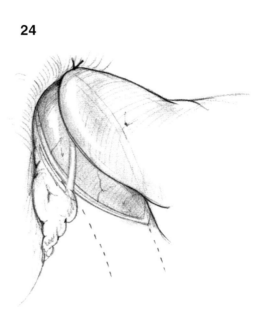

25

Anterior
partial wrap

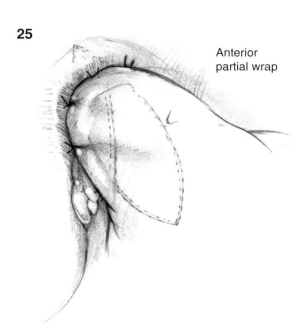

Toupet Fundoplication

26

270° posterior wrap

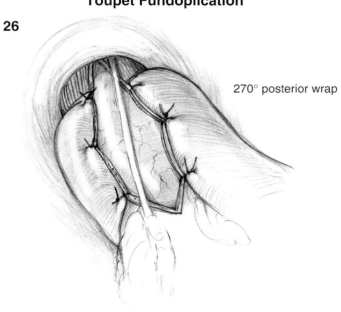

CHAPTER 17

Epiphrenic Diverticulectomy with Myotomy and Fundoplication

INDICATIONS Epiphrenic diverticula usually protrude from the right wall of the esophagus just above the gastroesophageal (GE) junction (**FIGURE 1**). They are usually associated with esophageal motility disorders, either diffuse esophageal spasm or achalasia. Even when preoperative esophageal motility does not detect a hypertensive nonrelaxing lower esophageal sphincter (LES), the treatment of choice for these lesions includes esophageal myotomy and diverticulectomy. Small, low-lying epiphrenic diverticula can be managed from the abdomen through the diaphragmatic hiatus. Large-mouth diverticula (greater than 3 cm) and those more than 3 cm above the hiatus should be approached through a right thoracoscopic approach as described in chapter 12. The chronically inflamed tissue often found adjacent to a diverticulum and the limited exposure of the mediastinum through an abdominal approach makes the transdiaphragmatic approach to large diverticula technically difficult and more hazardous than is necessary.

Symptoms of epiphrenic diverticula include frequent regurgitation, chest pain, regurgitation of partially digested food, and halitosis. These symptoms are often indistinguishable from the symptoms of achalasia, but because both conditions will be treated simultaneously, it is not necessary to make such distinctions.

PATIENT PREPARATION Once the diagnosis of an epiphrenic diverticulum has been made with a barium swallow, the underlying motility disorder should be identified with esophageal manometry. Occasionally it is difficult to differentiate esophageal spasm from vigorous achalasia; however, with either condition, esophageal myotomy above the level of the diverticulum is indicated.

One of the more important steps in patient preparation (often overlooked) is preoperative endoscopy and diverticulum lavage. Epiphrenic diverticula are often chronically impacted with food debris. If the diverticula are not evacuated prior to operation, food debris will be caught in the staple line, leading to its disruption. Although it is possible to do this endoscopic irrigation and evacuation on the operative table after general anesthesia is induced, we prefer to do this preoperatively in the endoscopy lab to minimize the distention of the gut with gas that may occur from the performance of intraoperative esophagoscopy.

PATIENT POSITIONING The patient is positioned supine with legs abducted as previously described for minimally invasive esophageal surgery (**FIGURE 2**).

DETAILS OF THE PROCEDURE The trocars are placed in a standard pattern as described for laparoscopic Nissen fundoplication (**FIGURE 3**). Likewise, initial dissection of the GE junction proceeds identically to that of the Nissen fundoplication as described in chapter 18.

1

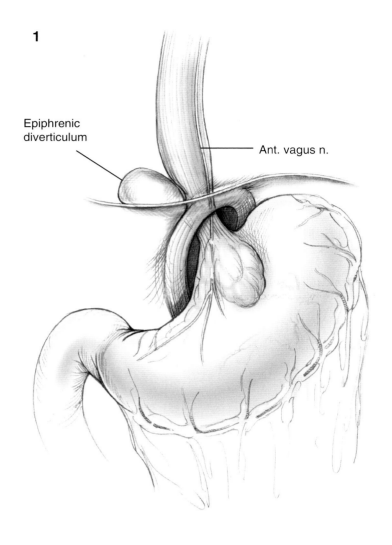

Epiphrenic
diverticulum

Ant. vagus n.

2

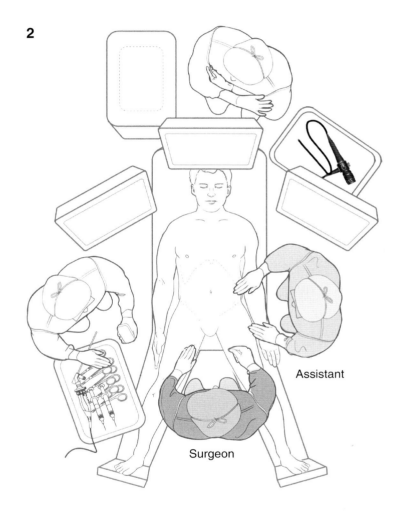

Assistant

Surgeon

3

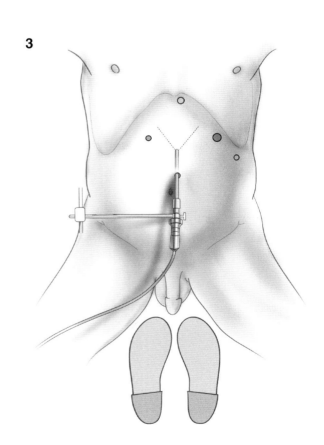

DETAILS OF THE PROCEDURE A Penrose drain is placed around the GE junction, the first assistant uses it to apply inferior traction on the lower esophagus, reducing it into the abdomen. Using blunt dissection and ultrasonic dissection or electrosurgery, the paraesophageal mediastinal tissues are gently teased apart. Because of the left turn of the esophagus at the GE junction, the diverticula generally lie to the right of the esophagus immediately above the upper end of the lower esophageal sphincter (**FIGURE 4**), Blunt dissection in the mediastinum defines the walls of the diverticulum, and an endoscope in the esophagus may help define the extent of the diverticulum. The diverticulum will not be covered with striated muscle, which makes it hard to distinguish from adjacent mediastinal tissue. If difficulty is encountered, an endoscope is placed into the diverticulum and transillumination used to identify the walls of the diverticulum. Gas may be placed in the diverticulum to further aid identification of the wall of the diverticulum. The wall is then bluntly dissected from the mediastinal tissue. With chronic food impaction in the diverticulum, there may be a fair amount of induration, inflammation, or fibrosis around the diverticulum, making this part of the operation difficult. If it appears that the upper reaches of the diverticulum cannot be obtained, we prefer to proceed directly to the myotomy portion of the operation and address the diverticulum through a right thoracoscopy. This second portion of the procedure may be performed immediately or in a delayed fashion, depending on the condition of the patient and the preoperative preparation.

For a small-mouthed diverticulum that can be completely mobilized through the hiatus, the diverticulum is resected with an articulating endoscopic stapler (**FIGURE 5**). Most diverticula can be addressed with a medium (3.5 mm) load of the stapler, but extraordinarily thick-walled diverticula may require the longer (4.8 mm) staple load. Occasionally the anterior or posterior vagus will lie across the neck of the diverticulum. Careful mobilization should be performed before diverticulectomy to avoid injuring this structure. A dilator in the true lumen of the esophagus or an endoscope helps prevent esophageal narrowing during transaction of the diverticula. The staple line is oversewn with interrupted sutures (**FIGURE 6**).

4

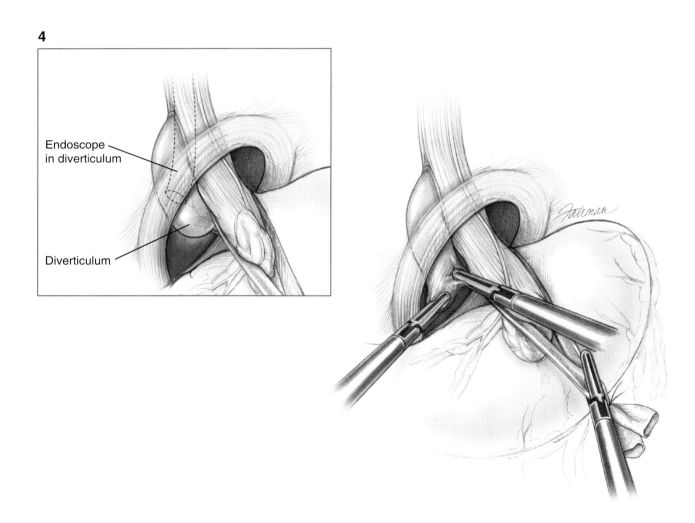

Endoscope in diverticulum

Diverticulum

5

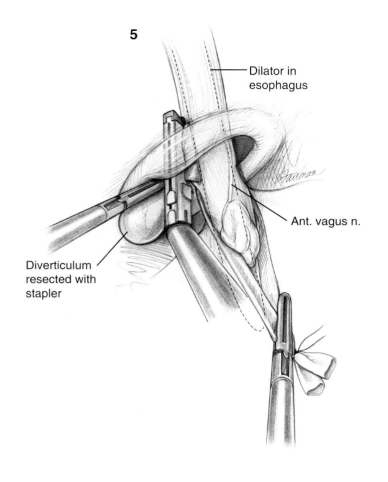

Dilator in
esophagus

Ant. vagus n.

Diverticulum
resected with
stapler

6

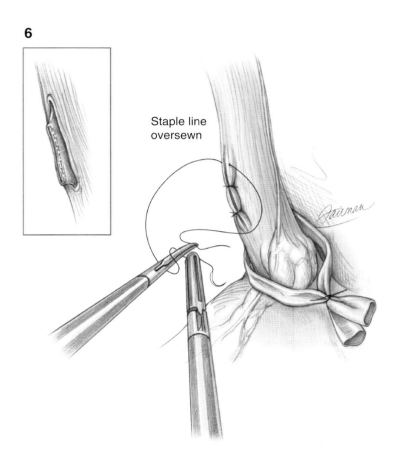

Staple line
oversewn

DETAILS OF THE PROCEDURE A Heller myotomy is then performed as described in chapter 16. This myotomy is routinely performed on the anterior left side of the esophagus, well away from the area of diverticulectomy. The superior end of the myotomy is taken to a point just above the neck of the diverticulum (**FIGURE** 7). Upon completion of both these procedures, the distal esophagus is filled with methylene blue through a nasogastric tube to make sure that no leaks are noted. A Toupet or Dor fundoplication should then be performed as described in chapter 16 (**FIGURE** 8).

POSTOPERATIVE CARE Both thoracoscopic and laparoscopic excision of epiphrenic diverticula have been performed for nearly 20 years. Although these entities are rare, experienced surgeons have noted a higher than expected rate of leak from these staple lines. For this reason we treat these lateral esophageal staple lines with care, including a 3-day rest from any PO nutrition, followed by water-soluble contrast swallow on postoperative day 5. Even with this cautious technique, we have seen some delayed leaks from staple lines.

If the large-mouth diverticulum has been approached through the hiatus, the Gastrografin swallow may show a residual "dog ear" of diverticulum at the superior end of the staple line. Small amounts of residual sac are rarely symptomatic; however, large amounts of retained diverticulum warrant a thoracoscopic approach if the patient does not have a complete resolution of preoperative symptoms. ■

7

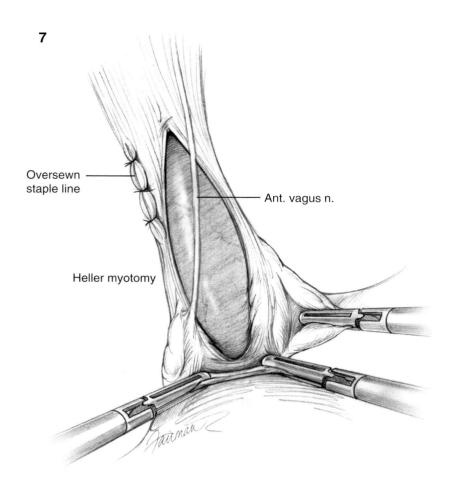

Oversewn staple line

Ant. vagus n.

Heller myotomy

8

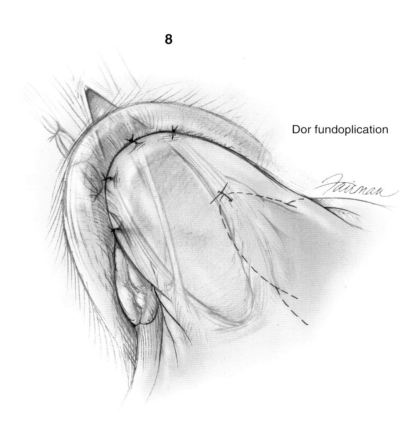

Dor fundoplication

TOTAL (NISSEN) FUNDOPLICATION

INDICATIONS Laparoscopic total or Nissen fundoplication is indicated for individuals with gastroesophageal reflux disease (GERD) that meets one of the following criteria: (1) GERD that is refractory to proton pump inhibition, (2) GERD that is incompletely responsive to proton pump inhibition, (3) GERD that is entirely responsive to proton pump inhibition, but patient choice or side effect profile merits consideration of antireflux surgery, (4) extraesophageal manifestations of GERD, and (5) complications of GERD (stricture, bleeding, aspiration, Barrett esophagus). Of these criteria, the patients who are most likely to achieve complete symptom relief are those who are responsive to medical therapy, who have esophageal symptoms of reflux (heartburn, regurgitation, chest pain), and those with a strongly positive pH study (see later discussion).

Contraindications are few, but the morbidly obese patient with gastroesophageal reflux may be better served with gastric bypass than with Nissen fundoplication. Although observational data demonstrate good outcomes in laparoscopic Nissen patients with a BMI up to 40, individuals who meet the indications for bariatric procedures (see Chapter 29) and who also have gastroesophageal reflux should be referred for a bariatric procedure rather than undergoing Nissen fundoplication.

PREOPERATIVE PREPARATION Before performing laparoscopic Nissen fundoplication, the patient must undergo anatomic and physiologic esophageal evaluation. This entails the performance of esophagogastroduodenoscopy (EGD), barium swallow, and esophageal motility study at a minimum. Although it is generally advisable to obtain an ambulatory 24-hour pH study in all patients before operation, this test may be omitted in individuals with esophageal symptoms of GERD, a response to proton pump inhibitors, and endoscopic evidence of esophageal injury. Multichannel intraluminal impedance (MII) measurement, especially when combined with pH measurement (MII-pH), may be the best tool to measure acid and non-acid reflux. Because of the nonspecific nature of esophageal symptoms, it is best not to perform laparoscopic Nissen fundoplication on patients with an anatomically normal esophagus, without confirming reflux using pH or impedance testing. Radionucleotide gastric emptying studies are indicated before laparoscopic antireflux surgery in patients with diabetes, previous gastric surgery, bezoars, or prominent nausea and vomiting symptoms.

Generally, the patient is continued on all preoperative medications until the morning of surgery. If possible, anticoagulants, antiplatelet agents, and nonsteroidal anti-inflammatory agents are discontinued. Glucose control should be optimized, and cardiopulmonary disease should be thoroughly evaluated with appropriate consultation and testing preoperatively. It is unnecessary to prep the colon for laparoscopic Nissen fundoplication.

ANESTHESIA General anesthesia with endotracheal intubation is necessary for this operation. Complete neuromuscular blockade is required. Intravenous antibiotics are not generally indicated. Before emergence from anesthesia, it is important that the patient be aggressively treated for postoperative nausea with ondansetron and phenergan or its equivalent. Some anesthesiologists also add low doses of steroids for their antiemetic effects. Last, if there has been little bleeding during the dissection, we also administer ketorolac at the end of the procedure to diminish postoperative pain.

POSITION Laparoscopic Nissen fundoplication is generally performed with the patient in the supine position with the legs extended and abducted 30 to 60 degrees so the surgeon can stand between the legs to perform the operation (**FIGURE 1**). Once the trocars are placed, steep reverse Trendelenburg position brings the operating trocars to the surgeon and allows gravity to retract the intestine from the operative field (**FIGURE 2**). Although many surgeons use the low lithotomy position to perform this operation, this position is less desirable, as peroneal nerve injury, deep vein thrombosis (DVT), and patient slippage while in reverse Trendelenburg position are increasingly frequent when stirrups are used. Additionally, some surgeons prefer to perform this operation without the legs abducted, operating from the left or from the right side of the patient. Although trocar positions have been adapted to perform fundoplication ergonomically from the side of the patient, the surgeon is addressing the hiatus obliquely if they stand at the side of the table. In the split-leg position, the assistant can stand to the left or the right side of the patient. If the assistant stands on the left side of the patient, they are able to hold the laparoscopic camera with their left hand (if a mechanical camera holder is not used) and operate an assisting trocar with their right hand. Optimally, the operative monitor is placed over the patient's head, fixed on a ceiling-mounted boom, and a monitor sits over the patient's right shoulder for the first assistant to view.

OPERATIVE PREPARATION A Foley catheter and an orogastric tube are placed after the induction of anesthesia. The upper abdomen of the patient from the nipple lines to the umbilicus is shaved with clippers after induction of anesthesia, and the abdomen is sterilely prepped.

INCISION AND EXPOSURE Laparoscopic Nissen fundoplication is performed with a five-port technique (**FIGURE 3**). Except in a pediatric population, we have obtained maximum flexibility by using two 10-mm ports and three 5-mm ports.

The operation begins with insufflation of the abdomen using the Veress needle technique placed through the umbilicus. Alternatively, some surgeons prefer to obtain primary access with open laparoscopy (Hasson technique) at the site of the operating laparoscope. If the patient has had a previous midline laparotomy in the region of the umbilicus, the abdomen is entered with the Veress needle at a point just below the left costal margin at the midclavicular line.

After obtaining a pneumoperitoneum, the primary puncture is placed 15 cm below the costosternal junction, slightly to the left of the midline. By placing the port to the left of midline and obliquely entering the abdomen—aiming toward the esophageal hiatus—the surgeon prevents the risk of postoperative port-site hernia, stays out of a fatty ligamentum teres, stays farther from the left lobe of the liver, and more accurately aligns the laparoscope with the trajectory of the esophagus (right to left) as it traverses the diaphragm.

Upon placement of the primary port, an angled (30- or 45-degree) laparoscope is introduced through this trocar and a brief abdominal survey is performed. All secondary trocars are placed under direct vision, and all trocar sites are infiltrated with 0.5% bupivacaine before the incision is made. The second trocar is introduced along the left costal margin 12 cm from the base of the sternum. This trocar is generally a 10-mm trocar, but a 5-mm trocar may be used, especially in children. The 10-mm trocar facilitates the passage of suture and suturing devices and is useful for the placement of endoscopic clips when necessary. The third trocar placed is a 5-mm trocar, generally placed 8 to 10 cm farther down the left costal margin than the second trocar. This trocar should not be placed farther lateral than the anterior axillary line and may be limited by the reflection of the left colon internally.

The fourth trocar, for liver retraction, will provide an entry track for a Nathanson liver retractor. This retractor is placed through the track created by a cutting 5-mm port that has been introduced and removed just inferior and left of the xiphoid, high in the epigastrium. The liver retractor is affixed to a mechanical arm fixed to the right side of the operating table (**FIGURE 4**).

Alternatively, the fourth trocar, for liver retraction, can be a 5-mm trocar placed on the right costal margin 12 to 15 cm from the sternal base. After placing this trocar, an articulated liver retractor is inserted and formed into position, then the left lobe of the liver is elevated maximally (**FIGURE 5**). The optimal position of the liver retractor allows access to the anterior arch of the hiatus as well as thoroughly defining the right crus of the diaphragm.

The fifth, and final, trocar is used for the surgeon's left hand and is placed along the right costal margin just inferior to the edge of the retracted left lobe of the liver. The point at which this trocar is placed is not determined by external anatomy, but by internal anatomy, and therefore may be somewhat variable in its superficial projection. It is generally desirable to have this trocar as high and as wide as is possible without going into the left lobe of the liver. This trocar should enter the abdomen to the left or through the round ligament and should be directed toward the hiatus for optimal ergonomics.

1

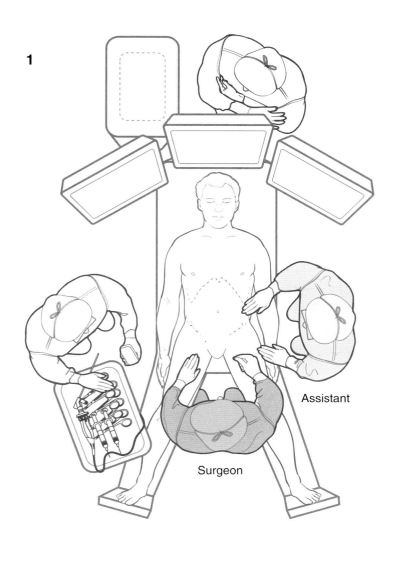

Assistant

Surgeon

2

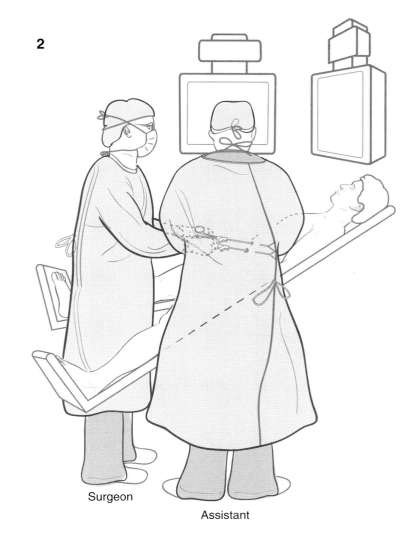

Surgeon

Assistant

3

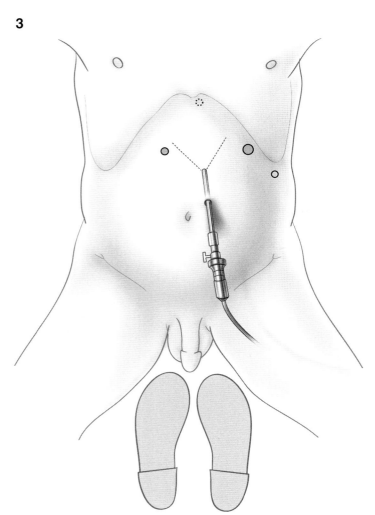

4

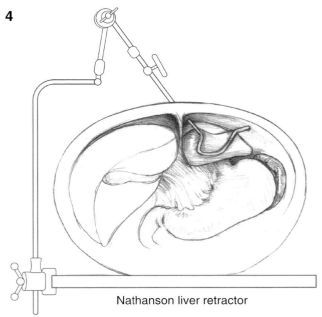

Nathanson liver retractor

5

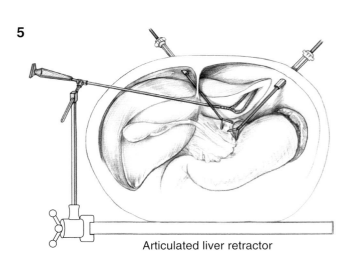

Articulated liver retractor

DETAILS OF THE PROCEDURE With the left lobe elevated, dissection commences by placing the assistant's grasper on the epiphrenic fat pad and retracting inferiorly and slightly toward the patient's left. This reduces any hiatal hernia present and puts the phrenoesophageal membrane on tension. The surgeon exposes the anterior surface of the caudate lobe and the right crus of the diaphragm by opening the gastrohepatic omentum above and below the hepatic branch of the vagus (**FIGURE 6**). Although it is desirable to preserve the hepatic branch of the vagus, many surgeons routinely divide it to obtain better access to the right crus of the diaphragm. After division of the gastrohepatic omentum above the hepatic branch of the vagus (pars flaccida), the surgeon places a blunt atraumatic grasper (Hunter grasper) beneath the phrenoesophageal ligament. This atraumatically establishes the plane between the esophagus and the diaphragm. This layer is then divided with electrosurgery or ultrasonic shears (**FIGURE 7**). The dissection proceeds around the arch of the hiatus and down the left pillar of the diaphragm as low as is easily visualized. Access to the mediastinum is obtained by placing two blunt graspers (closed) between the esophagus and the left crus of the diaphragm, then spreading horizontally (**FIGURE 8**). This is repeated on the right side of the esophagus in identical fashion. The anterior vagus nerve is generally affixed to the esophagus, and the posterior vagus nerve is not visible at this time. Dissection down the right crus of the diaphragm continues until the surgeon reaches its base, where the left crus is visualized emerging from behind the esophagus. Further horizontal two-handed spreading accomplishes a great deal of the dissection (**FIGURE 9**). This completes the preliminary phase of crural dissection.

The next phase of dissection includes the division of the short gastric arteries, and posterior mobilization of the stomach. The light cord of the angled laparoscope is rotated 30 degrees counterclockwise (11 o'clock position), and the surgeon grasps the greater curvature of the stomach at the level of the inferior pole of the spleen with an atraumatic grasper. The assistant grasps the greater omentum adjacent to the greater curvature of the stomach. The surgeon retracts the stomach to the patient's right and posteriorly while the assistant elevates the omentum anteriorly and to the patient's left (**FIGURE 10**). The ultrasonic shears are introduced, and entry to the lesser sac is gained by dividing the greater omentum adjacent to the greater curvature of the stomach. Several applications of the Harmonic scalpel may be necessary to gain access to the lesser sac on heavier patients. It is important that the short gastric vessels be visualized and completely occluded with the ultrasonic shears before the application of energy. Incomplete division of short gastric vessels will result in troublesome bleeding. As the dissection moves cephalad, the surgeon keeps moving the retraction point higher along the greater curvature, generally placing one jaw of the atraumatic grasper on the anterior wall of the stomach and the other jaw on the posterior aspect of the stomach. The assistant places one jaw of their grasper in the lesser sac, and one jaw in the greater sac to optimally retract the greater omentum.

When the surgeon begins to approach the superior pole of the spleen, a different retraction strategy is frequently required. The reflection of the peritoneum at the superior pole of the spleen widens the splenogastric omentum into several layers. In order to adequately expose this remote corner of the abdominal cavity, it is best for both surgeon and first assistant to retract on the stomach. The surgeon grasps the fundus of the stomach on the anterior surface and the first assistant grasps the fundus of the stomach on the posterior surface. The surgeon retracts anteriorly and to the right. The first assistant retracts posteriorly and to the right. This opens up the field at the superior pole of the spleen (**FIGURE 11**).

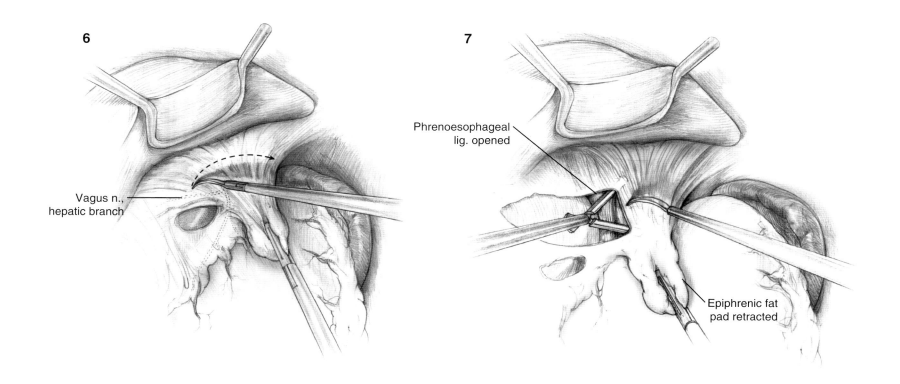

6

Vagus n., hepatic branch

7

Phrenoesophageal lig. opened

Epiphrenic fat pad retracted

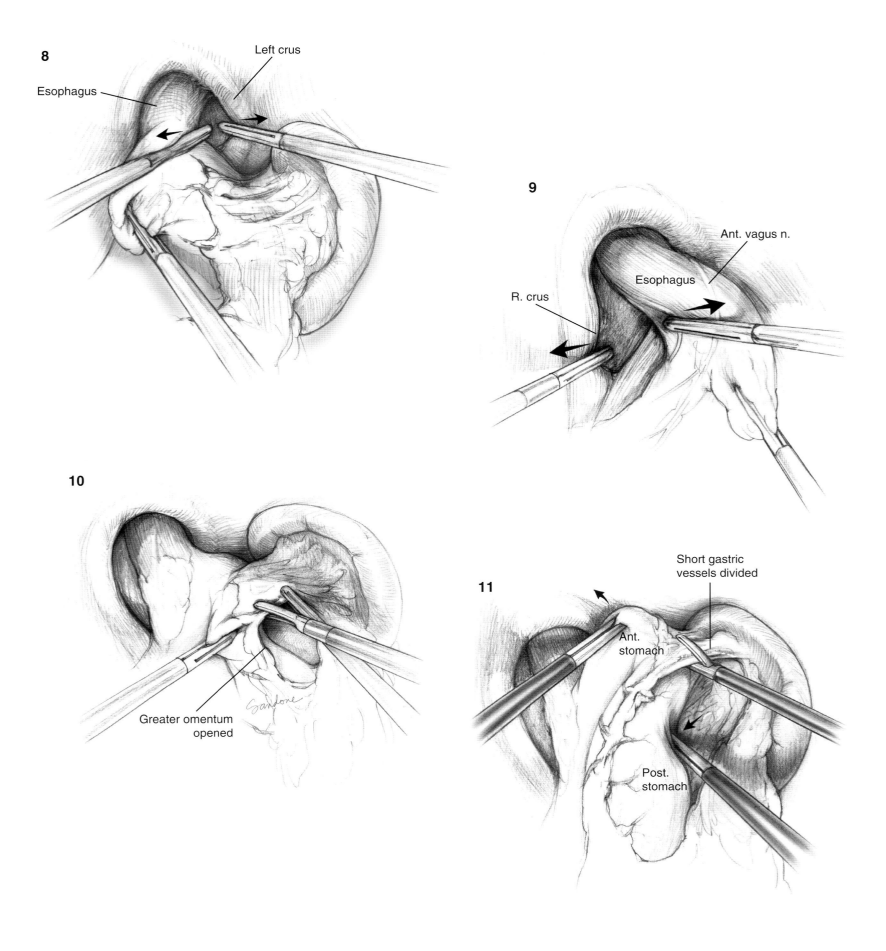

8

Esophagus

Left crus

9

R. crus

Esophagus

Ant. vagus n.

10

Greater omentum
opened

Sandone

11

Short gastric
vessels divided

Ant.
stomach

Post.
stomach

DETAILS OF THE PROCEDURE If a fatty greater omentum fills the lesser sac at the superior aspect of the spleen, obscuring the field of dissection, it may be necessary to reef up and retract the omentum inferiorly with a 90-cm 2-0 polypropylene suture (**FIGURE 12**). This suture can be brought out the abdominal wall through the trocar in the left anterior axillary line (**FIGURE 13A**). The trocar is withdrawn over a Hunter grasper and the suture is freed from the trocar as it emerges from the skin, then clamped to the adjacent drape to maintain inferior traction on the omentum (**FIGURE 13B**). One should not proceed in dissection of this tricky anatomic area without adequate exposure of the anterior wall of the stomach, the posterior wall of the stomach, and the superior pole of the spleen. The light cord of the laparoscope is rotated back to the 12 o'clock or the 1 o'clock position to visualize this region.

The next point of dissection is the posterior pancreaticogastric fold, which contains the posterior gastric artery. This fold is identified by medial retraction on the posterior body of the stomach, lower on the stomach than was necessary to expose the tip of the spleen. Medial and occasionally anterior retraction of this posterior wall lifts the posterior stomach away from the posterior retroperitoneum, exposing a consistent band from the superior surface of the pancreas (near the splenic artery) to the posterior aspect of the stomach (**FIGURE 14**). This band is divided with the ultrasonic shears, marching in a cephalad direction toward the base of the left crus of the diaphragm. The posterior gastric artery encountered in this bundle is divided with the ultrasonic shears. When the base of the left diaphragmatic crus is reached, dissection proceeds anteriorly along the left crus of the diaphragm, dividing all attachments between the left crus and the gastroesophageal (GE) junction. The best retraction for this region often requires the surgeon to grab the epiphrenic fat pad with an atraumatic grasper in the left hand and retract anteriorly and to the right while the first assistant maintains posteromedial retraction on the posterior wall of the stomach (**FIGURE 15**). The mediastinum to the left and posterior to the esophagus is thus entered. When the left crus is followed posteriorly, one reaches the right crus (previously dissected). If this maneuver is difficult, it is sometimes desirable to return to the right side of the esophagus and follow the right crus of the diaphragm farther posteriorly. The most important point here is that the posterior window behind the esophagus is not achieved by blunt dissection or passage of a blunt instrument, but by division of the peritoneal and neurovascular attachments between the diaphragm and the GE junction around the entire hiatal aperture. It is at this point that the posterior vagus nerve usually becomes visible from either the left or right side of the esophagus, lying adjacent to the posterior esophagus.

At this point, most surgeons will pass a Penrose drain around the GE junction. For most dissections, a 10-cm length of ¼-inch Penrose drain is most appropriate. The two ends of the drain are held by the assistant anteriorly while the surgeon places an Endoloop or two endoclips on the drain to hold the ends together (**FIGURE 16**). The assistant then replaces their atraumatic grasper with a more aggressive grasper, which will not slip off the drain and can be ratcheted down to maintain this attachment. The assistant retracts the GE junction caudally and slightly to the patient's left. This allows access to the mediastinum on the right side of the esophagus. The surgeon then mobilizes the distal esophagus from the posterior mediastinum with a combination of blunt dissection and ultrasonic shears (used conservatively on arterial blood supply to the esophagus). Most periesophageal attachments can be divided bluntly by tearing between two graspers without risking thermal injury to either vagus nerve.

The extent of mediastinal dissection is variable, depending on the length of the intraabdominal esophagus. It is only necessary to perform mediastinal dissection as high as is necessary to achieve a "tension-free" intraabdominal esophageal length of 2½ to 3 cm. The best way to assess tension-free intraabdominal length is to remove the assistant's grasper from the Penrose drain and perform a trial closure of the diaphragm posteriorly with two graspers. A dissecting instrument or ruler may be used to measure the length of esophagus remaining below the diaphragm at rest (**FIGURE 17**). Sometimes it may be necessary to dissect as high as the inferior pulmonary vein to achieve this length, and occasionally even with extensive mediastinal mobilization it is impossible to achieve 2½ cm of intraabdominal esophagus. It is at this point that one considers Collis gastroplasty, which is described in Chapter 21. Occasionally, it is necessary to remove the epiphrenic fat pad with a Harmonic scalpel to visualize the GE junction and assure oneself of adequate intraabdominal esophageal length.

Once it has been determined that adequate length of the intraabdominal esophagus has been attained, attention is directed toward diaphragmatic closure. There are many acceptable ways to close the diaphragm, and it is unlikely that any two surgeons perform this closure identically. It is generally agreed that the diaphragm should be closed up to the posterior aspect of an anteriorly retracted esophagus, that the "bites" of the diaphragm should be large, and that crural closure should be performed with nonabsorbable suture. Beyond that there is a great deal of variability among surgeons, including the type of nonabsorbable suture used, the type of needle holder or mechanical suturing device, the shape of the needle, and the method of knot tying.

Generally, the diaphragm is closed with interrupted pledgeted sutures of permanent braided suture on an atraumatic round needle. These sutures are placed 5 to 10 mm apart, require deep bites of the left and right crura of the diaphragm, and are tied intracorporeally (see Chapter 4). Because crural failure and recurrent hiatal hernia is one of the primary failure modes of this operation, 1-cm square felt pledgets are used to buttress the diaphragmatic closure (**FIGURE 18**).

12

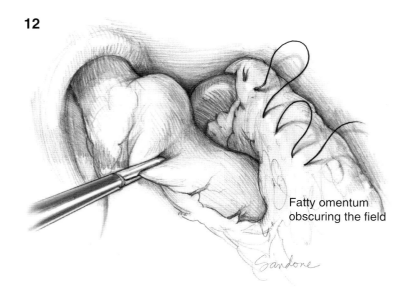

Fatty omentum obscuring the field

13

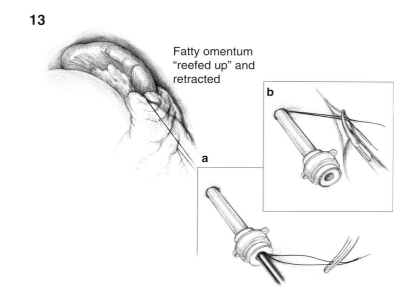

Fatty omentum "reefed up" and retracted

a

b

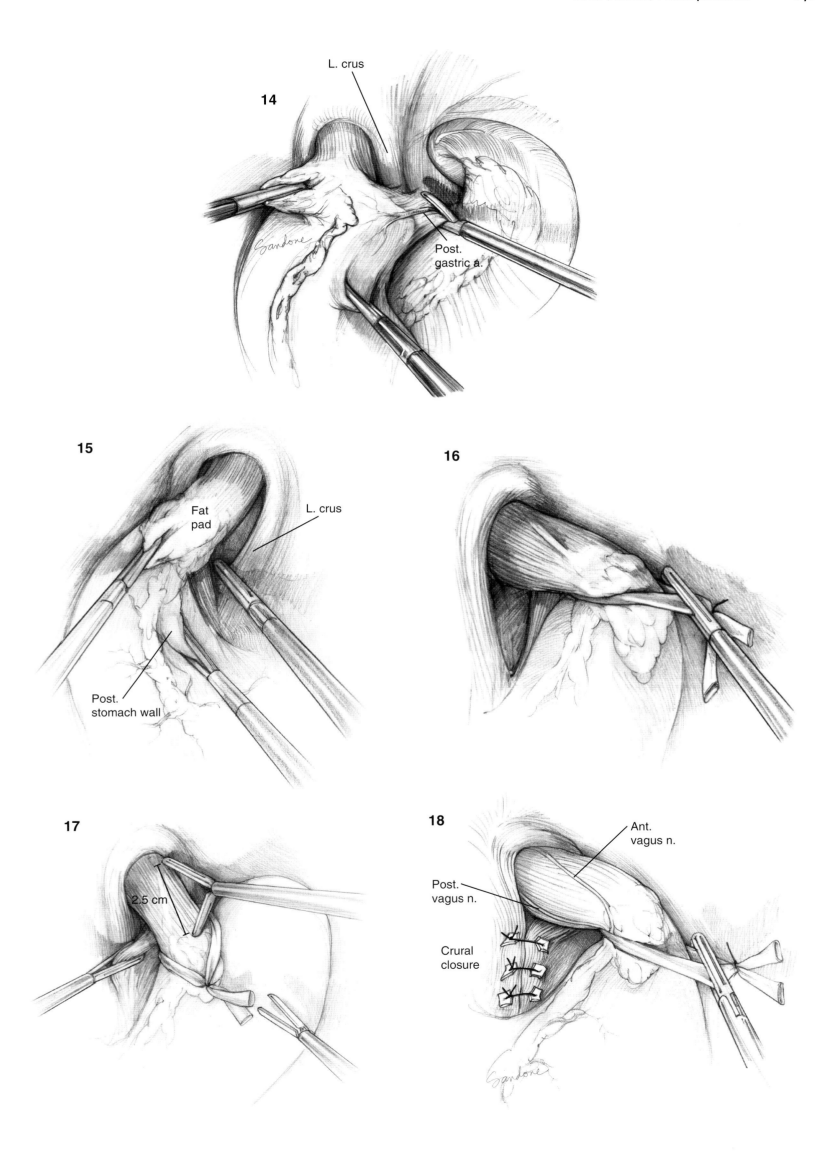

14

L. crus

Post.
gastric a.

15

Fat
pad

L. crus

Post.
stomach wall

16

17

2.5 cm

18

Ant.
vagus n.

Post.
vagus n.

Crural
closure

DETAILS OF THE PROCEDURE Upon completion of the crural closure, an atraumatic grasper is placed right-to-left behind the GE junction. The grasper is withdrawn, pulling the posterior aspect of the gastric fundus behind the esophagus (**FIGURE 19**). To avoid twisting the fundoplication, it is important that the posterior wall be used. Some surgeons choose to mark the ideal point for the suture line on the posterior stomach. The posterior wall is walked hand-over-hand backward down toward the angle of His to make sure that a point high on the fundus has been chosen. A "shoeshine" maneuver is then performed by sliding the two proposed points of fixation back and forth behind the esophagus (**FIGURE 20**).

At this point, the orogastric tube is removed and a large dilator (54 to 60 French) is passed orally under direct vision into the stomach. To avoid perforation of the esophagus, several safety steps can be employed. First, close communication between the anesthetist and surgeon is mandatory during dilator passage. The anesthetist should alert the surgeon to the distance of the tip of the dilator from the incisors marked on the side of the dilator. In addition, we generally pass a small dilator (36–40 French) first to make sure that there is unobstructed passage into the stomach. Whereas the smaller dilators will tend to fold back on themselves before perforation, larger, stiffer dilators will perforate if they run into an irregular stricture or diverticulum. Equally important, the inferior traction on the Penrose drain must be released and the laparoscope pulled back as the tip of the dilator passes into the stomach.

Once the dilator has been placed, the fundoplication is constructed. The type of wrap is dependent on preoperative manometric studies. Typically a total or 360-degree fundoplication (Nissen fundoplication) will be performed in patients with normal and ineffective esophageal motility. Alternatively, a posterior (Toupet) or anterior (Dor) partial fundoplication is performed in individuals in whom motility is absent (e.g., scleroderma or achalasia).

Although there is some variability in the construction of a Nissen-type fundoplication, most surgeons use a two- or three-stitch technique incorporating full-thickness bites of the stomach and partial-thickness bites of the esophagus on all stitches. The position for the first stitch is chosen by pulling the two limbs of the gastric fundus together at the 10 to 11 o'clock position on the esophagus. There should be no circumferential tension on the fundus with this maneuver. If there is tension, another point on the stomach, closer to the greater curvature, is chosen. Once the suture positions are chosen, the first stitch of permanent braided suture is introduced through the 10-mm trocar, and the needle is passed first through the left limb of the fundus, then through the esophagus (2.5 cm above the GE junction), then through the right limb of the fundus (**FIGURE 21**). A sliding slip knot is placed and slid down as described in Chapter 4. As the knot is slid into place, the two halves of the fundus are pulled into their final position The "floppiness" of the fundoplication is tested by placing a closed Hunter grasper between the dilator and the fundoplication to the left of the esophagus, and distracting the fundoplication away from the esophagus. This maneuver should allow 1-cm worth of redundancy (the size of an index finger) between the fundoplication and the esophagus (**FIGURE 22**). If the fundoplication is too loose or too tight, the first stitch is removed and another is placed. Subsequent stitches should be placed no more than 1 cm apart, thus creating an anterior distance between the top and bottom of the fundoplication that is 2 cm in length. It is important to place the superior stitch first, and the inferior stitch last, just above the GE junction. We generally place all three esophageal sutures to the right of the anterior vagus nerve (**FIGURE 23**).

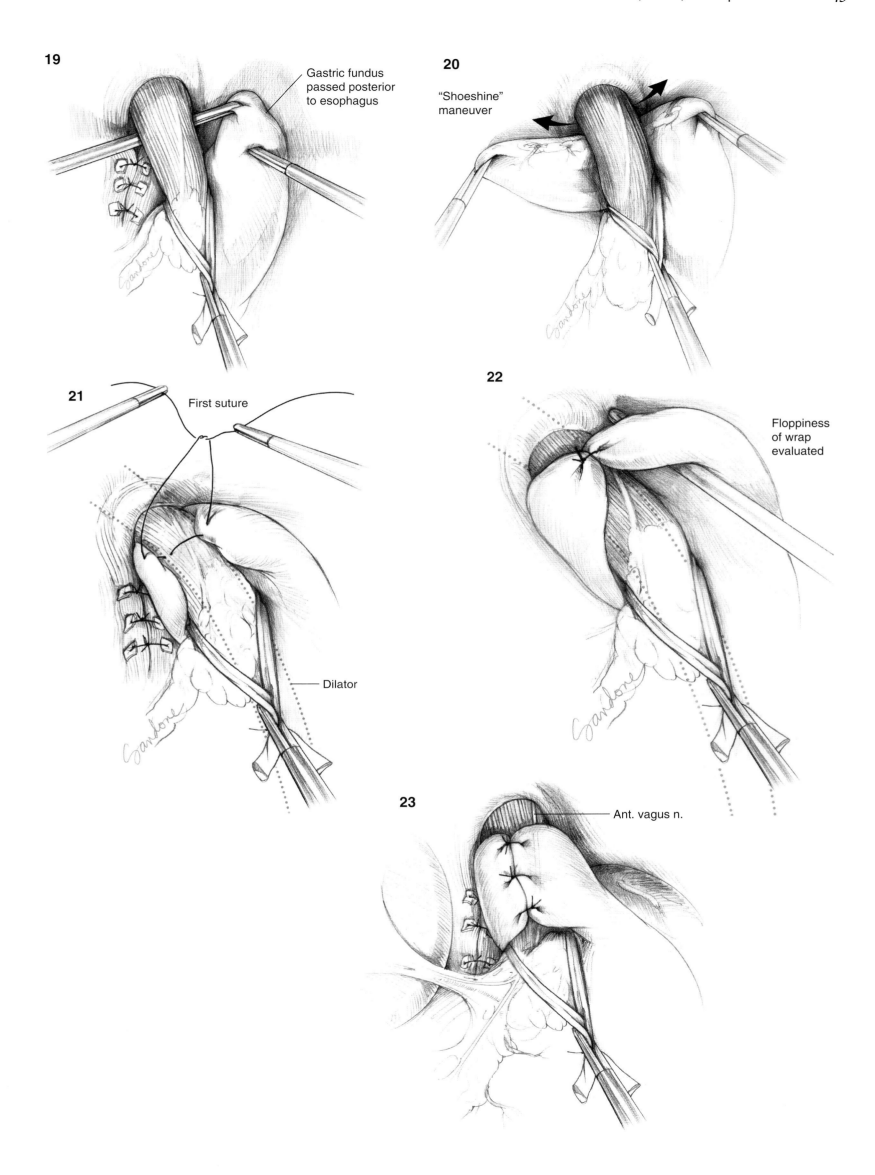

19

Gastric fundus passed posterior to esophagus

20

"Shoeshine" maneuver

21

First suture

Dilator

22

Floppiness of wrap evaluated

23

Ant. vagus n.

DETAILS OF THE PROCEDURE Although this completes the "standard" Nissen fundoplication, we generally place an additional suture posteriorly between the esophagus and the fundoplication to avoid posterior fundoplication slippage (**FIGURE 24**). The dilator is then removed, the table is flattened, and the fundoplication is placed in its anatomic position beneath the diaphragm (**FIGURE 25**). On rare occasion it is necessary to tack the fundoplication to the diaphragm to maintain its optimal positioning. It is questionable whether such suturing decreases postoperative failure, however. Completion upper endoscopy allows the surgeon to ensure proper valve configuration, a series of stacked coils, sitting just above the GE junction.

CLOSURE The abdomen is thoroughly irrigated and all fluid removed, the Penrose drain is removed, and the small amount of blood that accumulates between the spleen and diaphragm is evacuated. The liver retractor is removed under direct vision, as is each of the trocars. We do not close the trocar sites in the upper abdomen, 11 mm in diameter or less, and have not seen hernia complications resulting. The skin is reapproximated with a subcuticular suture and Steri-Strips or reapproximated with tissue glue.

POSTOPERATIVE CARE Essential elements of postoperative care include aggressive treatment of nausea with ondansetron and other agents. Pain relief is usually obtained with intravenous ketorolac and judicious use of narcotics. The Foley catheter is removed in the recovery room, and the patient transferred to the inpatient ward or a short-stay unit. The vast majority of surgeons and patients prefer at least an overnight stay to ensure pain control and resumption of a diet. Upon arrival to the unit, the patient is started on a clear liquid diet and advanced to a full liquid diet the next day. Because of distal esophageal edema, we have used a conservative dietary approach that includes 5 days of full liquids, followed by a modified esophageal diet for 3 weeks that avoids breads, meats, and raw vegetables. With strict adherence to this dietary protocol, few patients complain of postoperative dysphagia. Without such aggressive management, food impaction, nausea, retching, and wrap disruption have been reported.

In addition, we urge patients to resume activities of daily living immediately, but avoid events involving intraabdominal straining (particularly heavy lifting) for 6 to 8 weeks to minimize the likelihood of acute paraesophageal herniation of the fundoplication. This latter complication is the most immediately life-threatening complication that can occur to these patients, especially if unrecognized. An unrecognized fundoplication herniation may result in gastric fundus necrosis, mediastinitis, and empyema. The most fundamental caveat in postoperative care is that any patient who fares poorly for any reason (increasing pain, tachycardia, tachypnea, pleural effusion, fever, retching, or confusion) should be immediately studied with a barium swallow to rule out esophageal perforation or herniation of the fundoplication. Most catastrophes following laparoscopic fundoplication are treatable without great patient morbidity if they are recognized and treated early. ■

24

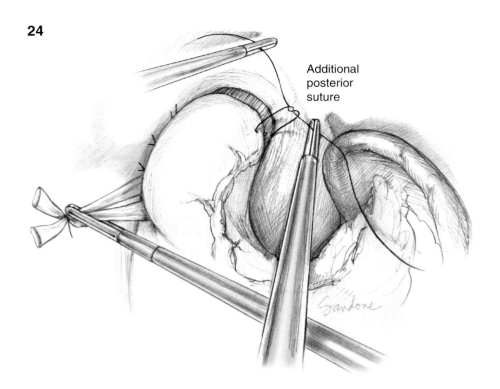

Additional
posterior
suture

25

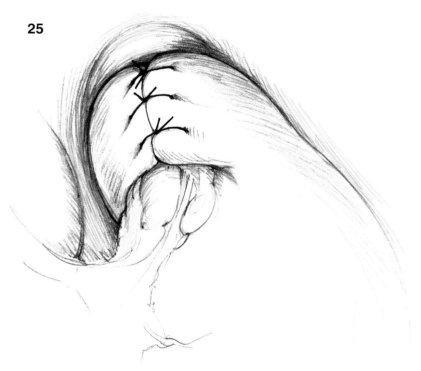

CHAPTER 19 · PARTIAL FUNDOPLICATION

INDICATIONS The complete encirclement of the lower esophageal sphincter with the fundus of the stomach is very effective in stopping gastroesophageal reflux. A greater understanding of the complex physiologic relationship that exists in normal swallowing, esophageal motility, and gastric reservoir function has suggested that a 360-degree fundoplication may not be optimal for all patients. Many different forms of partial fundoplication exist, differing in the technical details of wrap construction and the part of the esophagus covered. The Dor and Toupet fundoplications represent anterior and posterior versions of a partial fundoplication, respectively. Despite their differences, the overall goals of restoring intraabdominal esophageal length and reinforcing the lower esophageal sphincter remain constant.

The indications for partial fundoplication are no different from the indications for total fundoplication. The decision to perform partial fundoplication is based more on patient factors and esophageal physiology than on the severity of gastroesophageal reflux disease (GERD). The indications include: (1) GERD that is refractory to proton pump inhibition, (2) GERD that is incompletely responsive to proton pump inhibition, (3) GERD that is entirely responsive to proton pump inhibition, but patient choice or side effect profile merits consideration of antireflux surgery, (4) extraesophageal manifestations of GERD, and (5) complications of GERD (stricture, bleeding, aspiration, Barrett esophagus). Specific indications for the use of a partial fundoplication as opposed to a total fundoplication include: (1) patients with esophageal motility disorders in addition to GERD, (2) patients who have failed previous Nissen fundoplication due to significant postoperative dysphagia, (3) as an adjunct to laparoscopic Heller myotomy to prevent gross reflux, and (4) severe aerophagia and gas symptoms in a patient with well-documented GERD.

PREOPERATIVE PREPARATION, ANESTHESIA, AND PATIENT POSITIONING All are identical to that performed in laparoscopic Nissen fundoplication described in chapter 18. The patient is placed in a split-leg position with both arms tucked (**FIGURE 1**).

INCISION AND EXPOSURE The initial trocar setup and exposure for both Dor and Toupet partial fundoplication proceed in fashion identical to that for the Nissen fundoplication or Heller myotomy (**FIGURE 2**). Some surgeons do not mobilize the greater curvature of the stomach, dissect the posterior esophageal space, or take down the short gastric vessels with the performance of a Dor fundoplication. We believe that this dissection is imperative to perform a fundoplication without tension on the fundus of the stomach or fundic distortion. The detailed technique of esophageal mobilization and short gastric vessel division are found in Chapter 18. Once the posterior window has been made behind the esophagus, a Penrose drain is passed as described in the Nissen fundoplication chapter (**FIGURE 3**).

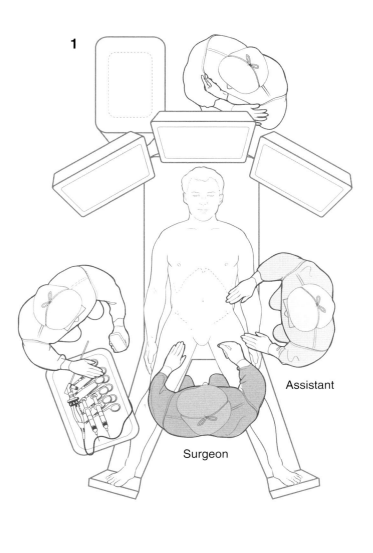

Assistant

Surgeon

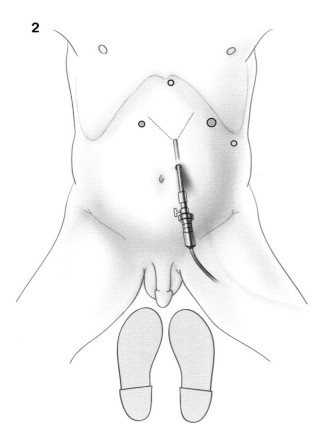

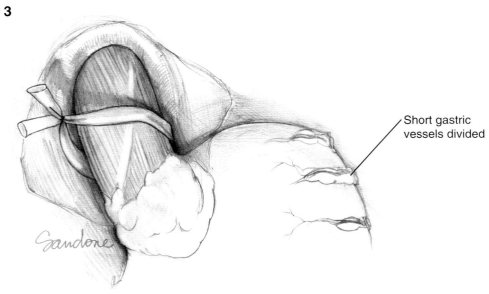

Short gastric
vessels divided

ANTERIOR PARTIAL (DOR) FUNDOPLICATION The anterior partial fundoplication creates a flap valve using the greater curvature of the stomach folded anterior to the intraabdominal portion of the distal esophagus. In the Heller myotomy procedure, the anterior wrap serves to cover the myotomy. A 56 to 60 French esophageal dilator is carefully advanced into the stomach.

The first step in this fundoplication is to roll the fundus of the stomach around to the anterior surface of the distal esophagus. This is done with two blunt atraumatic graspers, which will place the greater curvature vessels into the 12 to 1 o'clock position (viewing the esophagus as a clock face from the foot of the patient). The fundus should sit very comfortably in this position without any lines of tension. Once the final position of the fundoplication has been projected, the fundus is released and suturing begins.

Anterior partial fundoplication is performed with 5 to 7 braided, nonabsorbable sutures. The first stitch is placed on the greater curvature of the fundus approximately 3 cm distal to the angle of His and sutured to the midpoint of the left crus (**FIGURE 4**). The second stitch approximates the superior portion of the fundus—just posterior to the line of short gastric vessels—to the left side of the crural arch. Two additional sutures are placed across the crural arch, completing the "hanging" of the fundus from the arch. The last one or two sutures of the fundoplication incorporate the fundus of the stomach with the right crus of the diaphragm. When the fundoplication is complete, the entire anterior wall of the esophagus is covered by the fundoplication (**FIGURE 5**). The dilator is removed.

**4   Anterior Partial
    (Dor) Fundoplication**

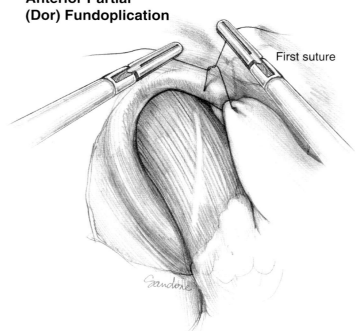

First suture

5

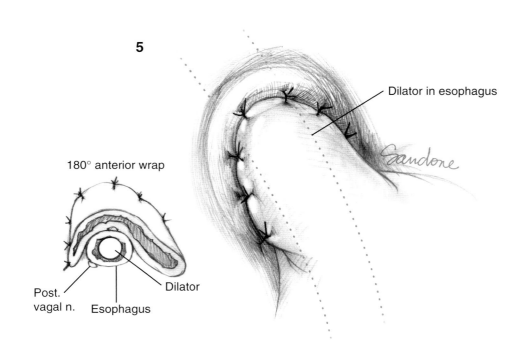

Dilator in esophagus

180° anterior wrap

Post.
vagal n.   Dilator

Esophagus

POSTERIOR PARTIAL (TOUPET) FUNDOPLICATION After complete mobilization of the stomach and esophagus, a Penrose drain is passed as described in the Nissen fundoplication chapter (**FIGURE 6**). If a large crural defect is present, it may be closed as described in Chapter 20. Upon completion of the crural closure, an atraumatic grasper is placed right to left behind the gastroesophageal junction. The grasper is withdrawn, pulling the posterior aspect of the gastric fundus behind the esophagus. To avoid twisting the fundoplication, it is important that the posterior wall be used. Some surgeons choose to mark the ideal point for the suture line on the posterior stomach. The posterior wall is then walked hand-over-hand backward down towards the angle of His to make sure that a point high on the fundus has been chosen. A "shoeshine" maneuver is then performed by sliding the two proposed points of fixation back and forth behind the esophagus (**FIGURE 7**).

The assistant then grasps the right aspect of the posterior wrap and distracts it to the left, demonstrating the crura posteriorly. Two interrupted sutures are then placed from the right wrap to the right crus (**FIGURE 8**). The final suture on this side is to the top of the right crus. A 56 French esophageal dilator is placed into the stomach prior to suturing the anterior portion of the wrap. This dilator serves as a guide to visualize the 10 and 2 o'clock esophageal position corresponding to a 270-degree wrap. The right side of the wrap is sutured to the 10 o'clock position, and the left side sutured to the 2 o'clock position (**FIGURE 9**). The wrap length should measure approximately 3 cm upon completion (**FIGURE 10**). If the posterior wrap is performed in conjunction with a Heller myotomy, the esophageal sutures are taken through the edges of the myotomy. This serves to hold the myotomy open. The dilator is removed.

CLOSURE The abdomen is thoroughly irrigated, the Penrose drain is removed, and the small amount of blood that accumulates between the spleen and diaphragm is evacuated. The liver retractor is removed under direct vision, as is each of the trocars. We do not close the trocar sites in the upper abdomen, 11 mm in diameter or less, and have not seen hernia complications resulting. The skin is reapproximated with a subcuticular suture and Steri-Strips or reapproximated with tissue glue.

POSTOPERATIVE CARE Essential elements to postoperative care include aggressive treatment of nausea intraoperatively with ondansetron and other agents. Pain relief is usually obtained with intravenous ketorolac and judicious use of narcotics. The Foley catheter is removed in the recovery room, and the patient is transferred to the inpatient ward. The vast majority of surgeons and patients prefer at least an overnight stay to ensure pain control and resumption of a diet. Upon arrival to the inpatient ward, the patient is started on a clear liquid diet and advanced to a full liquid diet the next day. Because of distal esophageal edema, we have used a conservative dietary approach that includes 5 days of full liquids, followed by a modified esophageal diet for 3 weeks that avoids breads, meats, and raw vegetables. With strict adherence to this dietary protocol, few patients complain of postoperative dysphagia. Without such aggressive management, food impaction, nausea, retching, and wrap disruption have been reported.

In addition, we urge the patients to resume activities of daily living immediately, but avoid events involving intraabdominal straining (particularly heavy lifting) for 6 to 8 weeks to minimize the likelihood of acute paraesophageal herniation of the fundoplication. This latter complication is the most immediately life-threatening complication that may occur to these patients, especially if unrecognized. An unrecognized fundoplication herniation may result in gastric fundus necrosis, mediastinitis, and empyema. Last, the most fundamental caveat in postoperative care is that any patient who fares poorly for any reason (increasing pain, tachycardia, tachypnea, pleural effusion, fever, retching, or confusion) should be immediately studied with a barium swallow to rule out esophageal perforation or herniation of the fundoplication. Most catastrophes following laparoscopic fundoplication are treatable without great patient morbidity if they are recognized and treated early. ■

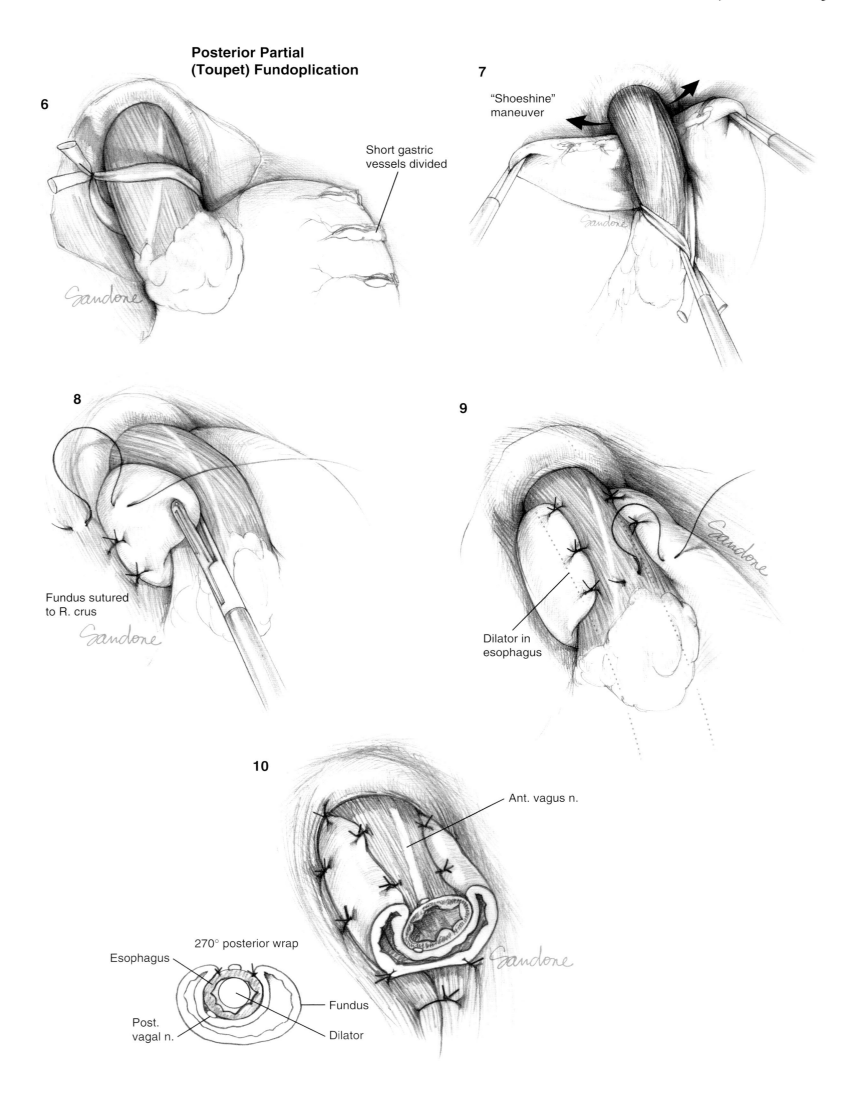

Posterior Partial (Toupet) Fundoplication

6

Short gastric vessels divided

7

"Shoeshine" maneuver

8

Fundus sutured to R. crus

9

Dilator in esophagus

10

Ant. vagus n.

270° posterior wrap

Esophagus

Post. vagal n.

Fundus

Dilator

CHAPTER 20

REPAIR OF PARAESOPHAGEAL HERNIA

INDICATIONS Laparoscopic repair of giant hiatal hernias, also known as paraesophageal hernias, is indicated for individuals with a symptomatic type II or III paraesophageal hiatal hernia. Symptoms are variable, including gastroesophageal reflux disease (GERD), dysphagia, chest or abdominal pain, or anemia. The patient must also be a candidate for a transabdominal approach to the hiatus, which excludes those with uncorrectable coagulopathy, contraindications to laparotomy, or a hostile abdomen, as well as patients who have had several prior failed laparoscopic operations, in which case an open procedure should be strongly considered.

PREOPERATIVE PREPARATION Before undergoing laparoscopic paraesophageal hernia repair, anatomic and physiologic esophageal evaluation should be performed. This entails the performance of esophagogastroduodenoscopy (EGD), barium swallow, and esophageal manometry. A 24-hour pH test is not needed, as all patients will receive a fundoplication, either total or partial, depending on the adequacy of motility. The remainder of preoperative preparation and intraoperative anesthetic management is similar to that for Nissen fundoplication (see Chapter 18).

POSITION Laparoscopic esophageal procedures are typically performed with the surgeon standing between the patient's abducted legs and with the patient in a steep reverse Trendelenburg position. The assistant typically stands on the patient's left side (**FIGURE 1**). Initiation of the pneumoperitoneum, placement of trocars, and liver retraction are all similar to that for laparoscopic Nissen fundoplication (see Chapter 18) (**FIGURE 2**).

DETAILS OF THE PROCEDURE After exposing the area of the esophageal hiatus by liver elevation, the surgeon and assistant reduce the intrathoracic stomach by hand-over-hand manipulation using atraumatic graspers. The gastrohepatic omentum is divided with the ultrasonic shears, including division of the hepatic branch of the vagus nerve for optimal exposure of the right crus of the diaphragm. The most important aspect of the operation is to gain entry into the proper plane between the peritoneum and endothoracic fascia (**FIGURE 3**).

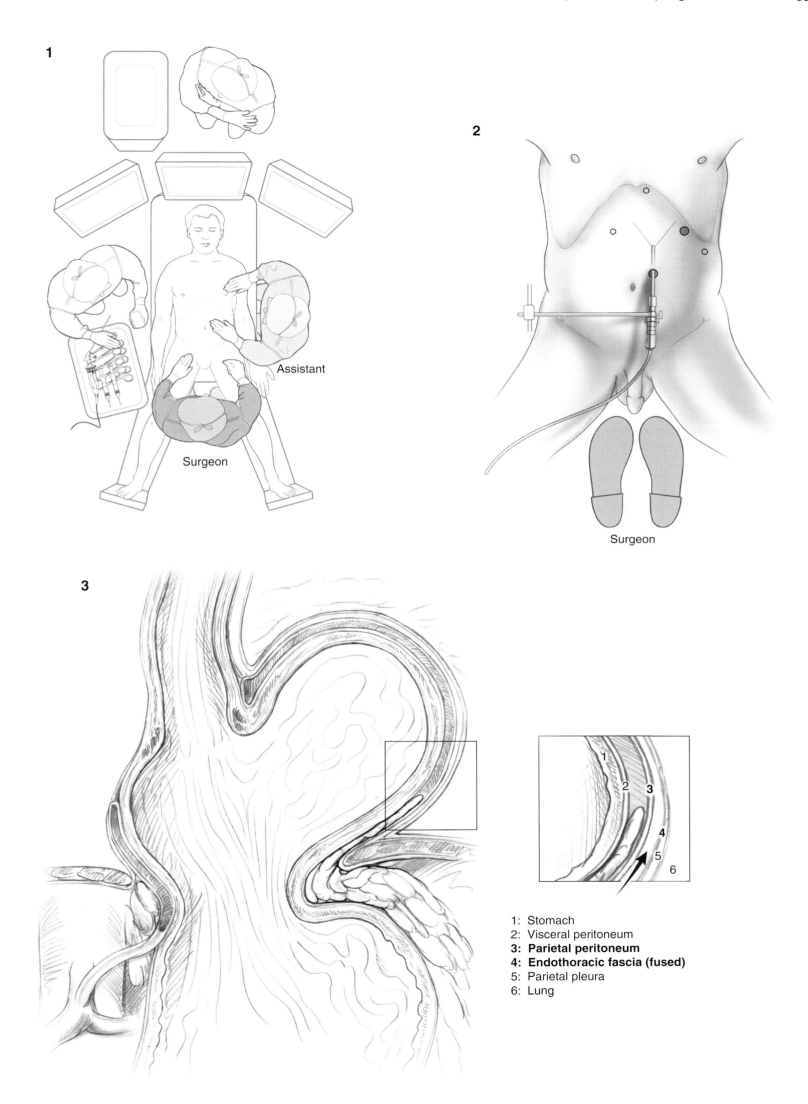

1: Stomach
2: Visceral peritoneum
3: Parietal peritoneum
4: Endothoracic fascia (fused)
5: Parietal pleura
6: Lung

DETAILS OF THE PROCEDURE Typically a large paraesophageal hernia contains two distinct sac elements. The anterior hernia sac is an extension of the abdominal peritoneum (greater sac of the abdomen) while the posterior hernia sac is an extension of the lesser sac (**FIGURE 4 INSET**). To reduce the anterior sac, the assistant grasps the stomach along the high lesser curve and retracts it to the patient's left (**FIGURE 4**). This maneuver often reveals that large amounts of fat and vessels of the lesser curvature of the stomach, including the left gastric artery, have been drawn into the mediastinum. In this case dissection of the anterior sac proceeds from the left crus. The Harmonic shears is used to divide the peritoneal sac just medial to the crural muscle, developing a plane between the sac and the mediastinal structures (**FIGURE 5**). After an incision has been made in the sac, the assistant aggressively retracts the sac caudad and to the patient's right. The surgeon then uses blunt sweeping strokes to dissect the sac toward the left lateral surface of the proximal stomach and esophagus. The correct plane is confirmed when the posterior aspect of the muscle fibers of the crus are visible. The plane is virtually avascular and should allow blunt cleavage of the sac from the mediastinal structures. The surgeon continues to divide the peritoneal sac around the medial circumference of the anterior portion of the hiatus and bluntly dissects the sac down toward the abdominal cavity. Throughout the entire dissection, the assistant continues to "choke up" on the hernia sac, placing appropriate traction at the point where the surgeon is working. This maneuver will facilitate further reduction of the stomach and herniated contents into the abdomen. Continuing this dissection to the right, the sac is divided around the anterior two thirds of the esophageal hiatus. At the point when visualization of the right crus of the diaphragm becomes clearer, it will be necessary to start the same dissection plane from the base of the right crus proceeding anteriorly (**FIGURE 6**). During this dissection, careful attention should be maintained as the esophagus comes into view within the mediastinum. Attention should focus on the position of the anterior and posterior vagus nerves to protect them from harm. As the anterior sac is reduced, these nerves are dissected along their lateral aspects such that they remain alongside the esophagus.

Although the short gastric vessels have been lengthened by the fundus being transposed into the thorax, the vessels are divided to enter the proper plane adjacent, and posterior to, the stomach. The gastrosplenic ligament is divided using the ultrasonic shears (**FIGURE 7**).

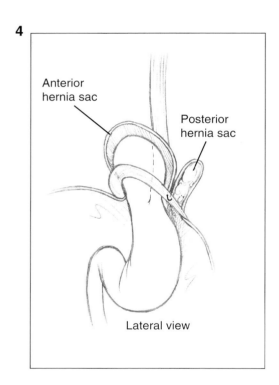

4

Anterior
hernia sac

Posterior
hernia sac

Lateral view

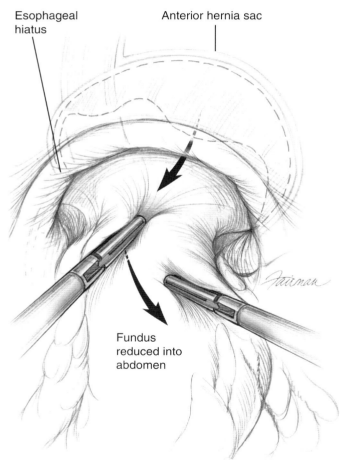

Esophageal
hiatus

Anterior hernia sac

Fundus
reduced into
abdomen

5

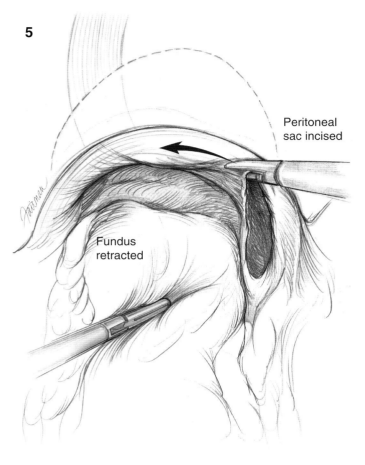

Peritoneal
sac incised

Fundus
retracted

6

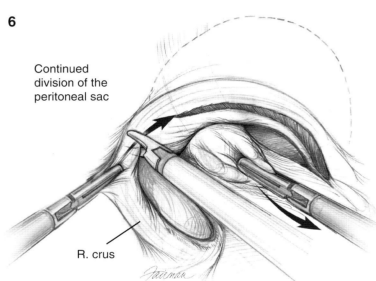

Continued
division of the
peritoneal sac

R. crus

7

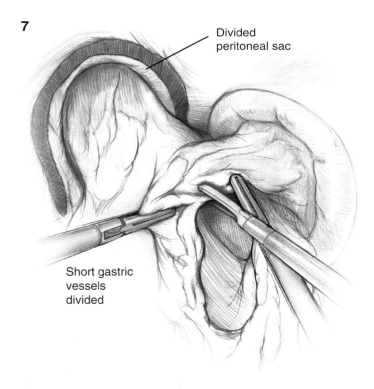

Divided
peritoneal sac

Short gastric
vessels
divided

DETAILS OF THE PROCEDURE This dissection is continued toward the highest short gastric vessels. The peritoneum posterior to and on the left side of the gastroesophageal junction is divided along the medial border of the base of the left crus to release the posterior sac elements. Working from both sides, the final attachments of the sac to the base of the right crus of the diaphragm are likewise divided and the sac mobilized into the peritoneal cavity (**FIGURE 8**). There are usually additional adhesions between the sac and the aorta. These can be easily divided with the ultrasonic shears while protecting the esophagus by retracting it anteriorly using an open-jawed Hunter dissector. At this point, all of the adhesions connecting the sac to the crura and mediastinum have been divided; the hernia sac will be hanging from its remaining medial attachments to the gastroesophageal junction and anterior esophageal wall.

While the assistant places caudad retraction on the sac at the gastroesophageal junction, a Penrose drain (15 cm) is placed around the esophagus. The esophagus is mobilized as high into the mediastinum as is possible without risking injury. The esophagus should never be directly grasped. The goal is to mobilize adequate esophagus such that at least 3 cm of the distal esophagus resides within the abdominal cavity in the absence of traction being placed on it.

The excessive hernia sac is excised, including any ischemic-appearing tissue or redundant sac that will hinder further manipulation. The hernia sac is placed on traction and divided (bivalved) just to the left of the anterior vagus nerve using the ultrasonic shears (**FIGURE 9**). The portion of the sac to the left of the anterior vagus nerve is excised as close to the stomach and esophageal walls as can be comfortably done without risking visceral injury. The excised sac is removed through the left upper quadrant 10-mm port.

At this point of the operation, if there is concern for damage to the esophagus, intraoperative endoscopy can be performed and insufflation of the stomach under saline can be used to look for "bubbling" indicating a leak. The position of the gastroesophageal junction is then determined. After the complete dissection, the gastroesophageal junction should remain well within the abdominal cavity without tension, and both vagus nerves should be identified. If there is inadequate esophageal length, a laparoscopic lengthening procedure is performed (see Chapter 21).

Attention is turned to the closure of the diaphragmatic crura. The goal is to close the crura such that they touch the walls of the empty esophagus. The posterior aspect is closed first with interrupted sutures of heavy-gauge braided material. Exposure to the retroesophageal hiatus is afforded by manipulation of the Penrose drain. Multiple, closely spaced sutures are placed starting posteriorly and working anteriorly. Pledgets are placed to prevent fraying of the muscles. Usually the crura can be closed without excessive tension using pledgeted sutures alone. Sometimes, sutures must also be placed anterior to the esophagus to complete the closure. At other times, the hiatal opening is large enough that primary closure is not possible without undue tension, virtually ensuring failure of the procedure. Various approaches have been used to create a tension-free closure of an enlarged hiatal opening. These include performing a relaxing incision lateral to the crura while using a biosynthetic material to close the defect.

The use of mesh to reinforce the crural closure is a controversial subject, and many techniques have been postulated. A variety of prosthetic materials have been used, from decellularized human or porcine tissue to various biopolymers, to pure synthetics, including PTFE and polypropylene.

A notched strip of prosthetic material 1.5 cm by 5 cm can be placed in lieu of the highest pledgeted stitch. This reinforced closure is secured with a double-arm mattress suture and parachuted into position. One centimeter of room should be left between the prosthetic material and the esophagus (**FIGURE 10**).

Alternatively, the base of a "U"-shaped biologic mesh can be oriented posterior to the esophagus so that the arms of the "U" extend up each side of the crural arch. The biosynthetic mesh can then be fixed in place with tissue "glue" or sewn in place with several absorbable sutures such that it lies flat against the diaphragm without tension (**FIGURE 11**).

A fundoplication is then performed using interrupted sutures of heavy-gauge braided material. A Nissen fundoplication is performed in those with adequate esophageal motility (**FIGURE 12**). Additional sutures may be placed between the fundoplication and the diaphragm or between the posterior aspect of the lesser curvature of the stomach and the arcuate ligament, similar to the Hill repair. Gastropexy sutures or gastrostomy tubes to stabilize the stomach, although classically employed, are no longer deemed necessary in most cases.

CLOSURE The remainder of the operation is similar to that as described for the Nissen fundoplication. The ports are removed with closure of any port sites larger than 10 mm in size. A nasogastric tube is not routinely used, and the Foley catheter is removed in the operating room or recovery room, or on the ward.

POSTOPERATIVE CARE Postoperative care is similar to that for Nissen fundoplication. The patient is generally hospitalized overnight and treated with intravenous antinauseants and nonsteroidal anti-inflammatory drugs. Ice chips and clear liquids are allowed the evening of surgery and a full liquid or soft diet the following morning. If no untoward events have occurred, the patient may be discharged late on the morning of the day after the operation. If the repair has been difficult, a barium swallow serves as a good "quality control" step before starting a diet. Should the patient retch or vomit in the immediate perioperative period, a barium swallow should be performed to rule out disruption of the repair. The patient is maintained on a soft diet for 4 to 6 weeks. ■

8

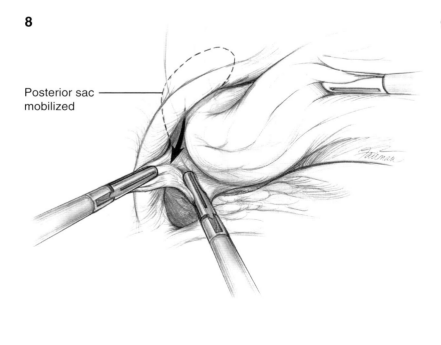

Posterior sac mobilized

9

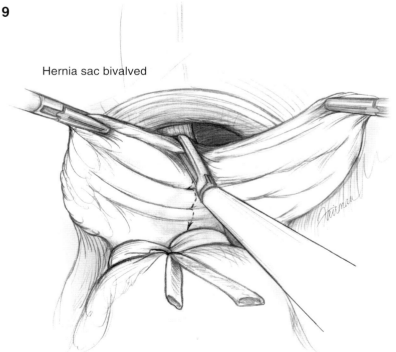

Hernia sac bivalved

10

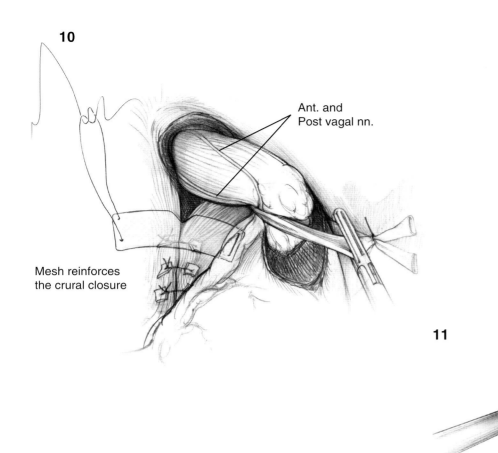

Ant. and
Post vagal nn.

Mesh reinforces
the crural closure

Alternate:
U-shaped mesh glued in position

11

12

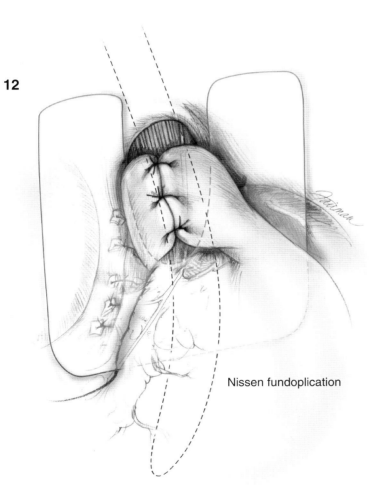

Nissen fundoplication

CHAPTER 21

WEDGE GASTROPLASTY FOR SHORT ESOPHAGUS (COLLIS GASTROPLASTY)

INDICATION A variety of minimally invasive surgical techniques have been described to treat the acquired short esophagus. These include the use of circular and linear staplers, passed through the left chest, through the right chest, and through a small epigastric incision. For the most part, these techniques have been discarded in favor of the laparoscopic wedge gastroplasty, also known as wedge fundectomy, or wedge Collis gastroplasty.

The indication for wedge gastroplasty for esophageal lengthening is the need to establish sufficient intraabdominal esophageal length to perform a fundoplication. Predictors of esophageal shortening include large hiatal hernia, Barrett esophagus, esophageal stricture, severe GERD or failed hiatal hernia repair with transdiaphragmatic migration of the stomach. It is not clear that any one of these conditions is more predictive of shortening than another, but certainly a combination of factors (Barrett and stricture and large hernia) increases the likelihood that the esophagus will be short. Accurate diagnosis of the short esophagus can only occur intraoperatively, after thorough esophageal mobilization has been carried high in the mediastinum, to the level of left inferior pulmonary vein.

Following maximal transhiatal mediastinal dissection of the esophagus, the left and right crura are brought together with graspers and all inferior tension on the gastroesophageal (GE) junction is released. If the GE junction, as marked by the superior border of the epiphrenic fat pad, retracts to within 2.5 cm of the closed hiatus, esophageal shortening can be diagnosed.

POSITION Collis gastroplasty is most often performed within setting of a laparoscopic Nissen fundoplication. This is generally performed in the supine position with the legs extended and abducted 30 to 60 degrees so the surgeon may stand between the legs to perform the operation (**FIGURE 1**). Trocars are set up identically to the laparoscopic fundoplication (**FIGURE 2**).

DETAILS OF THE PROCEDURE After complete mobilization of the esophagus, the decision to perform a Collis gastroplasty is usually made before the hiatal defect is closed. There are two reasons for this. First, the open hiatus will best accommodate the tip of the endoscopic stapling device, whereas the closed hiatus may make it more difficult to complete the high end of the staple line. Second, there is minimal contamination of the upper abdomen with this technique; exposing the staple line to pledgets or mesh risks contamination of these foreign bodies. On the other hand, it is sometimes difficult to assess the true length of the intraabdominal esophagus until the crura are completely closed. For this reason it is occasionally necessary to perform Collis gastroplasty after crural closure.

The first step in performance of a laparoscopic wedge Collis gastroplasty is removal of the epiphrenic fat pad (**FIGURE 3**). Removal of the fat pad proceeds down onto the angle of His and subsequently around the back of the esophagus such that the GE junction is cleared for a circumference of 180 degrees, leaving the fat only on the right side of the esophagus, near the lesser curvature vessels. It is unnecessary to remove the fat pad on the right side of the esophagus and may risk bleeding from branches of the left gastric artery. In addition, clearance of the epiphrenic fat pad on the right side of the GE junction would risk harm to the vagal trunks as they move to the right of the esophagus at the GE junction. The final confirmation of a short esophagus is made if the Penrose drain and the angle of His retract to the level of the hiatal arch when all inferior tension is removed.

Once the fat pad has been removed, a 48 French Maloney dilator is passed into the stomach. A point 2.5 cm inferior to the angle of His at the outside edge of the dilator is measured and marked with a single tap of the electrosurgical device. This point marks the target of the horizontal staple line, and the inferior end of the vertical staple line. This additional 2.5 cm is ample length to provide a length of tubular esophagus for performance of a short floppy fundoplication (**FIGURE 4**).

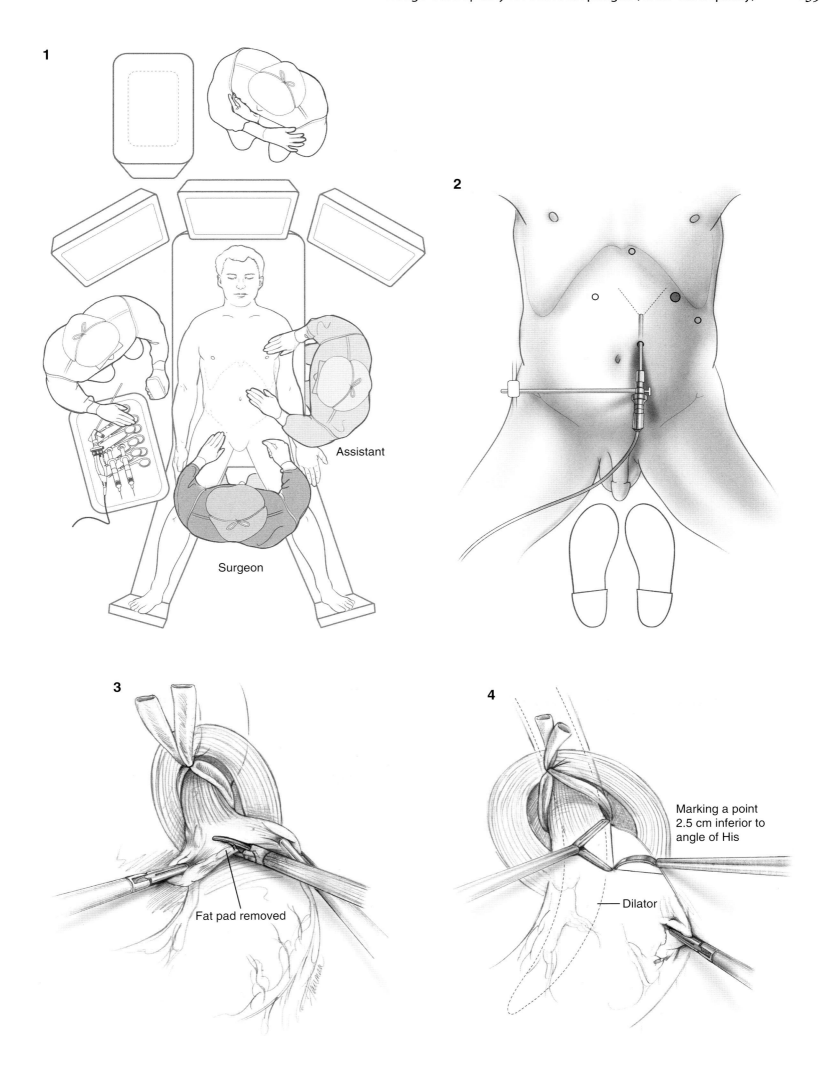

1

2

Assistant

Surgeon

3

Fat pad removed

4

Marking a point
2.5 cm inferior to
angle of His

Dilator

DETAILS OF THE PROCEDURE Through the 12-mm trocar placed along the left costal margin at the mid-clavicular line (see trocar placement for Nissen fundoplication), a roticulating 45-mm endoscopic stapler is placed with a blue staple load. The anvil blade is passed behind the stomach against the posterior wall, and the staple cartridge sits in front of the stomach along the anterior wall. The stapler is angled maximally to the patient's right. With their left hand the surgeon grasps the stomach at the angle of His, and the first assistant grasps a point approximately 5 cm from the angle of His along the greater curvature and flattens the angle of His by pulling inferiorly. The articulated stapler is positioned such that the horizontal staple line is directed toward the previously marked target point adjacent to the dilator (**FIGURE 5**). This first staple line is usually inadequate to reach the dilator, and a second firing of the 45-mm stapler may be necessary. A 60-mm stapler can be used; however, the tight working conditions in the upper abdomen make the longer stapler somewhat clumsy. A second horizontal firing of the stapler follows the same course as the first, with a trajectory again aimed for the point previously marked. Retraction for the second firing of the stapler is attained by the surgeon grabbing the superior staple line and lifting anteriorly at the same time the assistant grabs the inferior horizontal staple line and pulls laterally and anteriorly (**FIGURE 6**). With the second firing of the stapler, the dilator is usually encountered. As one closes the stapler, the dilator is pushed out of the jaws of the stapler. The horizontal staple line is not complete until this sensation of pushing the dilator out of the jaws of the stapler has been observed. Failure to bring the staple line up against the dilator will result in a boggy gastric tube.

The gastric tube is construction completed with a single vertical firing of the 45-mm endoscopic stapler using the blue cartridge (**FIGURE 7**). Occasionally a single firing of the GIA does not fully divide the angle of His. Although the temptation is to cut this small remaining bridge of tissue with scissors, experience dictates the firing of another staple to ensure that a small hole in the GE junction will not occur. The small wedge of stomach created by the stapler firings is removed through a large trocar.

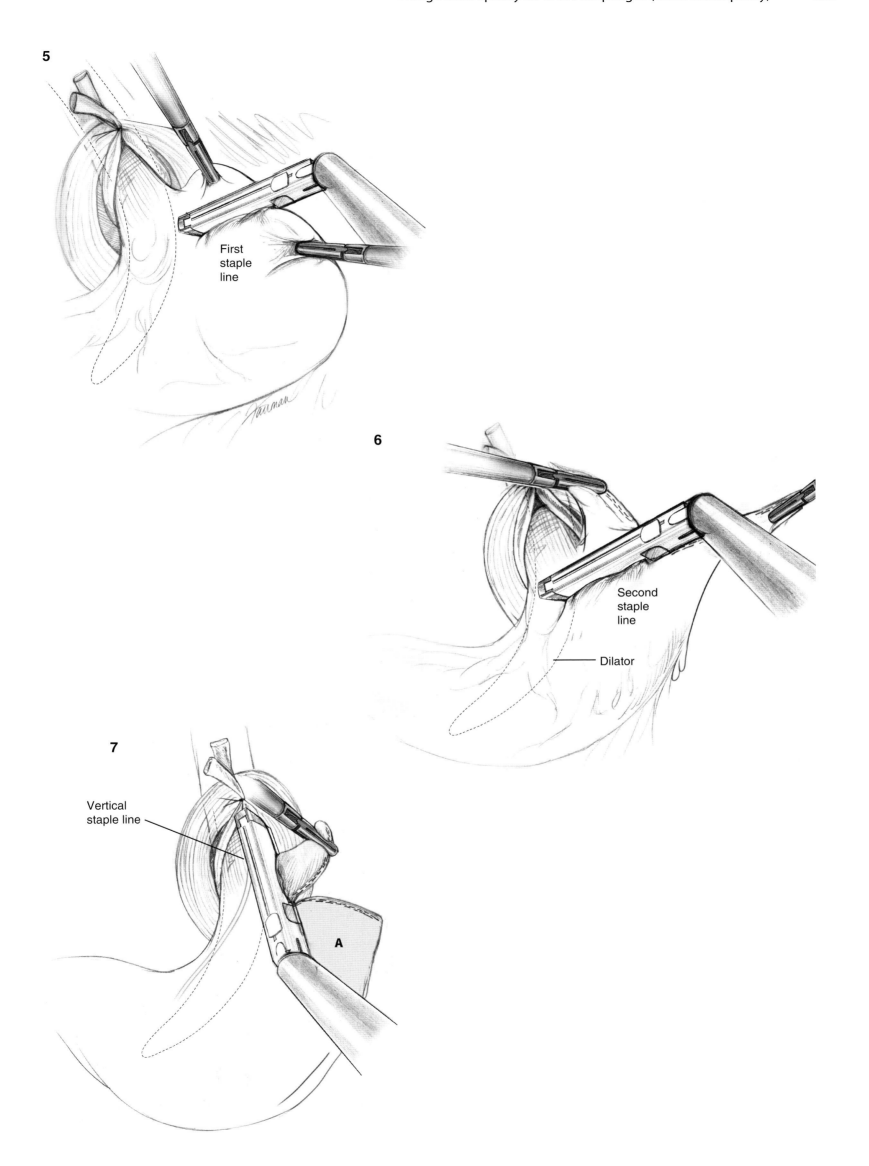

5

First
staple
line

6

Second
staple
line

Dilator

7

Vertical
staple line

A

DETAILS OF THE PROCEDURE The fundoplication is performed in the identical fashion to that described in the Nissen fundoplication chapter. The apex of the horizontal staple line will sit at the point of the superior or middle suture of the Nissen fundoplication and may be "tucked in" (**FIGURE 8**). With this technique, the vertical staple line is covered by the fundoplication and the horizontal staple lies adjacent to the esophagus. This places both staple lines against tissue and confines contamination if a small leak should occur.

The most critical step in creation of a Collis gastroplasty is to ensure that the first bite of the Nissen fundoplication is on the native esophagus and not on the newly created gastric tube (**FIGURE 9**). If the fundoplication is "wrapped" entirely around the gastric tube, a slipped Nissen has been created and the portion of the neoesophagus above the fundoplication will dilate significantly, allowing the fundoplication to become a point of esophageal outlet obstruction. Placing the highest fundoplication suture on the native esophagus leaves no opportunity for the creation of a "pseudo-antrum" above the fundoplication. Major critics of the Collis gastroplasty have often failed to observe this important nuance, which is necessary to obtain to good results. Following the completion of the fundoplication, the dilator is removed and the operation is completed as described in the Nissen fundoplication chapter (**FIGURE 10**).

Before removing trocars, it is important to return the patient to a level position and make sure the fundoplication fills the space immediately below the diaphragm. If a great deal of exposed esophagus lies within the abdominal cavity, the fundoplication may have been placed too low. Under these circumstances, the fundoplication is taken apart and reconfigured higher on the esophagus.

POSTOPERATIVE CARE A nasogastric tube is rarely needed after this procedure, but the patient is kept NPO until postoperative day 1, at which time a Gastrografin study is performed as a quality control measure to make sure that contrast readily passes into the stomach and that there are no leaks. Although esophageal edema is common, complete GE junction obstruction warrants reexploration immediately. ■

8

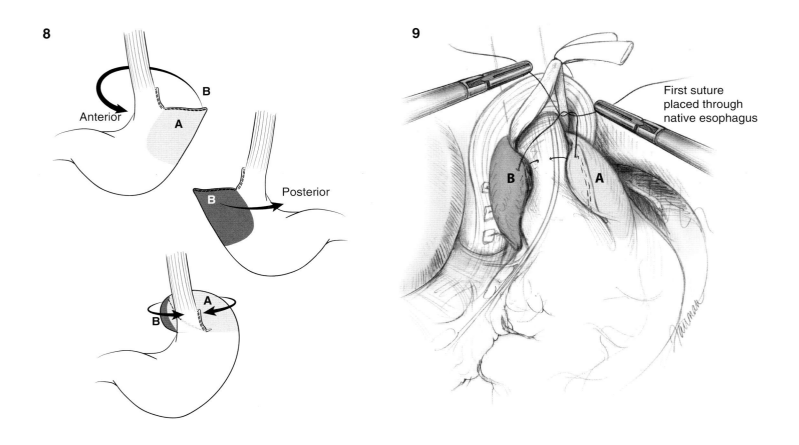

9

First suture placed through native esophagus

10

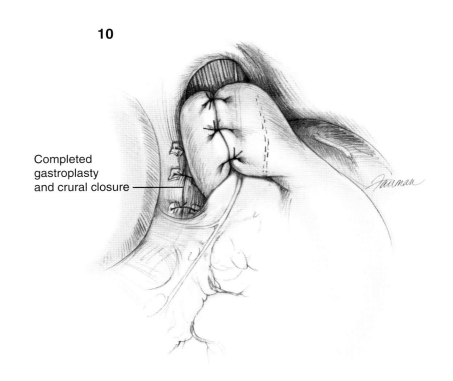

Completed gastroplasty and crural closure

Transhiatal Esophagectomy

INDICATIONS Transhiatal esophagectomy (THE) is indicated when two- or three-field transthoracic esophagectomy is unnecessary or when patient condition suggests that thoracotomy is risky. In patients with very early stage esophageal cancer, in which extended lymph node dissection is not necessary, i.e., Barrett esophagus with high grade dysplasia; or T1a esophageal cancer, THE is indicated. The frequency of lymph node (LN) metastases with T1b cancer warrants two- or three-field esophagectomy in the otherwise healthy patient with esophageal cancer. Lower esophageal adenocarcinoma or gastroesophageal (GE) junction cancer of more advanced stage can also be addressed with THE in the patient at excessive risk of complication after thoracotomy. Advanced cancers of the mid-esophagus should not be addressed with THE, as the midesophageal dissection is essentially blind, and therefore unsafe with THE. Benign indications for esophagectomy may be addressed with THE, with one caveat. The megaesophagus associated with end-stage achalasia is extremely vascular. Attempts to "strip" this esophagus from its mediastinal bed may result in large-volume bleeding. Direct transthoracic dissection (open or with thoracoscopy) is advisable in this setting (**FIGURE 1**).

PREOPERATIVE PREPARATION Patients undergoing minimally invasive esophagectomy must be carefully evaluated prior to surgery. The evaluation of a suspected malignancy includes a thorough staging workup. This should include computed tomography (CT) of the chest, abdomen, and pelvis; an esophagogastroduodenoscopy (EGD); a bronchoscopy for mid- to upper esophageal tumors; an endoscopic ultrasound; and a combined CT and positron emission tomography (PET) scan to provide clinical staging for all locally advanced tumors. Occasionally laparoscopic and/or thoracoscopic staging is needed to confirm or rule out extraesophageal metastases, but this is not routinely necessary. Cardiopulmonary risk stratification and optimization is pursued for all patients. Functional testing includes stair climbing and/or a 6-minute walk. Physiologic evaluation includes pulmonary function tests, an echocardiogram, and a stress test. Patients are placed on an exercise program, and smoking cessation is mandatory. In addition, all patients meet with a dietician preoperatively to promote nutritional optimization. In patients who are diabetic, tight control of serum blood glucose is achieved several weeks prior to surgery. Screening colonoscopy and visceral angiography are obtained in selected cases where there is a concern that the stomach will not be an adequate conduit for reconstruction. If there is any concern about other comorbidities, appropriate consultation is obtained preoperatively. Patients at high risk for arrhythmia or myocardial ischemia are placed on perioperative beta blockers. Anticoagulants, nonsteroidal anti-inflammatory agents, and antiplatelet agents are discontinued approximately 7 days prior to surgery if possible. Other preoperative medications are continued until the morning of surgery.

ANESTHESIA AND PATIENT POSITIONING Prophylactic antibiotics are administered and antiembolism pneumatic stockings are placed before the induction of general anesthesia. Preoperatively, cervical range of motion should be evaluated to gauge the patient's ability to tolerate varying degrees of extension necessary for completion of a cervical anastomosis. A single-lumen endotracheal tube is inserted. Two large-bore IVs or a central venous catheter is placed. If a central venous line is required, a right-sided subclavian or internal jugular approach should be used to maintain access to the left neck for the anastomosis. A radial artery line and Foley catheter are placed. On-table upper endoscopy is routinely performed to assess the location and extent of the tumor, the length of Barrett involvement, and the suitability and extent of the gastric conduit. This information solidifies preoperative planning for the surgical technique to be used. A nasogastric (NG) tube is passed into the stomach and placed on low continuous suction. A body warmer is applied after the final positioning, padding the pressure points, and securing the patient to the operating table.

The patient is placed in a supine split-legged position with padded leg straps and foot rests. This positioning allows for the patient to be placed into steep reverse Trendelenburg position, which improves exposure of upper abdominal anatomy. A large gel roll is placed transversely beneath the shoulder to facilitate extension of the neck. All pressure points are properly protected and padded. The surgeon stands between the patient's legs with the first assistant located at the patient's left, and the second assistant or scrub nurse stands at the patient's right (**FIGURE 2**).

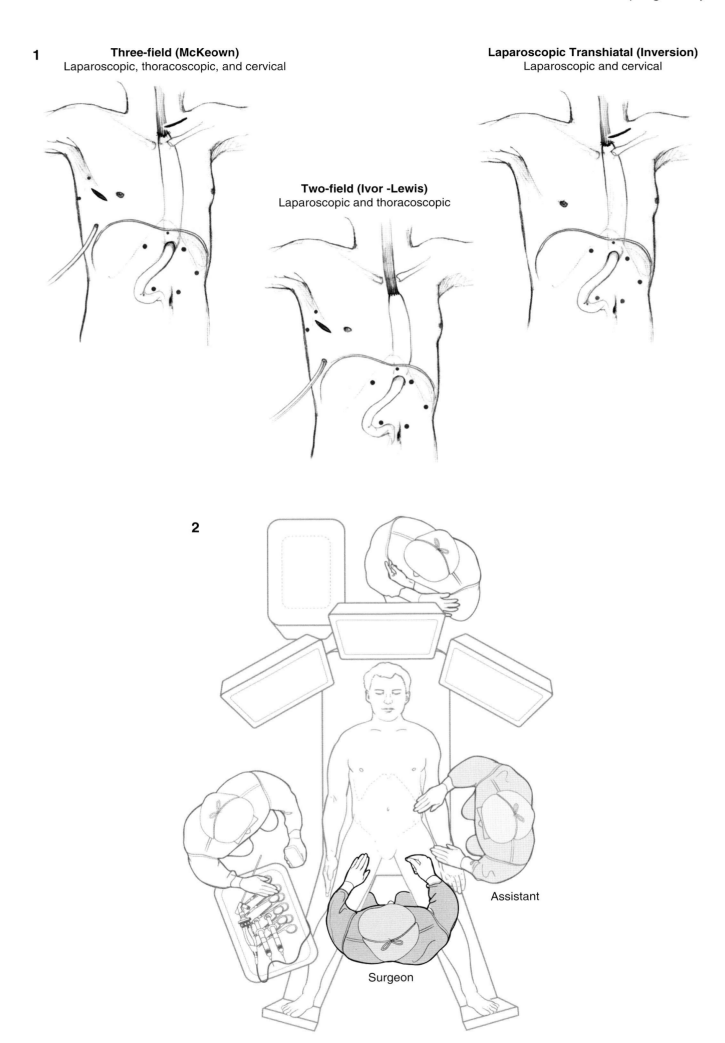

1

Three-field (McKeown)
Laparoscopic, thoracoscopic, and cervical

Two-field (Ivor -Lewis)
Laparoscopic and thoracoscopic

Laparoscopic Transhiatal (Inversion)
Laparoscopic and cervical

2

Assistant

Surgeon

PORT PLACEMENT The laparoscopic portion of the esophagectomy procedure is performed with a six-port technique. Three 5-mm ports, two 11- or 12-mm ports, and one 15-mm port are used (**FIGURE 3**). Precise localization of the laparoscopic ports is made according to the patient's body habitus. Although in patients with previous abdominal surgery the port placement may require a creative approach, the definitive port distribution generally approximates that for the Nissen fundoplication, but is 1 to 3 cm lower to allow access to the greater curvature of the stomach. Paradoxically, dropping the trocar positions lower is more important on thin individuals, as the diaphragms tend to be lower and flatter, moving the stomach a bit more inferiorly.

A CO_2 pneumoperitoneum is created using the Veress or Hasson technique as previously described in Chapter 2. The upper limit of insufflation pressure is set at 15 mmHg. The primary port is placed approximately 17 cm below the xiphoid to the left of the umbilicus. This placement facilitates alignment with the esophageal hiatus and its oblique entry into the abdominal cavity. The primary port serves as the location for the camera. The entire abdomen is closely examined for evidence of metastatic cancer, which may have not been detected with CT scan.

Subsequent upper abdominal ports should be placed high enough that the upper abdomen can be reached with the surgical instruments, but low enough to reasonably allow work along the greater curve of the stomach, the gastroepiploic arcade, and the pylorus. A 12-mm port is placed under direct vision approximately 12 cm lateral to the tip of the sternum, 3 cm inferior to the left costal margin. This port provides access for the surgeon's right hand. A third trocar is placed 8 cm lateral to the one previously described, along the same subcostal line. This 5-mm trocar serves as the primary port site for the first assistant. The fourth site of access is created immediately to the left of the xiphoid process for placement of the liver retractor. A 5-mm cutting trocar is used to create a passageway for the Nathanson liver retractor, which is placed through the track of the trocar (percutaneously) once the trocar is removed. The left lobe of the liver is elevated, and the Nathanson liver retractor is attached to a table-mounted holder (**FIGURE 4**). The fifth port is placed inferior to the right costal margin to the right of the falciform ligament. This 12-mm port provides access for the surgeon's left hand and for the endoscopic stapling device when the gastric conduit is created. This port site should be placed as far lateral as possible, without compromising access to the esophageal hiatus and posterior mediastinum. The sixth port site is placed in the patient's right midabdomen and is tailored based on internal anatomy. This 5-mm port provides access for the second assistant's instrument. It is through this port that the assistant elevates the gastric antrum during mobilization of the greater curvature.

3

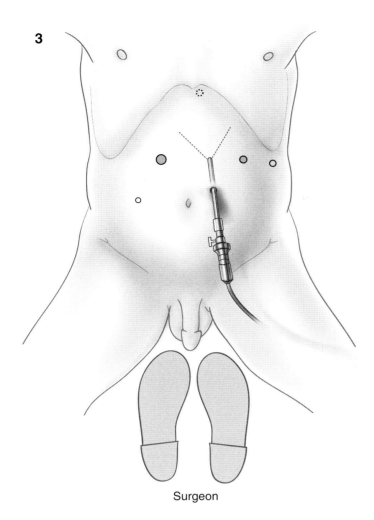

Surgeon

4

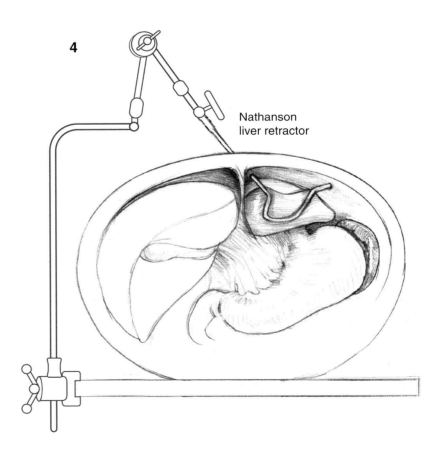

Nathanson
liver retractor

Esophageal and Gastric Mobilization The laparoscopic dissection starts by dividing the gastrohepatic ligament toward the right crus of the diaphragm with the ultrasonic dissector. The hepatic branch of the vagus nerve is divided. The first assistant grasps the epiphrenic fat pad and places the phrenoesophageal membrane on tension. The right crus is exposed and dissected from the top of the hiatus to the decussation with the left crus. This plane is then developed cephalad along the left crus to create a retroesophageal window (**FIGURE 5**). Care is taken during the early steps of the dissection to avoid entry into either thoracic cavity with subsequent loss of pneumoperitoneum. If early entry into either thoracic cavities occurs, a chest tube should be placed to suction to make sure both lungs are allowed to fully expand and all CO_2 is removed as it enters. We have also found that lowering the insufflating pressure in the abdomen minimizes the transdiaphragmatic air leak. In many cases, an adequate laparoscopic view can be maintained with insufflating pressures in the range of 8 to 12 mmHg.

Dissection is then taken to the superior portion of the esophageal hiatus toward the upper portion of the left crus. In this area, division of the upper phrenogastric attachments toward the highest short gastric vessels will help with mobilization of the spleen and cardia area away from the diaphragm. This generally makes division of the upper short gastric vessels easier.

At this point, attention is directed toward the greater curve of the stomach just opposite the inferior pole of the spleen. This anatomic landmark approximates the end of the left gastroepiploic arcade and the beginning of the short gastric vessels.

The assistant grasps the greater omentum adjacent to the greater curvature of the stomach and elevates it anteriorly and laterally. With the surgeon's left hand, the anterior wall of the stomach is retracted medially and posteriorly, toward the spine. The Harmonic scalpel is used to divide the gastrosplenic ligament and the intervening splenic vessels, entering the lesser sac in the progress (**FIGURE 6**). As the highest short gastric is approached, both surgeon and first assistant retract the stomach. The surgeon grasps the fundus of the stomach on the anterior surface, and the first assistant grasps the fundus of the stomach on the posterior surface. The surgeon retracts anteriorly and to the right. The first assistant retracts posteriorly and to the right. This opens up the field at the superior pole of the spleen (**FIGURE 7**). The retroesophageal plane is cleared more thoroughly as the greater curve of the stomach is rolled toward the right crus. All tissue posterior to the esophagus is cleared from the diaphragm (at the union of crura and over the preaortic fascia) and maintained en bloc with the esophagogastric junction. This includes the division of the posterior gastric artery, a branch of the splenic artery (**FIGURE 8**). As the GE junction is lifted and rolled to the right, the superior border of the pancreas and the splenic artery are visualized. As the surgeon proceeds along the left crus posteriorly, continuity is established with the right-sided dissection at the base of the right crus, and thus the posterior esophageal window is created. A Penrose drain is passed around the esophagus and secured with an Endoloop.

5

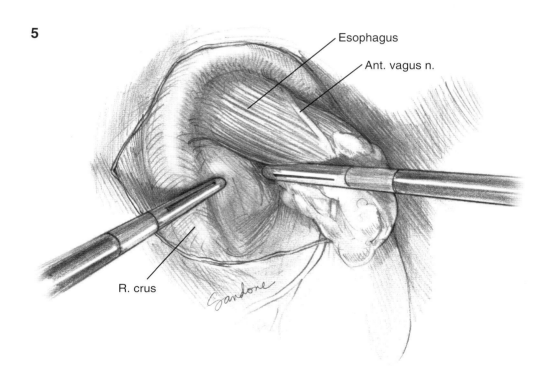

Esophagus

Ant. vagus n.

R. crus

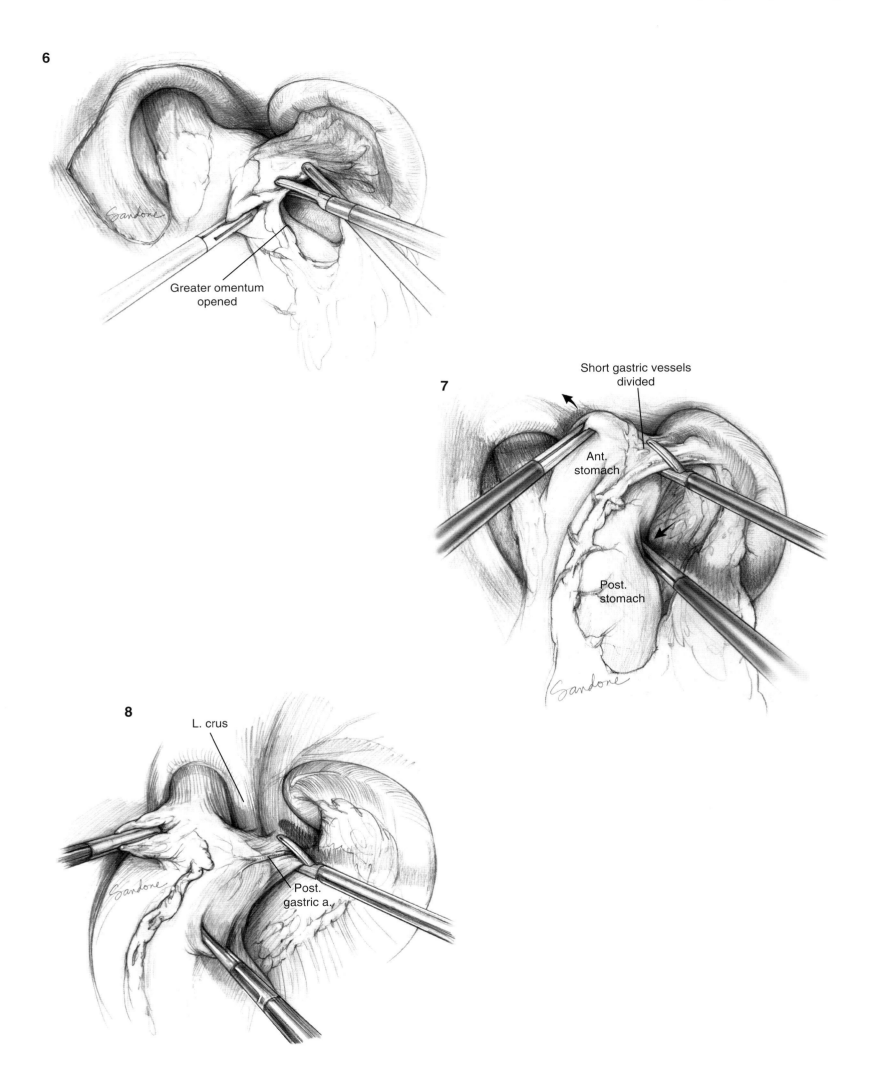

6

Greater omentum
opened

7

Short gastric vessels
divided

Ant.
stomach

Post.
stomach

Gandone

8

L. crus

Post.
gastric a.

Gandone

Esophageal and Gastric Mobilization The degree of central lymph node (LN) dissection is dependent on the indication for esophagectomy. When THE is performed for Barrett esophagus with high-grade dysplasia or benign disease, LN dissection is unnecessary. The peritoneum overlying the base of the left gastric vessels is opened to the base of the crura (**FIGURE 9**). A similar dissection behind the left gastric vessels, to the base of the diaphragm, thins out the pedicle adequately for stapling with a vascular load of the linear stapler (**FIGURE 10**).

When esophagectomy is performed for esophageal cancer, a complete dissection of LN stations 7, 8, 9, and 11 is performed, along the hepatic artery and the splenic artery at the superior pancreatic border. To expose this region for dissection, the first assistant slides an atraumatic grasper beneath the stomach to the left of the left gastric artery and elevates the stomach anteriorly. This places tension on the left gastric vessels and allows visualization in the retrogastric region. The second assistant may need to retract inferiorly (and gently) on the superior border of the pancreas to expose the LN basins along the hepatic and splenic arteries (**FIGURE 11**). In the course of this dissection, the left gastric vein is identified and divided with clips. The left gastric artery is divided at the level of the celiac trifurcation after clipping. Alternatively, the artery can be divided with the vascular load of a linear cutting stapler. The stapler can be placed through either upper abdominal port, whichever gives the best view of the closed stapler (**FIGURE 12**).

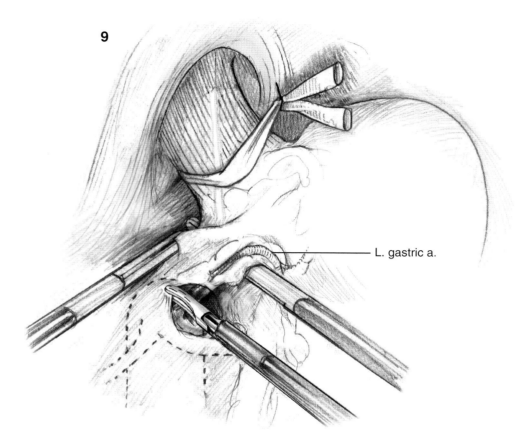

9

L. gastric a.

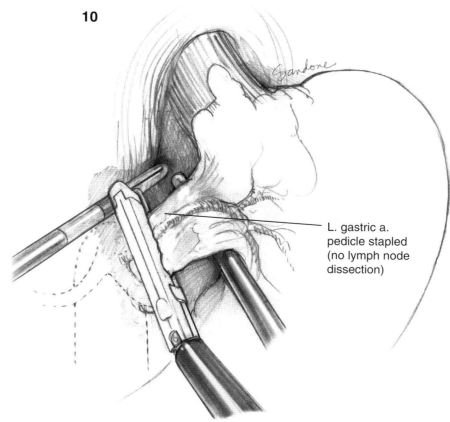

10

L. gastric a. pedicle stapled (no lymph node dissection)

11

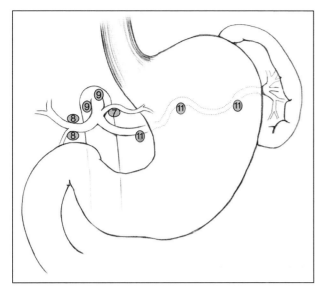

Lymph node dissection

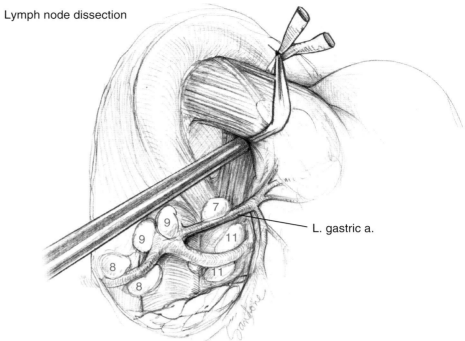

L. gastric a.

12   Left gastric a.

Splenic a.

Hepatic a.

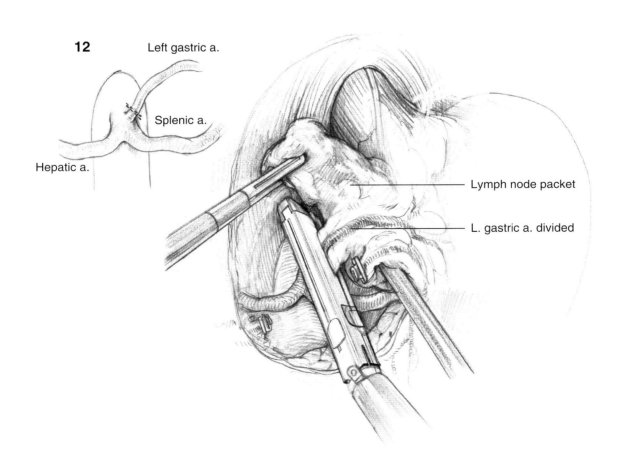

Lymph node packet

L. gastric a. divided

Esophageal and Gastric Mobilization The dissection along the greater curve is continued distally, dividing the left gastroepiploic artery and continuing through the gastrocolic omentum down the greater curvature toward the pylorus, outside of the right gastroepiploic arcade. This arcade must be identified and preserved, as it constitutes the major source of blood flow to the gastric tube. In addition, the transverse mesocolon may be fused to the gastrocolic omentum, putting the middle colic vessels at risk of injury by the unsuspecting surgeon. The first and second assistants grasp the body and antrum of the stomach, respectively, and retract in a superior and anterior direction. This movement serves to place the gastrocolic ligament on tension, displaying the gastroepiploic vessels and omentum to be divided (**FIGURE 13**). It is important to ensure that the entire gastrocolic omentum is divided all the way to the hepatic flexure, as undissected attachments between the pylorus and proximal transverse colon will limit a tension-free pull-up of the neoesophagus. At this point it becomes necessary for both assistants to grasp the posterior aspect of the stomach to facilitate mobilization of the posterior gastric wall away from the anterior surface of the pancreas (**FIGURE 14**). There are four potential pitfalls in this dissection: (1) injury to the transverse colon (especially in cases where diverticulosis is present); (2) injury to the transverse colon blood supply, especially when there is fusion of the greater omentum and transverse mesocolon; (3) gastric perforation secondary to overly aggressive retraction; and, perhaps most importantly, (4) injury to the right gastroepiploic vessels along the greater curvature of the stomach, or the gastroduodenal artery as it passes posterior to the duodenal bulb. The posterior gastric and duodenal dissection is completed at the point when the pulsations of the gastroduodenal artery are visualized. Care should be taken to preserve enough tissue to keep a healthy arcade without leaving excess tissue that will result in too much bulk on the gastric tube.

The dissection along the greater curve continues across the duodenum to the hepatoduodenal attachments. These are divided along the lateral duodenum and gallbladder area to complete the Kocher maneuver. This portion of the dissection is ergonomically easier if the surgeon moves their left-handed grasper to the lowest right-sided trocar, allowing an assistant on the right side of the table to elevate the gallbladder and the assistant on the left side of the table to retract the pylorus and proximal duodenum to the left (**FIGURE 15**). The Kocher is complete when the third portion of the duodenum is visualized as it curves back centrally and the pylorus is easily elevated to the diaphragmatic hiatus. If gentle lifting of the pylorus does not allow an easy, tension-free reach to the right crus, further duodenal and infrapyloric mobilization should be performed.

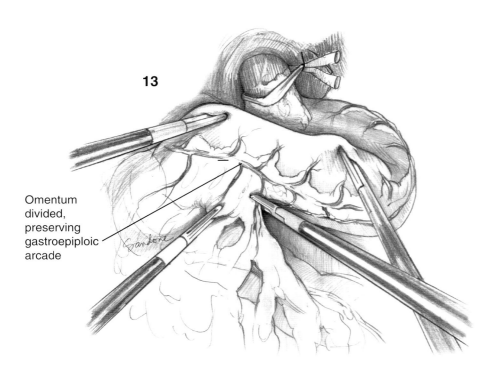

13

Omentum
divided,
preserving
gastroepiploic
arcade

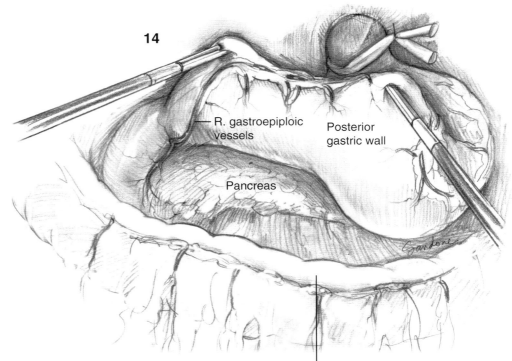

14

R. gastroepiploic
vessels

Posterior
gastric wall

Pancreas

Transverse colon

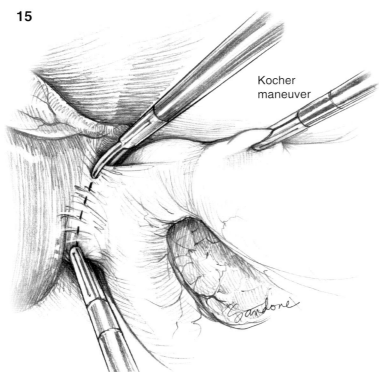

15

Kocher
maneuver

Creation of the Gastric Tube The NG tube is pulled back to a position within the thoracic esophagus, no more than 40 cm from the nasal ala. A site 2 to 4 cm proximal to the pylorus is identified on the gastric lesser curvature, sparing two or three branches of the right gastric artery. At the point selected, the lesser omentum is divided down to the substance of the stomach with the ultrasonic dissector in preparation for stapling. The right gastric artery is divided at the point where the conduit will be started. The surgeon and first assistant orient the stomach for conduit creation, working through the left upper and right lower ports (surgeon) and the left lower port (first assistant). The surgeon is responsible for orienting the lesser curvature for the stapler. The first assistant places another atraumatic grasper along the greater curve and gently stretches and flattens the stomach as the site for each stapler firing is chosen. The endoscopic tri-stapling device with a purple cartridge (or other equivalent stapler) is introduced through the 12-mm port site located in the patient's right upper abdomen. The first load is fired in a perpendicular orientation to the lesser curve and parallel to the greater curvature (**FIGURE 16**). Serial stapling is performed by the second assistant standing on the patient's right side to create a conduit approximately 3 to 4 cm wide. As the gastric tube stapling progresses cephalad, the first assistant's traction point is moved up the greater curvature to keep the tube "on stretch," lengthening it. Meanwhile, the surgeon is providing countertraction by pulling the staple lines toward the right lower quadrant and into the jaws of the stapler, with atraumatic graspers in both hands. The goal is to make the stomach appear like a taut tabletop before each firing of the stapler (**FIGURE 17**). In patients with cancer, once the neoesophagus is completed, the distal margin on the specimen side is sent for frozen section examination. This tissue is obtained with an endoscopic stapler to avoid opening the proximal stomach, usually at the far end of the staple line, nearest to the GE junction.

Attention is turned to the distal esophageal mobilization. With the first assistant grasping the Penrose drain, the esophagus and stomach are retracted inferiorly and slightly to the patient's left. The distal esophagus is circumferentially mobilized with its accompanying lymphatic tissue. The posterior mediastinum is cleared of all tissue to visualize the pericardium anteriorly, the right and left pleura laterally, and the surface of the aorta posterolaterally. Lymph nodes and periesophageal fat are generally left with the specimen but may be individually removed if they separate from the specimen during dissection. When high-grade dysplasia or benign disease is the diagnosis, the dissection may stay closer to the esophagus. Dissection is carried cephalad as far as safe visualization allows. At the completion of this lower mediastinal dissection, the anterior and posterior vagus nerves are divided with the Harmonic scalpel, critical to the removal of the esophagus (**FIGURE 18**).

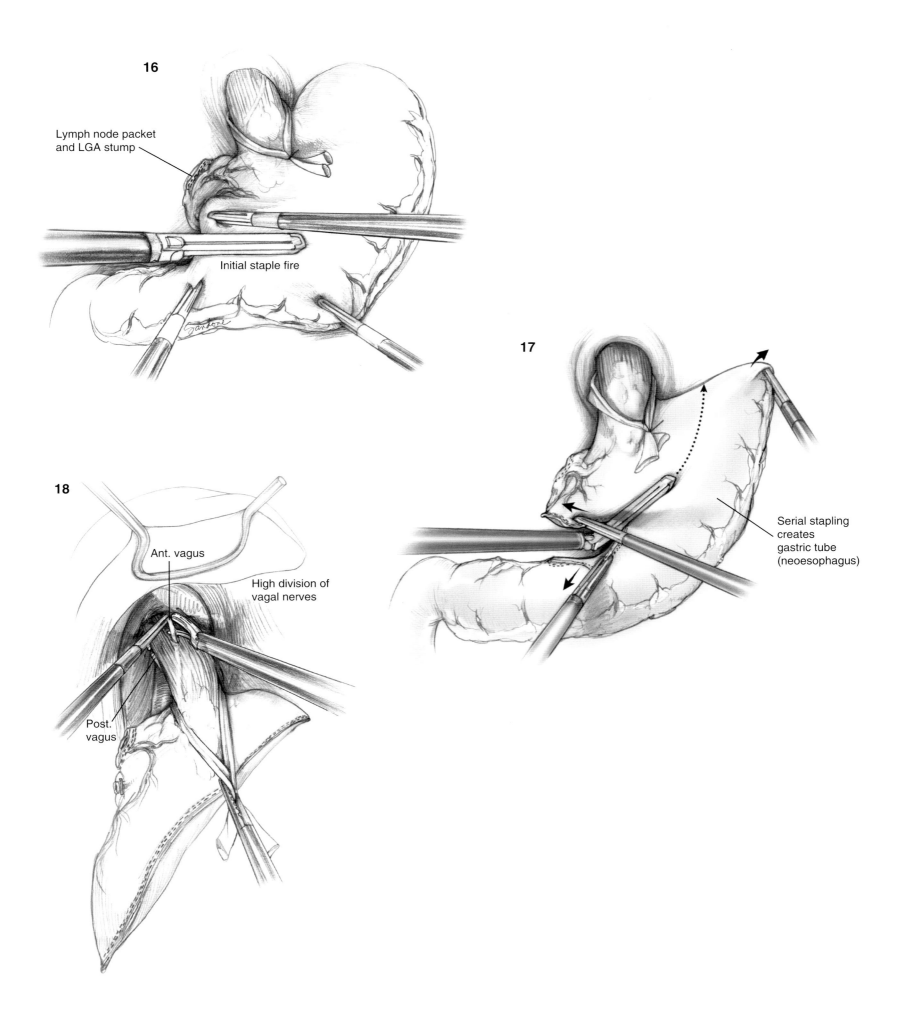

16

Lymph node packet and LGA stump

Initial staple fire

17

Serial stapling creates gastric tube (neoesophagus)

18

Ant. vagus

High division of vagal nerves

Post. vagus

Pyloroplasty or Pyloromyotomy At this point pyloroplasty can be performed (**FIGURES 19 AND 20**). We preferentially perform pyloromyotomy. A suture is placed across the pyloric muscle superiorly and elevated by the second assistant through the right upper quadrant port. With the heel of an "L" hook, the serosa overlying the pylorus is scored (**FIGURE 21**). The hook is then slipped along the gastric mucosa, beneath the pyloric muscle, which is elevated and divided with the hook (**FIGURE 22**). The pyloromyotomy is spread open with an atraumatic grasper, which allows visualization of the base of the gastric and duodenal mucosa, ensuring that all muscle fibers have been divided (**FIGURE 23**). If the mucosa is perforated, the pyloromyotomy is converted to a pyloroplasty.

19

Pyloroplasty   **20**

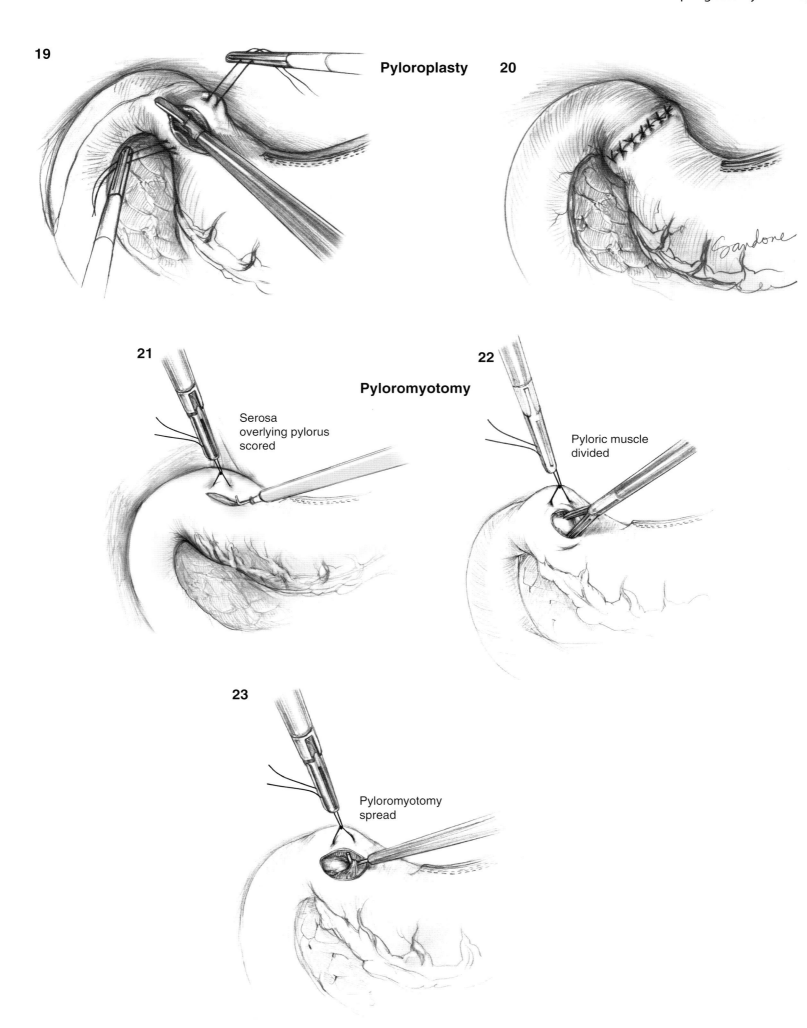

21

Pyloromyotomy   **22**

Serosa
overlying pylorus
scored

Pyloric muscle
divided

23

Pyloromyotomy
spread

CERVICAL PHASE

Position For the cervical esophageal mobilization, the surgeon stands on the patient's left side with the neck extended by a gel roll beneath the shoulders (**FIGURE 24**). A first assistant stands on the patient's right side.

Exposure of the Cervical Esophagus A 5-cm transverse incision is made in the left neck approximately one fingerbreadth above the clavicle (**FIGURE 25**). The subcutaneous tissue and platysma muscle are divided using electrocautery, thereby exposing the anterior border of the sternocleidomastoid muscle. Subplatysmal flaps are elevated to the level of the thyroid cartilage superiorly and the clavicle inferiorly. The field is held open with skin hooks. A blunt, self-retaining retractor (Weitlaner retractor) is applied to the skin edges medially and the sternocleidomastoid muscle laterally. The omohyoid muscle will be identified running in a transverse plane across the wound. This muscle is divided, exposing the internal jugular vein. The lateral border of the sternothyroid and the sternohyoid muscles are grasped with Allis clamps, sequentially, and a Kittner is used to free the muscle bellies, posteriorly. The branches of the ansa cervicalis nerve, inserting into the lateral aspect of the sternothyroid muscle, are divided with bipolar electrosurgery. Both muscles are divided over a right-angle clamp below the inferior pole of the thyroid, to maximize exposure of the esophagus.

Next, the left lobe of the thyroid gland is carefully grasped with one or two Babcock clamps and retracted medially (**FIGURE 26**). Should the middle thyroid vein or inferior thyroid artery limit access to the esophagus, they are ligated with fine silk suture and divided. During this portion of the procedure, the surgeon's and assistants' fingers are used for retraction. We avoid using any metal retractors deep in the neck, to avoid traction injury on the recurrent laryngeal nerve or the vagus nerve (**FIGURE 27**).

At this point, the superior mediastinum should be easily accessed by placing a finger along the anterior spine and using blunt dissection to open this space. With the assistant's index finger rotating and retracting the trachea medially, and the surgeon retracting the carotid sheath laterally with the index finger of their left hand, the esophagus and recurrent laryngeal nerve become apparent. After sharply incising the fine attachments posterolateral to the tracheoesophageal groove, the anterior wall of the esophagus can be mobilized away from the membranous trachea, using blunt dissection. This is continued in superior and inferior directions, so as to increase esophageal mobility. The lateral and posterior aspects of the esophagus are mobilized with blunt dissection using a Kittner and a finger. Once the esophagus is circumferentially mobilized, an umbilical tape is passed around the esophagus with a finger or a renal pedicle clamp (**FIGURE 28**). Further blunt dissection between the esophagus, trachea, spine and superior mediastinal structures is carried inferiorly as far as the finger will reach.

Despite the thorough dissection through the hiatus, from below, and through the thoracic inlet, from above, the midportion of the esophagus will still be attached. In the absence of cancer, inflammation, or fibrosis, this portion of the esophagus may be "stripped" out using a vein stripper. Although the esophagus may be removed with antegrade or retrograde "stripping," antegrade inversion is our preference, as it preserves the GE junction and does not expose the inside of the esophagus or stomach to the abdomen, mediastinum, or abdominal wall, eliminating the possibility of cancer seeding or infection of the operative field. We describe both techniques here.

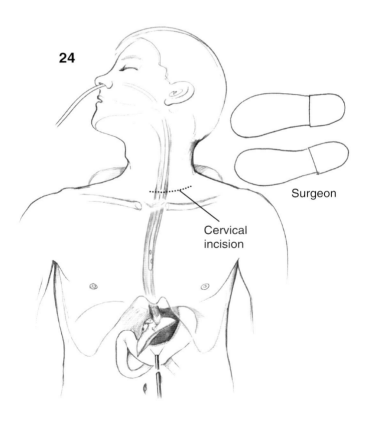

24

Surgeon

Cervical
incision

25

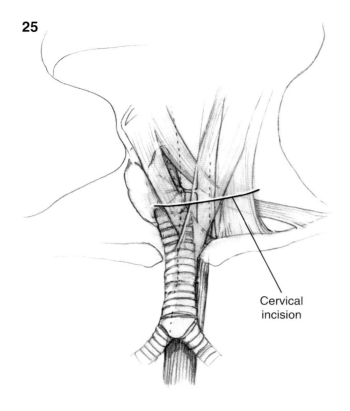

Cervical
incision

26

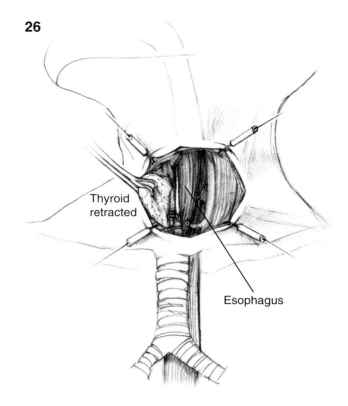

Thyroid
retracted

Esophagus

27

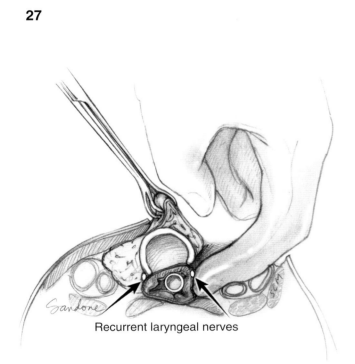

Recurrent laryngeal nerves

28

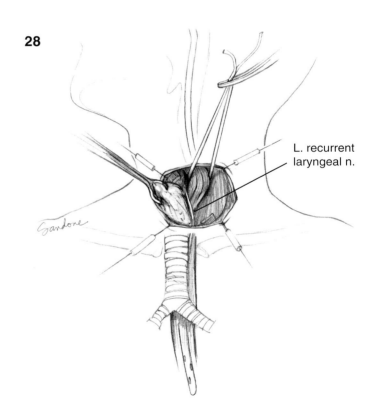

L. recurrent
laryngeal n.

Antegrade Inversion After maximal inferior dissection of the esophagus, a stay suture is placed through the lateral esophageal wall as low as is possible. The NG tube is pulled back so it sits just above the point of the esophagus to be divided. The cervical esophagus is divided above the suture with the endoscopic stapler, preserving as much length of cervical esophagus as is possible. A second stay suture is placed at the far end of the staple line, and a small esophagotomy is made midway along the staple line for the passage of the vein stripper (**FIGURE 29**).

The vein stripper is passed distally until it is visible with the laparoscope in the devascularized lesser curvature gastric remnant. The vein stripper is guided to the tip of this remnant. A suture is placed through the esophageal wall and around the vein stripper (**FIGURE 30**) to eliminate leaks from the esophagotomy and to prevent the vein stripper from tearing through the esophageal wall.

A medium-sized vein stripper "olive" is attached to the cervical end of the vein stripper and a long o-silk suture is tied just beneath the olive before inversion (**FIGURES 31–33**). This suture will preserve the mediastinal track of the esophagus after the esophagus has been extracted. The far end of this suture is secured with a hemostat so that it will not be accidentally pulled into the mediastinum during esophageal extraction.

Antegrade Inversion Technique

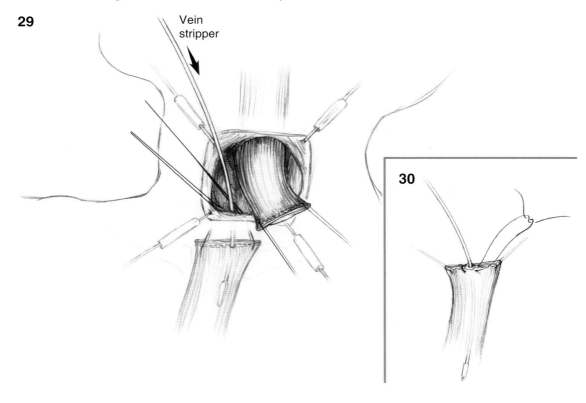

29   Vein stripper

30

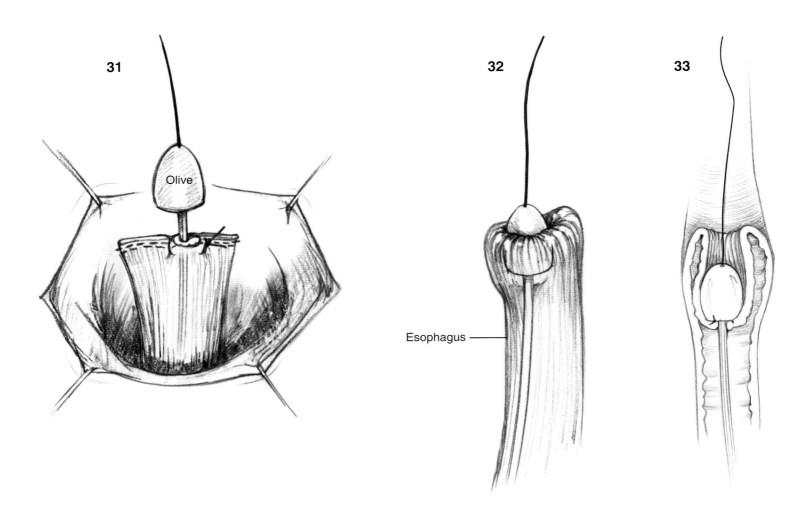

31   Olive

32   Esophagus

33

Antegrade Inversion The tip of the gastric remnant, with the vein stripper in it, is pulled out the left subcostal port site (**FIGURE 34**). It is necessary to enlarge this port site with scalpel and electrosurgical division of the fascia to allow the specimen to be extracted. The port is removed as the specimen is pulled out, and the tip of the stomach is secured between two hemostats. The wound is protected with sponges, and the tip of the gastric staple line is opened with scissors to retrieve the tip of the vein stripper.

The two stay sutures are removed from the divided esophagus in the neck, and inferior traction on the vein stripper starts the stripping process (**FIGURE 35**). As the "rolling edge" of the inversion reaches the diaphragm, it may be possible to laparoscopically visualize the vagal trunks if they have not been previously divided (**FIGURE 35, INSET**). Once the inverted esophagus emerges through the hiatus, connected to the neck only by the silk suture, traction on the vein stripper stops, and the entire specimen is pulled through the abdominal wall, en bloc (**FIGURE 36**). The silk suture is divided and the distal end is returned to the abdomen. In this fashion, the devascularized gastric remnant serves as a wound protector as well as a conduit for the vein stripper, ensuring that the wound will not be contaminated with viable tumor cells. The suture maintains the esophageal tract from the neck to the hiatus (**FIGURES 37 AND 38**).

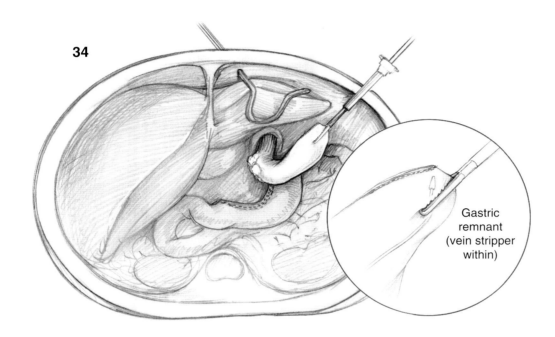

34

Gastric remnant (vein stripper within)

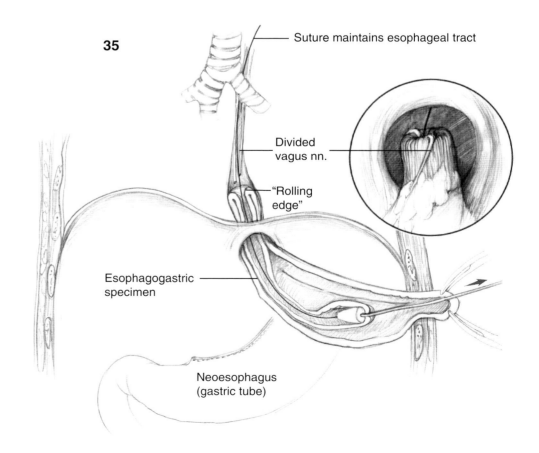

35

Suture maintains esophageal tract

Divided vagus nn.

"Rolling edge"

Esophagogastric specimen

Neoesophagus (gastric tube)

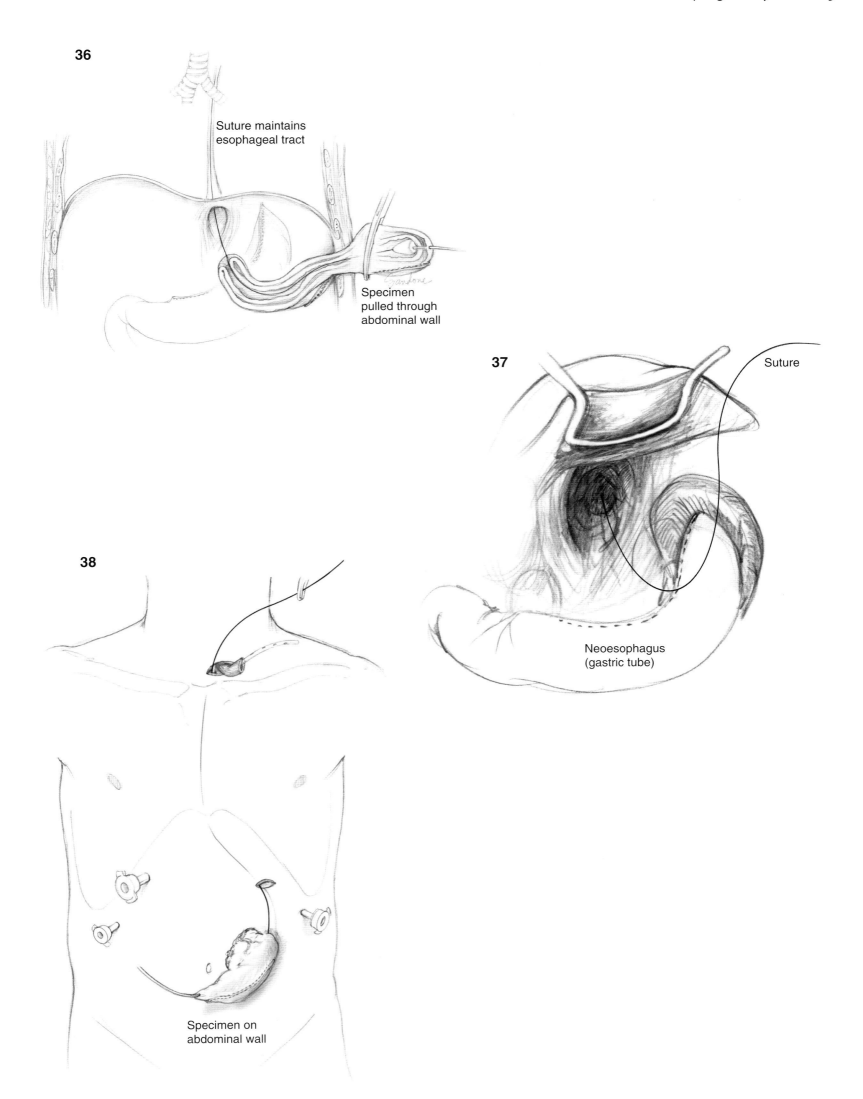

36

Suture maintains
esophageal tract

Specimen
pulled through
abdominal wall

37

Suture

Neoesophagus
(gastric tube)

38

Specimen on
abdominal wall

Antegrade Inversion At the cervical incision, a 28 French chest tube is "bridled" to the long mediastinal suture and pulled down into the abdomen (**FIGURE 39**). A clamp is placed on the end of the chest tube to prevent loss of the pneumoperitoneum. The chest tube is guided into the posterior mediastinum, while the surgeon pulls on the silk suture from below. The tube is maneuvered into the abdomen, and the proper anatomic space is maintained for gastric pull-up. The tip of the neoesophagus is sutured to the end of the chest tube with two 0-silk sutures (**FIGURE 40**). Proper orientation of the neoesophagus is verified prior to pull-up. The chest tube is gently withdrawn through the cervical incision as the surgeon and first assistant assist from below (**FIGURE 41**). Once the neoesophagus can be palpated within the superior mediastinum, it is grasped and gently pulled into the cervical wound.

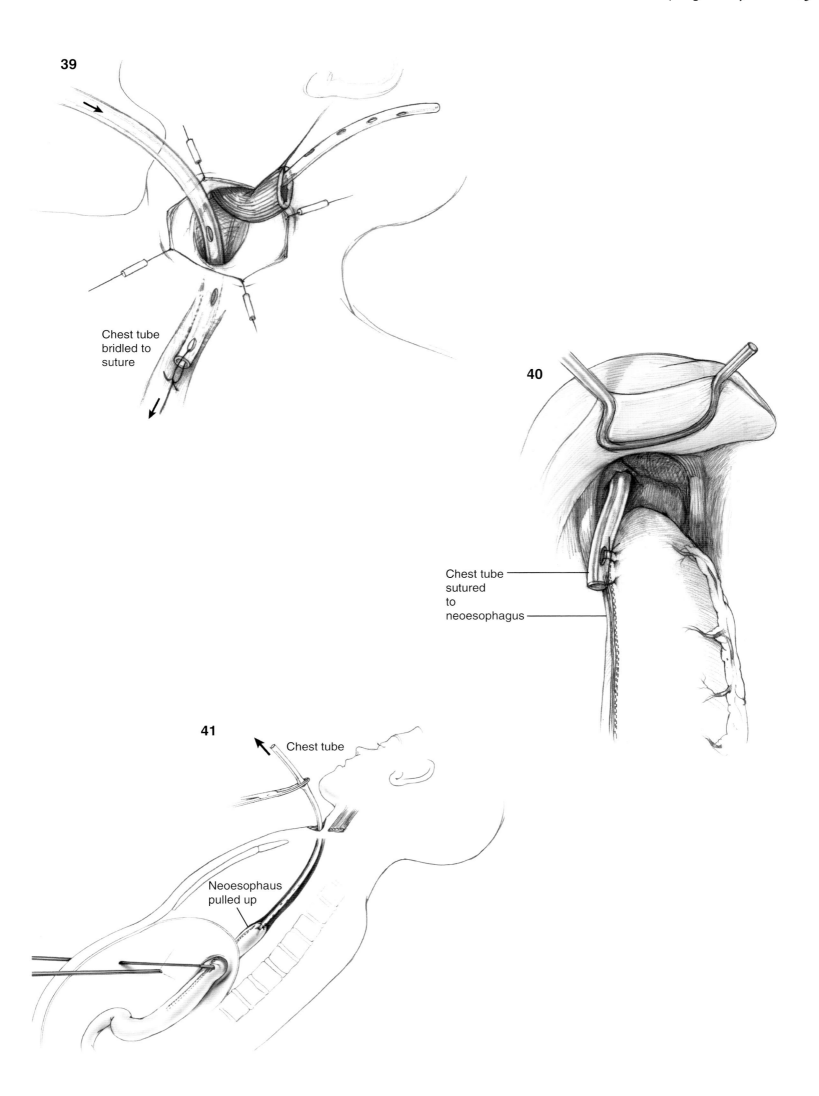

39

Chest tube bridled to suture

40

Chest tube sutured to neoesophagus

41

Chest tube

Neoesophaus pulled up

Cervical Anastomosis The method of anastomosis can be hand sewn, side-to-side stapled, or end-to-side stapled. We perform a stapled, end-to-side cervical anastomosis as described by Orringer. The staple line of the lesser curvature resection site is maintained toward the right. If the tip of the conduit is redundant or ischemic, it is removed with an linear stapling device. The staple line may be oversewn with interrupted sutures.

A traction suture is placed on the neoesophagus at the inferior aspect of the cervical incision to elevate it to the skin level. A second stay stitch is placed in the anterior wall of the remaining esophagus to keep it oriented correctly. The staple line on the residual esophagus is removed and the NG tube is pulled out and tucked out of the way. By lowering the cut end of the remaining esophagus to the conduit, the site of anastomosis is defined. A 1.5-cm gastrotomy is created on the anterior wall of the stomach, adjacent to the greater curvature, and just above the gastric stay stitch. Two sutures are used to line up the posterior corner of the divided esophagus to the edges of the gastrotomy. A 45-mm-long linear stapling device (purple cartridge or equivalent) is introduced into the esophagus and gastrotomy. The thinner anvil of the stapler is inserted through the gastrotomy, and the cartridge side is placed within the esophagus. The traction sutures are drawn inferiorly as the stapler is advanced (**FIGURE 42**). It is critical that the posterior wall of the esophagus and anterior wall of the stomach be appropriately aligned and that the gastric conduit staple line not be included in the esophagogastrostomy. The stapler is fired and the anastomosis is inspected for hemostasis. The NG tube is carefully passed through the anastomosis and positioned distally in the gastric conduit, bridging the diaphragm (**FIGURE 43**). This is done under laparoscopic visualization. The gastrotomy and esophagotomy are closed in two layers, with 3-0 monofilament absorbable suture in a running fashion, followed by interrupted Lembert sutures (**FIGURE 44**).

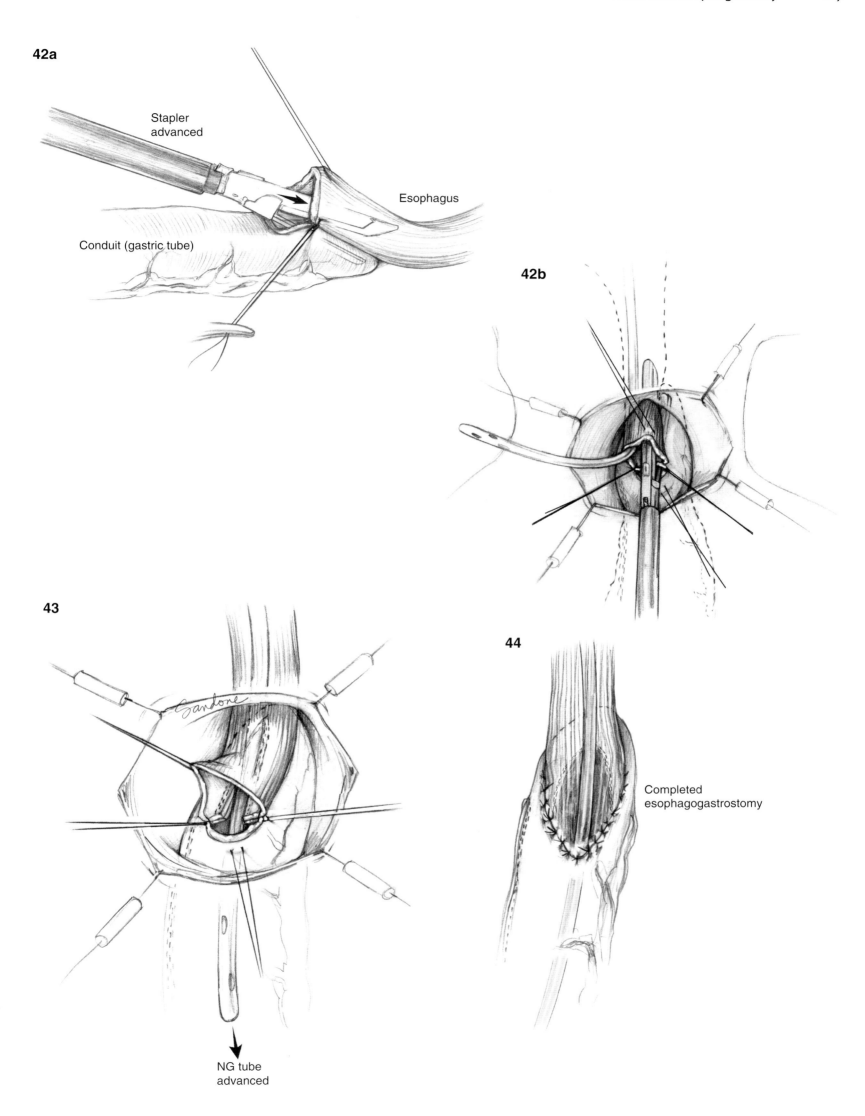

42a

Stapler
advanced

Esophagus

Conduit (gastric tube)

42b

43

44

Completed
esophagogastrostomy

NG tube
advanced

Cervical Anastomosis The esophagus and anastomosis are returned to the posterior mediastinum behind the trachea, the field is irrigated, and a Jackson-Pratt (JP) drain is placed alongside the anastomosis for several days to remove all serosanguinous fluid from the operative field (**FIGURE 45**). The platysma is reapproximated with a running absorbable suture, and the skin is closed with a running monofilament absorbable subcuticular suture. A jejunostomy tube is placed and all abdominal incisions are closed (**FIGURE 46**). It is necessary to perform fascial closure on the port site from which the specimen was extracted, but all other port sites may be managed with skin closure only.

Retrograde Inversion (Alternative) The retrograde inversion of the esophagus was the first technique to be developed, as it provides excellent visualization of the mediastinal dissection, but the shortcomings of this approach, mentioned earlier, limit its use to non-neoplastic indications for esophagectomy.

Once the mediastinal dissection is complete, the NG tube is pulled back and the esophagogastric junction (EGJ) is divided with an endoscopic stapling device placed through the right upper quadrant 15-mm port

(**FIGURE 47**). The free piece of stomach is removed in a specimen bag and sent to pathology.

The esophagus is mobilized in the neck as previously described. Two 3-0 silk sutures are placed in the distal cervical esophagus, and it is elevated into the wound. A small cervical esophagotomy is created and a vein stripper is passed distally (**FIGURE 48**). The vein stripper is advanced until the tip can be seen protruding at the staple line of the EGJ division site. The ultrasonic shears are used to create a small enterotomy in the middle of the EGJ staple line, and the vein stripper is passed through this opening and withdrawn through the 12-mm right upper abdominal port site. The 12-mm port is completely removed, and the medium-sized "olive" is attached to the end of the vein stripper. In addition, a 100-cm silk suture is tied to the end of the vein stripper. The vein stripper and silk suture are placed back into the peritoneal cavity, and the 12-mm port is replaced. With the first and second assistants grasping the staple line and retracting inferiorly, the staple line and enterotomy site is reinforced with a 0-silk horizontal mattress suture (**FIGURE 49**).

The vein stripper is gently withdrawn through the cervical esophagotomy, beginning the outside-to-in inversion of the distal esophagus (**FIGURES 50–52**).

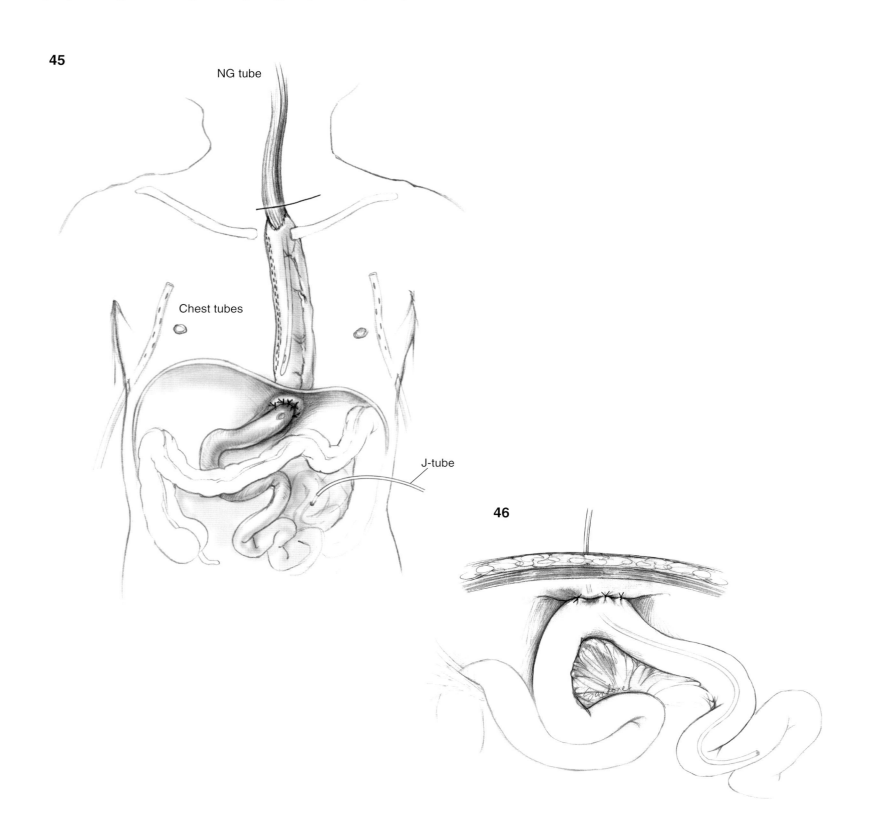

45

NG tube

Chest tubes

J-tube

46

Retrograde Inversion Technique

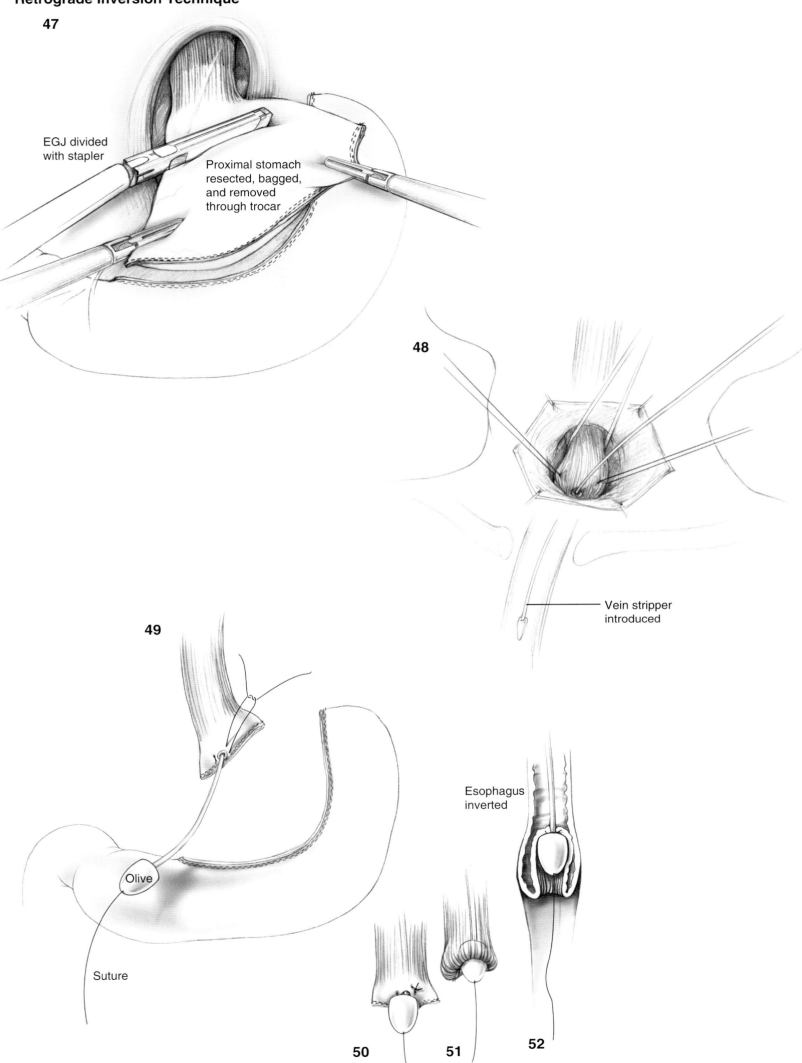

47

EGJ divided with stapler

Proximal stomach resected, bagged, and removed through trocar

48

Vein stripper introduced

49

Olive

Suture

Esophagus inverted

50   **51**   **52**

Retrograde Inversion (Alternative) It may be necessary to use bariatric-length instruments and laparoscope as the inversion proceeds into the high posterior mediastinum (**FIGURE 53**). The rolled edge of the esophagus can be grasped and mediastinal attachments can be divided under direct vision (**FIGURE 54**). These points of attachment can be accentuated by moving the vein stripper in and out in small increments (**FIGURE 55**).

Once the end of the vein stripper reaches the cervical esophagus, the cervical esophagotomy is extended distally to provide passage for the bulky specimen on the end of the vein stripper (**FIGURE 56**). Blunt transcervical finger dissection will facilitate the completion of the inversion part of the procedure. The cervical esophagus is divided at the site of the inversion (**FIGURE 57**). The length of the silk suture, which has been brought up to the neck with the inversion, should be preserved. The proximal margin of the esophagus is identified and sent for intraoperative histologic examination. The cervical anastomosis and closure is performed as previously described. ■

53

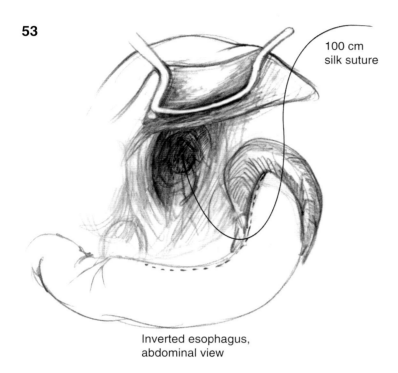

100 cm
silk suture

Inverted esophagus,
abdominal view

54

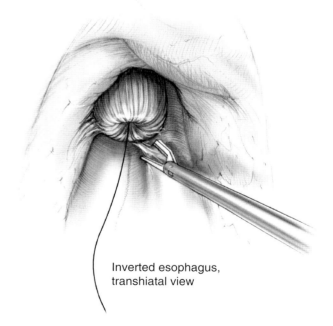

Inverted esophagus,
transhiatal view

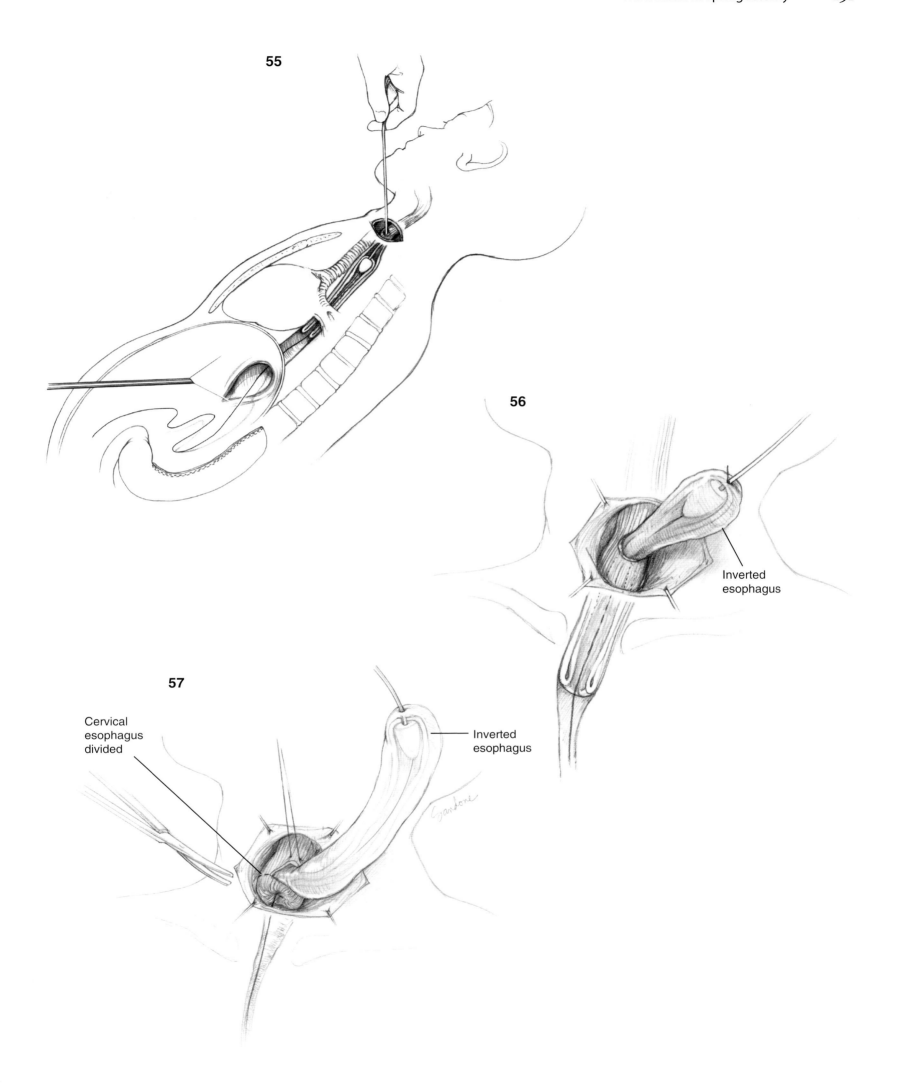

55

56

Inverted
esophagus

57

Cervical
esophagus
divided

Inverted
esophagus

CLOSURE OF PERFORATED DUODENAL ULCER

INDICATIONS The laparoscopic approach is indicated in patients with a suspected or confirmed perforation of a duodenal ulcer. It is a suitable alternative to the standard open Graham patch repair, except in cases of prior upper abdominal surgery. Simple closure of the perforation is indicated for patients with ongoing instability, delayed presentation, or prohibitive medical comorbidities.

Rarely is "definitive" ulcer surgery indicated, but it may be considered for those who are *Helicobacter pylori* negative, do not use nonsteroidal anti-inflammatory agents (NSAIDs), and have well-documented recurrent peptic ulcer disease. In the absence of gastric outlet obstruction, the operation of choice is highly selective vagotomy. In the presence of gastric outlet obstruction, antrectomy and reconstruction or gastrojejunostomy may be considered.

PREOPERATIVE PREPARATION These patients classically present with a history of previously diagnosed peptic ulcers or may report long-term use of NSAIDs. A plain film radiograph may show free air. The diagnosis may be confirmed with an upper gastrointestinal radiograph with water-soluble contrast, not barium. However, a prolonged workup to confirm a diagnosis may be counterproductive, as early surgical intervention is usually warranted.

The patient should have good intravenous access and be adequately resuscitated. Appropriate antibiotic coverage should be given preoperatively.

ANESTHESIA General anesthesia with endotracheal intubation is necessary for this operation. Complete neuromuscular blockade is required. Given the incidence of concurrent gastritis in these patients, the use of ketorolac for pain control should be avoided in the postoperative period.

POSITION The patient is positioned supine in modified lithotomy with arms tucked at the sides. The surgeon stands between the legs, and the assistant stands to the left side of the patient. The operative monitors are placed above the patient's head (**FIGURE 1**).

OPERATIVE PREPARATION A Foley catheter and orogastric tube are placed after the induction of anesthesia. The abdomen of the patient from the nipple lines to the pubis is shaved with clippers after induction of anesthesia, and the abdomen is sterilely prepped.

DETAILS OF PROCEDURE

Trocar Position Because the abdominal wall is thinnest in the region of the umbilicus, this operation commences with insufflation of the abdomen using the Veress needle technique placed through the umbilicus. Alternatively, initial access may be achieved using the Hasson technique at the umbilicus.

The procedure may be performed with a three-trocar technique (**FIGURE 2**). A 10-mm cannula for the endoscope is placed at the umbilicus. Depending on the size of the patient and distance to the stomach, the camera port may need to be placed more cephalad along the midline. A 5-mm port is placed in the right subcostal region at the midclavicular line, and an additional 10-mm port is placed in the left subcostal region at the midclavicular line. If the liver is adherent to the site of perforation, an additional trocar at the subxiphoid position may be necessary for placement of a Nathanson or fan-type retractor to elevate the liver.

The patient is placed in a moderate reverse Trendelenburg position to allow the small bowel and colon to slide away from the stomach. A thorough exploration and lavage of the abdomen is performed to rule out other causes of pneumoperitoneum, such as perforated diverticulitis.

The site, size, and probable cause of the perforation should be noted. A large perforation that extends to the posterior surface of the duodenum may be difficult to repair adequately using the laparoscopic approach. If the perforation is in the stomach, the possibility of gastric malignancy or lymphoma should be considered.

The perforation is closed with three or more nonabsorbable interrupted sutures placed at least 7 mm from the edges of the perforation (**FIGURE 3**). The sutures should be tied as they are placed, but the tails are left uncut at 3 to 4 cm long. A portion of the omentum is laid over the site of perforation, and the suture tails are tied above the omental patch to secure it in place (**FIGURES 4 AND 5**).

The perforation site is irrigated to remove any remaining debris. Methylene blue may be instilled into the stomach through the nasogastric tube to confirm complete closure of the perforation. A drain may be placed if desired.

POSTOPERATIVE CARE The nasogastric tube should initially be left in place on low continuous suction to allow for decompression of the stomach. It is removed as soon as output is decreased and any abdominal distension is resolved. Perforation and leakage of gastric contents into the peritoneal cavity may cause the equivalent of a chemical burn, and these patients may develop a significant inflammatory response and third-spacing of fluid. Aggressive fluid resuscitation is warranted. Intravenous antibiotics are maintained until the patient becomes afebrile. It is essential to check serology for *H. pylori*, and triple therapy is initiated once the patient tolerates oral intake. Acid suppression with a proton pump inhibitor should be continued in patients with complicated peptic ulcer disease. ■

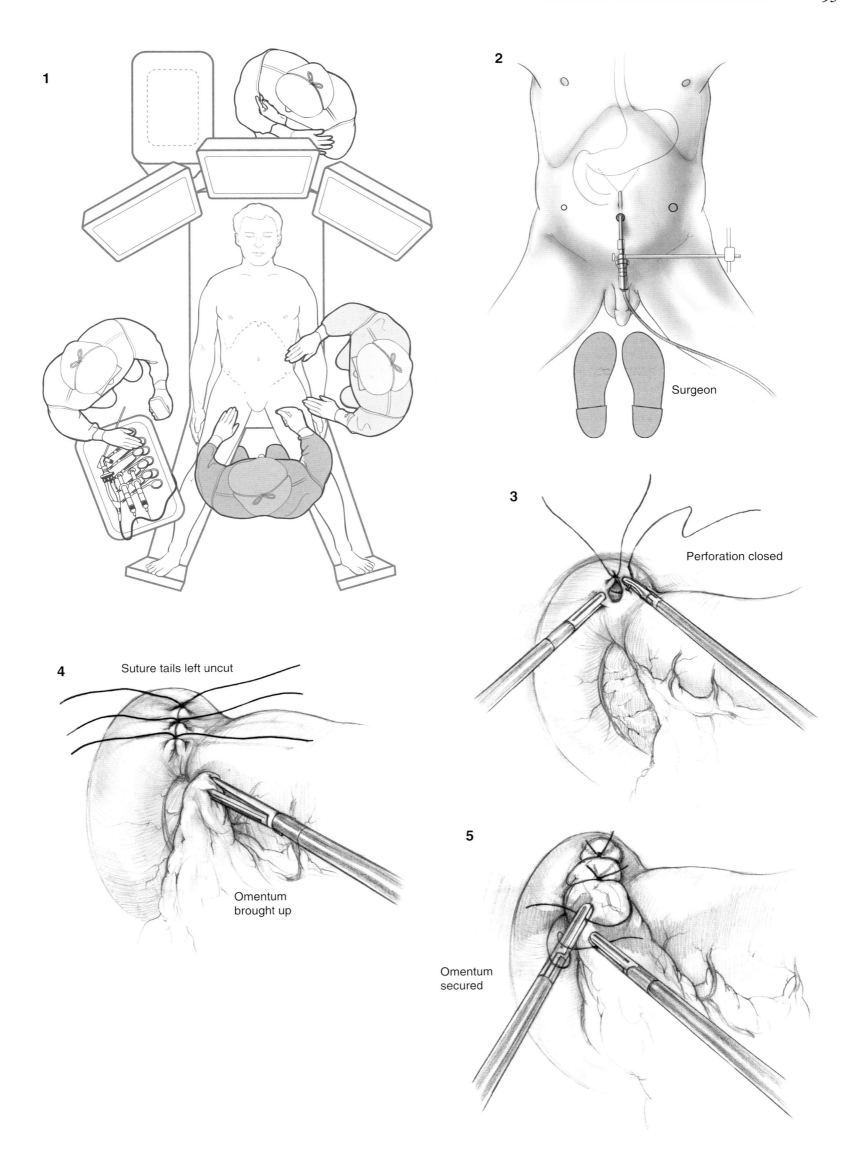

1

2

Surgeon

3

Perforation closed

4 Suture tails left uncut

Omentum
brought up

5

Omentum
secured

PYLOROPLASTY

INDICATIONS Laparoscopic pyloroplasty is most frequently performed as an adjunct to laparoscopic Nissen fundoplication for patients with gastroesophageal reflux and delayed gastric emptying, and may be used in conjunction with laparoscopic esophagectomy. Most frequently, pyloroplasty is indicated in esophagectomy, but may be indicated in iatrogenic gastric emptying disorders, where a previous operation has damaged the vagus nerve and created impaired gastric emptying. Because Nissen fundoplication, by itself, improves gastric emptying, pyloroplasty is reserved for those with profound emptying disorders manifest by residual food in the stomach on endoscopy and/or solid phase emptying that is twice the upper limit of normal ($T_{1/2} \geq 150$ min). Other indications for pyloroplasty include gastroparesis outside the setting of fundoplication, or in a patient who has a very functional Nissen fundoplication but evidence of profound gastroparesis. For patients undergoing laparoscopic esophagectomy, pyloroplasty will improve gastric conduit emptying; however, it may accelerate gastric emptying sufficiently to create dumping and diarrhea, and may increase bile reflux.

PREOPERATIVE PREPARATION Patients with symptoms of delayed gastric emptying (e.g., bloating, early satiety, postprandial upper abdominal pain, vomiting) deserve evaluation with a 4-hour solid (or dual) phase nuclear medicine gastric emptying study. In addition, upper endoscopy should be performed on any patient being evaluated for pyloroplasty. Food remaining in the stomach after an overnight fast is not unusual in patients with gastroparesis. Anatomic abnormalities of the pylorus such as gastric outlet obstruction from peptic ulcer disease must be ruled out, as a pyloroplasty in the presence of chronic or acute inflammation may lead to serious complications.

ANESTHESIA General anesthesia is used. A preoperative antibiotic is administered. For isolated pyloroplasty, invasive monitoring may not be necessary, but when associated with a more complex operation such as esophagectomy, invasive monitoring is required.

POSITION When pyloroplasty is combined with Nissen fundoplication or esophagectomy, the patient is positioned with their arms tucked and their legs abducted. Because the pylorus is not a midline structure, an isolated pyloroplasty may be best approached with the surgeon standing on the left side of the patient working in a triangulated fashion toward the pylorus, somewhat similar to the approach for laparoscopic cholecystectomy. Regardless of the patient position, pneumatic compression boots are applied and a first-generation cephalosporin is given intravenously (**FIGURE 1**).

INCISION AND EXPOSURE When part of a Nissen fundoplication, the pyloroplasty is usually performed by introducing an additional 5-mm trocar just to the patient's right of the umbilicus which can be used for the surgeon's left hand (**FIGURE 2A**). When performed as a stand-alone procedure, the laparoscopic pyloroplasty is performed from the patient's left side with the left hand (5-mm trocar) through a umbilical approach, the camera is positioned to the left of the midline, and the right hand along the left costal margin, to create the classic diamond approach to the pylorus (**FIGURE 2B**). Although a fourth trocar may be placed for use by the assistant and the liver retractor may occasionally be necessary, most frequently pyloroplasty can be done by a single operating surgeon with a camera holder (human or mechanical).

DETAILS OF THE PROCEDURE An atraumatic grasper is placed in the surgeon's left hand and ultrasonic shears are placed in the surgeon's right hand. A 30 or 45-degree laparoscope is used through the trocar between the surgeon's hands. The pylorus is identified at the point in which the antrum becomes narrow. The muscular ring of the pylorus can be palpated even with laparoscopic instruments, and the vein of Mayo is seen draining inferiorly. If there is any doubt about the location of the pylorus, on-table endoscopy with transillumination of the stomach is very effective for confirming location before an incision is made.

1

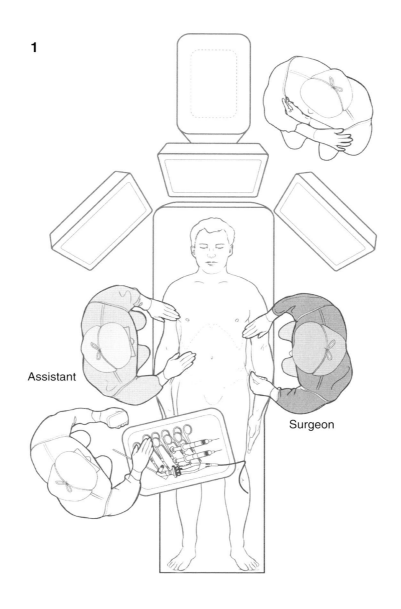

Assistant

Surgeon

2a

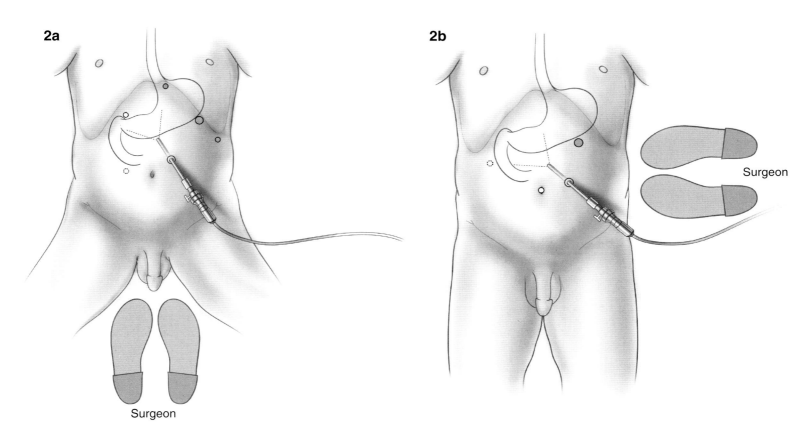

Surgeon

2b

Surgeon

DETAILS OF THE PROCEDURE Starting 1 cm on the gastric side of the pylorus in the midpoint of the ring, the active blade of the ultrasonic scissors is touched to the gastric serosa in the high-amplitude "cutting" mode. With gentle pressure on the serosa, the active blade will penetrate into the stomach quickly, at which point the shears are closed toward the duodenum, perpendicular to the pyloric ring, and ultrasonic energy is again applied (**FIGURE 3A**). It is generally quite easy to determine when the thickened pyloric muscle has been divided, as the very thin walled duodenum is easily distinguishable. The incision is taken no more than 1 cm onto the duodenum, leaving a total length of gastrotomy and duodenotomy of 3 cm (**FIGURE 3B**).

The duodenotomy and gastrotomy are then closed in the opposite direction. There are many ways to sew this closed, but the pyloroplasty can generally be closed with five or six nonabsorbable sutures. The first suture, a 2-0 six-inch silk or braided nylon, is placed in the midpoint of the closure. The suture starts at the farthest corner of the gastrotomy and goes to the farthest corner of the duodenotomy, aligning the midpoint of the closure (**FIGURE 4**). If this suture were tightened, it would be difficult to place additional sutures. Thus a single square knot is created but not slid down tight. The needle is cut off and removed from the abdomen. Next, a stitch is placed in the superior most corner of the pyloroplasty using identical suture type. The gastric wall and gastric mucosa are gathered with the first pass of the needle. The needle is passed either forehand or backhand through the duodenal wall immediately adjacent to the cut pyloric muscle. Again, two overhand knots are thrown to create a square knot, but this too is not tightened and the needle is removed. The third suture is applied halfway between the midpoint of the pyloric closure and the superior end. Again, this suture takes a full-thickness bite of the stomach wall and a full-thickness bite of the duodenum wall. A sliding slip knot is created, and this knot is tightened to pull the upper edges of the pyloroplasty together (**FIGURE 5A**). The knot is completed by throwing another square knot on top of the first, and the suture is cut. The suture at the superior end of the pyloroplasty is slid down to oppose the upper end of the pyloroplasty. The knot is then converted back to a square configuration and an additional square knot is thrown atop this. The suture ends are divided and removed. At this point, the only suture that has not been tightened down is the middle suture, which will ultimately define the midpoint of the pyloric closure. Although it seems logical not to tighten any of the sutures until they are all placed, it becomes very confusing to keep suture ends oriented if they are all left long. The strategy described in this chapter prevents this problem.

The lower end of the pyloric closure is addressed in the same fashion as the superior end. The fourth suture placed is a full-thickness bite of the stomach wall adjacent to the pylorus at the inferior end of the closure, which exits with a full-thickness bite of the duodenum again immediately adjacent to the pyloric muscle. A sliding slip knot is placed and the needle is removed. A fifth suture, halfway between the two loose sutures, is placed full-thickness to the gastric wall and then full-thickness to the duodenum. As before, this suture is tied down snugly with two square knots. The inferiormost suture is slid down and converted to a square knot, and an additional square knot is placed atop this (**FIGURE 5B**). This leaves only the middle suture still loose. At this point it is easy to assess whether the middle suture will, by itself, adequately close the remaining gap of the pyloroplasty. If the single suture appears adequate, it can be slid down, converted, and a square knot placed atop it. If there is any concern about defects existing, one or two additional sutures can be placed before the first suture is tightened. This completes the pyloroplasty (**FIGURE 6**). The pyloroplasty should be tested by installation of methylene blue through a nasogastric (NG) tube or with intraoperative endoscopy. The endoscopic appearance of the pyloroplasty, especially in its edematous form, is often a bit discouraging to the surgeon who is expecting to see a wider gastric outlet created. With the disappearance of edema over the first few weeks, the desired result is often a much larger aperture.

CLOSURE Assuming all trocars are no more than 10 mm and are above the umbilicus, it is generally not necessary to place fascial closure sutures unless—with a very thin patient—the fascial defect can readily be appreciated and closed with an 0-Vicryl suture.

POSTOPERATIVE CARE At the completion of the procedure, patients are given a potent intravenous antiemetic, and ketorolac is administered for postoperative pain control as well. The NG tube may be discontinued in the operating room, or it may be left for 1 or 2 days to ensure gastric decompression. It is generally a good idea to prove the patency of the pyloroplasty with a water-soluble contrast radiograph on the second or third postoperative day before resuming an oral diet. ∎

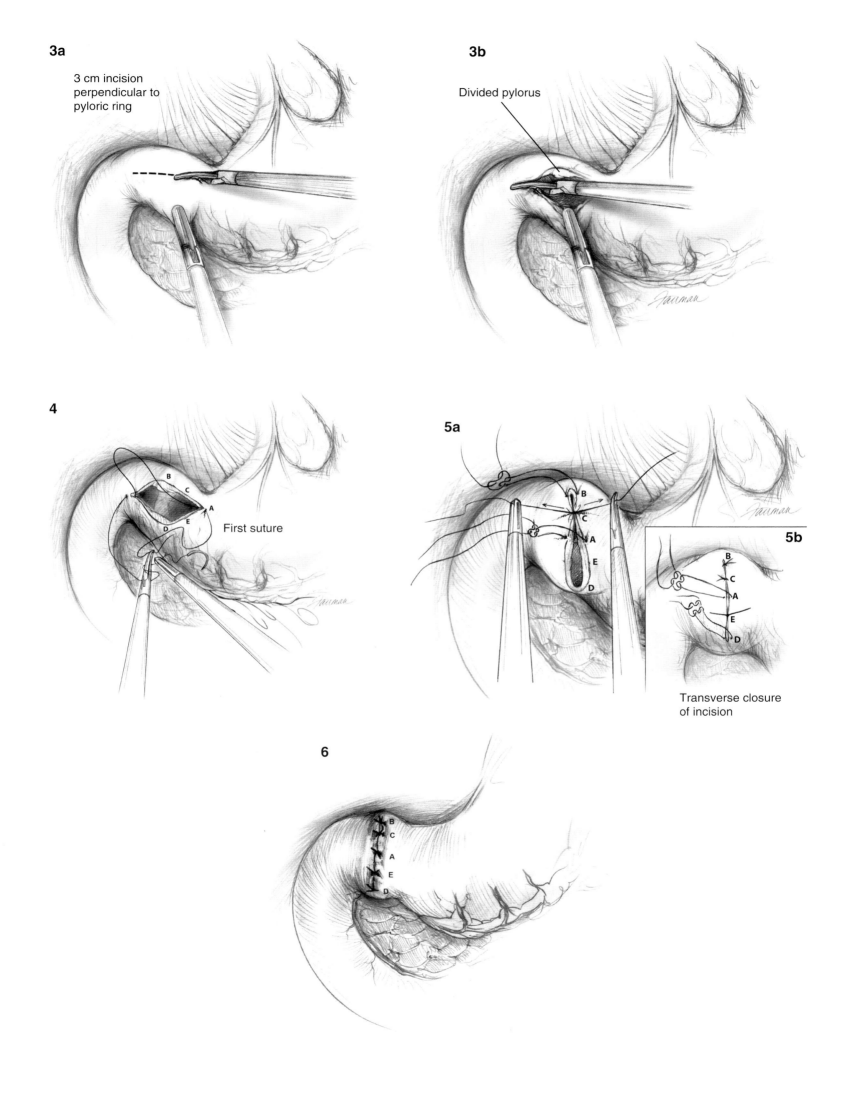

3a

3 cm incision
perpendicular to
pyloric ring

3b

Divided pylorus

4

First suture

5a

5b

Transverse closure
of incision

6

WEDGE RESECTION OF GASTRIC SMOOTH MUSCLE TUMORS

INDICATIONS Gastric smooth muscle tumors may either be leiomyomas or gastrointestinal stromal tumors. The gastrointestinal stromal tumors are characterized by their larger size (usually >1 cm), by the number of mitoses, and by the presence of a C-Kit mutation on exon 9 or 11. Although the differentiation between leiomyoma and gastrointestinal stromal tumor (GIST) is a relatively new distinction, it has some importance from a surgical perspective, as GISTs have a greater propensity for recurrence and must be resected with a margin of normal stomach circumferentially. On the other hand, leiomyomas, which are most common in the esophagus, can also be found in the proximal stomach. These can be treated with either wedge resection or an endogastric "shelling out" when they are small and symptomatic (see Chapter 38). Asymptomatic lesions less than 1 cm can generally be observed.

The minimally invasive resection of GISTs requires good clinical judgment. Although there is no specific size of GIST that defines the need for an open (vs. laparoscopic) resection, most surgeons use 6 cm in the largest dimension of the tumor as the upper limit of safety for minimally invasive resection. As the tumors get larger, the need for a large counterincision to remove the tumor intact negates much of the benefit of the laparoscopic approach. Larger tumors pose a greater risk for local and regional recurrence, making the laparoscopic approach less appealing.

GISTs may occur anywhere in the stomach, but are more common proximally. In order to safely remove a GIST with a wide local resection, the surgeon must have excellent access to the tumor and the normal surrounding stomach. Particularly difficult places to remove these tumors are in the region of the gastroesophageal junction, on the high posterior wall of the stomach, and on the lesser curvature of the stomach. Thankfully, most such tumors are located in a more favorable position closer to the greater curvature. Pre-pyloric GISTs are rare but are probably best addressed with a sleeve resection of the antrum with hand-sewn or stapled laparoscopic B1 reconstruction.

PREOPERATIVE PREPARATION Before addressing the gastric smooth muscle tumor, several imaging studies are necessary. The primary imaging test necessary is esophagogastroduodenoscopy (EGD) to determine the exact location of the lesion in the stomach, and to demonstrate that the lesion is submucosal and not a mucosa-based lesion such as gastric cancer. The next study should be an upper abdominal computed tomography (CT) scan to define the intra- and extragastric components of the tumor as well as to determine whether the tumor is localized or not. With disseminated disease, resection of the primary tumor is not indicated unless it is actively bleeding or obstructing the stomach. Last, endoscopic ultrasound with fine-needle aspiration may be obtained to prove that the tumor harbors spindle cells and to determine, through specialized stains, if the lesion is a GIST or leiomyoma.

ANESTHESIA General anesthesia is usually used, and perioperative antibiotics are administered.

POSITION The patient position is somewhat dependent on the location of the tumor. For high gastric tumors, the surgeon stands between the legs as with a Nissen fundoplication (**FIGURE 1**).

For pre-pyloric pathology, the surgeon stands on the patient's left side and use trocar positions similar to those described for pyloroplasty (see Chapter 24).

INCISION AND EXPOSURE For the high gastric and greater curvature tumors, the port positions for the Nissen fundoplication work quite well (**FIGURE 2**). The left subcostal port for the surgeon's operating hand should be a 12-mm trocar to allow passage of the Endo GIA stapler. It is often helpful to have an upper GI endoscope available to assess the stomach upon completion of the gastric repair. For a pre-pyloric GIST that will be treated with a local resection, the trocar positions described for the pyloroplasty will work quite well.

1

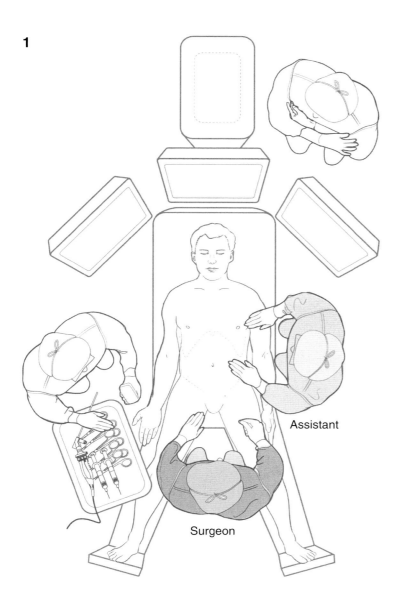

Assistant

Surgeon

2

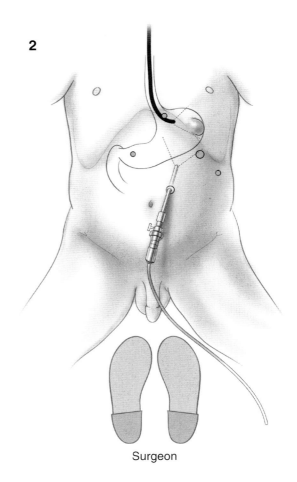

Surgeon

DETAILS OF THE PROCEDURE Working through the two uppermost tro-cars, and standing between the legs, the surgeon identifies the site of the tumor with direct visual inspection. If the tumor is close to the GE junction, it will probably be necessary to raise the left lobe of the liver with a Nathanson type liver retractor (see Chapter 2). If the tumor involves the greater curvature of the stomach or sits on the posterior wall of the stomach, it will be necessary to take down short gastric vessels to adequately expose the tumor. Sometimes it is helpful to put an Endoloop around the external projection of the tumor as a handle for the first assistant to pull the tumor up and away from the stomach (**FIGURES 3A AND 3B**). Once the tumor is elevated, an endoscopic linear stapler with the 3.8- or 4.5-mm staples (green or blue load) is fired below the tumor, maintaining a 1-cm margin from the edges of the tumor. Several staple loads may be necessary to keep a clear margin around the tumor (**FIGURES 4A AND 4B**). Care should be taken to ensure that the resection of a large tumor does not narrow the stomach. When the tumor has been effectively wedged off the stomach, it is placed in a specimen bag and retrieved via a 12-mm port (**FIGURE 5**). This port will often need to be upsized for tumors larger than 1½ cm in diameter. Under these circumstances incision extension is probably the best way to allow extraction of the GIST. The gastric closure is then tested with an endoscope, which not only will confirm that there are no leaks, but will determine that the stomach is of adequate width and patency.

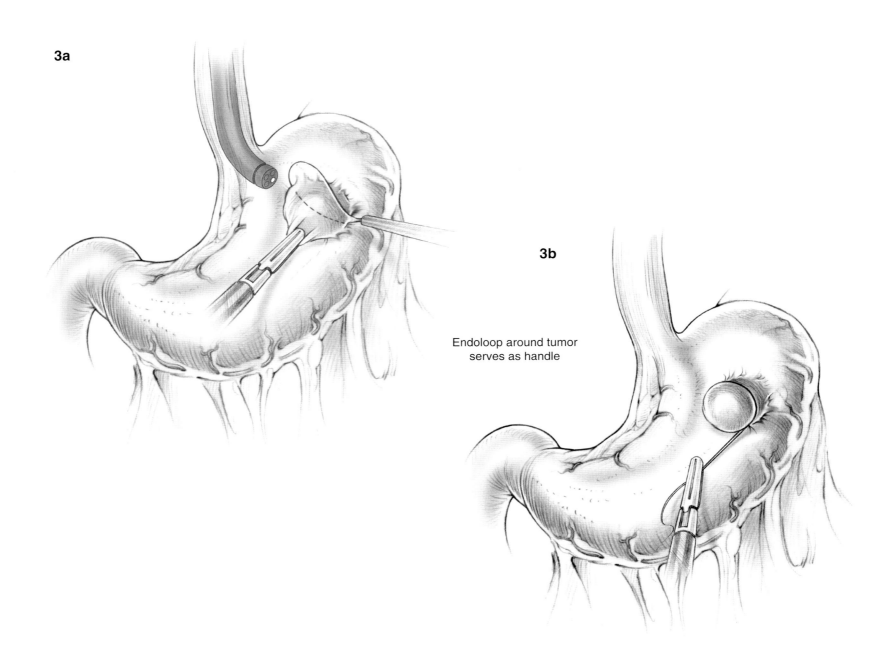

3a

3b

Endoloop around tumor
serves as handle

4a

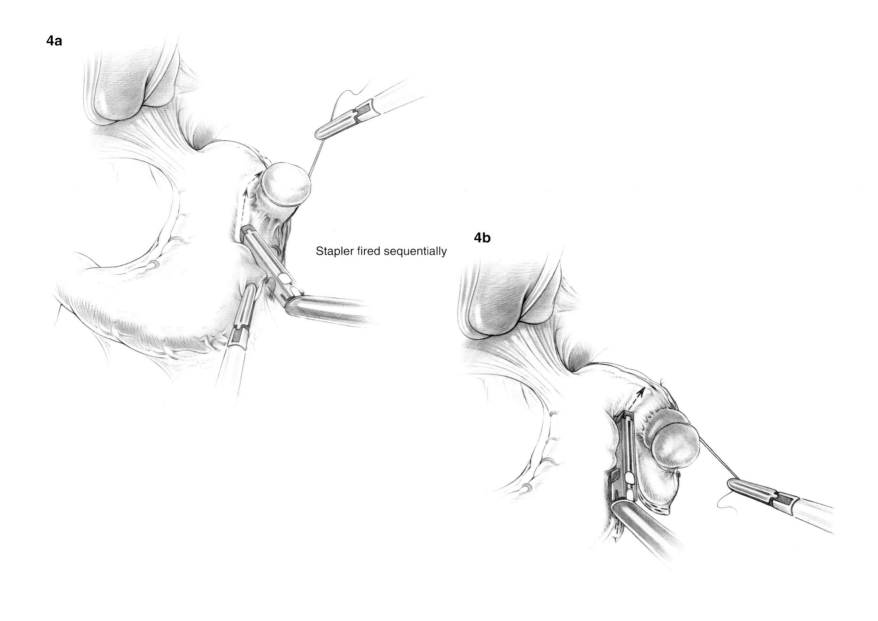

Stapler fired sequentially

4b

5

Tumor placed in
specimen bag

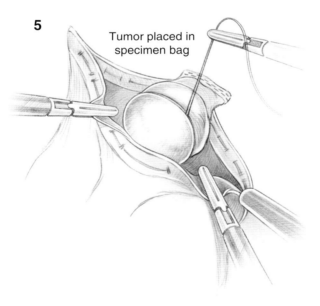

Full Thickness Resection If the tumor is close to the gastroesophageal junction or the pylorus, such that a stapled resection would compromise the lumen at either of these points a non-stapled full-thickness resection technique can be employed. In this technique the primary resection is accomplished by marking the gastric wall with electrosurgery 1 cm away from the tumor in a 360-degree pattern. Using the Harmonic scalpel, the tumor is excised from the stomach with the 1-cm margin of normal tissue (**FIGURE 6**). This defect is closed in a two-layer fashion with a running internal suture of 2 or 3-0 Vicryl followed by a running second layer of 2-0 silk or a synthetic braided suture (**FIGURE 7**). After closure, the stomach should be tested for leaks with methylene blue through a nasogastric tube or endoscopy with air insufflations of the stomach. The tumor is placed in a specimen bag, as above, and removed through a trocar site.

POSTOPERATIVE CARE Given the nature of the partial gastrectomy, it may be tempting to leave the patient NPO until the ileus has resolved; however, clear liquids are generally tolerated shortly after the operation, and discharge may be complete on the first or second postoperative day. It is prudent to obtain a Gastrografin upper GI examination before the patient leaves the hospital. ■

6

Full thickness resection

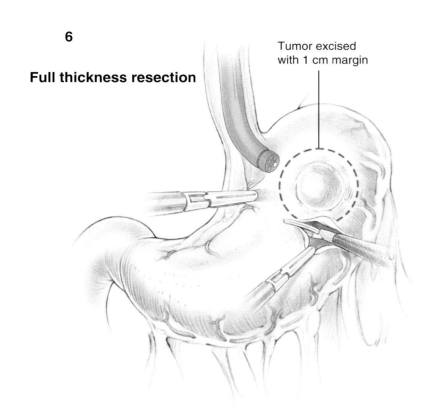

Tumor excised
with 1 cm margin

7

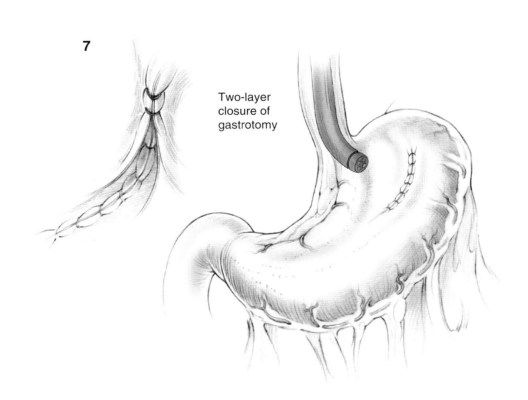

Two-layer
closure of
gastrotomy

GASTRECTOMY WITH ROUX-EN-Y RECONSTRUCTION

INDICATIONS Gastrectomy is most often performed for gastric cancer or peptic ulcer disease. The complexity of the operation needs to be matched with the expertise of the surgeon. Wedge resection of a small gastric tumor (e.g., leiomyoma) falls on the simpler end of the complexity spectrum and can be performed by most well-trained minimally invasive general surgeons. Total gastrectomy with J-pouch reconstruction and D2 lymph node dissection for proximal gastric cancer falls on the more difficult end of the complexity spectrum and should be performed by experts in minimally invasive surgery for upper GI malignancy. This chapter addresses the more complex procedures, subtotal and total gastrectomy, with extensive (D2) lymph node dissection, the international "standard" for gastric cancer surgery. D2 dissection requires removal of lymph node stations along the celiac trunk, left gastric, splenic, and hepatic arteries. Familiarity with regional lymph node anatomy and the international naming conventions is critical to adequate lymph node harvest and subsequent staging (**FIGURE 1**). The final anatomy of the subtotal gastrectomy with Roux en Y gastrojejunostomy is shown (**FIGURE 2**).

Subtotal Gastrectomy

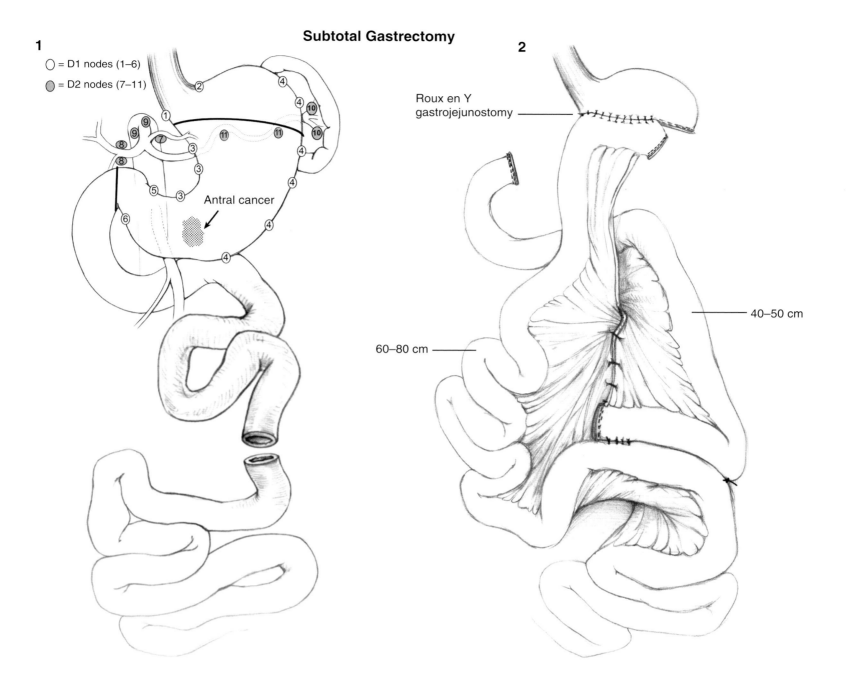

PATIENT SELECTION, STAGING, AND PREOPERATIVE PREPARATION
A complete preoperative upper GI endoscopic examination is necessary in all patients to characterize gastric pathology and identify synchronous pathology. Cancer staging also requires pre-treatment computed tomography (CT) scanning, endoscopic ultrasonography, and diagnostic laparoscopy with peritoneal washings. Positron emission tomography (PET) scanning may be useful, but is less frequently performed with gastric cancer than with thoracic malignancies. Prior to treatment, multidisciplinary discussion (tumor board) should occur. In many cases of advanced malignancy, preoperative (neoadjuvant) chemotherapy with or without radiation therapy may be indicated. Restaging with CT scanning, at a minimum, should precede operation.

A full cardiopulmonary evaluation should be considered. Stair climbing or a 6-minute walk test may be as valuable as noninvasive cardiac imaging. Patients should continue all preoperative medications until the morning of surgery, with the exception of aspirin, nonsteroidal anti-inflammatory agents, warfarin, or heparin. Mechanical bowel preparation is generally not necessary. Intraoperative esophagogastroduodenoscopy may aid in localizing pathology and determining the limits of resection, as well as completion examination of the anastomosis for patency and integrity (i.e., negative leak test). Intraoperative laparoscopic hepatic ultrasound may be necessary, depending on the indication for operation and the results of preoperative imaging studies.

ANESTHESIA General anesthesia with complete neuromuscular blockade is required for laparoscopic gastrectomy. Intravenous antibiotics directed against intestinal flora are administered preoperatively. A nasogastric tube is placed into the stomach to low wall suction.

OPERATIVE PREPARATION A urinary catheter should be placed. The upper abdomen is shaved with clippers from the nipple lines to the umbilicus after induction of anesthesia, and the abdomen is sterilely prepped.

PATIENT AND SURGEON POSITIONING The patient is positioned supine with the legs split. Monitors are positioned at the head of the bed to enable visualization by the surgeon and first assistant. The surgeon stands between the patient's legs for the gastric and duodenal dissection, while the assistant may stand on the patient's left or right (**FIGURE 3**). The surgeon may move to the patient's right for construction of the Roux limb and jejunojejunostomy, while the assistant stands on the patient's left. After placement of the initial trocar, steep reverse Trendelenburg positioning optimizes exposure of the upper abdomen for the gastric and duodenal dissection.

INCISION, TROCAR PLACEMENT, AND EXPOSURE Laparoscopic gastrectomy requires access to the stomach and proximal duodenum, as well as to the proximal jejunum for creation of the Roux-en-Y limb. Trocar placement should accommodate both of these fields of dissection. The surgeon will usually move from a position between the legs to the right side of the stomach, as the operation moves from gastric dissection to small bowel preparation (**FIGURES 4 AND 5**).

A Veress needle placed at the umbilicus achieves pneumoperitoneum. Alternatively, depending on surgeon preference, an open (Hasson) technique or a visual dilating trocar can be used to enter the abdomen. A 10-mm trocar is placed approximately 18 to 20 cm below the xiphoid process in the midline, usually just above or below the umbilicus, depending on body habitus. An angled (30- or 45-degree) laparoscope is used for both construction of the Roux limb and dissection of the stomach and duodenum. Two 12-mm trocars are placed. The first one in the right subcostal position just lateral to the midaxillary line that accommodates the surgeon's left hand. The second one is placed in the right lower quadrant in the mid-axillary line that accommodates the surgeon's right hand for the jejunojejunostomy. A 5-mm trocar is placed in the left subcostal position, approximately 4 to 5 cm below the costal margin in the lateral abdominal wall under direct visualization. This port serves as an assistant trocar for both the Roux limb construction and the gastric and duodenal dissection. A 12-mm trocar is placed in the left upper quadrant approximately 12 cm left of the xiphoid and 2 to 4 cm below the costal margin and accommodates the surgeon's right hand for the gastric and duodenal dissection. The surgeon's left hand manipulates instruments placed through the right subcostal trocar for the proximal stomach dissection, and through the right lower quadrant trocar for the distal gastric and duodenal dissection. A 5-mm port can be placed in the subxiphoid position to facilitate entry of the Nathanson liver retractor if necessary (**FIGURES 4 AND 5**).

3

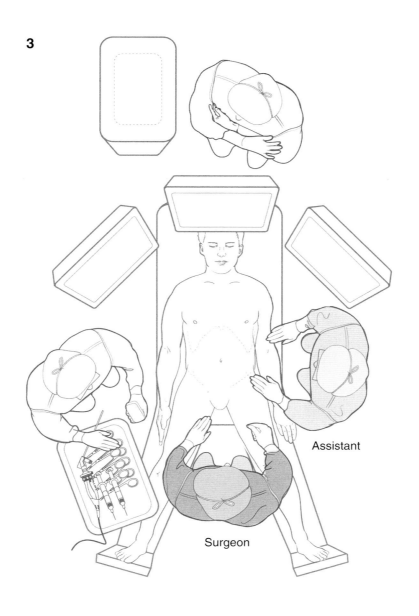

Assistant

Surgeon

4   Position for gastric dissection   **5   Position for construction of Roux limb**

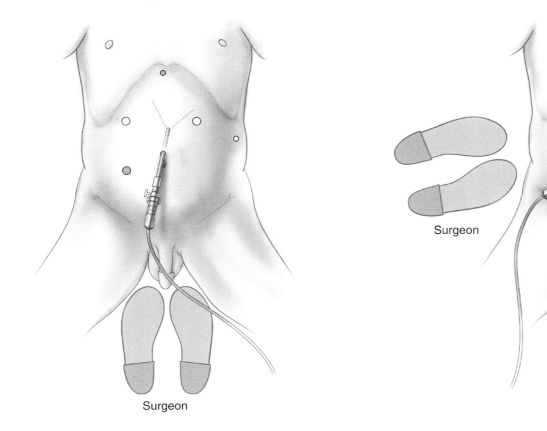

Surgeon

Surgeon

DETAILS OF PROCEDURE

Gastric and Duodenal Dissection Prior to beginning the dissection, a thorough laparoscopic exploration of the abdomen should be performed to identify any coexisting pathology and, in the case of gastric cancer, to determine the presence of metastatic disease. Laparoscopic hepatic ultrasound should be performed if appropriate.

Assuming laparoscopic exploration identifies no contraindications to proceeding with the operation, laparoscopic gastrectomy begins with the gastric dissection. The first maneuver is entry into the lesser sac. For most advanced cancer, the omentum should be removed from the transverse colon using the Harmonic scalpel (**FIGURE 6**). Reflection of the omentum cephalad after this dissection is completed should provide access to the lesser sac. For a small antral cancer, subtotal gastrectomy is the procedure of choice. In this situation the short gastric vessels are spared and will be the blood supply of the gastric remnant. For all other locally advanced gastric cancers, total gastrectomy is the procedure of choice. In this situation, the short gastric vessels are divided with the Harmonic scalpel.

Dissection of the left gastric pedicle is next performed. By elevating the gastric cardia, anteriorly, the left gastric artery and vein are put on stretch. The peritoneum overlying the junction of left gastric and celiac arteries is opened, and lymph nodes in this region (station 7) are left with the stomach. Celiac (station 9) and hepatic artery (station 8) lymph nodes may be removed at this point as shown, but the D2 dissection is easier to complete after the stomach has been removed. The left gastric artery and vein are divided flush with the celiac artery with a 30-cm vascular cartridge of the linear stapler (**FIGURE 7**).

The distal gastric dissection is next performed by elevating the omentum and greater curve of the stomach ventrally to demonstrate the right gastro-epiploic pedicle and posterior antrum. The gastroepiploic pedicle is divided at its origin with the linear stapler (vascular load, 30 mm) thereby removing subpyloric lymph nodes (station 6) (**FIGURE 8**).

6

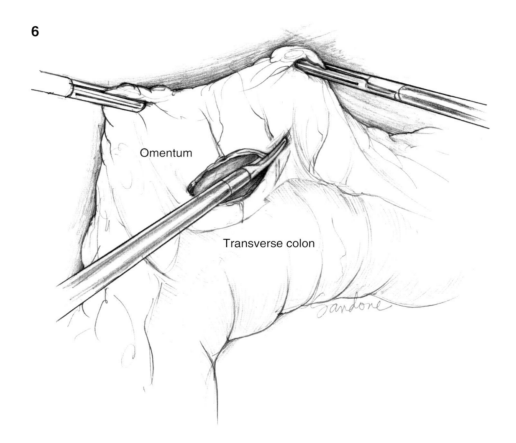

Omentum

Transverse colon

7

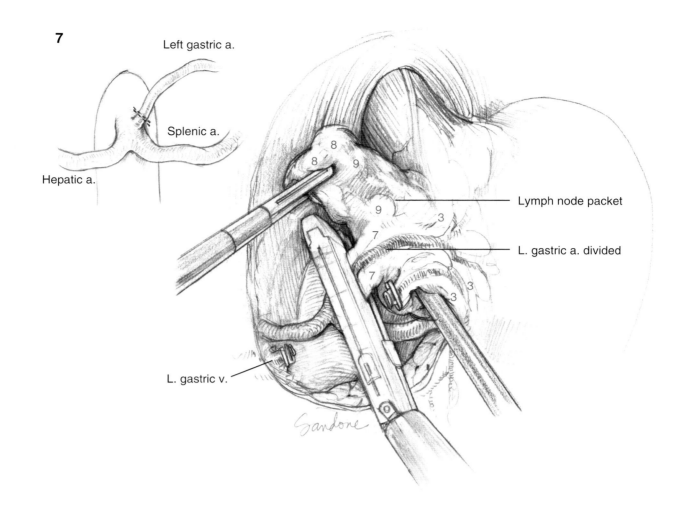

Left gastric a.

Splenic a.

Hepatic a.

Lymph node packet

L. gastric a. divided

L. gastric v.

8

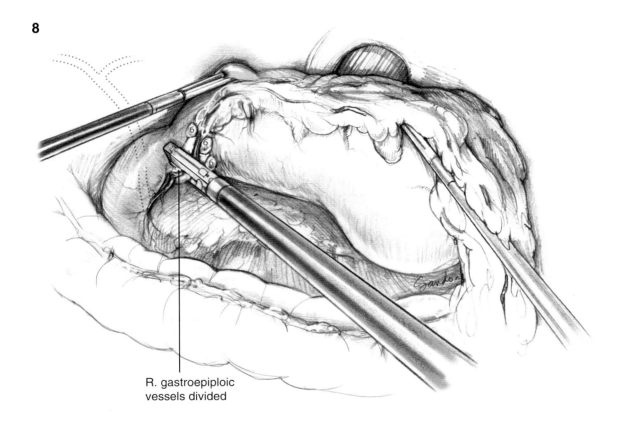

R. gastroepiploic
vessels divided

Gastric and Duodenal Dissection Elevation of the antrum and duodenum ventrally allows for a circumferential duodenal dissection that begins along the inferior aspect of the duodenum and is carried posteriorly between the duodenum and the pancreas. During the course of this dissection, the gastroduodenal artery may be encountered and should be dropped distally by hugging the posterior surface of the duodenum. Once the dissection is carried 2 to 3 cm distal to the pylorus, the duodenum is divided with an articulating 45-mm linear cutting stapler with 3.5-mm staples (**FIGURE 9**). It is important to ensure that all oral and nasogastric tubes are withdrawn prior to stapling the duodenum. The pylorus is usually easily identified with visual inspection and palpation with instruments. Any difficulty in identifying the pylorus should prompt intraoperative endoscopic confirmation of the location of the pylorus prior to division of the duodenum.

After dividing the duodenum, the remaining tissues of the gastrohepatic ligament attached to the lesser curve are divided with the ultrasonic shears. Other than the right gastric vessels, there are usually no remaining large vessels in this tissue.

Subtotal Gastrectomy Once the proximal duodenum has been divided, a point of proximal division on the stomach is chosen. Depending on the situation, intraoperative endoscopy may assist in determining the proximal resection margin. In order to avoid narrowing the gastroesophageal (GE) junction, a large (50–60 French) dilator may be passed by mouth into the proximal stomach. An articulating linear cutting stapler with medium-length (3.5-mm) staples is passed through the left or subcostal trocar and articulated to divide the stomach from the tip of the spleen to the right side of the GE junction (**FIGURE 10**). Serial firings of the stapler are required to transect the upper stomach, after which the specimen is usually easily extracted in a laparoscopic specimen bag through one of the 12-mm trocar sites. Gentle dilation of the trocar site is usually all that is required to remove the specimen from the abdomen, but incision extension may be necessary. Proximal and distal specimen margins are sent to pathology for frozen section analysis.

9

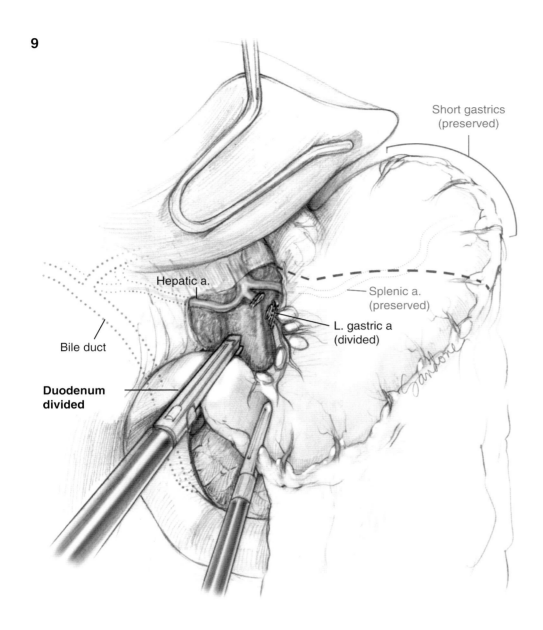

Short gastrics
(preserved)

Hepatic a.

Splenic a.
(preserved)

L. gastric a
(divided)

Bile duct

**Duodenum
divided**

10

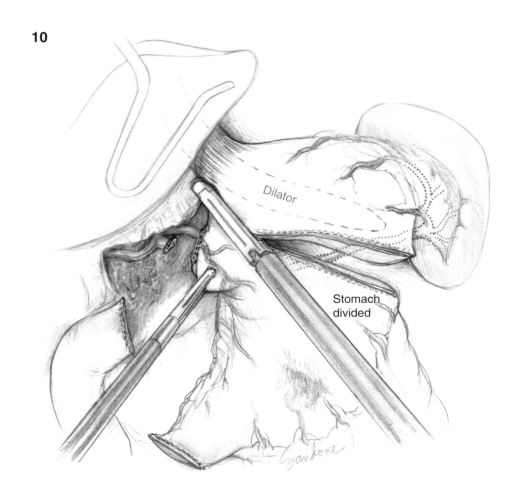

Dilator

Stomach
divided

D2 Lymph Node Dissection With the stomach removed, the remainder of the D2 lymph nodes can be removed, by extending the ultrasonic dissection of the celiac artery to its base (station 9), then following the splenic artery to the hilum, removing all lymph nodes from station 11. Nodes in the splenic hilum (station 10) do not require removal for distal gastric cancers, as they rarely harbor malignancy. Lymph nodes from each station are removed separately directly through a 12-mm trocar, or bagged if the specimen is too large for such extraction. Last, the hepatic artery is followed to the porta hepatis, removing station 8 lymph nodes (**FIGURE 11**).

Total Gastrectomy With midbody, proximal, or diffuse cancers, a total gastrectomy will be needed for all but the smallest tumors (**FIGURE 12A**). An articulating linear cutting stapler with medium-length (3.5-mm) staples is passed through the left subcostal trocar and articulated to divide the esophagus just above the GE junction (**FIGURE 12B**). A short lower midline incision is made, and a wound protector is placed. The gastric remnant and omentum are removed through this port, which will be converted to a gel port later in the case to facilitate J pouch creation and esophagojejunostomy. Proximal and distal specimen margins are sent to pathology for frozen-section analysis. A D2 lymphatic dissection is then performed, as described earlier.

Lymph node dissection for subtotal gastrectomy

11a

11b

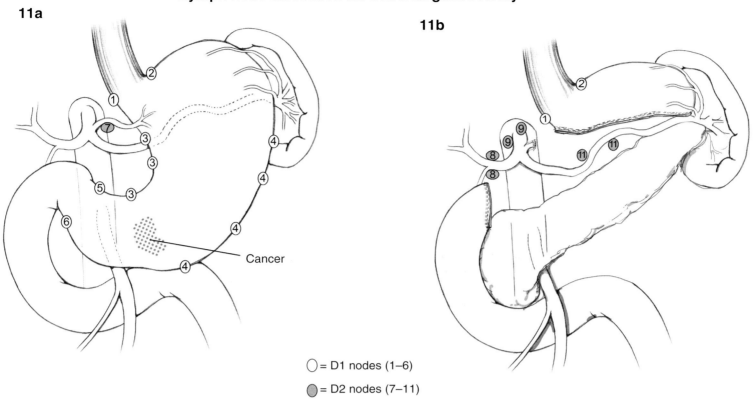

Cancer

◯ = D1 nodes (1–6)

⬤ = D2 nodes (7–11)

Lymph node dissection for total gastrectomy

12a

12b

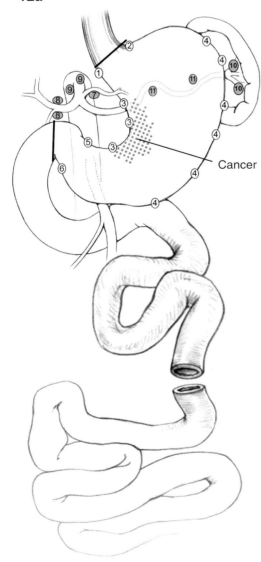

Cancer

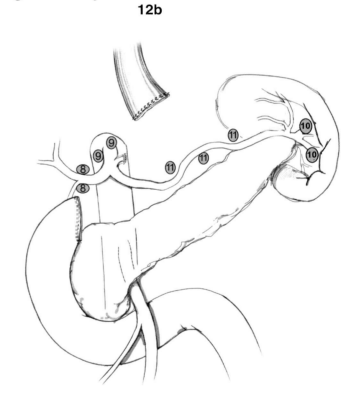

Roux-en-Y Gastrojejunostomy (Subtotal Gastrectomy) Reconstruction after subtotal gastrectomy may be performed with a loop gastrojejunostomy (Bilroth II reconstruction) or a Roux-en-Y gastrojejunostomy. With more extensive gastric resections, a loop gastrojejunostomy usually results in excessive tension on the gastrojejunal anastomosis, which may be avoided with an antecolic Roux limb reconstruction. Roux limb reconstruction may also reduce the risk of subsequent bile reflux gastritis, but may increase the risk of anastomotic ulceration and slow upper GI transit.

Construction of the Roux-en-Y limb begins with identification of the ligament of Treitz. The transverse colon is elevated cephalad by the assistant, and the surgeon sweeps the entire small bowel caudad. Correct identification of this point is critical. The ligament of Treitz can usually be directly visualized at the root of the colonic mesentery with gentle hand-over-hand caudad retraction of the proximal jejunum. The ligament of Treitz has been reached when it is impossible to progress up the jejunum more proximally, as the jejunum dives beneath the superior mesenteric artery to become the duodenum. The jejunum is next traced distally from the ligament of Treitz approximately 40 to 50 cm. Measurement of the bowel can be performed with a premeasured umbilical tape placed in the abdomen, or simply by visual estimation. The jejunum is divided with a 45-mm linear cutting stapler with 2.5-mm staples at the chosen point (**FIGURE 13**). A 4 cm length of Penrose drain is sutured to the distal jejunum, to identify it as the Roux limb. The jejunal mesentery is divided with a single firing of a linear cutting stapler with 2.5-mm staples. The mesenteric split relieves tension on the jejunal limb. If tension remains excessive after division with one staple firing, further division of the mesentery should be undertaken with a second stapler firing. Hemorrhage is rarely encountered while dividing the mesentery and can usually be controlled by oversewing the bleeding mesenteric edge. It is important to divide the mesentery equidistant from both transected ends of jejunum to avoid devascularizing either limb. The distal end of the jejunum is then traced 60 to 80 cm distally, keeping the Roux limb to the patient's right, and the biliary or afferent limb to the patient's left.

A jejunojejunostomy is created 60 to 80 cm along the Roux limb. Placement of two stay sutures between the cut end of the transected proximal jejunum and the point on the jejunum 60 cm distally allows for manipulation of the bowel during creation of a side-to-side linear stapled anastomosis. Electrosurgery is used to create enterotomies in each limb of intestine, and an articulating linear cutting stapler with 2.5-mm staples is inserted through the right subcostal trocar into the limbs of the jejunum and fired, creating the anastomosis (**FIGURE 14**). The resultant defect from the stapled anastomosis is closed in two layers using a running 2-0 braided absorbable suture, followed by interrupted 2-0 serosal sutures. The mesenteric defect is closed with one or two figure-of-eight sutures or running suture placed between the cut edge of the mesentery on the biliary limb and the mesentery of the Roux limb. Exposure of this defect is easily achieved by having the assistant elevate the jejunojejunostomy (**FIGURE 15**).

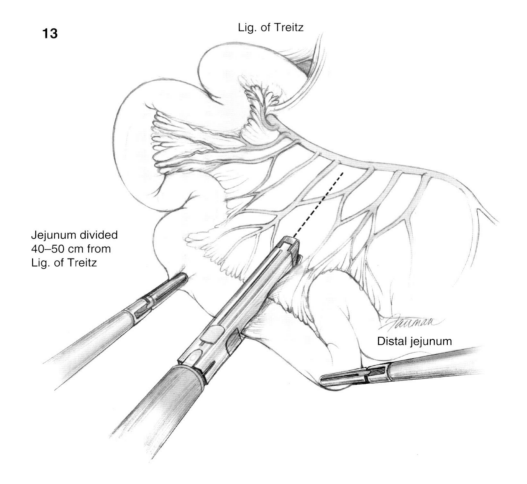

13

Lig. of Treitz

Jejunum divided
40–50 cm from
Lig. of Treitz

Distal jejunum

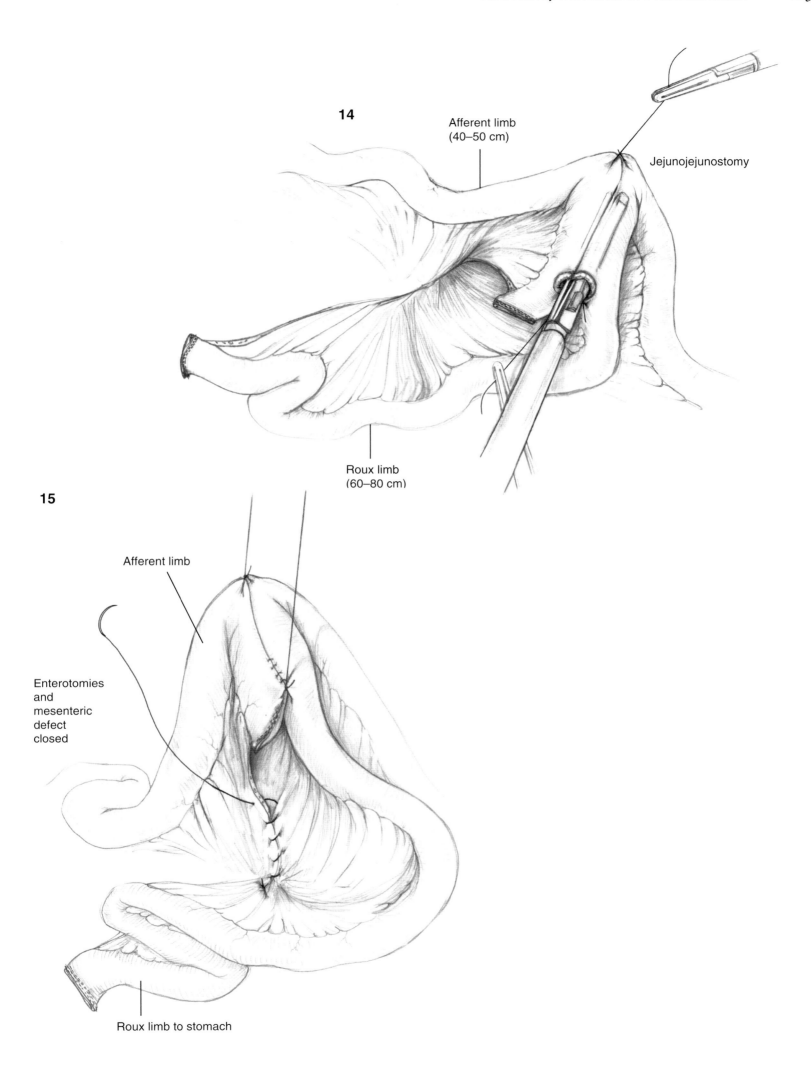

14

Afferent limb
(40–50 cm)

Jejunojejunostomy

Roux limb
(60–80 cm)

15

Afferent limb

Enterotomies
and
mesenteric
defect
closed

Roux limb to stomach

Roux-en-Y Gastrojejunostomy (Subtotal Gastrectomy) The end-to-side gastrojejunal anastomosis is created in a similar fashion to the just-described jejunojejunostomy, using a linear stapled technique. The Roux limb is brought up antecolic to the proximal remnant stomach and traced back to the jejunojejunostomy to ensure that the limb is not twisted as it is brought cephalad. If the Roux limb was kept to the patient's right and afferent limb to the left, then the staple line on the end of the Roux limb should face the patient's left. The Roux limb is sutured to the staple line of the gastric pouch using a running 2-0 nonabsorbable suture. Both ends of the suture are preserved to allow manipulation of the anastomosis by the surgeon and assistant.

Once this posterior layer is completed, the anastomosis is created with a 45-mm blue- or purple-load linear cutting stapler. A small gastrotomy is made anterior to the staple line of the pouch with the ultrasonic shears, and an adjacent enterotomy is made in the Roux limb. These only need to be large enough to admit the jaws of the linear stapler. The stapler is placed into each lumen, closed, and fired (**FIGURE 16**). The stapler is carefully removed and the common opening is inspected to make sure the internal staple lines are hemostatic. The nasogastric tube is passed through the anastomosis into the jejunum prior to suturing the gastroenteric defect. The enterotomy is then closed in two continuous layers. The inner layer of suture should be absorbable. After the inner layer is completed, an outer Lembert layer of nonabsorbable suture completes the anastomosis (**FIGURE 17**). The Penrose drain identifying the Roux limb is removed, and the long sutures are cut.

16

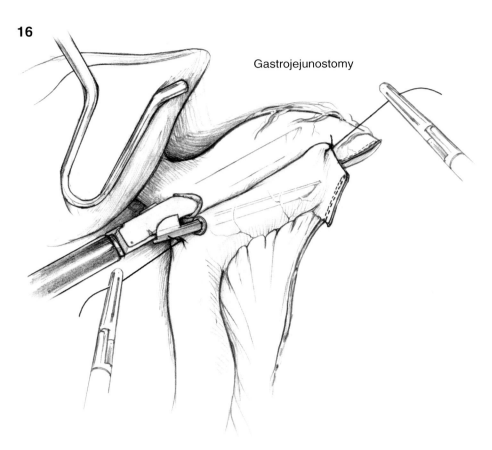

Gastrojejunostomy

17

Final configuration of
subtotal gastrectomy

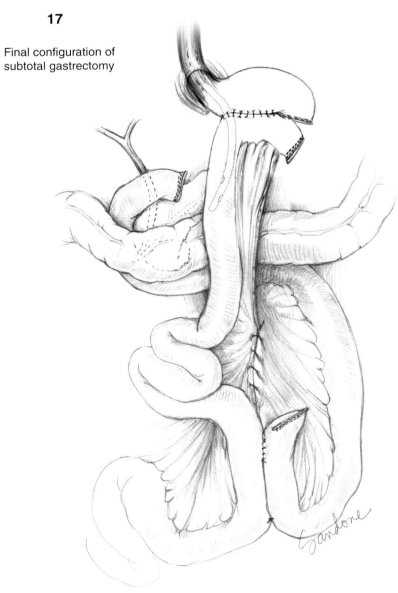

Roux-en-Y Esophagojejunostomy with J Pouch (Total Gastrectomy)
The creation of the Roux limb for J-pouch esophagojejunostomy starts in an identical fashion to Roux-en-Y gastrojejunostomy. Once the jejunum is divided, it is pulled through the hand port previously used to remove the stomach and folded back on itself to create a 15-cm jejunal pouch. A 2-0 polypropylene purse-string suture is placed at the apex of the J, and an enterotomy is made with electrosurgery. Two to three firings of the linear cutting stapler join the two walls of the jejunum, creating the pouch (**FIGURE 18**). Additional length on the Roux limb is required to ensure the ability to reach the esophagus without tension. As a result, final construction of the jejunojejunostomy should follow construction of the pouch and assessment of its ability to reach the esophageal hiatus. The jejunojejunostomy is then created outside of the wound protector, but otherwise identical to that illustrated in Figures 13 and 14.

Next a 21- or 25-mm circular stapler anvil is introduced into the esophagus through the mouth with a specialized introducer and the post is brought through a small hole at the end of the esophageal staple line (**FIGURE 19**). Lacking this device, the esophageal staple line can be cut off and the anvil secured in the distal end of the esophagus with a purse-string suture.

The jejunal pouch is brought back out the hand port, the proximal jejunal staple line is opened, and the circular stapler handle is first passed through the detached gel membrane of the gel port and then introduced into the pouch through the newly opened end of the J-pouch. The tip of the stapler is brought through the middle of the purse-string defect at the apex of the pouch, and the sharp tip is extended (**FIGURE 20**). The pouch and circular stapler are slipped back into the abdomen, and pneumoperitoneum is reestablished. The camera is moved to the left upper quadrant

trocar. The stapler is docked with the anvil and fired. Interrupted sutures may be placed between the esophagus and jejunum to decrease the chance of anastomotic leak. A nasogastric tube is inserted across the anastomosis under direct visualization with the tip of the tube positioned in the jejunal pouch. The opening in the tip of the jejunal pouch is closed a with a linear stapling instrument (**FIGURE 21**).

It is important to perform routine intraoperative endoscopy or methylene blue leak tests of the esophagojejunal or gastrojejunal anastomosis. To perform this evaluation, the Roux limb is occluded distal to the anastomosis using a laparoscopic bowel grasper. Clean sponges are packed around the anastomosis, and one ampule of methylene blue diluted in 200 to 500 mL of saline is infused into the stomach by gravity drainage via a nasogastric tube. The operative field and sponges are examined for extravasated methylene blue. Any leaks are repaired by oversewing, and a repeat test is performed to confirm successful repair. A jejunostomy tube for early postoperative feeding can by placed distal to the jejunojejunostomy, if desired. Usually this measure is reserved for patients undergoing total gastrectomy or esophagectomy, and those in whom current or future nutrition is in question. This procedure is described in Chapter 13.

POSTOPERATIVE CARE Postoperative care after laparoscopic gastrectomy follows basic surgical management principles. Nasogastric tube decompression of the remnant stomach is performed for 1 to 3 days, depending on outputs and bowel function, although no data exist supporting prolonged nasogastric decompression. Some surgeons prefer to avoid postoperative nasogastric tube decompression altogether. After return of bowel function, patients are advanced to a postgastrectomy diet, consisting of small, frequent meals. ∎

18   Total Gastrectomy

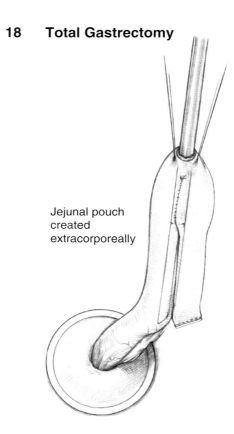

Jejunal pouch
created
extracorporeally

19

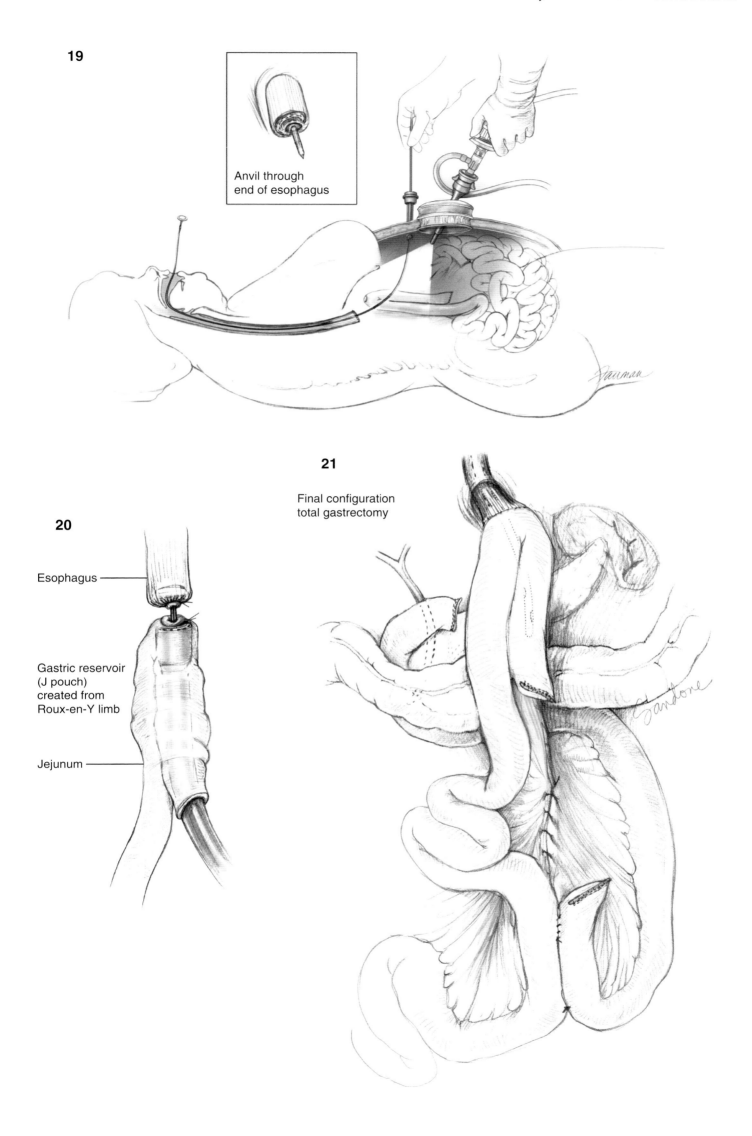

Anvil through
end of esophagus

20

Esophagus

Gastric reservoir
(J pouch)
created from
Roux-en-Y limb

Jejunum

21

Final configuration
total gastrectomy

SECTION IV
MINIMALLY INVASIVE ENTERAL ACCESS

Gastrostomy Tube Placement

INDICATIONS Placement of a gastrostomy tube is indicated for feeding or prolonged gastric decompression. The laparoscopic approach is indicated when a percutaneous endoscopic gastrostomy (PEG) cannot be placed or is contraindicated. This includes situations such as an obstructing oropharyngeal or esophageal lesion, or when interposition of the colon or omentum over the stomach makes the blind percutaneous approach unsafe. Patients with prior upper abdominal surgery may have adhesions that would render a laparoscopic approach difficult. Such patients may require placement of the gastrostomy tube under direct visualization using open techniques.

Patients who require gastrostomy tube placement are often debilitated and malnourished, and the laparoscopic approach is particularly advantageous for this population.

PREOPERATIVE PREPARATION If enteric feeding is only needed for a short interval, placement of a nasoenteric tube should be considered as an alternative. Distal obstruction, delayed gastric emptying, and gastroesophageal reflux are contraindications to gastric feeding. In patients with a risk of aspiration, placement of a jejunal feeding tube may be warranted.

ANESTHESIA General anesthesia with endotracheal intubation is necessary for this operation. Complete neuromuscular blockade is required. Nausea control with ondansetron and a second agent is beneficial. If there has been little bleeding during the dissection, ketorolac is given at the completion of the procedure to diminish postoperative pain.

POSITION The patient is positioned on a spit-leg bed with arms tucked at the sides. The surgeon stands between the patient's legs, and the assistant stands to the left side of the patient. The operative monitor is placed above the patient's head (**FIGURE 1**). A Foley catheter and orogastric tube are placed after the induction of anesthesia. The abdomen of the patient from the nipple lines to the pubis is shaved with clippers after induction of anesthesia, and the abdomen is sterilely prepped.

DETAILS OF PROCEDURE

Trocar Position The operation commences with insufflation of the abdomen using the Veress needle technique at the umbilicus. Alternatively, initial access can be achieved using the Hasson technique at the umbilicus.

The procedure is performed with a two-trocar technique. The proposed site of the gastrostomy is marked on the skin, at least two fingerbreadths below the left costal margin. A 5-mm (or 10-mm) cannula for a 5-mm (or 10-mm) laparoscope is placed at the umbilicus. Depending on the size of the patient and distance to the stomach, the camera port may need to be placed more cephalad along the midline. In a small patient a 5-mm laparoscope is adequate, but in a large patient a 10-mm scope may be necessary for adequate imaging. A 5-mm port is placed in the right subcostal region at the midclavicular line. An additional 5-mm port may be placed in the left subcostal region for assistance, if necessary (**FIGURE 2**).

1

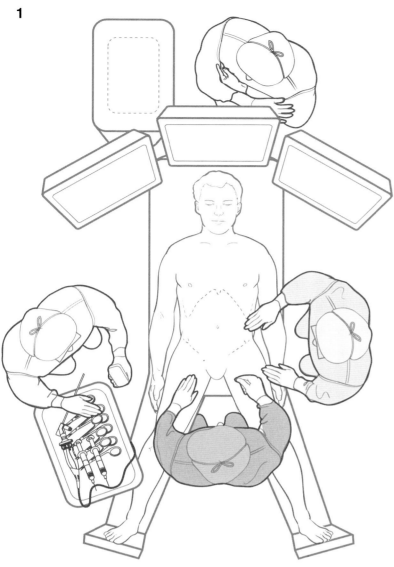

2

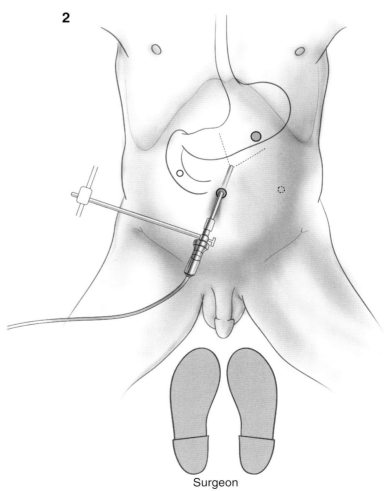

Surgeon

Gastrostomy Tube Placement The patient is placed in a moderate reverse Trendelenburg position to allow the small bowel and colon to slide away from the stomach. The anterior wall of the body of the stomach is grasped at least 8 cm away from the pylorus and brought up to the left upper anterior wall at the proposed gastrostomy tube site. If there is undue tension, another portion of the stomach should be selected. The pneumo-peritoneum pressure is decreased to 6 to 8 mm Hg to make it easier to elevate the stomach to the abdominal wall.

After local anesthetic is administered and a small nick made in the skin, a T-fastener needle is brought through the abdominal wall and the anterior wall of the stomach **(FIGURE 3)**. Before deploying each T-fastener, air should be injected into the needle to confirm insufflation of the stomach. This ensures that the T-fastener will not be placed through the back wall of the stomach or in a submucosal plane. Elevation of the anterior wall is essential throughout this procedure to prevent injury to the back wall of the stomach.

A total of four T-fasteners are placed in a diamond pattern **(FIGURE 4)**. To optimize retraction and visualization, the first T-fastener should be placed laterally and superiorly away from the endoscope. The second and third T-fasteners are placed at the superior medial and inferior lateral position. The final fastener is placed inferior medially closest to the endoscope. The T-fasteners are then lifted, but not yet permanently secured, to ensure proper fixation and elevation of the anterior gastric wall.

A small incision is made in the skin between the T-fasteners. A 14-gauge needle is passed through this incision into the stomach. Air should again be insufflated to confirm intraluminal position of the needle tip. A 0.35-mm guidewire is advanced through this needle and threaded at least 15 cm into the stomach **(FIGURE 5)**. Using the Seldinger technique, dilators are sequentially passed over the guidewire to dilate the tract **(FIGURE 6)**. A 16 to 18 French gastrostomy tube is then passed into the stomach, and the guidewire is removed **(FIGURE 7)**. The balloon of the gastrostomy tube is filled and the tube retracted to its final position. The T-fasteners are secured over bolsters to maintain the stomach in apposition with the anterior abdominal wall. The gastrostomy tube is secured to the skin with sutures or a Silastic footplate **(FIGURE 8)**.

POSTOPERATIVE CARE The gastrostomy tube should initially be kept to gravity drainage to allow for decompression of the stomach. Feeding through the tube may be started the morning after surgery, and advanced to goal over the next 48 hours. If bolsters are used (as shown in these drawings) they should be removed between 7 and 14 days from placement. Latex tubes should be changed every 3 months, and Silastic tubes should be replaced every 6 to 9 months. A "button" appliance may be used to replace the tube after a track has formed, after at least 3 weeks to a month. ■

3

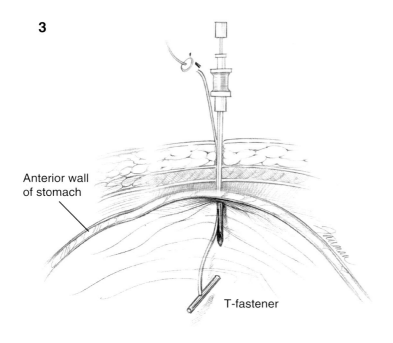

Anterior wall
of stomach

T-fastener

4

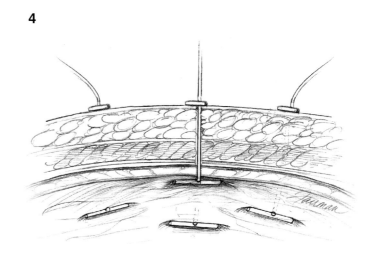

5

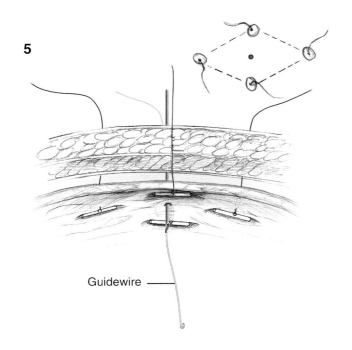

Guidewire

6

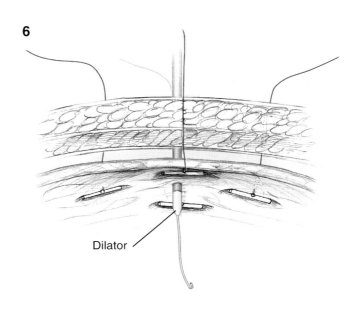

Dilator

7

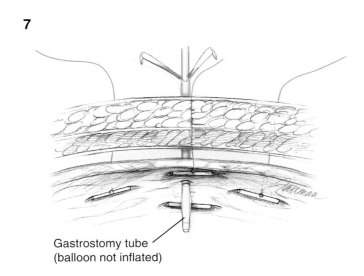

Gastrostomy tube
(balloon not inflated)

8

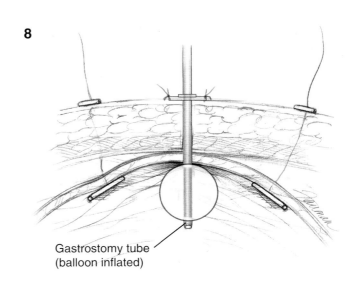

Gastrostomy tube
(balloon inflated)

JEJUNOSTOMY TUBE PLACEMENT

INDICATIONS Whenever possible, nutrition should be delivered through enteral routes. The past two decades have seen a shift in treatment approaches from open techniques to a predominance of laparoscopically and endoscopically placed feeding tubes. Beginning in the early 1990s, the technique for laparoscopic feeding jejunostomy tube (J-tube) placement has undergone numerous revisions and refinements, providing a safe and expedient form of enteral access.

Patients with complex surgical and medical problems benefit greatly from adequate nutritional support. Enteral feeding is often required for patients with significant recurrent aspiration, intraabdominal trauma, long-term ventilatory support, esophageal or gastric dysmotility, and complications following abdominal operations that render the upper GI tract undesirable or inaccessible for enteral access. In addition to patients with long-term enteral feeding requirements, the surgeon anticipating a delay in oral intake after complex abdominal procedures may elect to place a jejunostomy tube for early postoperative feeding.

PATIENT POSITIONING The patient should be placed in the supine position. General anesthesia with a naso- or orogastric tube for stomach decompression is required. All pressure points are carefully protected. The operating surgeon stands on the patient's right with the assistant on the patient's left. The primary monitor should be over the patient's left shoulder, with an additional monitor for the assistant at the right shoulder (**FIGURE 1**).

DETAILS OF PROCEDURE The future tube position is chosen and marked in the left midabdomen, near the lateral edge of the rectus muscle. The site should be at least 4 cm from the costal margin and well above the patient's usual belt line. A pneumoperitoneum to 15 mm Hg pressure with CO_2 is obtained through the umbilicus with a Veress needle. If the jejunostomy is to be performed as a stand-alone procedure, the first port is a 5-mm camera port placed to the right of the umbilicus, approximately 15 cm from the jejunostomy tube entrance site. Two other ports are placed in the right abdomen above and below the primary port (**FIGURE 2**). Both secondary ports should be 5-mm. Care is exhibited to place all trocars lateral to the right epigastric artery. If the J-tube is performed as a complementary procedure to a more involved laparoscopic procedure, the port positions chosen for that procedure may be used for the jejunostomy tube placement. However, if visualization of the ligament of Treitz or bowel manipulation is difficult, additional trocars should be placed to improve the safety and ease of the operation.

Several techniques have been used successfully to allow laparoscopic J-tube placement. The T-fastener method to attach the jejunum to the abdominal wall is essentially a combination percutaneous Seldinger technique with laparoscopic guidance.

The transverse colon is elevated cephalad and anteriorly. The ligament of Treitz is identified. The jejunum is traced distally from the ligament of Treitz for a distance of at least 40 cm. The ideal location is the portion of jejunum with the longest mesentery. The target site for the placement of the T-fasteners is identified on the antimesenteric side of the jejunum. The assistant palpates the abdomen from the outside while observing the depression point internally to confirm the proposed tube position (**FIGURE 3**).

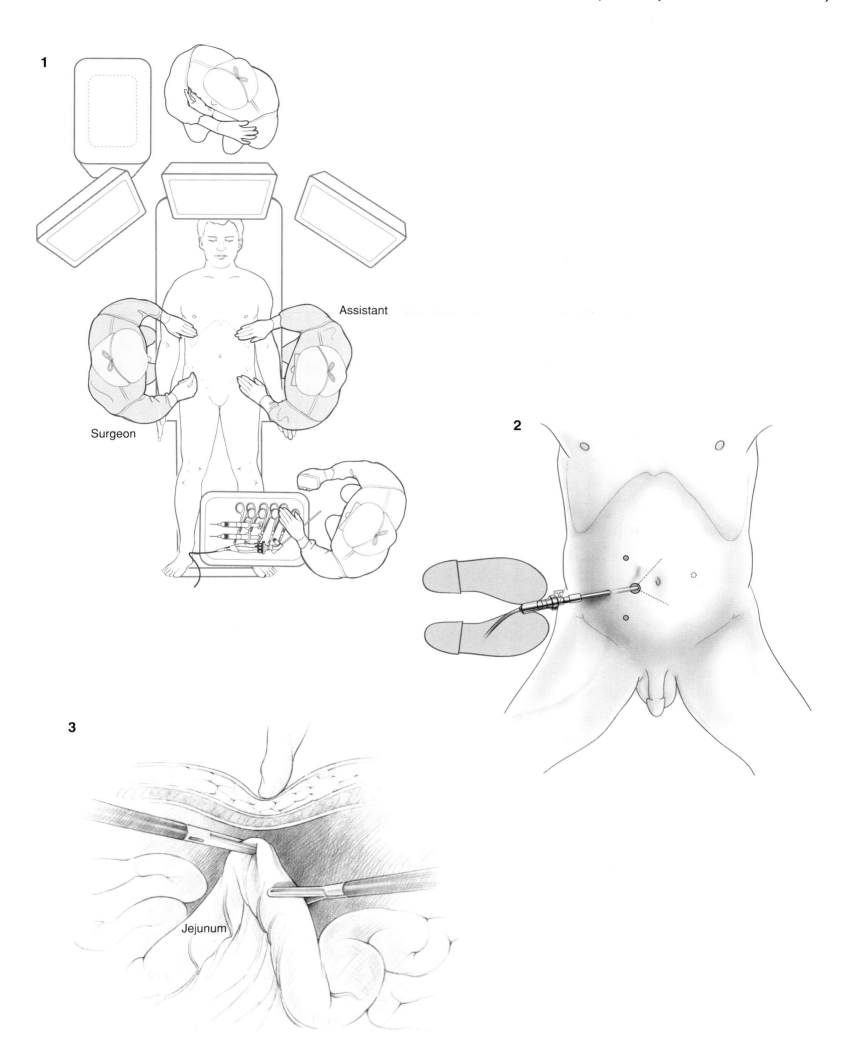

1

Assistant

Surgeon

2

3

Jejunum

DETAILS OF PROCEDURE   Local analgesia is administered with a 20-gauge needle, thoroughly injecting in all layers of the abdominal wall and creating a wheal on the peritoneal surface to again confirm position. With the operating surgeon gently holding the bowel near the abdominal wall at points proximal and distal to the enterotomy site, the assistant passes the T-fastener needle and places the first securing T-fastener. The first fastener is placed at the most proximal position in the middle of the bowel, akin to the 12 o'clock position on a clock (**FIGURE 4**). Air is injected through the needle to confirm that the needle tip position is intraluminal and not in the bowel wall prior to deployment. The same is done for the anchoring sutures at the 3 and 6 o'clock positions. Next, the large-bore needle is passed through the abdominal wall and into the jejunum, centering it in the middle of the 12 and 6 o'clock. The guidewire is passed through the needle, advancing at least 25 cm into the distal bowel lumen (**FIGURE 5**). The needle is carefully removed, leaving the guidewire behind. The dilating catheter and sheath are passed over the wire into the jejunum and directed into the distal jejunal limb (**FIGURE 6**). After the tract is adequately dilated, the wire and dilator are removed, and the jejunostomy tube is passed through the sheath (**FIGURE 7**) and advanced into the lumen (**FIGURE 8**). Additional coordination may be required as the tube is advanced. It is imperative to make sure that the tip of the tube is passed distally, not proximally. The operating surgeon may need to straighten or otherwise manipulate the bowel in order to facilitate tube passage. Other techniques that may prevent the tube from coiling or passing aborally include gently milking the tube through the bowel and/or injecting saline through the tube to provide lubrication. If resistance is encountered, the tube may need to be repositioned.

The sheath is carefully peeled away, leaving the catheter in the lumen. The operating surgeon can help guide the tube further into the jejunum using atraumatic graspers if necessary. The final anchoring suture is placed at the 9 o'clock position (**FIGURE 9**). Once the tube is properly positioned, the assistant gently pulls on the fastening sutures and, under direct laparoscopic visualization, the bowel is cinched up to the peritoneum (**FIGURE 10**). Decreasing insufflation pressure to a maximum of 8 mm Hg lowers the abdominal ceiling, bringing it closer to the jejunum. Care should be taken not to strangulate the bowel while ensuring an adequate seal against the peritoneal surface. We favor not using further anchoring sutures either proximal or distal to the T-fasteners.

Before camera and port removal, the operating surgeon must ensure that the bowel is not kinked or twisted. The tube is secured at skin level by crimping the metal clips to the suture above the supplied bolsters. Additional anchoring sutures affixing the tube to the skin should be placed to avoid accidental early tube dislodgement.

ALTERNATE APPROACHES   If specific kits are unavailable, laparoscopic approaches can still be successfully employed using other instrumentation. The bowel can be fixed to the abdominal wall with intracorporeally placed sutures in the same configuration as the T-fasteners. Alternatively, transfacial sutures can be placed using a percutaneous grasping type needle device to secure the jejunum to the abdominal wall in the same diamond configuration. Other percutaneous Seldinger-type introducers may be used for introducing any type of jejunostomy tube desired. The technique of "needle catheter jejunostomy" can be employed. This technique does not require attaching the small bowel to the abdominal wall, but uses a very small tube that may be more easily plugged or dislodged.

POSTOPERATIVE CARE   Feeding should be instituted slowly and advanced to goal while the patient is carefully monitored. We use only "trophic levels" of tube feeding (10–20 mL/hr) until the postoperative ileus has audibly resolved. Although 24-hour around-the-clock feedings are usually initialized, the patient can be rapidly transitioned to 16-hour nocturnal feedings to allow greater daytime independence. The cotton bolsters are cut off flush with the skin level 7 to 14 days after tube placement, depending on the patient's nutritional status. Typically, feeding tubes can be replaced without too much difficulty once the tract has epithelialized (approximately 2–3 weeks after placement). It is prudent to confirm the intraluminal position of the replacement tube with a contrast radiograph before resuming tube feeds, unless the tract is very well epithelialized and tube changes have become frequent and facile.

Though established as a safe technique, laparoscopically placed J-tubes are not without potential pitfalls. Intolerance of feeding can lead to GI distress, bloating, flatulence, and diarrhea. Wound infection, GI content leakage around the skin site or intraperitoneally, and erosion of the skin at the tube site are potentially avoidable complications that should be addressed with diligent tube and wound care. Tube dysfunction including blockage, dislodgement, and breakdown over time may require tube replacement. Rare but potentially catastrophic complications include bowel perforation, infarction, and bowel obstruction due to volvulus or inspissation of concentrated formulas. ■

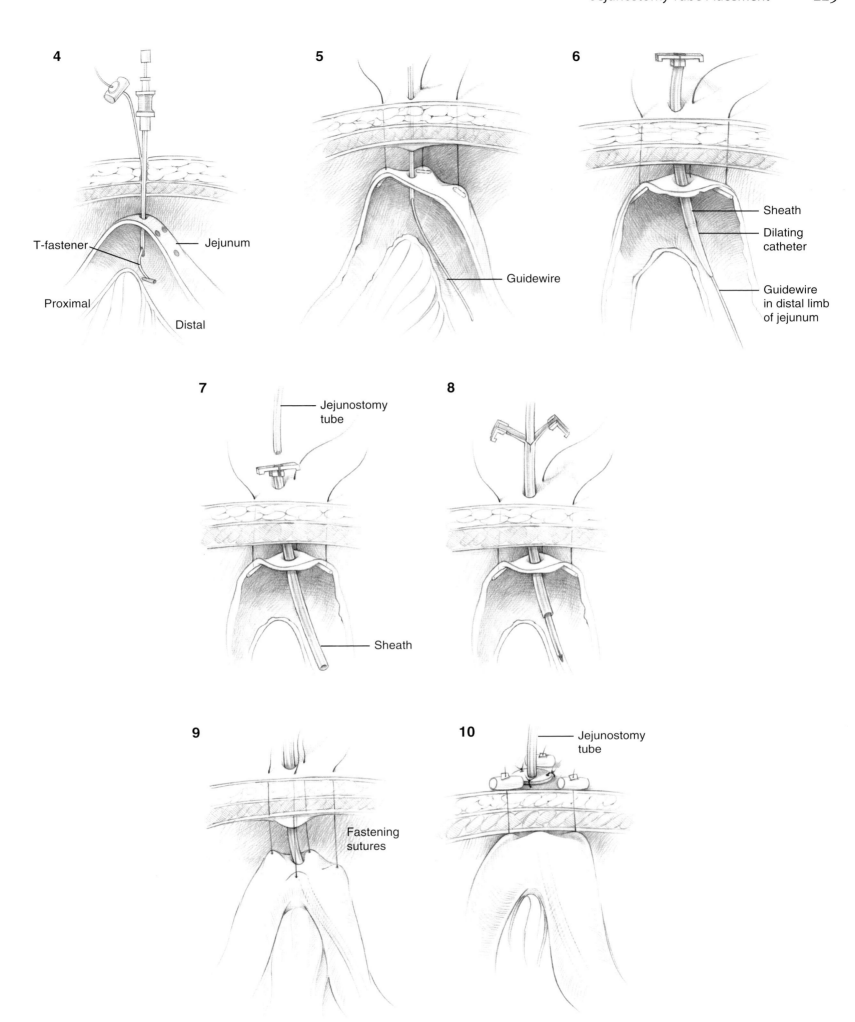

4

T-fastener

Jejunum

Proximal

Distal

5

Guidewire

6

Sheath

Dilating catheter

Guidewire in distal limb of jejunum

7

Jejunostomy tube

Sheath

8

9

Fastening sutures

10

Jejunostomy tube

SECTION V
MINIMALLY INVASIVE BARIATRIC SURGERY

ROUX-EN-Y GASTRIC BYPASS

INDICATIONS Laparoscopic Roux-en-Y gastric bypass (LRYGB) is indicated for patients who meet the 1991 NIH Consensus criteria for bariatric surgery. These indications include a body mass index (BMI) of 40 kg/m² or greater or 35 kg/m² or greater and the presence of serious obesity-related comorbidities. Additionally, patients must have failed attempts at nonsurgical weight loss such as supervised medical weight loss programs, behavioral therapy, or pharmacologic therapy. Comorbidities that are frequently associated with morbid obesity (and improve or resolve after gastric bypass) include obstructive sleep apnea, obesity hypoventilation syndrome, hypertension, diabetes, hyperlipidemia, degenerative joint disease, and gastroesophageal reflux disease. Other obesity-related comorbidities include venous stasis disease, migraine headaches, pseudotumor cerebri, asthma, infertility or menstrual problems, stress urinary incontinence, gout, and skin infections related to a pannus or skin folds.

PREOPERATIVE PREPARATION Bariatric surgery patients require an extensive preoperative evaluation to determine their anesthetic risk, to define the severity of known comorbidities, and to identify occult comorbid conditions such as sleep apnea, obesity hypoventilation syndrome, and coronary artery disease. This evaluation requires a multidisciplinary approach. The bariatric team should include dieticians, psychologists, and medical subspecialists who can optimize the patient's cardiovascular, pulmonary, and endocrine status prior to surgery. Patients with active substance abuse problems or uncontrolled psychiatric disorders are not candidates for bariatric surgery. Strong family and social support for the patient is important to achieving a successful outcome.

Patients who are preparing for bariatric surgery must be fully informed about all of the available surgical options. The choice of laparoscopic bariatric operations today include laparoscopic adjustable gastric banding, sleeve gastrectomy, gastric bypass, or a malabsorptive procedure such as biliopancreatic diversion (BPD) or BPD with duodenal switch. The risks and benefits of LRYGB should be discussed in detail with the patient and put into context with the other available bariatric procedures and other major laparoscopic operations performed today.

ANESTHESIA Laparoscopic RYGB requires a general anesthetic. The anesthesiologist must be prepared for a difficult airway in this patient population. The surgeon should be available during induction, intubation, and extubation should a surgical airway become necessary. Patients with sleep apnea and obesity hypoventilation syndrome are at particularly high risk for airway problems and should be continued on their continuous positive airway pressure (CPAP) devices postoperatively in the hospital. Antiemetics should be started in the operating room during the case and continued as needed postoperatively. Pain control is achieved with narcotic patient-controlled anesthesia for 1 or 2 days postoperatively and transitioned to oral pain medication in elixir form prior to discharge.

POSITION The patient is placed supine on the operating table with legs together and arms abducted. The weight limit for the operating room table should be confirmed with the manufacturer and should be sufficient for bariatric patients. A padded footboard is placed on the foot of the bed, and the patient's legs are secured together with the feet on the footboard. Adequate padding must be placed between the knees and calves prior to securing the legs together. A safety belt is placed low across the patient's hips. The arms are abducted no more than 90 degrees and padded before they are secured to the armboards. Before prepping and draping, the patient is placed in steep reverse Trendelenburg position and observed for stability on the operating table.

The primary surgeon stands to the patient's right. The first assistant stands across from the surgeon on the patient's left and the second assistant or camera operator stands to the left of the first assistant. The scrub nurse stands at the foot of the bed within arm's reach of the surgeon and first assistant. Video monitors are placed above the patient's head on the left and the right (**FIGURE 1**).

OPERATIVE PREPARATION A Foley catheter and orogastric tube are placed after induction of anesthesia. The surgeon must remember to have the anesthesiologist remove the orogastric tube from the stomach before the gastric pouch is created. The abdomen is prepped and draped to provide an adequate field should the patient be converted to laparotomy. The field should be draped far laterally to provide access for the liver retractor and first assistant's retraction ports.

INCISION AND EXPOSURE Abdominal access is obtained using a Veress needle in the supraumbilical position. The first port placed is a 10-mm camera port superior and to the right of the umbilicus. This will be the primary camera port for the remainder of the case and will give the necessary perspective for placement of the remaining ports. The four operating ports are placed under laparoscopic visualization. Intraperitoneal needle visualization and infiltration of local anesthetic allows the laparoscopist to identify the intraperitoneal site of trocar entry *before* trocar placement, as most trocar injuries from secondary trocars occur when the port is introduced out of the laparoscopic field of vision. The liver size, body habitus, and degree of adhesions present will dictate the exact position of the remaining ports but the location and port size is generally consistent. Typically, three 12-mm and one 5-mm ports are placed as shown (**FIGURE 2**). After all five ports are placed, laparoscopic inspection of the peritoneal cavity is completed.

Creating an adequate working space at the gastroesophageal (GE) junction is key to performing this operation safely. A 5-mm Nathanson liver retractor is placed in the subxiphoid position after completion of the jejunojejunostomy in advance of creating the gastric pouch.

DETAILS OF THE PROCEDURE

Antecolic Roux-en-Y The first step is to create the Roux limb and complete the jejunojejunostomy. The bed is maintained in the flat position during this part of the operation. The greater omentum is passed completely into the upper abdomen, and the transverse colon is retracted superiorly. A grasper is used by the assistant to retract the transverse mesocolon superiorly, and the surgeon identifies the ligament of Treitz. Any small bowel in the left upper quadrant is then pulled downward, and the proximal jejunum is placed in a "C" configuration to help orient the proximal and distal segments (**FIGURE 3**). The jejunum is then divided approximately 50 cm distal to the ligament of Treitz using a linear cutting stapler with a vascular load (**FIGURE 4**). The mesentery of the jejunum is further divided with one or two firings of the same stapler to provide sufficient length of mesentery for tension-free passage of the Roux limb to the gastric pouch. Care should be taken to ensure adequate blood supply on both sides of the staple line as the mesentery is divided. Immediately after the division of the small bowel, a short Penrose drain is sutured to the corner of the distal segment (Roux limb) to avoid confusing the Roux limb with the biliopancreatic limb later in the case.

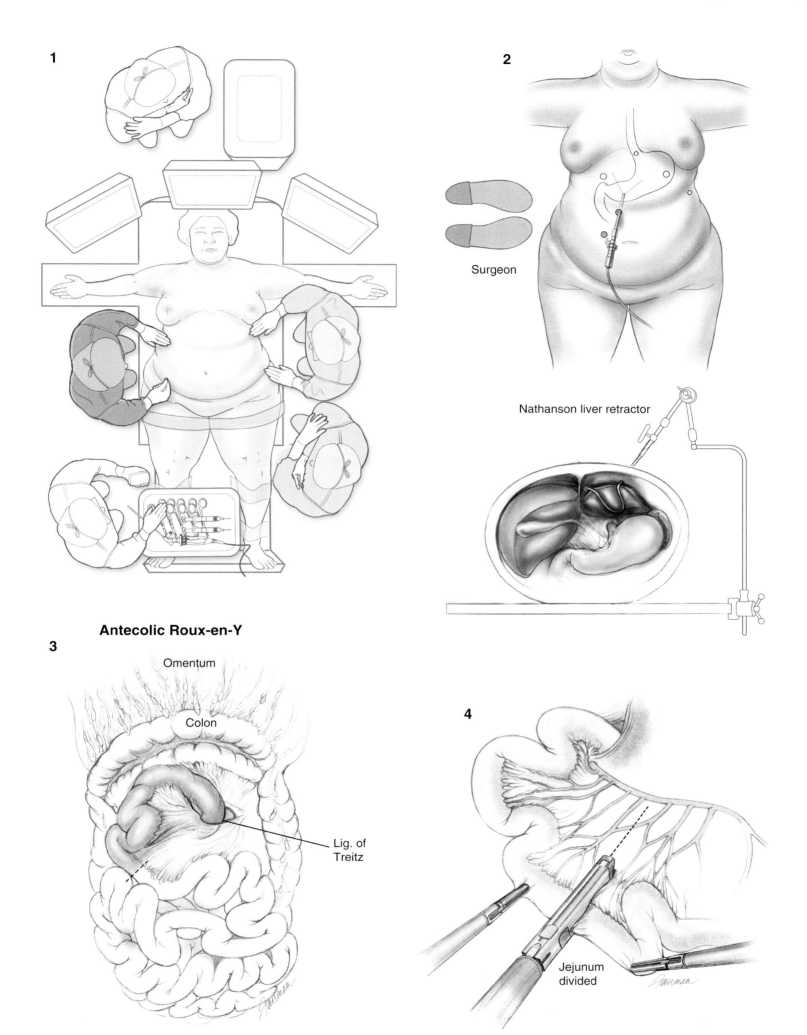

1

2

Surgeon

Nathanson liver retractor

Antecolic Roux-en-Y

3

Omentum

Colon

Lig. of Treitz

4

Jejunum divided

Antecolic Roux-en-Y The Roux limb is measured distally from the Penrose drain for a distance of at least 75 cm. (**FIGURE 5**). Increasing the length of the Roux limb from 75 cm to 150 cm or longer can improve weight loss in superobese patients (BMI > 50). The bowel should be gently straightened (not stretched) against a rigid measuring device such as a marked grasper to determine the proper Roux limb length. Once the appropriate length is measured, a suture is placed to approximate the end of the biliopancreatic limb and the Roux limb side by side.

The Bovie cautery is used to create an enterotomy in the biliopancreatic limb. An enterotomy is then made in the antimesenteric side of the adjacent Roux limb. This is offset from the first enterotomy (1–2 cm proximal) to provide easier access for the linear stapler. A side-to-side, functional end-to-end jejunojejunostomy is created using the linear stapler with a 45-mm vascular load (**FIGURE 6**). The common opening is closed with a running absorbable suture. Alternatively, a second stapler firing can be used after placing a stitch through the common lumen and using graspers at each corner, creating three points of fixation. If this method is used, care must be taken to avoid narrowing either lumen.

Once the jejunojejunostomy is completed, it is inspected for kinking or obvious staple line failures, and two reinforcing Lembert sutures are placed using 3-0 braided nonabsorbable suture. One reinforcing stitch is placed between the stapled end of the biliopancreatic limb and the Roux limb ("Brolin stitch"). The second ("crotch stitch") is placed at the other end of the anastomosis to relieve tension where the two bowel limbs separate. The mesenteric defect between the biliopancreatic and Roux limb is then closed with a running nonabsorbable suture (**FIGURES 7 AND 8**).

The omentum is divided to allow antecolic placement of the Roux limb. With the transverse colon still flipped upward, this step can be started where the omentum attaches to the transverse colon. As the omentum is divided with the ultrasonic shears, the two leaves are pulled downward and apart to create a path for the antecolic Roux limb. The Roux limb is passed upward to the gastric pouch between the leaves of the completely divided omentum in the antecolic and antegastric position (**FIGURE 9**). The attached Penrose drain provides an atraumatic handle for this maneuver. To minimize tension on the Roux limb during creation of the gastrojejunostomy, all of the Roux limb and the completed jejunojejunostomy (which can act like an anchor) should be delivered as far superiorly as possible.

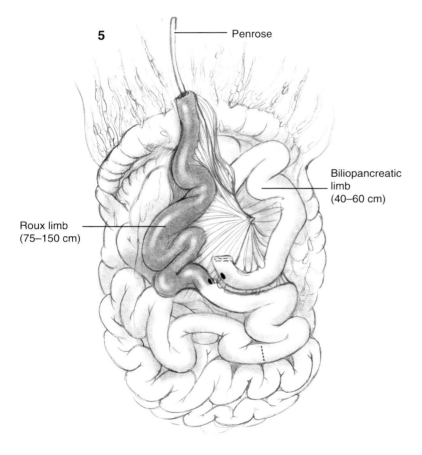

5   Penrose

Biliopancreatic limb (40–60 cm)

Roux limb (75–150 cm)

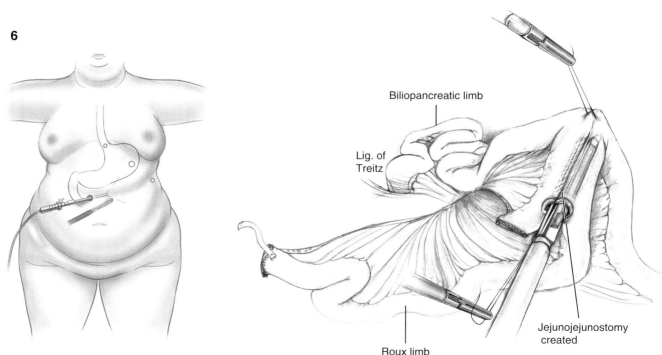

6

Biliopancreatic limb

Lig. of Treitz

Jejunojejunostomy created

Roux limb

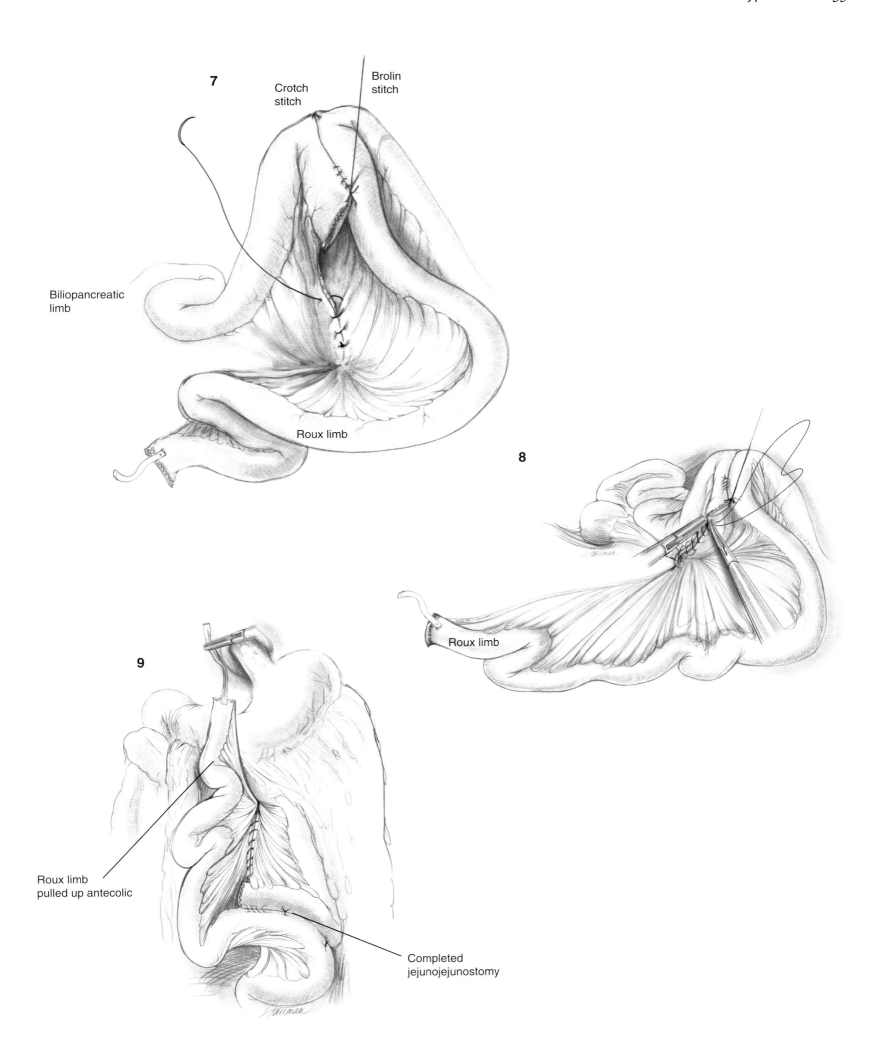

7

Crotch stitch

Brolin stitch

Biliopancreatic limb

Roux limb

8

Roux limb

9

Roux limb pulled up antecolic

Completed jejunojejunostomy

Creation of Gastric Pouch The patient is placed in steep reverse Trendelenburg position for this part of the operation. The dissection is started by creating a window in the clear space of the gastrohepatic ligament just below the hepatic branch of the vagus with the ultrasonic shears. The ideal size of the gastric pouch can be determined using a 30-cc gastric balloon inflated in the gastric fundus and pulled back against the GE junction. Once the lesser curvature is reached at the inferior end of the balloon, a retrogastric space is developed carefully using a combination of the Harmonic scalpel and blunt dissection. Once the space is entered, it is enlarged to allow the passage of a 45-mm medium thick linear stapler into the retrogastric space. The stapler is fired to start the construction of the pouch. The stomach can be tented up to expose any adhesions to the pancreas that require division. The linear stapler with a blue load is then placed horizontally across the lesser curvature of the stomach immediately below the balloon (**FIGURE 10A**). Once this firing is complete, blunt dissection can be used to create a path up to the angle of His. A blunt instrument with a roticulating tip is used to perform this maneuver. The fundus is pulled caudad by the assistant, and two or three more firings of the stapler are directed toward the angle of His to complete the gastric pouch (**FIGURE 10B**). The pouch should be 15 to 20 mL in size when completed. The pouch is dissected free from the left crus of the diaphragm with the ultrasonic scalpel to improve mobility and ensure complete separation from the excluded stomach. The excluded stomach is dissected away from the pouch. If any oozing is encountered during gastric pouch creation or mobilization, a sponge is placed in the abdomen and the area lateral to the angle of His is packed to improve visualization. The sponge should be removed after completion of the gastrojejunostomy.

Retrocolic Roux-en-Y In the early experience with this operation, most surgeons placed the Roux limb in the retrocolic, retrogastric position to avoid tension on the gastrojejunostomy. There is now a large experience with placing the Roux limb in the antecolic and antegastric position, and this is the preferred approach for most surgeons. There has been no increase in leak or stricture rates with the technically easier antecolic approach. Nevertheless, placement of the Roux limb in the retrocolic space may be necessary if the patient has adhesive disease or a foreshortened mesentery that prohibits antecolic placement. The need for retrocolic placement is usually determined after an attempt to bring the Roux limb antecolic to the gastric pouch has been unsuccessful. The retrocolic Roux limb can be delivered to the pouch in the antegastric or retrogastric position based on the amount of tension present.

To place the Roux limb in the retrocolic space, an opening is created in the transverse mesocolon approximately 4 cm to the left and 4 cm superior to the ligament of Treitz (**FIGURE 11**). This is done by tenting up the peritoneal surface of the mesocolon and dividing it with the ultrasonic shears. After the mesentery has been opened, careful blunt dissection is used to enter the less sac and the retrogastric space. A blunt roticulating grasper is used to create a path for the Roux limb. Once the path has been determined, the Penrose drain is used to pull the Roux limb through the mesocolic defect and behind the stomach. Once the Penrose emerges from behind the excluded stomach, it is grasped from above and an adequate length of Roux limb is delivered to the gastric pouch (**FIGURE 12**). Care is taken to ensure that the Roux limb is not twisted as it is passed to the pouch. After the retrocolic gastrojejunostomy is completed, the mesenteric defects are closed. This includes closing the mesocolic defect around the Roux limb as well as the space between the mesocolon and the Roux limb mesentery (Peterson's space) with running nonabsorbable suture. The mesenteric defect at the jejunojejunostomy is closed as described above.

Creation of Gastric Pouch

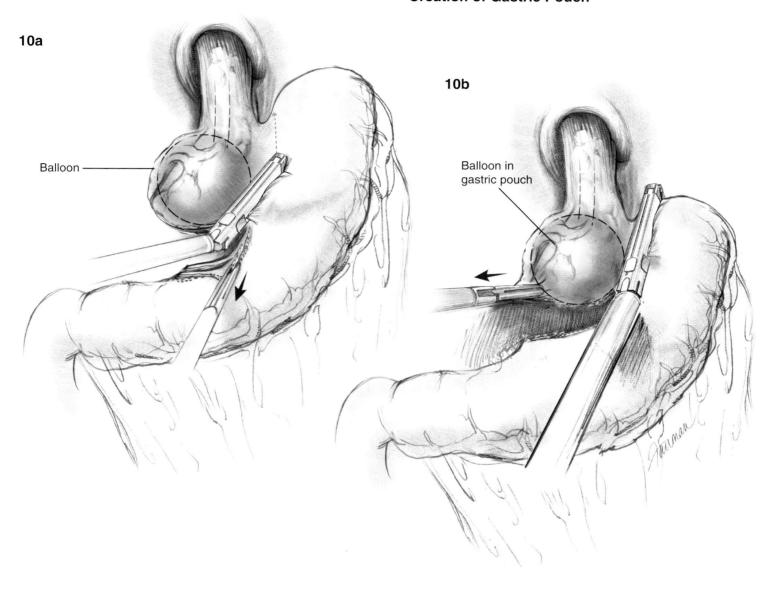

10a

Balloon

10b

Balloon in
gastric pouch

Retrocolic Roux-en-Y

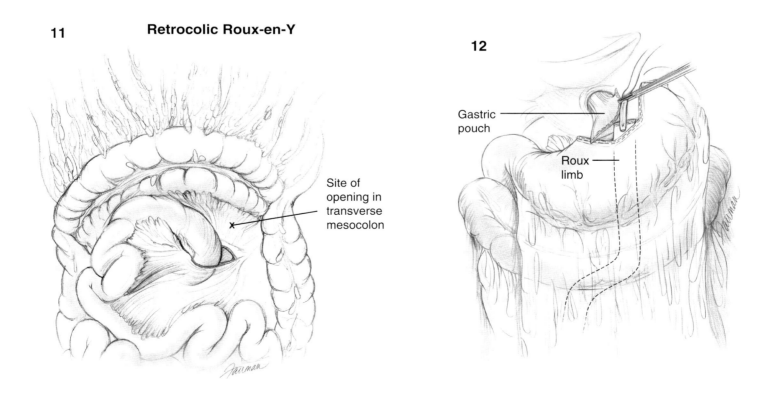

11

Site of
opening in
transverse
mesocolon

12

Gastric
pouch

Roux
limb

Hand-Sewn Gastrojejunostomy After the gastric pouch is created, the gastrojejunal anastomosis is completed. The hand-sewn technique uses a two-layer anastomosis over a 32 French orogastric tube. Though technically the most demanding technique, this method has the advantage of using less specialized equipment (staplers) and generally has a lower stricture rate than the circular stapled techniques.

The Roux limb is delivered to the gastric pouch without twisting or tension in an antecolic (or retrocolic) fashion. Interrupted 2-0 nonabsorbable sutures are used to approximate the Roux limb to the pouch. The staple line of the pouch can be incorporated into this posterior layer (**FIGURE 13**). A 32 French blunt orogastric tube is gently placed in the pouch and used to localize the site for the gastrotomy. A 12-mm gastrotomy and an adjacent 12-mm jejunotomy are made with the ultrasonic shears (**FIGURE 14**). A corner stitch of 3-0 absorbable suture is used to start the inner layer of the anastomosis. It is tied, and the suture is then brought back inside the anastomosis (**FIGURE 15**). The inner layer is run posteriorly and then completed anteriorly. Prior to completing this layer, the orogastric tube can be placed through the anastomosis to size the lumen and help prevent an inadvertent bite through the back wall of the anastomosis (**FIGURE 16**). After the inner layer is complete, an anterior outer layer of nonabsorbable Lembert sutures is placed (**FIGURE 17**). After the anastomosis is complete, the orogastric tube is removed and intraoperative endoscopy is performed. The anastomosis is inspected for patency and hemostasis. With the anastomosis submerged in saline and the Roux limb clamped closed, air insufflation is used to check for leaks (**FIGURE 18**).

13   Hand-sewn Technique

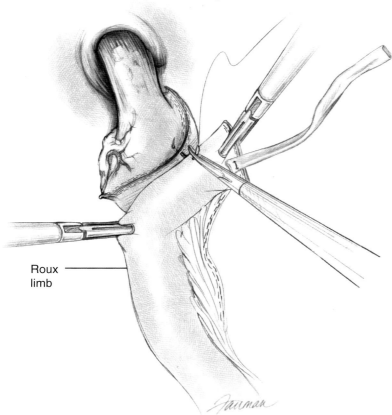

Roux
limb

14

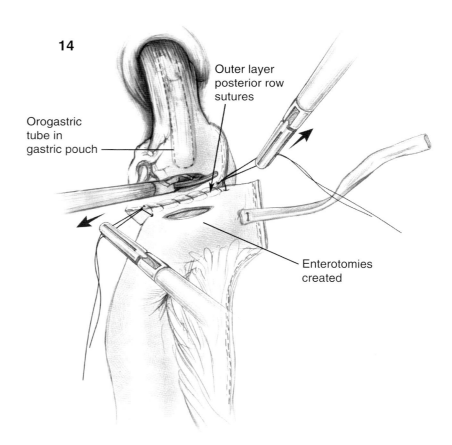

Outer layer
posterior row
sutures

Orogastric
tube in
gastric pouch

Enterotomies
created

15

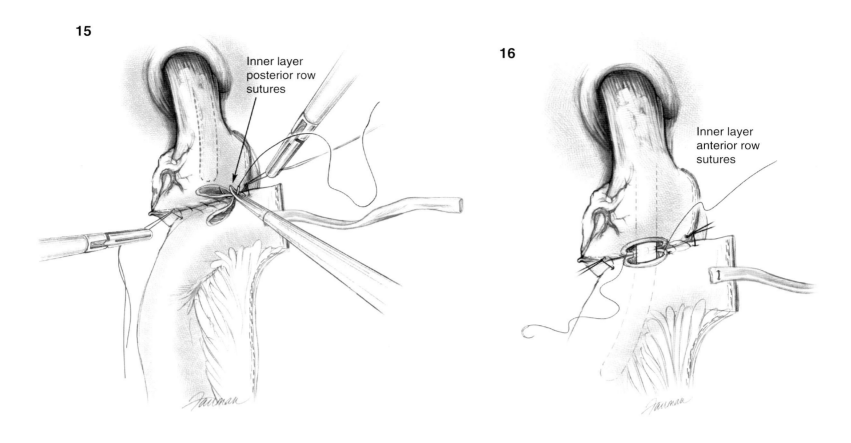

Inner layer
posterior row
sutures

16

Inner layer
anterior row
sutures

17

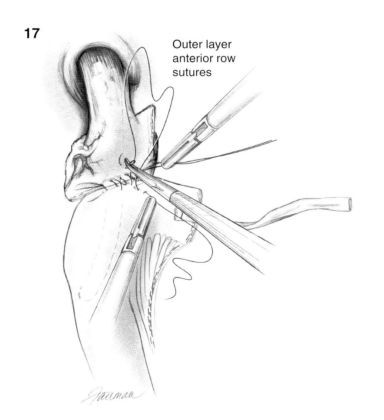

Outer layer
anterior row
sutures

18

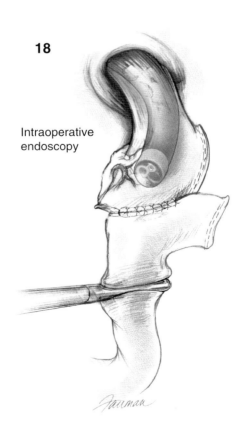

Intraoperative
endoscopy

Linear-Stapled Technique As an alternative to the handsewn technique, the gastrojejunostomy can be created using a stapler. After the jejunojejunostomy is completed and the gastric pouch is created, the Roux limb is delivered to the pouch using the attached Penrose drain as a handle. With the Roux limb positioned for anastomosis, the Roux limb is traced back to the jejunojejunostomy to make sure there are no twists in this bowel segment. The biliopancreatic limb should again be traced back to the ligament of Treitz to ensure that the Roux limb and not the pancreatobiliary limb will be stapled to the stomach. The Roux limb is sutured to the posterior wall of the gastric pouch using a running 2-0 nonabsorbable suture (**FIGURE 19**). Both ends of the suture are preserved to allow manipulation of the anastomosis by the surgeon and assistant.

Once this posterior layer is completed, the anastomosis is created with a 45-mm medium thick linear cutting stapler. A small gastrotomy is made anterior to the staple line of the pouch with the ultrasonic shears and an adjacent enterotomy is made in the Roux limb. These only need to be large enough to admit the jaws of the linear stapler. The stapler is placed 1.5 cm into each lumen, closed, and fired (**FIGURE 20**). The stapler is carefully removed, and the common opening is inspected to make sure the internal staple lines are hemostatic (**FIGURE 21**). The enterotomy is closed in two continuous layers over a 32 French orogastric tube. The inner layer of suture should be absorbable. After the inner layer is completed, an outer Lembert layer of nonabsorbable suture completes the anastomosis (**FIGURE 22**). The Penrose drain is removed and the long sutures are cut. The endoscope allows inspection for anastomotic bleeding at the time of the procedure and provides insufflation for leak testing. Alternatively, methylene blue can placed down the nasogastric tube (NGT) to evaluate for leak, although this test may be less sensitive.

19   **Linear Stapled Technique**

Roux limb

20

Enterotomies
created;
stapler inserted
and fired

21

22

Enterotomy
closed in
2 layers

Orogastric
tube

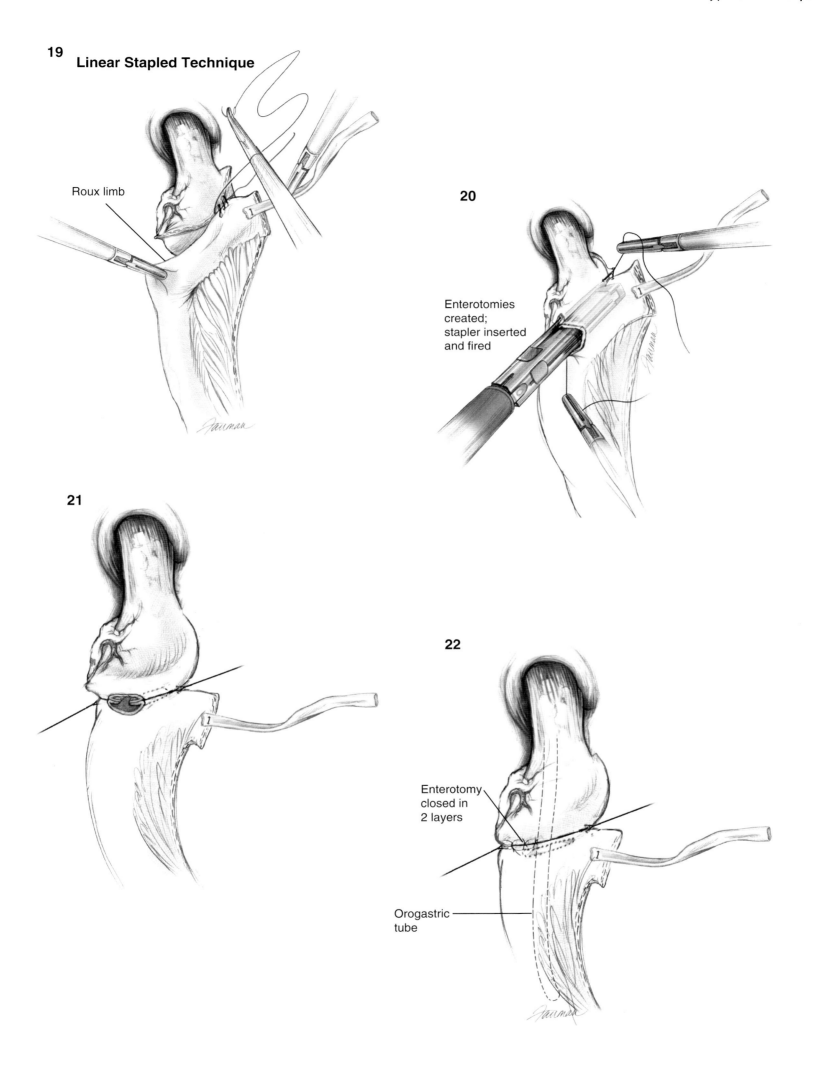

Circular Stapled Gastrojejunostomy, Transoral Method In this anastomotic technique, the small gastric pouch and jejunojejunostomy are created using linear staplers as described earlier. For the gastrojejunostomy, a 21-mm circular stapler anvil attached to a tube is placed transorally and pushed through a small gastrotomy in the posterior pouch (**FIGURE 23**). The surgeon should confirm with the anesthesiologist that the patient is completely paralyzed before pulling the anvil down through the oropharynx. The jaw is subluxed as the anvil is pulled into the esophagus (**FIGURE 24**). Once the anvil is in the gastric pouch with the shaft delivered through the gastrotomy, the orogastric tube is separated from the anvil and removed through a port. A left upper quadrant port is enlarged enough to permit entry of the circular stapler. The stapled end of the Roux limb is cut off to open the end of the Roux limb, and the EEA stapler is placed in the lumen of the bowel. The spike is pushed through the antimesenteric border of the Roux limb and the stapler is attached to the anvil, closed and fired to create the anastomosis (**FIGURE 25**). The open end of the Roux limb is closed with a firing of the linear stapler. To avoid leaving a large blind pouch at the end of the Roux limb, only about 2 cm of this "candy cane" limb should be left in place. The circular staple line is reinforced with circumferential interrupted sutures (**FIGURE 26**). The final configuration is shown (**FIGURE 27**).

Final Steps and Closure It is advisable to check for staple line bleeding and perform intraoperative leak testing of the gastrojejunostomy with an endoscope at the end of the case, regardless of the technique used. With the patient flat, the anastomosis is checked for air leaks by occluding the Roux limb distal to the gastrojejunostomy with a bowel clamp, submerging the anastomosis in saline, and insufflating the proximal Roux limb and gastric pouch with air using an endoscope. Any area of the anastomosis that bubbles with insufflation should be carefully localized and oversewn. Fibrin glue may also be applied to the anastomosis in such cases, or in revisional cases when the tissue is indurated. As the endoscope is withdrawn, the anastomosis is inspected for hemostasis. A Jackson-Pratt drain can be left near the anastomosis if concern for leak remains.

Cholecystectomy is performed at the time of LRYGB if the patient is found to have symptomatic cholelithiasis during the preoperative evaluation. A core liver biopsy may be performed if there is concern for non-alcoholic fatty liver disease. The biopsy needle is placed through a nick in the skin into the liver under laparoscopic guidance. The biopsy site is cauterized after the needle is removed from the liver. After the liver biopsy is completed, a final inspection is performed looking for bowel kinks or twists, staple line bleeding or failure, and retained sponges (if used during the gastric dissection). Port sites 10 mm or greater are closed with absorbable suture using a suture-passer.

POSTOPERATIVE CARE Patients are admitted to the bariatric surgical ward after recovering from anesthesia. Sequential compression devices are used throughout the perioperative period, and low-molecular-weight heparin is started within 24 hours postoperatively for venous thromboembolism (VTE) prophylaxis. VTE prophylaxis is extended after discharge for patients with a BMI > 55 or a history of VTE. Antiemetic therapy is started in the operating room and continued as needed on the ward. Patient-controlled analgesia is used for pain management. Essential preoperative medications are continued in intravenous form until the patient is started on liquids. Patients ambulate with assistance the evening of surgery, and frequent use of incentive spirometry is encouraged. Patients take nothing by mouth the night of surgery. A Gastrografin swallow the morning of postoperative day 1 may be obtained, but is not required. If the swallow study is negative for a leak, the patient is started on a clear liquid diet. Once the patient is tolerating liquids, medications are given in elixir form or pills are crushed. The majority of patients are discharged to home on postoperative day 2 when they meet discharge criteria (normal vital signs, regular ambulation, adequate pain control with oral analgesics, tolerating liquids).

Patients are monitored closely for tachycardia and tachypnea during the postoperative period. Anastomotic leaks and pulmonary embolism can have similar presentations in these patients, and a persistent heart rate above 120 beats per minute or shortness of breath mandate an evaluation. Peritoneal findings on physical exam are frequently absent in this patient population; radiologic studies should be performed early if there is suspicion of a leak. When clinical suspicion for a leak is high, laparoscopic reexploration should be performed in lieu of radiographic imaging.

Patients are advanced to a full liquid and then a soft diet over the first 4 to 6 weeks after surgery. Eventually small portions of solid food are well tolerated. Nutritional deficiencies such as iron, B$_{12}$, calcium and vitamin D and folate can occur after LRYGB. All patients should receive lifelong oral micronutrient supplementation and have levels monitored annually. ∎

23   Circular Stapled, Transoral Technique

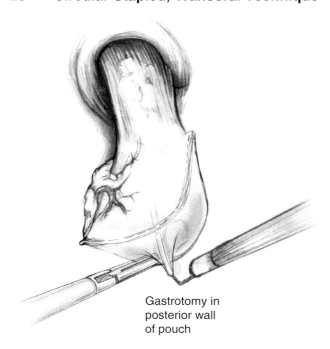

Gastrotomy in posterior wall of pouch

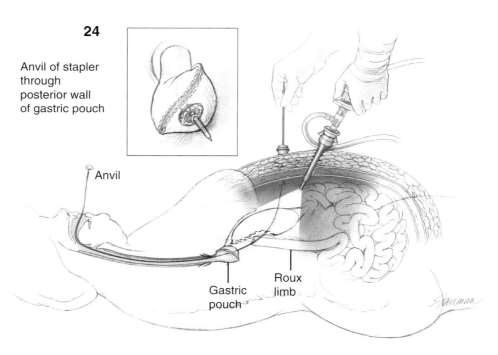

24

Anvil of stapler through posterior wall of gastric pouch

Anvil

Gastric pouch

Roux limb

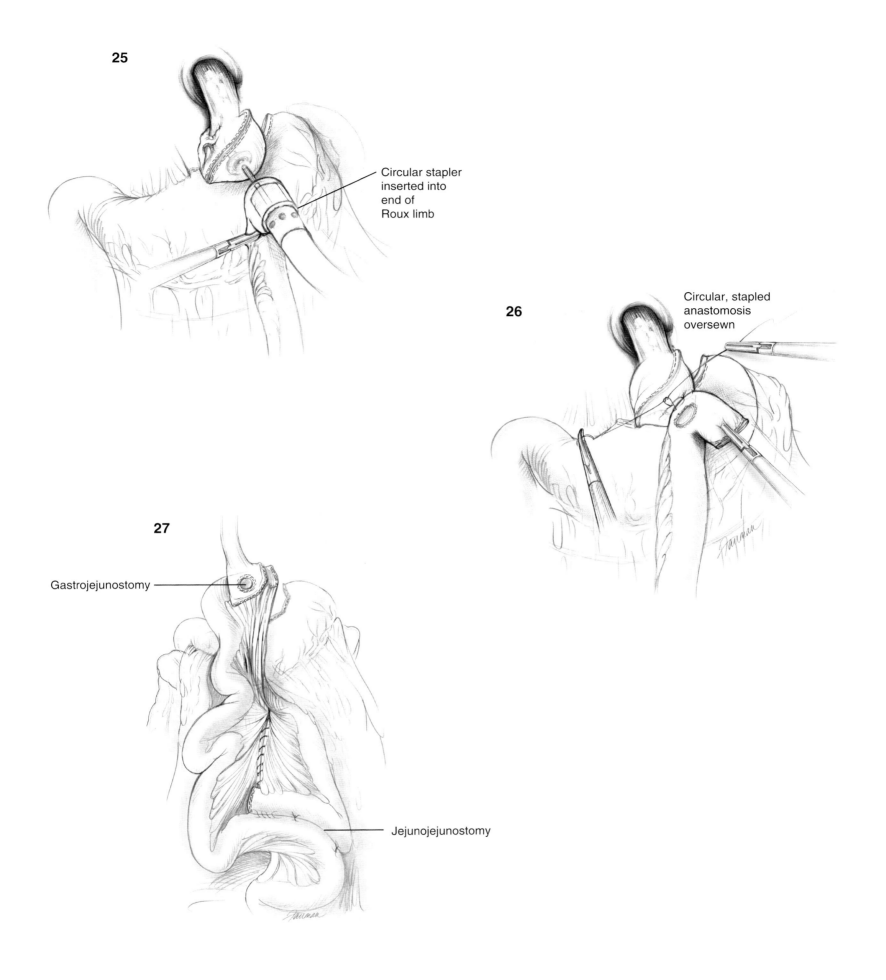

25

Circular stapler inserted into end of Roux limb

26

Circular, stapled anastomosis oversewn

27

Gastrojejunostomy

Jejunojejunostomy

GASTRIC BAND PLACEMENT

INDICATIONS Gastric banding involves the placement of a prosthetic band around the upper stomach, to create a small gastric pouch similar to gastric bypass, but without the need for transection or anastomosis of the gastrointestinal tract. Surgeons in Europe and Australia have accumulated significant experience with gastric banding over the past three decades. As data accumulate, it has become clear that weight loss and metabolic disease remission outcomes after gastric banding do not match those associated with gastric bypass or sleeve gastrectomy, and long-term morbidity requiring band explant may exceed 50%. Nonetheless, peri-operative major morbidity and mortality associated with gastric banding is 5–10-fold lower than that associated with gastric bypass and sleeve gastrectomy. As such, gastric banding, while waning in use, remains a component of the bariatric surgery armamentarium. Gastric band patients often require multiple fills of the band reservoir before weight loss begins, and they typically achieve maximal weight loss after 2 to 5 years. Patients who have difficulty with frequent postoperative visits may not be ideal band candidates, nor are patients who do not understand the postoperative care involved in gastric banding. Candidacy for gastric banding is dictated by National Institutes of Health (NIH) criteria for bariatric surgery and require patients to have a body mass index of at least 40, or at least 35 with a serious obesity-related comorbidity. In addition, patients should demonstrate a full understanding of the advantages and disadvantages of gastric banding, and a willingness to comply with postoperative care.

PREOPERATIVE PREPARATION Candidates for gastric banding should undergo a preoperative upper gastrointestinal series to identify the presence of hiatal hernia. Small hiatal hernias can be repaired at the time of gastric band placement. The presence of a large hiatal hernia, however, although not an absolute contraindication to gastric banding, should be considered carefully in a surgeon's early experience, because repair of such hernias in obese patients can be technically challenging. Patients with symptoms of gastroesophageal reflux disease should undergo 24-hour esophageal pH testing. Data are sparse, but most series report improvement of gastroesophageal reflux disease after gastric banding, although a minority of studies demonstrates worsening of symptoms. Similarly, patients with symptoms of esophageal motility disorders should undergo preoperative esophageal manometry. The presence of significant esophageal dysmotility should be considered a relative contraindication to gastric banding. Despite a paucity of data studying the effect of gastric banding on esophageal motility, concerns remain regarding the long-term effects of gastric banding on patients with severe esophageal dysmotility.

Patients should continue all preoperative medications until the morning of surgery, with the exception of aspirin, nonsteroidal anti-inflammatory agents, warfarin, or heparin. Mechanical bowel preparation is not necessary.

ANESTHESIA General anesthesia with complete neuromuscular blockade is required for laparoscopic gastric banding. Intravenous antibiotics directed against skin flora are often administered, although no data exist to support this practice. Aggressive prophylaxis of nausea prior to emergence from anesthesia is important, as postoperative retching or vomiting may disrupt the gastrogastric fundoplication or band position. Low-dose steroids may be useful in the prevention of perioperative nausea.

A urinary catheter may be placed, although after an initial experience, operative times are usually reduced to the point where this is unnecessary. A gastric balloon suction catheter is passed transorally into the stomach and placed to low wall suction. The upper abdomen is shaved with clippers from the nipples to the umbilicus after induction of anesthesia, and sterilely prepped in the routine manner.

POSITIONING The patient is positioned supine with closed legs and a footboard. The arms are abducted and secured to armboards. The surgeon stands on the patient's right, and the assistant stands on the patient's left. Monitors are positioned at the head of the bed (**FIGURE 1**).

INCISION AND EXPOSURE A Veress needle placed at the umbilicus achieves pneumoperitoneum. Alternatively, an open (Hasson) technique or a visual dilating trocar can be used to enter the abdomen at the left medial trocar position. Trocar positioning for gastric banding uses five trocars placed in the upper abdomen (**FIGURE 2**). A common error is placement of trocars too caudad to allow access to the hiatus. A 10-mm trocar should be placed 2 to 3 cm to the left of midline, approximately 10 to 12 cm below the costal margin, and will accommodate an angled (30- or 45-degree) laparoscope. This trocar should be placed first, as a misplaced (i.e., placed excessively caudad) laparoscope trocar is usually easily managed with a long and/or angled laparoscope. After placement of the initial trocar, steep reverse Trendelenburg positioning optimizes exposure of the upper abdomen. The remaining trocars are then placed with the operative field in view, allowing for optimal placement.

A 5-mm trocar is placed in the left lateral subcostal position, 2 to 3 cm below the left costal margin, to allow the assistant's grasper to reach the hiatus. Next, a 5-mm trocar is used to create a fascial defect directly under the xiphoid process through which a Nathanson liver retractor is placed. Placement of the liver retractor and exposure of the hiatus can usually be accomplished at this point, with only the left subcostal assistant's trocar in place. Once hiatal exposure is achieved, the remaining trocars are placed. A 5-mm trocar is placed in the right subcostal position, to allow direct passage of the surgeon's grasper from right to left posterior to the stomach. When placing this trocar, it is often helpful to visually confirm that an instrument passed through it will access the hiatus without interference from the right lobe of the liver. Although this trocar should be placed caudad enough to allow an instrument passed through it to clear the liver as it traverses the abdomen, placement of this trocar too caudad is a common mistake, as is placement too medial. When placed too caudad, an instrument passed through this trocar will not approach the hiatus at the proper angle to pass posterior to the stomach from the base of the right crus to the angle of His. When placed too medial, dissection and suturing will be difficult, as this trocar will be too close to the right medial trocar, which is also used for suturing. The right medial 15-mm trocar accommodates insertion of the band device into the abdomen and is placed 2 to 4 cm to the right of the patient's midline, approximately 2 to 4 cm below the costal margin. This trocar is the site at which the band access port will be sewn to the fascia of the abdominal wall. Placement of this trocar site too caudad will lead to a band port that is difficult to access because of the greater amount of abdominal wall fat in the lower abdomen. This trocar should therefore be placed such that when the abdomen is fully desufflated, the trocar incision where the band access port will lie is 2 to 4 cm below the right costal margin, in an area where the abdominal wall is relatively thin. In patients with large or steatotic livers, an Endoflex retractor can be placed in addition to a Nathanson liver retractor. Ideal exposure permits visualization of the suprahiatal diaphragm, the caudate lobe beneath the pars flaccida, and the tip of the spleen.

DETAILS OF THE PROCEDURE

Preparation of the Band Device Various types and sizes of gastric bands are available. Specific indications for each may be obtained from the manufacturer.

Before commencing the operation, the band device is prepared. The band is flushed with saline while held inverted using a syringe fitted with the metal slip tip provided with the band, removing as much air as possible from the band. The band is then completely deflated, and the flat silicone tip is attached to the band tubing. The port is prepared by flushing with saline using the Huber-type needle provided with the device. Use of any other needle may damage the port (**FIGURE 3**). Gastric bands are not inflated at the time of placement, as this may predispose to early post–band placement obstruction. Band fills are performed no earlier than 6 weeks after surgery.

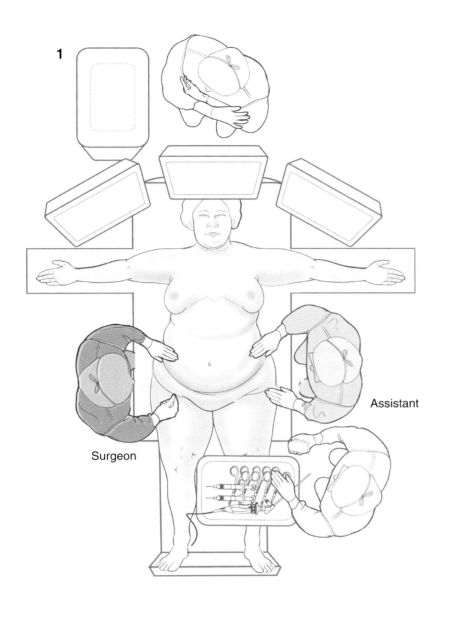

Surgeon

Assistant

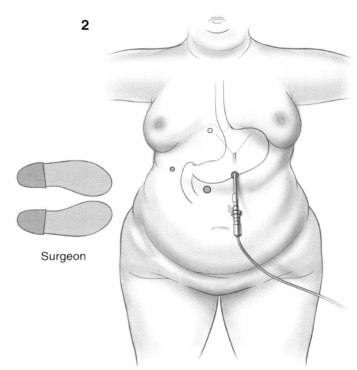

Surgeon

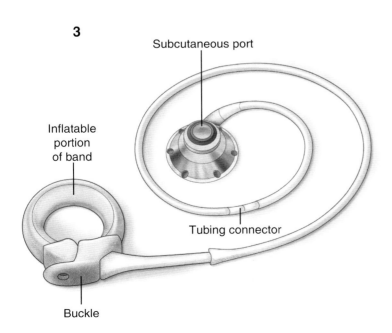

Subcutaneous port

Inflatable
portion
of band

Tubing connector

Buckle

Dissection Dissection commences at the angle of His. The peritoneum overlying the cardia of the stomach as it meets the left crus is opened. The goal of this maneuver is to allow easy passage of the surgeon's grasper from right to left posterior to the stomach through the areolar tissue between the cardia and the left crus. To accomplish this, the assistant retracts the apex of the omental fat caudad, while simultaneously pressing down on the greater curvature of the stomach, thus exposing the angle of His. The surgeon's left hand retracts the anterior gastric fat pad to the patient's right and slightly caudad, thus exposing the peritoneum overlying the angle of His. Using a combination of cautery and blunt dissection, the peritoneum attaching the cardia of the stomach to the left crus is opened (**FIGURE 4**). Sweeping a blunt dissector along the lateral aspect of the left crus after the peritoneum has been divided with cautery usually accomplishes this dissection easily.

The hiatus is next approached from the patient's right side. The pars flaccida is divided using cautery, exposing the fat pad overlying the right crus (**FIGURE 5**). A replaced or accessory left hepatic artery, if encountered, should be preserved if possible, although transection of such arteries is usually safe and only rarely associated with clinical sequelae. The surgeon grasps the fat overlying the right crus and retracts it to the patient's left, exposing the muscle fibers of the right crus. Once the right crus is exposed, the surgeon passes the overlying fat to the assistant's grasper, who continues to retract it to the patient's left, maintaining exposure. Clear visualization of the fibers of the right crus close to the base of its junction with the left crus is critical before proceeding further. Failure to properly identify the right crus can lead to perforation of the stomach during subsequent passage of the surgeon's grasper posterior to the stomach.

Once exposure of the right crus is achieved, a small nick is made in the peritoneum overlying the base of the right crus with cautery. The surgeon carefully passes a blunt grasper through the right lateral trocar at the base of the crus from the patient's right to left, posterior to the stomach (**FIGURE 6**). It is at this juncture that perforation of the stomach can occur. In addition to maintaining exposure, it is imperative that the grasper pass easily with no resistance. Any resistance encountered should prompt the surgeon to halt, regain exposure, and reassess positioning along the right crus. Some find this maneuver more easily performed with the gastric balloon inflated and the balloon cinched against the hiatus. Although this may aid in determining the appropriate point at which to pass a grasper, with experience this step may be unnecessary. The orogastric tube can be positioned just past the gastroesophageal junction, cephalad to the point where the grasper passes posterior to the stomach. Caution should be taken to avoid passage of the grasper too far to the patient's left, which may cause splenic injury; the grasper should be passed only far enough to reach the point where the peritoneum overlying the angle of His was taken down previously.

Once the grasper has been passed posterior to the stomach, the assistant releases the fat pad overlying the right crus, and attention is directed to the area of previous dissection at the angle of His. With the assistant gently retracting omentum and stomach caudad, the tip of the grasper should be visible exiting between the left crus and the cardia at the point where the peritoneum was divided previously. A thin film of transparent areolar tissue overlying the grasper may be present and can be cleared with gentle spreading of the grasper. If the tip of grasper is not visible, or appears to be covered with stomach serosa rather than areolar tissue, the grasper should be withdrawn and exposure of the right crus and passage of the grasper repeated. Any difficulty in passage of the grasper posterior to the stomach should prompt performance of a methylene blue test to identify a posterior gastric perforation.

4

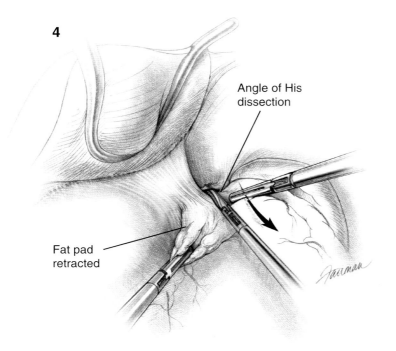

Angle of His
dissection

Fat pad
retracted

5

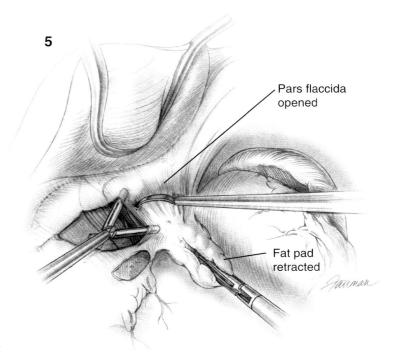

Pars flaccida
opened

Fat pad
retracted

6

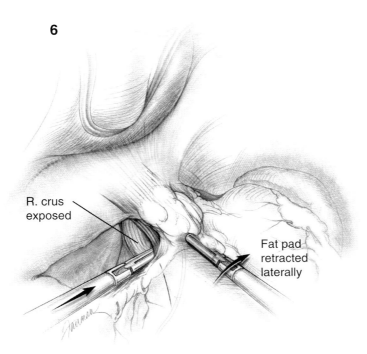

R. crus
exposed

Fat pad
retracted
laterally

Placement of Band At this point the band is inserted into the abdomen through the 15-mm trocar. This is best accomplished by removing the cap valve on the 15-mm trocar. The band is grasped with a laparoscopic grasper at the tip of the buckle, extended along the shaft of the grasper, and gently inserted into the abdomen. As the band is passed though the trocar, the leak from the trocar will lead to partial desufflation of the abdomen. Passage of the band into the abdomen must therefore be accomplished quickly but with care, so as not to injure underlying tissues. The tubing of the band is then inserted through the trocar, the trocar cap valve replaced, and the tubing reduced into the abdomen completely. At this point the band should be positioned in the abdomen so that the flat silicone tip can be easily accessed near the hiatus at the appropriate time, but the remainder of the band is caudad and removed from the operative field. Care should be taken at all times to avoid manipulation of the clear inflatable inner balloon of the band, to prevent inadvertent damage to the band that can lead to subsequent band leakage.

The assistant retrieves the flat tubing attached to the band and places it in the surgeon's grasper which has been passed posterior to the stomach. The surgeon then withdraws the grasper, pulling the band around the stomach posteriorly from left to right (**FIGURE 7**). The surgeon then passes the flat portion of the tubing through the end of the band. The buckle of the band is released from the posterior tissues so that the band can freely rotate around the upper stomach This is easily accomplished by simply rotating the band from the patient's right to left, pulling it through the posterior peritoneal tissue overlying the right crus (**FIGURE 8**). Occasionally, cautery of this overlying tissue is required to free the band. Application of cautery will not damage the band. The surgeon then draws the silicone tubing through the band buckle past the first flange, partially locking the band. At this point, consideration must be given to removing the gastric fat pad with cautery. If a large fat pad is present, if there is a significant amount of lesser curve fat, or if the band otherwise appears to be tight around the upper stomach, then the fat pad should be removed using cautery dissection. This may reduce the incidence of transient postoperative obstruction (**FIGURE 9**).

At this point, a methylene blue test for gastric perforation may be performed. This can be accomplished by gentle compression of the stomach distal to the band with the shaft of a grasper passed through the right lateral trocar, and instillation of methylene blue through the gastric balloon suction catheter positioned proximal to the band. A methylene blue test should be performed before fully locking the band, because a locked band that is snug around the upper stomach may obscure a leak, leading to a false-negative methylene blue test. Routine methylene blue tests are recommended in a surgeon's early experience. After experience is acquired, many surgeons reserve such tests only for situations in which difficulty is encountered with band placement. Identification of a gastric perforation requires removal of the band and an attempt at repair, which is often not possible because of the posterior location of such perforations. In this instance placement of drains and administration of parenteral nutrition is indicated.

7

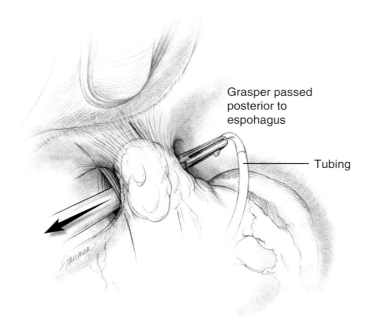

Grasper passed
posterior to
espohagus

Tubing

8

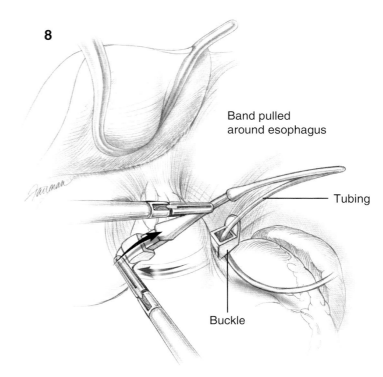

Band pulled
around esophagus

Tubing

Buckle

9

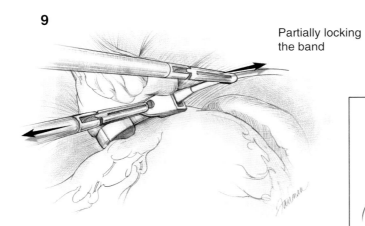

Partially locking
the band

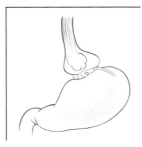

Gastrogastric Fundoplication Attention is directed to creation of the gastrogastric fundoplication over the band. Construction of a proper fundoplication is critical to preventing band slippage and erosion, and to ensure correct positioning of the band below the gastroesophageal junction. Band slippage is better termed band prolapse. In most cases, the left lateral redundant fundus prolapses above the band and becomes incarcerated. The gastrogastric fundoplication should incorporate as much redundant fundus as possible to prevent prolapse. A braided permanent suture is generally used. The fundoplication must also incorporate gastric tissue above the band, to ensure that the band stays just below, rather than at, the gastroesophageal junction. Failure to incorporate gastric serosa above the band into the fundoplication may lead to placement of the band at the gastroesophageal junction. Removal of the anterior gastric fat pad often aids in visualization of the gastric serosa above the band.

The assistant retracts the apex of the omentum caudad, exposing the upper fundus. The surgeon places a stitch in the serosa of the lateral-most fundus below the band and lifts it above the band to test the wrap. The wrap should be snug but not tight. Readjustment of the stitch should be performed if too much or too little fundus is incorporated. The stitch is next taken on the stomach above the band, while the assistant, grasping the band tubing just below the buckle, gently retracts the band caudad and to the patient's right, exposing the proximal stomach above the band (**FIGURE 10**).

Once the first stitch is placed, it is left untied while the surgeon fully locks the band, pulling the second flange through the band buckle. The band cannot be unlocked after this point. Placement of the first stitch before fully locking the band simplifies exposure and identification of gastric serosa above the band, ensuring a gastrogastric, rather than esophagogastric, fundoplication. Once locked, the surgeon should ensure that the band rotates freely around the stomach. The the first stitch is then tied. One to three more stitches are placed between the fundus and the gastric pouch above the band, taking care not to puncture the band with the needle. Gentle retraction of the band caudad and to the patient's right by the assistant exposes the gastric pouch above the band and ensures correct placement of these sutures. The fundoplication should not be carried over the buckle of the band, as this may be associated with higher rates of erosion. Generally, three or four stitches are sufficient to create an adequate fundoplication (**FIGURE 11**).

Closure and Placement of Band Port After completion of the fundoplication, the liver retractor is removed, and the band tubing is withdrawn through the 15-mm trocar, which is subsequently removed. The remaining trocars are also removed, and the abdomen desufflated. The use of radially expanding trocars generally avoids the need for fascial closure. However, the 15-mm trocar site may need to be closed if a hernia appears imminent.

The band tubing is cut at its junction with the flat silicone tip, which is discarded. The band access port is attached to the tubing and sewn to the fascia of the anterior abdominal wall using a permanent monofilament suture. It is important to reduce redundant tubing into the abdomen through the trocar site, and to ensure that no kinks are present in the tubing that may impede subsequent band fills. It is critical to sew the band access port directly to the fascia to prevent access port twisting and rotation (**FIGURE 12**). The access port is sewn in place such that the tubing always exits the same side of each patient (shown here exiting to the patient's right). This consistency prevents injury to the tubing during subsequent fills. The subcutaneous tissue is closed over the port, followed by a skin closure using a subcuticular suture. An occlusive dressing is placed, and the skin incisions over the remaining trocar sites are closed.

POSTOPERATIVE CARE Routine upper GI imaging is performed upper gastrointestinal series in all patients on the first postoperative day to confirm correct band position and free flow of contrast through the band. Failure of contrast to flow freely through the band may indicate improper band position, transient postoperative obstruction due to edema or excessive fat around the upper stomach, or a gastric perforation. A properly positioned band should lie parallel to the transverse plane (i.e., the lumen of the band should not be visible on an anteroposterior film) and should be angled toward the patient's left shoulder. Gastric perforation may present with failure of contrast to pass through the band, usually accompanied by contrast extravasation. This latter finding may be obscured by the band itself, and thus reexploration should be considered in patients who demonstrate signs consistent with perforation, such as fever or significant abdominal pain. Transient postoperative obstruction usually resolves spontaneously within 1 to 3 days. The use of diuretics may hasten resolution. Repeat laparoscopy with fat pad removal in patients with transient postoperative obstruction can be performed if this was not performed at the time of initial operation.

If the upper gastrointestinal study demonstrates proper band position and free flow of contrast through the band with no evidence of leak, then patients are advanced to a clear, then full liquid diet and may be discharged on postoperative day 1 or 2. Discharge of patients on the day of surgery should be considered only after successful initial experience has been accumulated. Patients are maintained on a full liquid diet for 2 weeks after surgery, and then advanced to a dry, low-fat, high-protein diet.

Band fills are performed based on weight loss and satiety. The first fill should occur no earlier than 6 weeks after surgery, to allow formation of a pseudocapsule around the access port. This practice may lower the risk of port infections. Band fill guidelines are available from the manufacturer. ∎

10

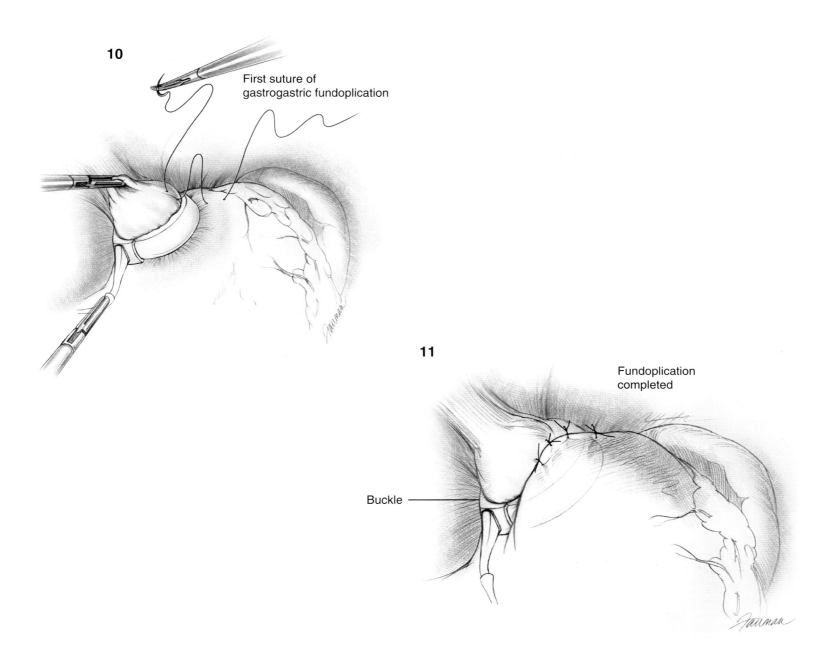

First suture of
gastrogastric fundoplication

11

Fundoplication
completed

Buckle

12

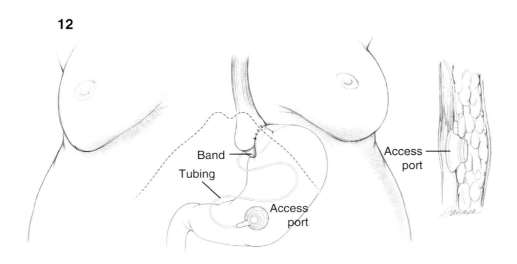

Band

Tubing

Access
port

Access
port

"Sleeve" Gastrectomy and Duodenal Switch

INDICATION Traditionally, biliopancreatic diversion with lateral "sleeve" gastrectomy and biliopancreatic diversion has been performed as a single or staged procedure for patients categorized as "superobese." The technical challenges of performing the procedure laparoscopically combined with the associated severe nutritional deficiencies have made this combined procedure less popular in recent years. Initially offered as the first part of the staged procedure prior to weight loss, the sleeve gastrectomy has become increasingly popular as a stand-alone procedure. Reports of excellent weight reduction have become increasingly common in the literature, resulting in the acceptance of the procedure by the American Society of Metabolic and Bariatric Surgery as a surgical option in select patients. Although many minimally invasive surgeons consider it to be technically less challenging to perform, the risk of leak from the long gastric staple line, gastric dysmotility, and treatment failure due to delayed dilation of the stomach should warrant caution among inexperienced bariatric surgeons.

The biliary pancreatic diversion creates a malabsorptive state in which bile and digestive enzymes within a long afferent intestinal limb contact food within a "common channel" measuring only 100 cm. The alimentary limb of the Roux-en-Y measures only 250 cm from its anastomosis with the duodenum to the cecum. The small intestine is normally 600 cm long (with some variation), so in this operation, the total length of the small intestine is shortened to about 40% of normal, but the length of the "common channel," where digestion of complex fats and proteins occurs, is only 1/6 or 16% of normal. When combined with the lateral gastrectomy, the procedure accomplishes dramatic weight loss by creating both severe restrictive and malabsorptive conditions.

PREOPERATIVE PREPARATION Bariatric surgery patients require an extensive preoperative evaluation to determine their anesthetic risk, to define the severity of known comorbidities, and to identify occult comorbid conditions such as sleep apnea, obesity hypoventilation syndrome, and coronary artery disease. This evaluation requires a multidisciplinary approach. The bariatric team should include dieticians, psychologists, and medical subspecialists who can optimize the patient's cardiovascular, pulmonary, and endocrine status before surgery. Patients with active substance abuse problems or uncontrolled psychiatric disorders are not candidates for bariatric surgery. Strong family and social support for the patient is important to achieving a successful outcome.

Patients who are preparing for bariatric surgery must be fully informed about all of the available surgical options. The choice of laparoscopic bariatric operations today include laparoscopic adjustable gastric banding, sleeve gastrectomy, gastric bypass, or a malabsorptive procedure such as biliopancreatic diversion (BPD) or BPD with duodenal switch (BPDS). The risks and benefits of lateral sleeve gastrectomy and duodenal switch should be discussed in detail with the patient and put into context with the other available bariatric procedures and other major laparoscopic operations performed today.

ANESTHESIA Laparoscopic sleeve gastrectomy with or without duodenal switch requires a general anesthetic. The anesthesiologist must be prepared for a difficult airway in this patient population, and anesthesia backup should be immediately available throughout the case. The surgeon should be available during induction, intubation, and extubation should a surgical airway become necessary. Patients with sleep apnea and obesity hypoventilation syndrome are at particularly high risk for airway problems and hypoxia and should be continued on their continuous positive airway pressure (CPAP) devices postoperatively in the hospital. Antiemetics should be started in the operating room during the case and continued as needed postoperatively. Pain control is achieved with narcotic patient-controlled anesthesia for 1 or 2 days postoperatively and transitioned to oral pain medication in elixir form prior to discharge.

POSITIONING The patient is placed supine on the operating table with legs together and arms abducted. A padded footboard is placed on the foot of the bed and the patient's legs are secured together with the feet on the footboard. Adequate padding must be placed between the knees and calves prior to securing the legs together. The arms are abducted no more than 90 degrees and padded before they are secured to the arm boards. Prior to prepping and draping, the patient is placed in steep reverse Trendelenburg position and observed for stability on the operating table. The weight limit for the operating room table should be confirmed with the manufacturer and determined to be sufficient before the patient is placed on the table.

The primary surgeon stands to the patient's right. The first assistant stands across from the surgeon on the patient's left, and the second assistant or camera operator stands to the left of the first assistant. The scrub nurse stands at the foot of the bed within arm's reach of the surgeon and first assistant. Video monitors are placed above the patient's head on the left and the right (**FIGURE 1**).

OPERATIVE PREPARATION A Foley catheter and orogastric tube are placed after induction of anesthesia. The surgeon must remember to have the anesthesiologist remove the orogastric tube from the stomach before the gastric pouch is created. The abdomen is prepped and draped to provide an adequate field should the operation be converted to laparotomy. The field should be draped far laterally to provide access for the liver retractor and first assistant's retraction ports.

Trocar Placement The primary (camera) port should be in the midline, slightly cephalad to the umbilicus. In a patient with a very large belly (android fat distribution), the xiphoid should be used as the major landmark. The camera can be placed 20 to 25 cm caudad to the xiphoid. This position will allow adequate views of the ileocecal junction, the duodenum, and the greater curvature of the stomach. Two 12-mm trocars are placed, one in the left upper quadrant and one in the left midabdomen. These two trocars are used to manipulate the stomach during gastric resection and small bowel during creation of the alimentary limb, common channel, and duodenoenterostomy when applicable (**FIGURE 2A**). The left lower quadrant port is not necessary when only a sleeve gastrectomy is performed (**FIGURE 2B**). A 5-mm trocar is placed in the right upper quadrant. This trocar can be used by the assistant to help position the stomach during a sleeve resection or assist in the creation of the alimentary limb and common channel during BPDS. A fourth 12-mm trocar is placed in the right middle quadrant to assist in making the lateral gastrectomy. A 5-mm trocar is placed in the subxiphoid position to allow insertion of a Nathanson liver retractor.

1

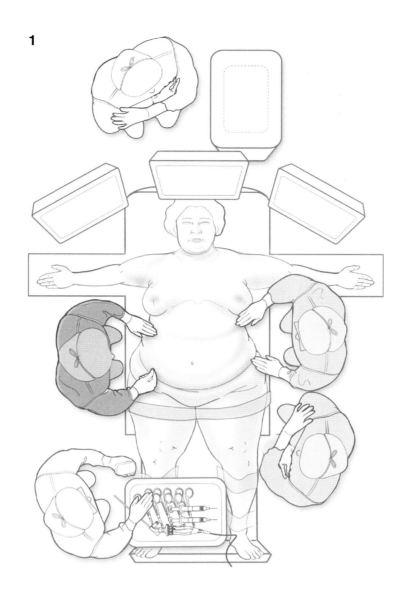

Trocar Placement for Sleeve Gastrectomy with Duodenal Switch

2a

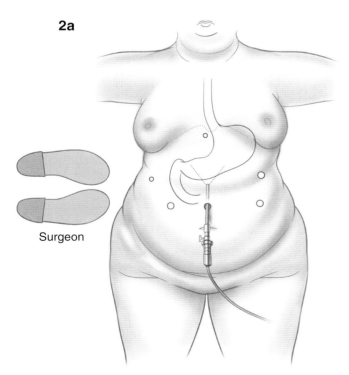

Surgeon

Trocar Placement for Sleeve Gastrectomy without Duodenal Switch

2b

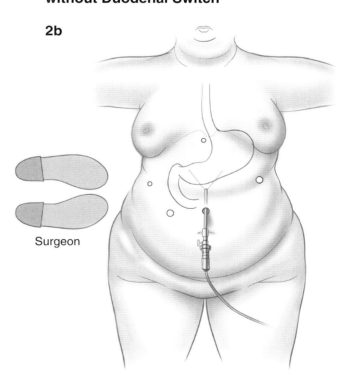

Surgeon

DETAILS OF THE PROCEDURE

Sleeve Gastrectomy The liver is elevated using a Nathanson liver retractor in the subxiphoid position. The conduct of the operation starts with devascularization of the greater curvature of the stomach, 6 cm proximal to the pylorus, with an ultrasonic dissector (**FIGURE 3**). The dissection hugs the stomach, preserving the right and left gastroepiploic arteries. The short gastric arteries are divided. The anterior epiphrenic fat pad is mobilized from the gastroesophageal junction and reflected to the patient's right to expose the angle of His (cardiophrenic angle). A 34 French bougie dilator is passed and situated against the lesser curvature of the stomach (**FIGURE 4**).

Division of the stomach is begun approximately 6 to 10 cm from the pylorus using serial firing of the intermediate-to-thick-tissue endoscopic stapler, following the curve of the dilator (**FIGURES 5A AND 5B**). Subsequent stapler firings are carried up to the angle of His (**FIGURE 6**). Prosthetic staple line reinforcements can be used to buttress staple lines, if desired. Alternatively, the staple line can be oversewn with an interrupted or running suture (**FIGURE 7**). The key critical element of the gastric resection is the creation of a narrow gastric tube eliminating most of the fundus. The resected lateral gastric segment is placed in a specimen bag and removed at the end of the case.

3

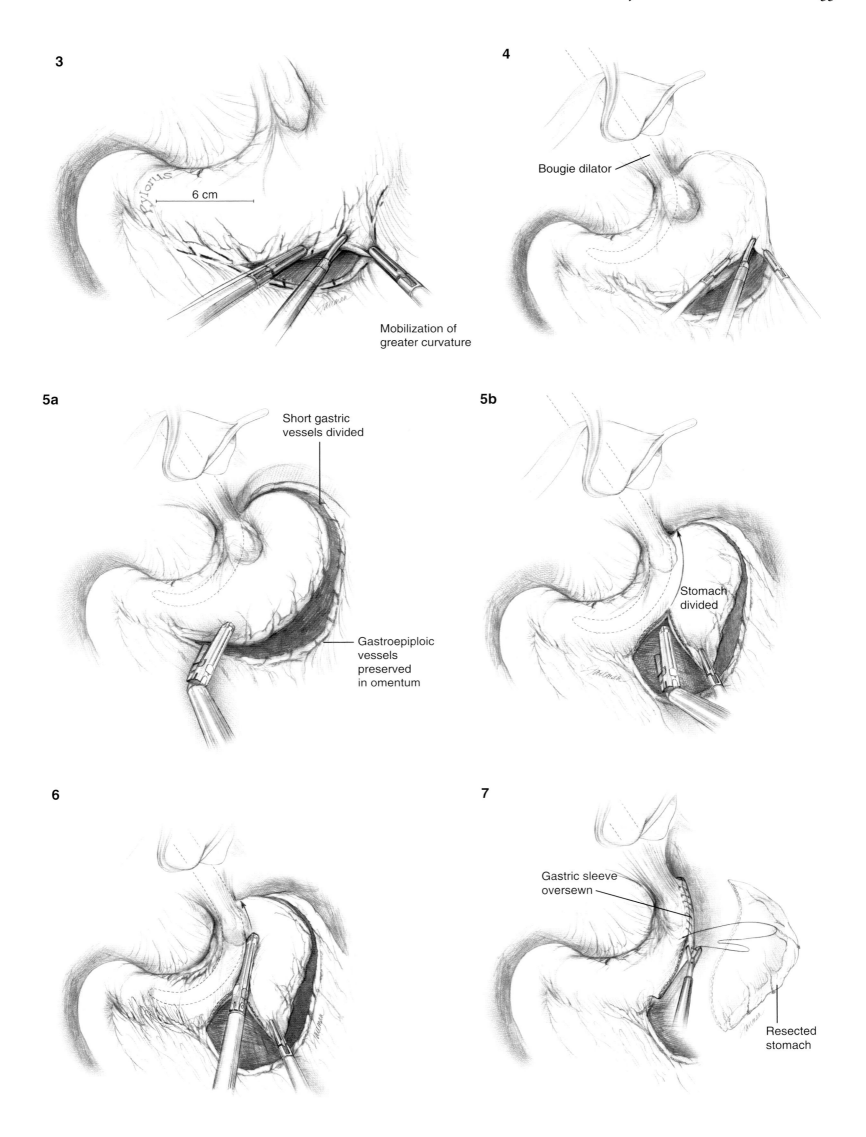

6 cm

Mobilization of
greater curvature

4

Bougie dilator

5a

Short gastric
vessels divided

Gastroepiploic
vessels
preserved
in omentum

5b

Stomach
divided

6

7

Gastric sleeve
oversewn

Resected
stomach

Duodenal Switch An additional 12-mm port is placed in the left midabdomen, and attention is turned to the right lower quadrant. The surgeon moves to the patient's left side (**FIGURE 8**). This portion of the operation may be divided into several steps: creation of a 150-cm alimentary limb and a 100-cm common channel, division of the duodenum, and anastomosis of the alimentary limb to the duodenum.

Creation of the common channel and the biliopancreatic limb is performed with the surgeon on the left side of the patient with the camera looking into the right lower quadrant. With the bed positioned in Trendelenburg and tipped left side down, the omentum is retracted cephalad exposing the cecum. The terminal ileum is identified at its junction with the colon. The small bowel is run 100 cm proximal to this point. A 10-cm segment of suture or umbilical tape can assist in the accuracy of this step (**FIGURE 9**). A marking suture is placed 100 cm proximal to the ileocecal valve to mark the point where the biliary limb will be connected to the alimentary limb (**FIGURE 10**). This 100-cm segment of ileum will be the common channel. From the 100-cm mark, the surgeon continues to run the bowel proximally an additional 150 cm. The bowel is divided with a linear stapler at this point, 250 cm proximal to the ileocecal valve (**FIGURES 11A AND 11B**).

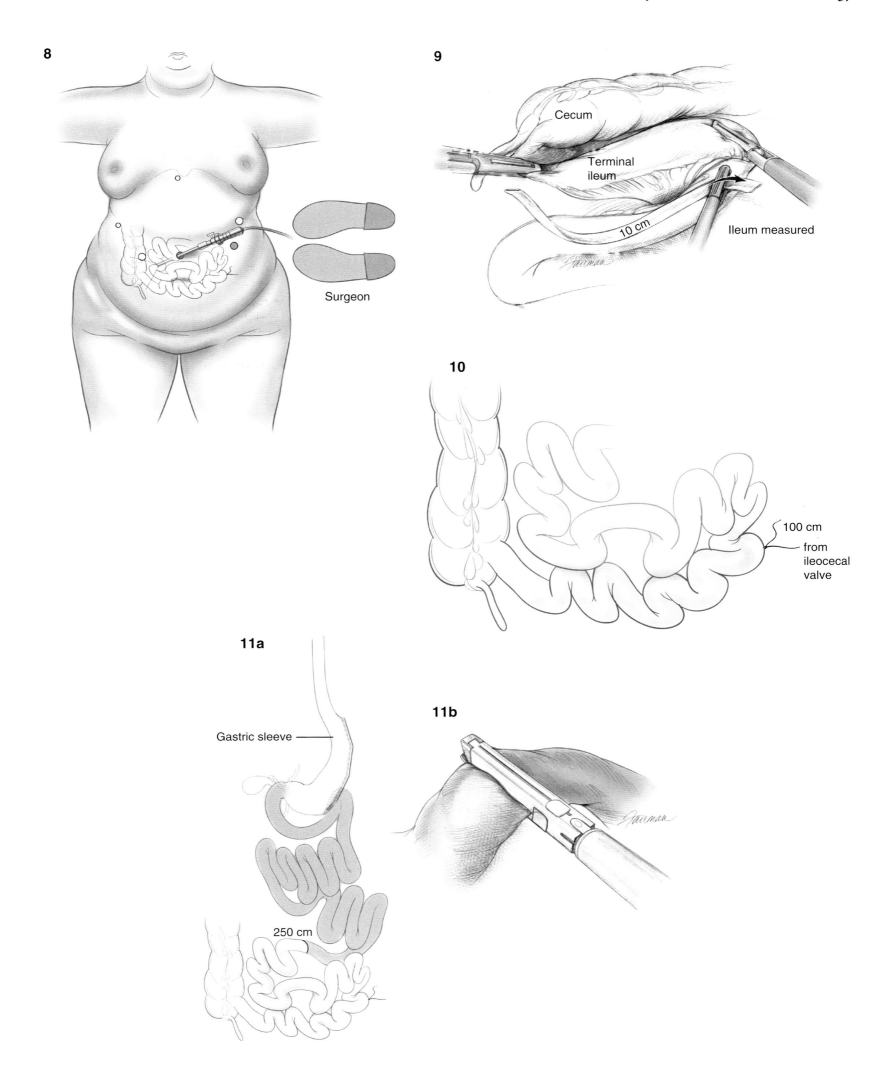

8

Surgeon

9

Cecum

Terminal
ileum

10 cm

Ileum measured

10

100 cm
from
ileocecal
valve

11a

Gastric sleeve

250 cm

11b

Duodenal Switch The distal end (alimentary limb) is marked with a suture to ensure that it will not be confused with the proximal end (biliary limb) **(FIGURE 12)**. The biliary limb (the proximal end of the small intestine) is then brought down along the alimentary limb to the point where the suture had been previously placed (100 cm proximal to the ileocecal valve) **(FIGURE 13)**.

  The biliary limb is anastomosed to the ileum (now common channel) in a side-to-side fashion using a linear stapler. In creation of the side-to-side intestinal anastomosis, it is important to keep the alimentary limb on the patient's right side and the biliary limb on the patient's left side. The staple line of the biliary limb should face the direction of the ileocecal valve to ensure continuity of intestinal peristalsis. Tacking sutures are used to align the intestinal limbs prior to anastomosis **(FIGURE 14)**. Using the electro-surgical hook, enterotomies are made in the biliary and distal alimentary limbs. The enterotomies are enlarged to allow passage of a 45-mm linear stapler **(FIGURE 15)**.

  A linear stapler is introduced into the enterotomies and fired **(FIGURE 16)**. The resulting defect in the anastomosis is closed in two layers with a 2-0 absorbable suture **(FIGURES 17 AND 18)**.

12

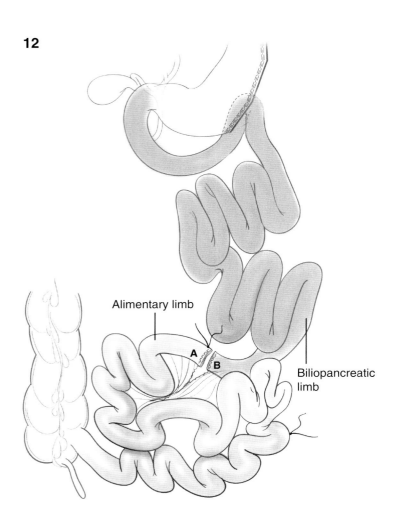

13

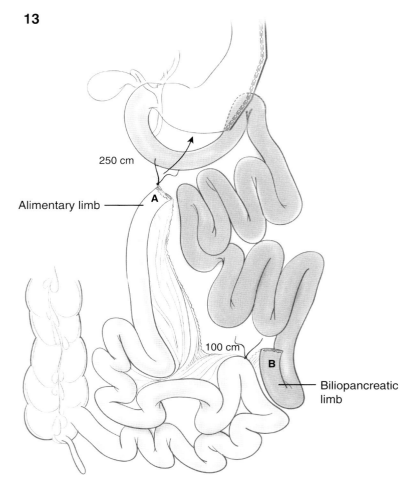

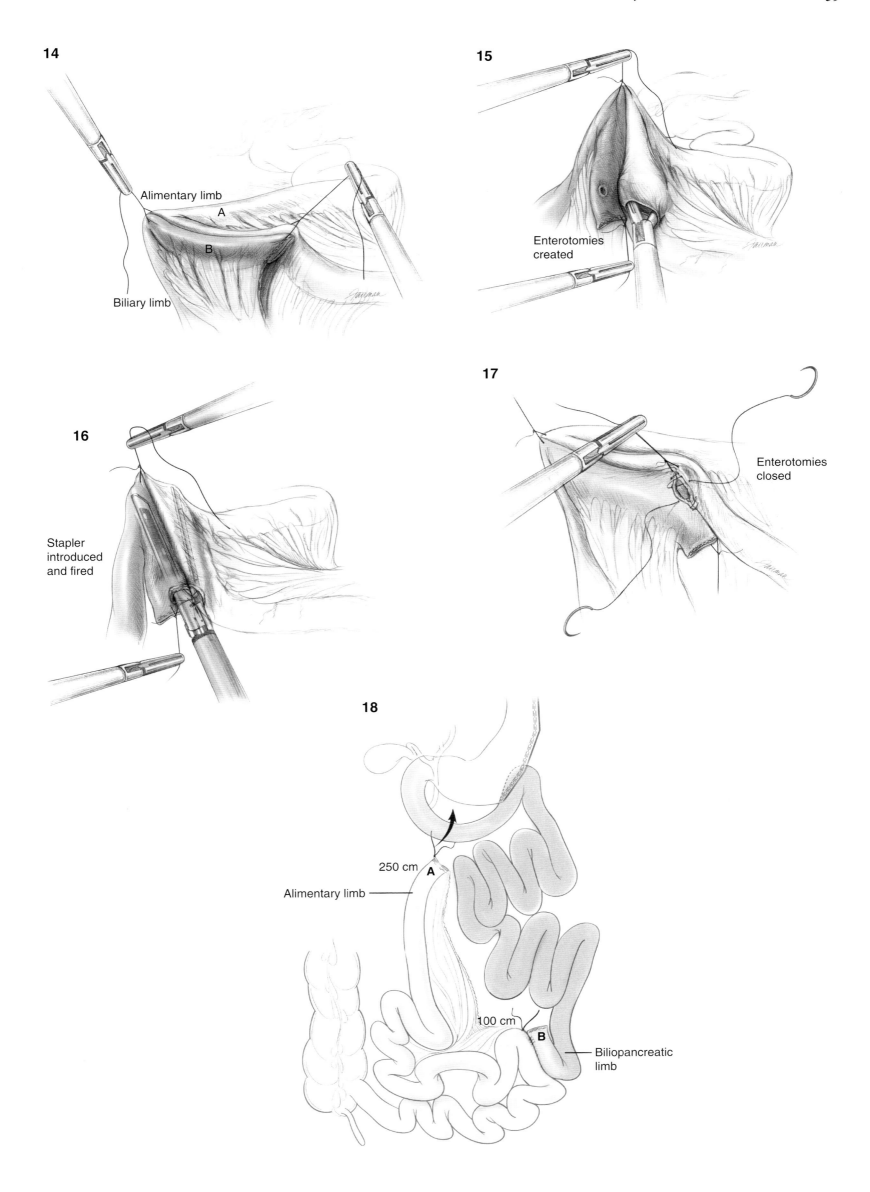

14

Alimentary limb

A

B

Biliary limb

15

Enterotomies
created

16

Stapler
introduced
and fired

17

Enterotomies
closed

18

250 cm **A**

Alimentary limb

100 cm **B**

Biliopancreatic
limb

Duodenal Switch Attention is turned to the duodenum. The pylorus can usually be identified as a waist at the distal end of the stomach or carefully palpated with a dissector. Once identified, dissection is initiated on the gastric side of the pylorus and carried about 4 cm distal to the pylorus (**FIGURE 19**).

The proper dissection plane is most easily developed on the greater curvature of the stomach, and then can be carried on to the duodenum. A small amount of dissection on the cephalad side of the duodenum is required to complete circumferential mobilization. Dissection of the duodenum at this level should be performed with caution, as there can be many small perforating vessels between the duodenum and pancreas. Insertion of an esophageal dissector will facilitate blunt dissection in the retroduodenal

space, allowing completion of the circumferential dissection (**FIGURE 20**). The duodenum is transected 2 to 4 cm distal to the pylorus using a 60-mm medium thickness linear stapler (**FIGURE 21**). After transection, the stomach and proximal duodenum are relatively mobile, enabling the alimentary limb to be brought up in an antecolic fashion to create the duodenoenterostomy (**FIGURE 22**).

The duodenoenterostomy is performed in either a sutured or stapled end-to-side fashion. The alimentary limb is first secured to the duodenum with a posterior row of interrupted braided absorbable sutures. An electrosurgical hook is used to create enterotomies in the stomach and duodenum (**FIGURE 23**).

19

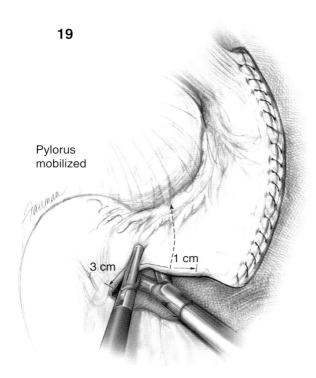

Pylorus mobilized

3 cm

1 cm

20

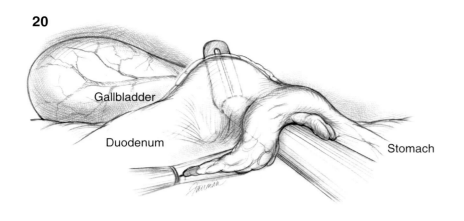

Gallbladder

Duodenum

Stomach

21

Pylorus

Duodenum
divided

22

Divided
duodenum

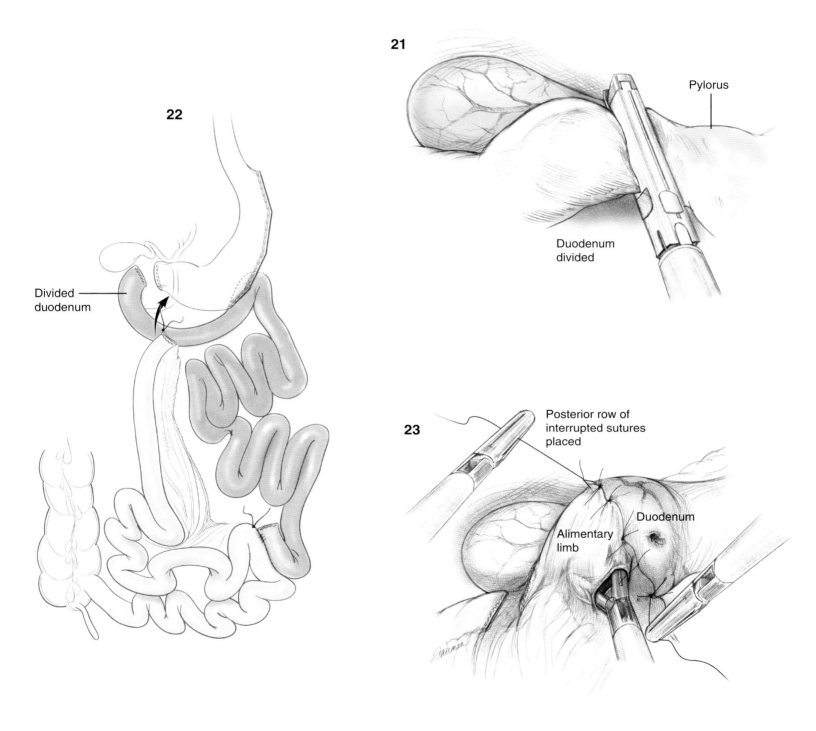

23

Posterior row of
interrupted sutures
placed

Duodenum

Alimentary
limb

Duodenal Switch A 45-mm medium thickness linear stapler is introduced into the enterotomies and fired (**FIGURE 24**). The final enterotomy is closed in two layers with a braided absorbable 2-o suture. The anastomosis is completed with an anterior row of interrupted sutures (**FIGURE 25**). Methylene blue is then infused through an orogastric tube, or endoscopy can be used, to evaluate the anastomosis for leaks.

If the sleeve gastrectomy and duodenal switch were performed concurrently, the surgeon must remember to remove the resected gastric remnant through one of the larger ports (**FIGURE 26**).

POSTOPERATIVE CARE Patients are admitted to the bariatric or general surgical ward after recovering from anesthesia. Sequential compression devices are used throughout the perioperative period, and low-molecular-weight heparin is started within 24 hours postoperatively for venous thromboembolism (VTE) prophylaxis. VTE prophylaxis is extended for 30 days after discharge for patients with a BMI > 55 or a history of VTE. Antiemetic therapy is started in the operating room and continued as needed on the ward. Patient-controlled analgesia is used for pain management. Essential preoperative medications are continued in intravenous form until the patient is started on liquids. Patients ambulate with assistance the evening of surgery, and frequent use of incentive spirometry is encouraged. Patients take nothing by mouth the night of surgery. A Gastrografin upper GI x-ray (UGI) may be obtained the morning of postoperative day 1 but is not required. If the UGI study is negative for a leak, the patient is started on a clear liquid diet. Once the patient is tolerating liquids, medications are given in elixir form or pills are crushed. Patients are monitored closely for tachycardia and tachypnea during the postoperative period. Anastomotic leaks and pulmonary embolism can have similar presentations in these patients, and a persistent heart rate above 120 beats per minute or shortness of breath mandate an evaluation. Peritoneal findings on physical exam are frequently absent in this patient population, and radiologic studies should be performed early if there is suspicion of a leak. When clinical suspicion for a leak is high, laparoscopic reexploration should be performed in lieu of radiographic imaging.

The majority of patients are discharged to home on postoperative day 2 when they meet discharge criteria (normal vital signs, regular ambulation, adequate pain control with oral analgesics, tolerating liquids). Patients are advanced to a full liquid and then a soft diet over the first 4 to 6 weeks after surgery. After that, small portions of solid food are usually well tolerated.

Because it is a malabsorptive operation, patients suffer from often-severe diarrhea and excessive foul-smelling gas. Deficiencies of nutrients such as iron, B_{12}, and folate are typical. Therefore, all patients should receive lifelong oral micronutrient supplementation and have vitamin and mineral levels monitored annually. ■

24

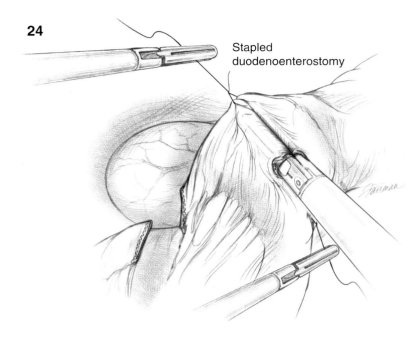

Stapled
duodenoenterostomy

25

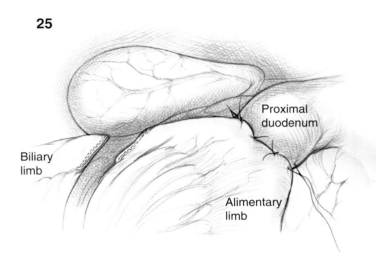

Proximal
duodenum

Biliary
limb

Alimentary
limb

26

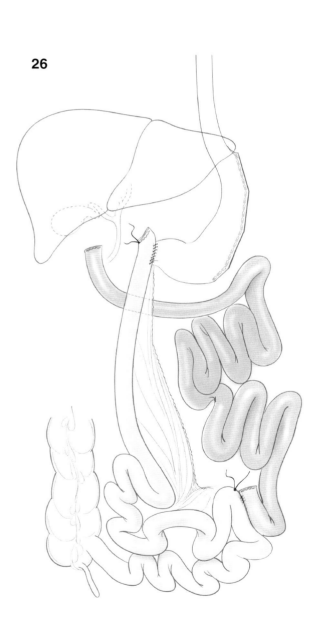

Section VI
MINIMALLY INVASIVE HEPATOPANCREATOBILIARY SURGERY

LAPAROSCOPIC CHOLECYSTECTOMY

INDICATIONS The most common indication for laparoscopic cholecystectomy (LC) is symptomatic cholelithiasis. Classic biliary colic is characterized by severe right upper quadrant (RUQ) postprandial and nocturnal pain radiating to the right scapula and epigastrium, associated with nausea, and an ultrasound showing gallstones. This constellation of symptoms and signs is found in more than 50% of patients referred for cholecystectomy. Other presentations include acute cholecystitis (fever, leukocytosis, RUQ peritoneal irritation), acalculous cholecystitis, choledocholithiasis, cholangitis, and biliary dyskinesia. It is rarely necessary to remove asymptomatic gallstones.

Contraindications to the laparoscopic approach include previous right upper quadrant surgery, severe chronic liver disease, gallbladder necrosis, suspected gallbladder cancer, or massive bowel distention (ileus). Patients with previous laparotomy may have few intraabdominal adhesions, or the adhesions may be dense. Because it is difficult to predict the presence of these adhesions, this is procedure often started laparoscopically, then converted to laparotomy if 30 minutes have passed without completing the dissection of the cystic duct and artery.

PATIENT POSITIONING The patient is positioned supine on a fluoroscopic operating table. It is often necessary to reverse the table to make sure the post will not be in the way of an operative fluoroscopic cholangiogram. Ideally both arms are tucked, but the right arm may be left out. Leaving the left arm extended on an armboard will often interfere with the C arm, so is not recommended (**FIGURE 1**).

OPERATIVE PROCEDURE A carbon dioxide pneumoperitoneum is obtained through a periumbilical incision with a Veress needle or an open laparoscopy technique. A 10-mm port is placed adjacent to the umbilicus, and a 30-degree forward oblique-viewing laparoscope is introduced. Under laparoscopic visualization, another 10-mm port is placed through the epigastrium. This port starts in the midline, but is then angled to the right to enter the peritoneal cavity at the inferior edge of the liver, just to the right of the falciform ligament, at the "corner" created by the reflection of the peritoneum onto the right side of the falciform ligament. Two 5-mm trocars are placed in the right subcostal region. The first of these is just to the right of the gallbladder fundus, as visualized laparoscopically. The surface projection of this point is usually 2 to 5 cm below the right costal margin, just lateral to the midclavicular line (MCL). The fourth and last trocar is placed in the anterior axillary line, at about the level of the umbilicus. In thin patients this port is moved inferiorly and in obese patients it is moved superiorly (**FIGURE 2**).

With an aggressive toothed 5-mm grasper ("gallbladder grasper") entering through the most lateral 5-mm port, the fundus of the gallbladder is grasped and pushed as far superiorly as possible (**FIGURE 3**). This maneuver elevates the undersurface of the liver, where the gallbladder sits, exposing the porta hepatis *en face* to a 30-degree laparoscope. The first assistant can maintain this retraction with their left hand while running the camera with their right hand. Alternatively a penetrating towel clip is passed though the handle of the clamp and the gallbladder grasper is pinned in position to the drapes or the patient's skin (**FIGURE 4**).

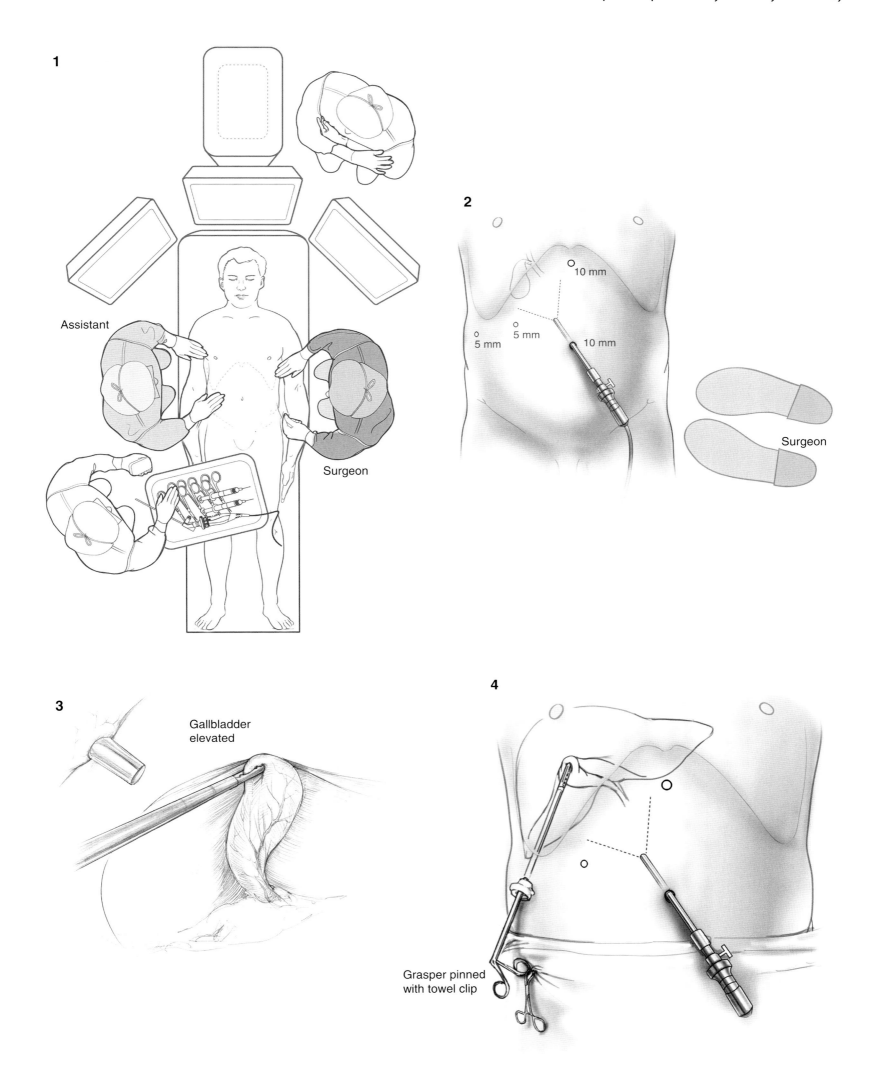

1

Assistant

Surgeon

2

10 mm

5 mm

5 mm   10 mm

5 mm

Surgeon

3

Gallbladder
elevated

4

Grasper pinned
with towel clip

OPERATIVE PROCEDURE With acute cholecystitis or hydrops of the gall-bladder, a tense, thick-walled gallbladder defies the jaws of the grasper. If this is the case, the gallbladder can be decompressed by making a hole in the fundus with the an electrosurgical hook, and the bile drained with a suction wand (**FIGURES 5A AND 5B**). The cholecystotomy is closed with an Endoloop, or the fundus grasper may be used to simultaneously close the hole and elevate the gallbladder.

Before commencing dissection, the relevant anatomy should be mentally reviewed (**FIGURE 6**). The cystic lymph node is a good landmark for the cystic artery, which nearly always sits immediately beneath the node and lymphatics. Whereas the cystic duct *always* emerges from the infundibulum of the gallbladder, the cystic artery has many variations, which can lead to troublesome bleeding or anatomic confusion if the surgeon is not aware of the many anatomic variations of arterial blood supply in this region (**FIGURE 7**).

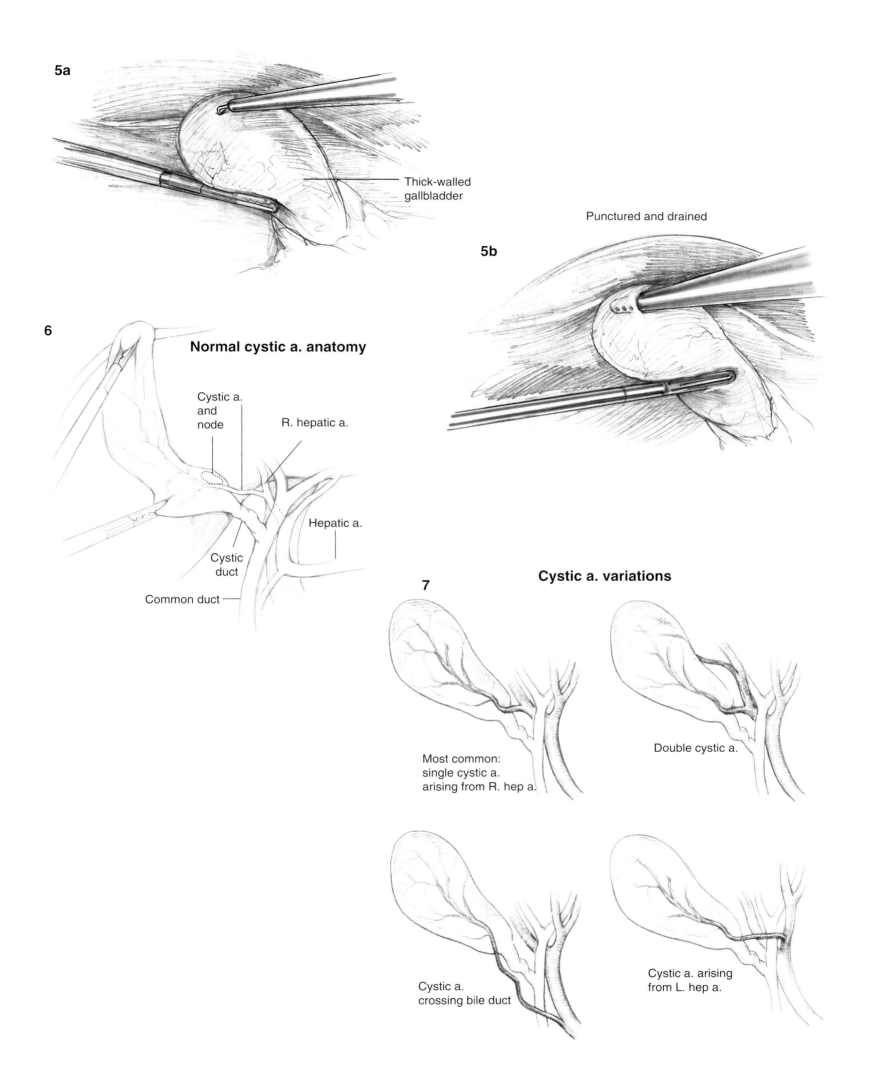

5a

Thick-walled
gallbladder

Punctured and drained

5b

6

Normal cystic a. anatomy

Cystic a.
and
node

R. hepatic a.

Hepatic a.

Cystic
duct

Common duct

Cystic a. variations

7

Most common:
single cystic a.
arising from R. hep a.

Double cystic a.

Cystic a.
crossing bile duct

Cystic a. arising
from L. hep a.

OPERATIVE PROCEDURE Working two-handed from the left-hand side of the table, the surgeon picks up the infundibulum of the gallbladder with an atraumatic grasper (Hunter grasper) in their left hand. With a Maryland grasper in their right hand, dissection commences by stripping the peritoneum and fat off the infundibulum, in the direction of the common bile duct (CBD) (**FIGURE 8**). Some advocate stripping without use of electrosurgery, but such technique will often create a bloody field of dissection, more so in acute cholecystitis. Bleeding in the porta hepatis darkens the operative field and obscures important anatomical cues, increasing the likelihood of CBD injury. The electrocoagulation trigger is tapped as the peritoneum is grasped, creating a localized cautery burn of the peritoneum before stripping. It is important that no electrosurgical current be delivered during the peritoneal stripping, to avoid accidental burn of the CBD or duodenum, which can lead to a delayed stricture or fistula.

The stripping continues counterclockwise (looking from below) around the infundibulum of the gallbladder to reach the posterior aspect of the gallbladder and cystic duct. This is accomplished by superior and medial rotation of the fundus with the surgeon's left hand (**FIGURE 9**). By moving the infundibulum up and down with the left hand and rotating the 30-degree laparoscope, the surgeon achieves a near-circumferential view of the gallbladder infundibulum as the dissection progresses. The Maryland grasper is then used to gently open up a small window between the cystic artery and cystic duct (**FIGURE 10**). Aggressive spreading in this region will cause unwanted bleeding, as the small vessels between cystic artery and duct are easily avulsed.

At this point in dissection, the Maryland grasper is replaced with an electrosurgical hook. The electrosurgical hook is passed through the window in Calot's triangle, the tip of the hook is directed toward the gallbladder, and the small vessels in this region are elevated and coagulated (**FIGURE 11**). Failure to obtain hemostasis during this dissection leads to poor visibility in the porta hepatis and a higher incidence of bile duct injury. This dissection clearly defines the inferior edge of the cystic artery and the superior wall of the cystic duct as it widens to become the gallbladder. Continued dissection up the convex surface of the gallbladder on the hepatic side of the cystic artery further opens up Calot's triangle.

The infundibulum of the gallbladder is then retracted anteriorly and to the left to open up the posterior aspect of Calot's triangle. With the peritoneum on stretch as the left hand pulls the gallbladder away from the liver, the hook is slid between the peritoneum and gallbladder posteriorly. The peritoneum is divided to further separate the gallbladder infundibulum from the liver (**FIGURE 12**).

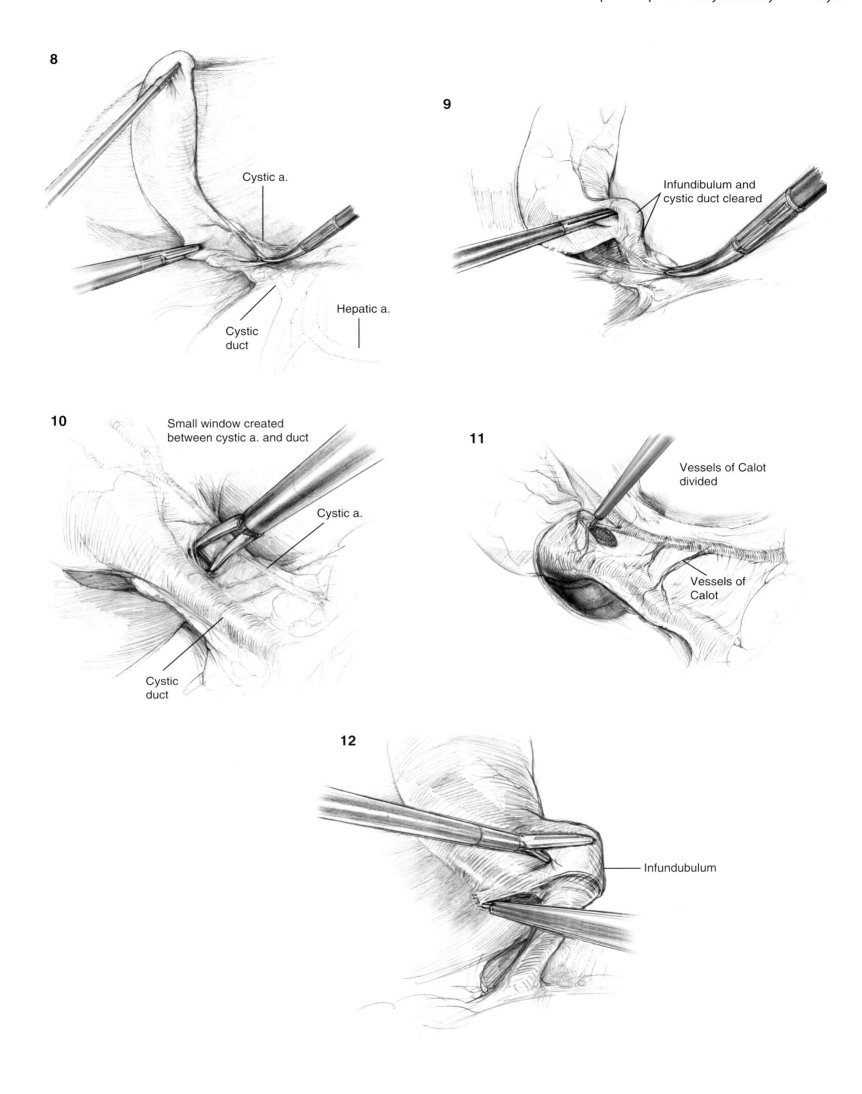

8

Cystic a.

Cystic duct

Hepatic a.

9

Infundibulum and cystic duct cleared

10

Small window created between cystic a. and duct

Cystic a.

Cystic duct

11

Vessels of Calot divided

Vessels of Calot

12

Infundubulum

OPERATIVE PROCEDURE The result of this dissection is that the gallbladder looks like a polyp on a stalk. When the infundibulum is retracted posterolaterally, the liver can be seen through the window in Calot's triangle created by dissection of the cystic artery and cystic duct, and by detaching the gallbladder infundibulum. This "view" has been termed the "critical view of safety" (**FIGURE 13**). Pedunculation of the gallbladder and obtaining the "critical view of safety" are prerequisites for the placement of clips and division of the cystic artery and cystic duct. After this dissection is complete and the anatomy confirmed by both members of the operating team, the first clip is placed on the infundibulum of the gallbladder, just as it narrows to become the cystic duct (**FIGURE 14**).

Cholangiography Intraoperative cholangiogram is used selectively by most surgeons, but should be within the skill set of all surgeons regardless of how infrequently it is used. Two methods of performing cholangiography are most popular:

1. Percutaneous cholangiography—Using a laparoscopic hook or Metzenbaum scissors, a small ductotomy is made in the cystic duct, just below the clip on the gallbladder infundibulum (**FIGURE 15A**). If the incision is more than 50% of the diameter of the cystic duct, the duct will spin, making cannulation difficult and risking avulsion. Through a small skin incision immediately below the 9th rib in the mid clavicular line, a specialized catheter with a needle introducer (Mixter catheter) or a large-bore IV catheter is placed (**FIGURE 15B**). A 4 or 5 French catheter is passed into the abdominal cavity, flushed with saline, then picked up with a Maryland grasper in the surgeon's right hand and placed in the cystic duct. The catheter is flushed with saline as the clip is slowly closed. When flushing becomes difficult, pressure on the clipper is terminated, which allows restoration of flow through the cholangiocatheter (**FIGURE 15C**).

   With appropriate lead shielding, 50% contrast agent is injected under fluoroscopic guidance. The cholangiogram is not complete without visualization of the duodenum, the left hepatic duct, and two ducts going to the right lobe of the liver (anterior and posterior sectoral ducts). Isolated right posterior sectoral bile duct injury may not be detected unless careful inspection of the intrahepatic biliary anatomy on the cholangiogram demonstrates the presence of two major right hepatic ducts. Upon completion of cholangiography, the clip is removed, the catheter is pulled out.

2. Cholangiography with the Olsen clamp—A specialized clamp accepting a cholangiocatheter down its central channel can be purchased from several manufacturers. The clamp is introduced through the mid clavicular trocar. The clamp is placed next to the ductotomy, and the catheter is advanced into the duct. The clamp is closed around the cystic duct to hold it in place during cholangiography (**FIGURE 15D**). Fluoroscopic cholangiography is performed as described above.

13   **Critical View of Safety**

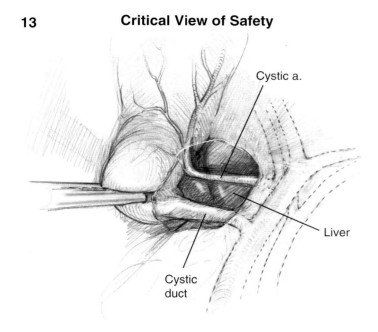

Cystic a.

Liver

Cystic
duct

14

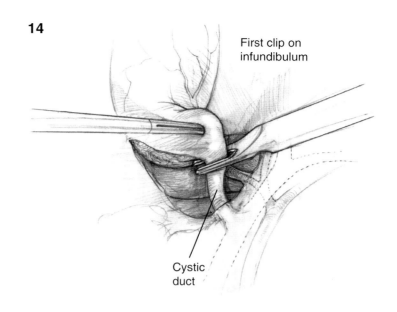

First clip on
infundibulum

Cystic
duct

Cholangiography, Percutaneous Technique

15a

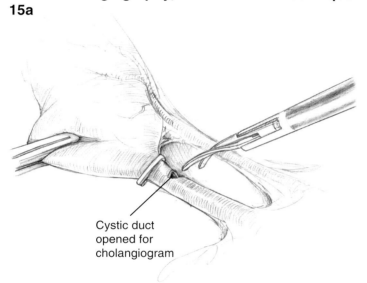

Cystic duct
opened for
cholangiogram

15b

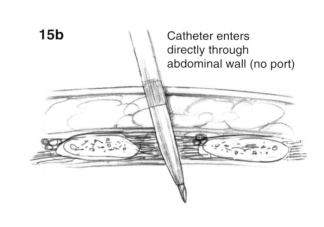

Catheter enters
directly through
abdominal wall (no port)

15c

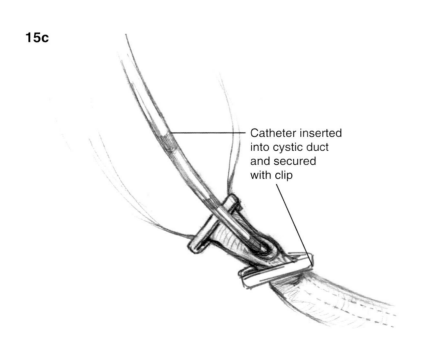

Catheter inserted
into cystic duct
and secured
with clip

15d   ### Cholangiography Using Olsen Clamp

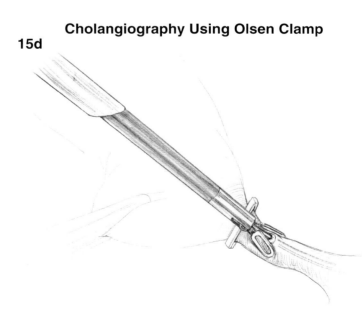

Completion of Cholecystectomy Following cholangiography, the cystic duct is secured with two clips, and is divided with scissors (**FIGURE 16**). Two clips are placed on the cystic artery near its origin, and one is placed distally near the gallbladder before dividing the cystic artery (**FIGURE 17**). If the cystic artery appears to be quite small, there may be a second cystic artery, often travelling in the gallbladder bed.

The gallbladder is "peeled" off the undersurface of the liver with the electrosurgical hook. Critical in this dissection is establishing countertraction with the surgeon's left hand pulling the gallbladder away from the liver bed. The hook can be used by "painting" electrical current at the interface of gallbladder and liver off the elbow of the hook (**FIGURE 18**) or by hooking beneath the connective tissue, distracting it and then applying electrical current (**FIGURE 19**).

The tip of the hook cautery should point away from the gallbladder to avoid inadvertent perforation. The "painting" technique is quicker, but has a higher risk of perforating the gallbladder than the "hooking" method. If a hole in the gallbladder occurs, it should be controlled with a suture, clip, or an Endoloop to prevent spilling stones into the abdominal cavity. As the gallbladder starts to come away from the liver, it may be challenging to maintain traction on the line of dissection. If the back of the hook is used to elevate the gallbladder, the surgeon's left hand can be "marched up" the hepatic surface of the gallbladder, grasping near the point of dissection to attain optimal tension along the line of dissection.

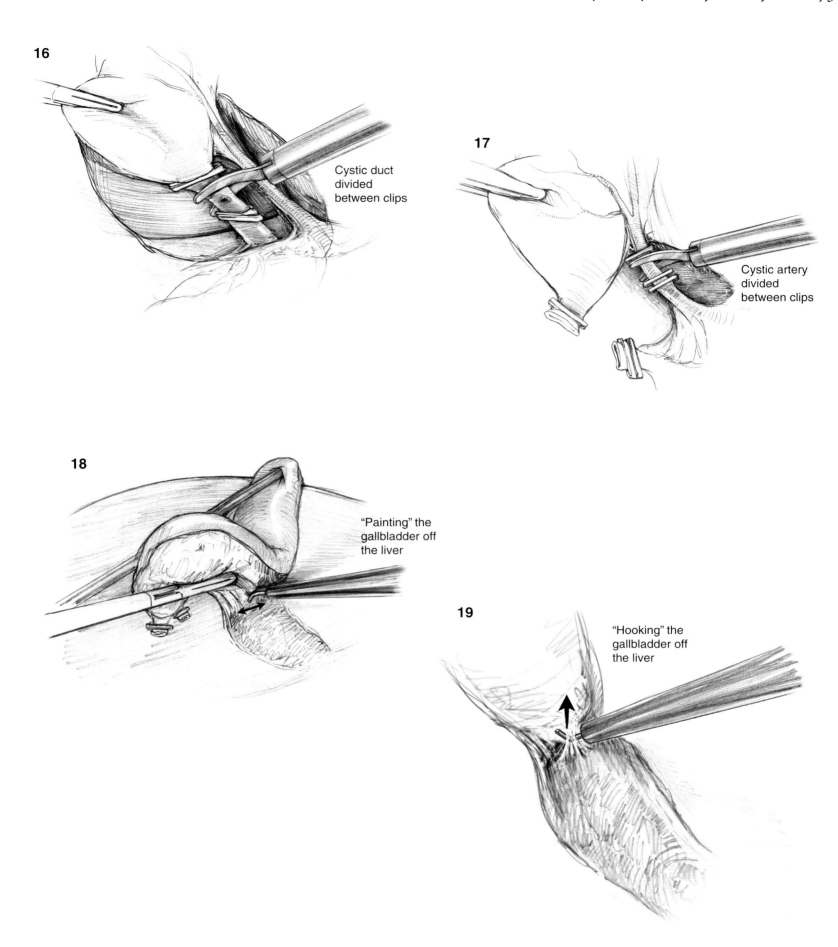

16

Cystic duct
divided
between clips

17

Cystic artery
divided
between clips

18

"Painting" the
gallbladder off
the liver

19

"Hooking" the
gallbladder off
the liver

Completion of Cholecystectomy When the gallbladder is nearly free of the liver, the infundibulum (cystic duct end) is passed superior to the liver edge and the remaining attachments are exposed by grabbing the right peritoneal edge with the assistant's grasper and the left peritoneal edge with the surgeon's left hand stretching the remaining peritoneal attachments between liver and gallbladder (**FIGURE 20**). Before finally separating liver and gallbladder, a visual inspection of the liver bed will reveal any bleeding from the liver bed. All oozing should be controlled with fulguration using electrosurgery at a high power (coagulation mode—setting of 80 watts) (**FIGURE 21**). If bile is collecting in the porta hepatis, a detailed inspection of the cystic duct stump and the liver bed is imperative to identify a source of the bile. If a source of bile cannot be identified, it is often safer to place a closed suction drain (Jackson-Pratt type) rather than attempting further dissection in the porta hepatis. Further dissection could convert a self-limited biliary fistula into a full-fledged common bile duct injury.

When the gallbladder is free of the liver, it should be removed in one of two fashions. If there is no sign of infection and the gallbladder has not been perforated during dissection, it is most cost-effective to remove the gallbladder through the umbilical trocar site (with camera guidance from the epigastric port). This site is chosen because incision extension (often necessary to remove a large stone burden) carries little risk of bleeding (**FIGURE 22**). Extending the epigastric incision by extending division of the rectus sheath and rectus muscle runs a greater risk of bleeding from the rectus muscle or superior epigastric artery. Rarely, if the gallbladder is damaged during dissection, or so inflamed that extraction might lead to disruption, a 10-mm specimen retrieval bag is used to remove the gallbladder (**FIGURE 23**). The umbilical port is generally used for gallbladder extraction. Upon removing the gallbladder, the right upper quadrant is examined and all fluid is removed from around the liver. If a port site has been enlarged, the fascia is closed with interrupted sutures of #1 braided absorbable suture, and the skin is reapproximated with absorbable suture or skin glue.

POSTOPERATIVE CARE Antiemetic and ketorolac are administered at the completion of the operation, and the patient is generally discharged later the same day. ■

20

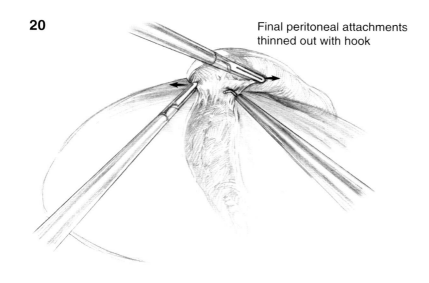

Final peritoneal attachments
thinned out with hook

21

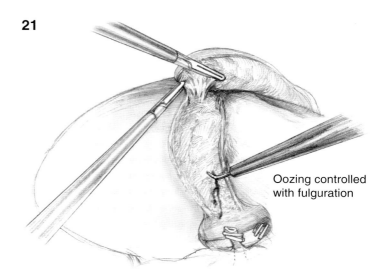

Oozing controlled
with fulguration

22

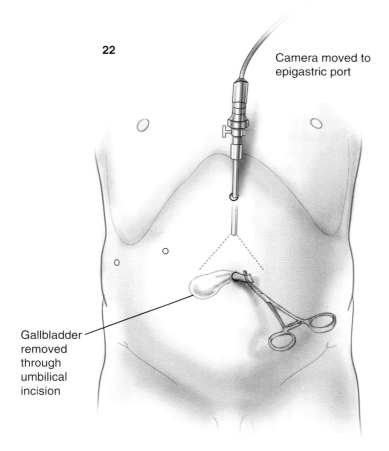

Camera moved to
epigastric port

Gallbladder
removed
through
umbilical
incision

23

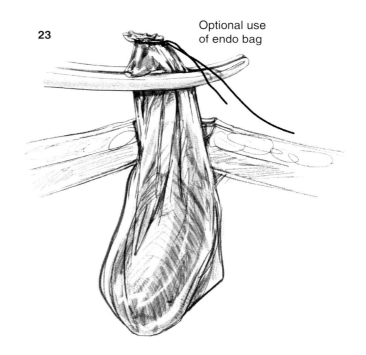

Optional use
of endo bag

SINGLE-INCISION CHOLECYSTECTOMY

HISTORY AND INDICATIONS Laparoscopic cholecystectomy is currently regarded as the procedure of choice for the treatment of symptomatic gallbladder disease. Current techniques include variations on a three- or four-port approach that are generally well tolerated by the vast majority of patients. However, postoperative abdominal, incisional, and shoulder pain still occurs in most patients and persists for a number of days after the procedure. To counter this, laparoscopic techniques continue to evolve in order to minimize scarring and accelerate recovery. Natural-orifice transluminal endoscopic surgery (NOTES), for example, is a technique first introduced in 2005 that attempts to address certain intraabdominal pathology by purely endoscopic techniques. Its application continues to be investigated at this time. Another technique, single-incision laparoscopic surgery (SILS), which was first reported in 1997 and further refined in 2008, has entered into mainstream clinical practice. SILS techniques have now been applied to a number of different procedures, but the most established application for this technique has been for cholecystectomy.

In general, SILS cholecystectomy can be considered in any patient found to be a candidate for the laparoscopic approach. It has been completed successfully in patients with body mass indexes (BMIs) up to 44.6 kg/m². Current data suggest that a small proportion (4%) of patients will need conversion to either a conventional laparoscopic cholecystectomy or open cholecystectomy, principally because of severity of gallbladder disease.

PREOPERATIVE CONSIDERATIONS

Patient Preparation Symptomatic gallbladder disease is the usual diagnosis prompting cholecystectomy, and suitable preoperative testing and patient preparation should be initiated at the time of diagnosis. The anticipated severity of the disease and other patient factors, such as morbid obesity or prior abdominal surgeries, should be considered before committing to a SILS approach, particularly if the surgeon is still within his or her learning curve. The patient should be consented for SILS, but both laparoscopic and open approaches should be discussed with them, including the more common complications such as bleeding, infection, and damage to intraabdominal structures.

Equipment and Instrumentation SILS cholecystectomy can be carried out using standard laparoscopic instruments, including atraumatic graspers and a hook electrocautery, with separate port entry at the umbilicus. However, there are now commercially available SILS-specific "all-in-one"

ports that incorporate three-port apertures into a molded or low-profile configuration. Use of these commercial SILS ports also mandates a custom roticulating grasper and dissector for the procedure because of the limitations in range of motion dictated by the port design (**FIGURE 1**).

A 5- or 10-mm, 30- or 45-degree laparoscope can be used. A bariatric-length 5- or 10-mm, 30-degree laparoscope provides sufficient length for the light stem to be positioned to minimize interference with the handle grips of the working instruments. There are also laparoscopes currently available that have the light stem connector positioned parallel to the laparoscope instead of perpendicular, as is the case with most current models. These facilitate easier conduct of the operation. Additional equipment includes

- Laparoscopic suction irrigator
- Maryland-style dissector
- Atraumatic gallbladder grasper
- L-hook
- Specimen retrieval bag
- 5-mm clip applier (9-mm clips)
- 0 nonabsorbable braided suture on a Keith needle

ANESTHESIA General anesthesia is required. Placement of an orogastric (OG) tube will facilitate decompression of the stomach. If antibiotics have not already been administered, this should be done prior to incision. A Foley catheter is required in order to decompress the bladder and decrease the risk of bladder injury.

ROOM SETUP AND POSITIONING The patient is positioned supine on the operating table with arms tucked in a position identical to the conventional laparoscopic approach. After general anesthesia is induced, a Foley catheter catheter is placed. The operating surgeon is positioned on the patient's left side to the right of the scrub nurse or technician. The assistant is positioned on the patient's right side.

Display monitors are positioned off the patient's right and left shoulders in line with the operating surgeon and assistant's line of sight (**FIGURE 2**).

OPERATIVE CONDUCT

Access and Port Placement There are a number of umbilical or periumbilical incisions that allow for the SILS port access. Depicted in this chapter a curvilinear 180-degree skin incision placed on the superior umbilical crease (**FIGURE 3**).

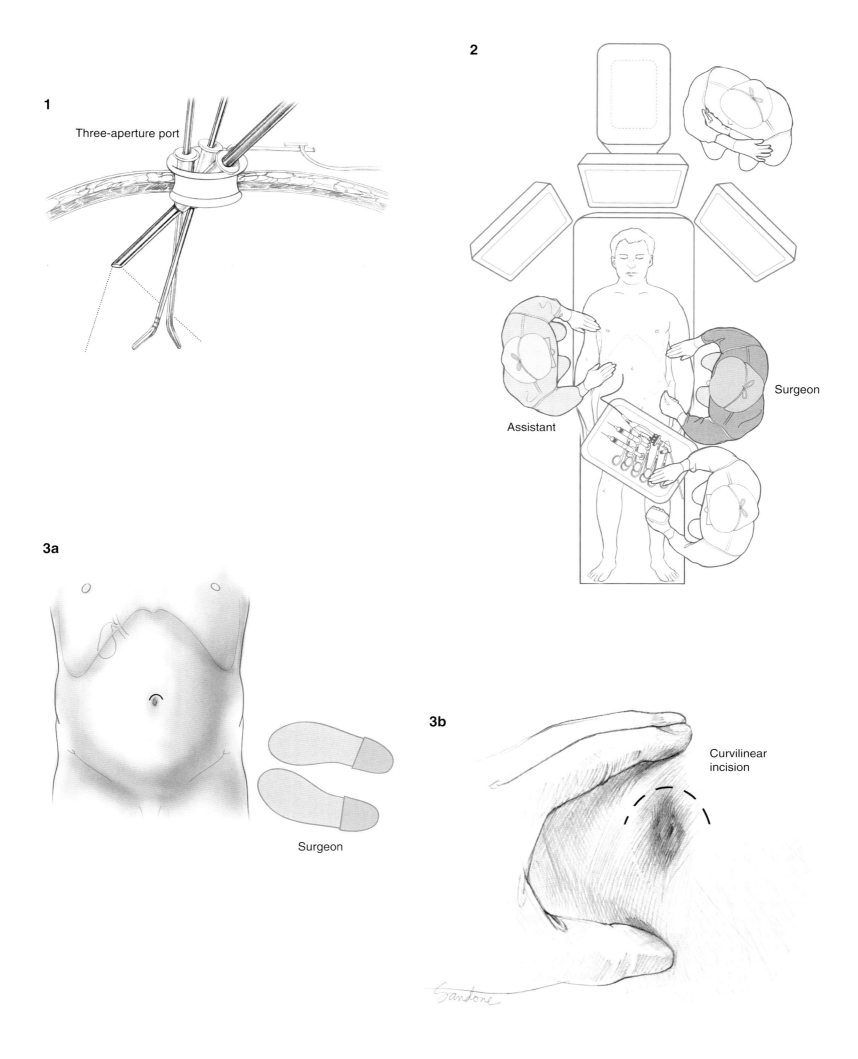

1

Three-aperture port

2

Assistant

Surgeon

3a

Surgeon

3b

Curvilinear incision

Sandone

Access and Port Placement Following the skin incision, the fascia is grasped and elevated as the preperitoneal space and peritoneum are encountered and incised sharply. Once the abdomen is entered, the complete incision is sized and should be able to accommodate the tips of the index and middle fingers. The SILS port is grasped on its inferior ring with a large curved clamp and lubricated well with surgical lubricant. The tip of the clamp and the anterior portion of the port are introduced into the incision at a 45-degree angle **(FIGURE 4)** and gently pushed into position while simultaneously lifting up on the abdominal wall. With gentle and sustained pressure, the interior ring of the SILS port will seat itself into the abdomen below the peritoneum, and the clamp can be released and removed. Three 5-mm laparoscopic ports are then introduced into the SILS port, and carbon dioxide (CO_2) insufflation is initiated through the insufflation cuff until a pneumoperitoneum of 12–14 mm Hg pressure is achieved. A 5-mm, 30-degree laparoscope is introduced through the uppermost port, and a cursory laparoscopic examination is made to assure that there are no immediate contraindications to proceeding. With the camera port established, an atraumatic grasper is introduced, and the liver edge is elevated in order to visualize the disease state of the gallbladder. The surgeon's experience and judgement should guide the decision to proceed with a SILS approach at this point. If there is evidence of severe inflammatory disease, the decision to convert to a traditional laparoscopic approach should be made based on the level of experience with SILS.

Conduct of the Operation If the decision is made to proceed with the SILS approach, retraction of the fundus of the gallbladder is necessary. On the back table, a braided nonabsorbable suture is passed on a Keith needle in a U-stitch fashion through the rubber gasket obtained from a 5-mL syringe, and a knot is tied to secure the gasket **(FIGURE 5, INSET)**. One of the 5-mm ports is changed out for a 12-mm one, and the needle, suture, and attached gasket are introduced into the abdomen. A laparoscopic needle holder grasps the needle with one hand while a laparoscopic gallbladder grasper is used to control the tip of the gallbladder with the other hand, and the needle is passed through the gallbladder, **(FIGURE 5)** then out through the abdominal wall at the right costal margin, where it is retracted and secured with a hemostat **(FIGURE 6)**. This elevates the gallbladder to allow dissection around the infundibulum.

At this point, the infundibulum of the gallbladder is grasped and retracted laterally (or superiorly) by the grasper in the operator's right hand.

The Maryland dissector is introduced through the left port, and dissection begins by removing the connective tissue overlying the infundibulum of the gallbladder. The remainder of the dissection is carried out in a fashion identical to a laparoscopic approach, including isolation of the cystic duct and artery and confirmation of the "critical view of safety." However, with the SILS approach, the dissection is more challenging due to the close grouping of the trocars at the umbilicus, the need to cross operating instruments inside the abdomen, **(FIGURE 7)** the lack of the commonly accepted sturdiness of SILS instruments, and the inability to completely retract the tip of the gallbladder in a cephalad fashion or manipulate the organ to assist with visualization or dissection. Difficulty in these areas generally decreases to an acceptable level as surgeon experience increases.

After the infundibular dissection is complete and anatomy verified, the cystic duct and artery are then secured using serial clip applications. Once the duct and artery are transected, the hook cautery is used to facilitate removal of the gallbladder from the liver bed **(FIGURE 8)**. When the gallbladder is free of all attachments, one of the 5-mm ports is swapped out for a 12-mm port to allow a specimen retrieval bag to be introduced into the abdomen. The retraction suture is cut at the level of the skin, and the gallbladder is placed in the bag. Care should be taken to ensure that the rubber gasket used in retracting the gallbladder is also inserted into the bag. A laparoscopic grasper is used to elevate the liver to visualize the gallbladder fossa for evidence of bleeding or bile pooling. A suction aspirator can be used through the remaining port to irrigate and evacuate the gallbladder fossa.

Specimen Removal and Closure The grasper and suction device are removed, then the SILS port and specimen bag are removed as one unit **(FIGURE 9)**. The fascial defect is closed with large interrupted sutures. The skin incision may be closed with tissue adhesive, absorbable subcuticular suture, or surgical staples.

POSTOPERATIVE CARE The OG tube and Foley catheter are removed at the end of the operation. Nausea and pain should be treated aggressively. Most patients are discharged to home on the day of surgery with prescriptions for pain medication and a stool softener. They should receive detailed instructions, including the procedure they have undergone, expected postoperative course, and instructions regarding medications and signs of possible complications. Routine follow-up care in the clinic occurs between 1 and 4 weeks postoperatively. ■

4

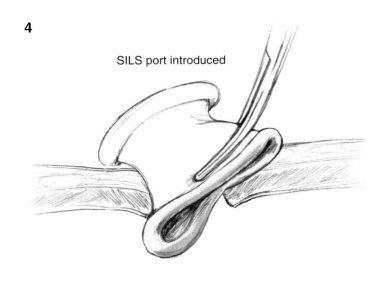

SILS port introduced

5 Bumper fashioned from syringe plunger

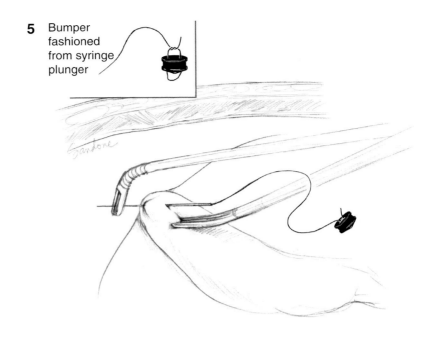

6 Gallbladder retracted through abdominal wall

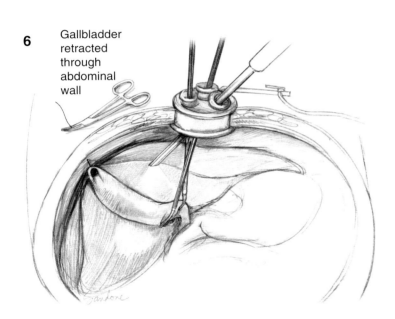

7

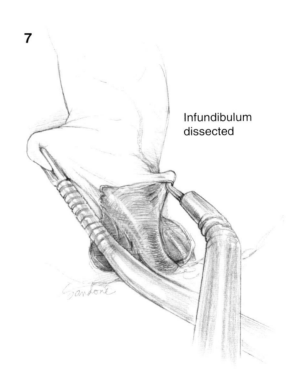

Infundibulum dissected

8

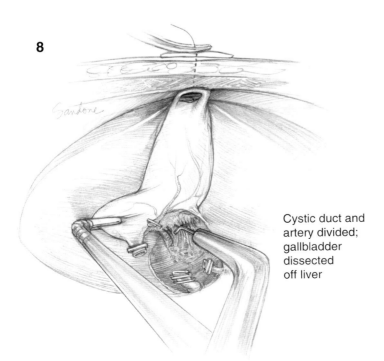

Cystic duct and artery divided; gallbladder dissected off liver

9

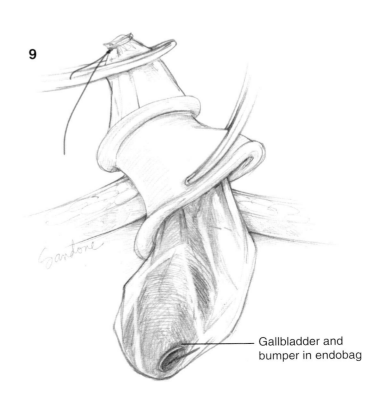

Gallbladder and bumper in endobag

COMMON BILE DUCT EXPLORATION

INDICATIONS Laparoscopic common bile duct (CBD) exploration (LCBDE) is indicated for all patients with known CBD stones at the time of laparoscopic cholecystectomy, but is most commonly used when an intraoperative cholangiogram or ultrasound exam demonstrates one or more filling defects in the CBD, presumed to be CBD stones. Following cholecystectomy, most CBD stones are addressed with endoscopic retrograde cholangiography and endoscopic sphincterotomy (ERC/ES) rather than LCBDE. Additionally, in the presence of acute cholangitis or acute pancreatitis from choledocholithiasis, ERC/ES has proven to be a safer strategy that open CBDE. Although no studies have randomized patients with acute cholangitis to LCBDE or ERC/ES, the benefits of urgent bile duct decompression can usually be achieved with an ERC/ES, followed by laparoscopic cholecystectomy (if not already performed) at a later date, when the acute illness has resolved.

Contraindications to LCBDE are few. In patients with an impacted stone, LCBDE may fail, requiring the placement of a T tube, followed by ERC/ES or a hybrid radiologic and endoscopic procedure. Additionally, the patient with portal vein thrombosis or other etiologies of portal hypertension may have extensive venous collateralization in the porta hepatis, making choledochotomy to remove stones very hazardous.

PATIENT PREPARATION LCBDE is performed as an adjunct to laparoscopic cholecystectomy in all but a few rare situations. The patient position and room setup are identical to those for laparoscopic cholecystectomy (**FIGURE 1A**). The fundus of the gallbladder remains elevated at the time of cholangiography and bile duct exploration (**FIGURE 1B**). The most important aspects of preparation are ensuring that the patient is on a fluoroscopy table, which will allow the C-arm to get under the patient without running into the table supporting column (**FIGURE 1C**). The second most important aspect of preparation is ensuring that a cart containing all LCBE equipment is close at hand.

Items necessary on the LCBDE cart include an endoscopic light source (for the choledochoscope), an endoscopic video camera, and an additional monitor if these items are not built into the room where laparoscopic cholecystectomy is being done. The central item for LCBDE is the 3- to 3.5-mm (diameter) flexible choledochoscope, kept sterile on the CBDE cart. The cart should have, at a minimum, the following items: hydrophilic guidewires (100 cm, 0.035-in. diameter), disposable scope introduction sheaths, 8-mm dilating balloons (for the cystic duct), 2.8 French flat wire baskets, and T tubes that can be placed over a guidewire. Helical stone baskets (3–4 French) with filiform tips are useful if fluoroscopic bile duct exploration is to be attempted instead of endoscopic choledochoscopy. Access to an electrohydraulic lithotripsy unit is valuable for the rare occasion where impacted stones cannot be dislodged.

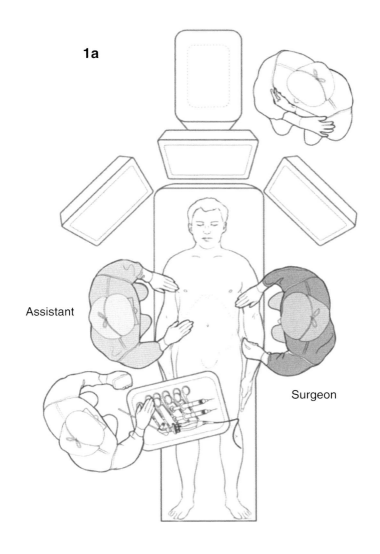

1a

Assistant

Surgeon

1b

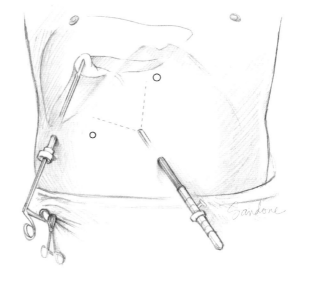

1c

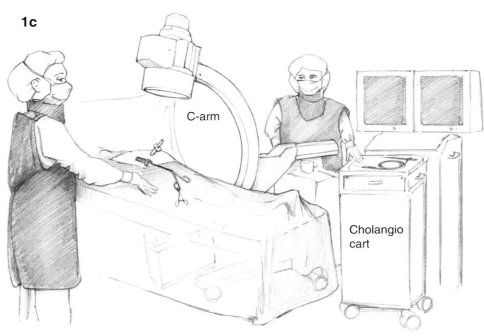

C-arm

Cholangio cart

OPERATIVE PROCEDURE LCBDE may be done through the cystic duct with fluoroscopic guidance or with choledochoscopic guidance, or it can be performed through a choledochotomy with endoscopic guidance. These techniques are, to a certain degree, complementary. The transcystic duct techniques are useful for distal CBD stones <6 mm in diameter (as measured by cholangiography or ultrasonography) in a nondilated or minimally dilated duct. Choledochotomy and direct CBD exploration is useful for common hepatic duct stones, stones >6 mm in diameter, or dilated CBDs, usually > 1.0 cm.

Laparoscopic Transcystic Fluoroscopic CBDE When a choledochoscope is not available or when a simple approach is desirable, this approach is applicable. Following the performance of percutaneous cholangiography (**FIGURE 2**) as described in chapter 32, the finding of one or several filling defects in the CBD prompts LCBDE.

The first step is to remove the clip from the CBD, but leave the cholangiogram catheter in place (**FIGURE 3**). A hydrophilic guidewire is passed through the cholangiogram catheter into the CBD, past the stones, and into the duodenum. The cholangiography catheter is then removed, leaving the guidewire in place. A helical stone basket is passed over the guidewire into the distal CBD. The guidewire may be removed to leave a channel for contrast injection, to confirm that the basket is not in the duodenum (**FIGURE 4**). The basket is opened in the distal CBD and pulled back slowly. When a stone is engaged, the basket is closed and removed through the cystic duct (**FIGURE 5**). The basket may be passed as many times as is necessary to remove all stones seen on cholangiography. A completion cholangiogram should be performed. If it demonstrates that all stones have been removed, the cystic duct is clipped and the cholecystectomy is completed. Baskets without channels for guidewires and cholangiography may be used, but with that technique the basketing is truly "blind" and the stone yield is lower (50%–60%).

This technique has two shortcomings: possible basket entrapment in the duodenum or CBD, and a failure rate to clear the duct of 30% to 40%. Nonetheless this distinctly "low-tech" approach has been appealing to many, especially those who are just beginning to perform LCBDE.

Transcystic Fluoroscopic CBDE

2

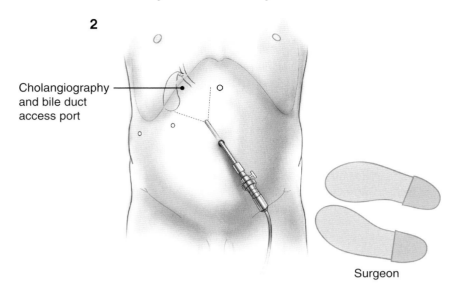

Cholangiography
and bile duct
access port

Surgeon

3

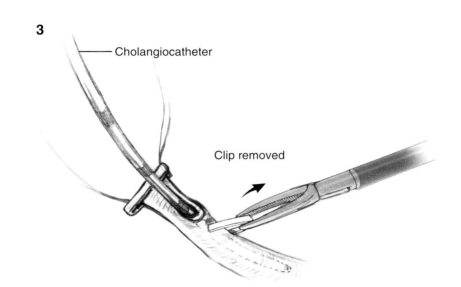

Cholangiocatheter

Clip removed

4

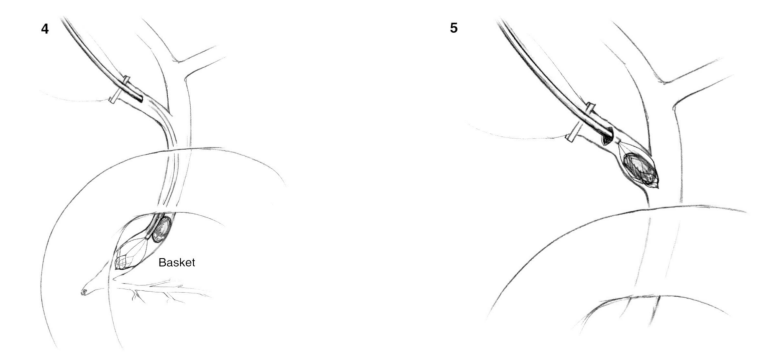

Basket

5

Laparoscopic Transcystic Endoscopic CBDE This is the most commonly used approach. It requires a greater array of equipment than fluoroscopic exploration, including the thin-caliber flexible choledochoscope (described earlier), a light source for the choledochoscope, video camera, monitor, and dilating balloons to enlarge the cystic duct to accommodate the scope.

The procedure starts in the same way as the fluoroscopic procedure with the placement of a guidewire through the cholangiocatheter and removal of the catheter. Next, a Berci plastic sheath is passed over the guidewire (**FIGURE 6**). This sheath, or introducer, allows the frequent in and out passage of the choledochoscope through the abdominal wall, and contains a diaphragm to prevent pneumoperitoneum leakage. Next, an 8 mm radial dilating balloon is passed over the guidewire and placed deep in the cystic duct with about 3 to 5 mm of balloon remaining out of the cystic duct (**FIGURE 7**). The purpose of cystic duct dilation is to allow ready access to the duct with the scope, and to facilitate extraction of CBD stones. The balloon is inflated and left in place for 5 minutes while the choledochoscope is set up. The choledochoscope is connected to an IV bag of sterile saline, to the light source, and to the video imaging system.

After 5 minutes, the dilating balloon is deflated and removed. Most commonly the guidewire is also removed, and the scope is introduced through the plastic introducer and placed into the cystic duct with a rubber-shod Maryland grasper. The choledochoscope can be passed over the guidewire. The tips of the Maryland grasper will damage the choledochoscope if they are not shod with short segments of a 10 French soft red rubber catheter before scope introduction (**FIGURE 8**). As soon as the scope is introduced, the saline irrigation is started through the operating channel (**FIGURE 9**). The anesthesiologist gives the patient 0.5 to 1 mg of glucagon to relax the sphincter of Oddi. The scope is passed under direct video imaging into the distal duct until the first stone is visualized.

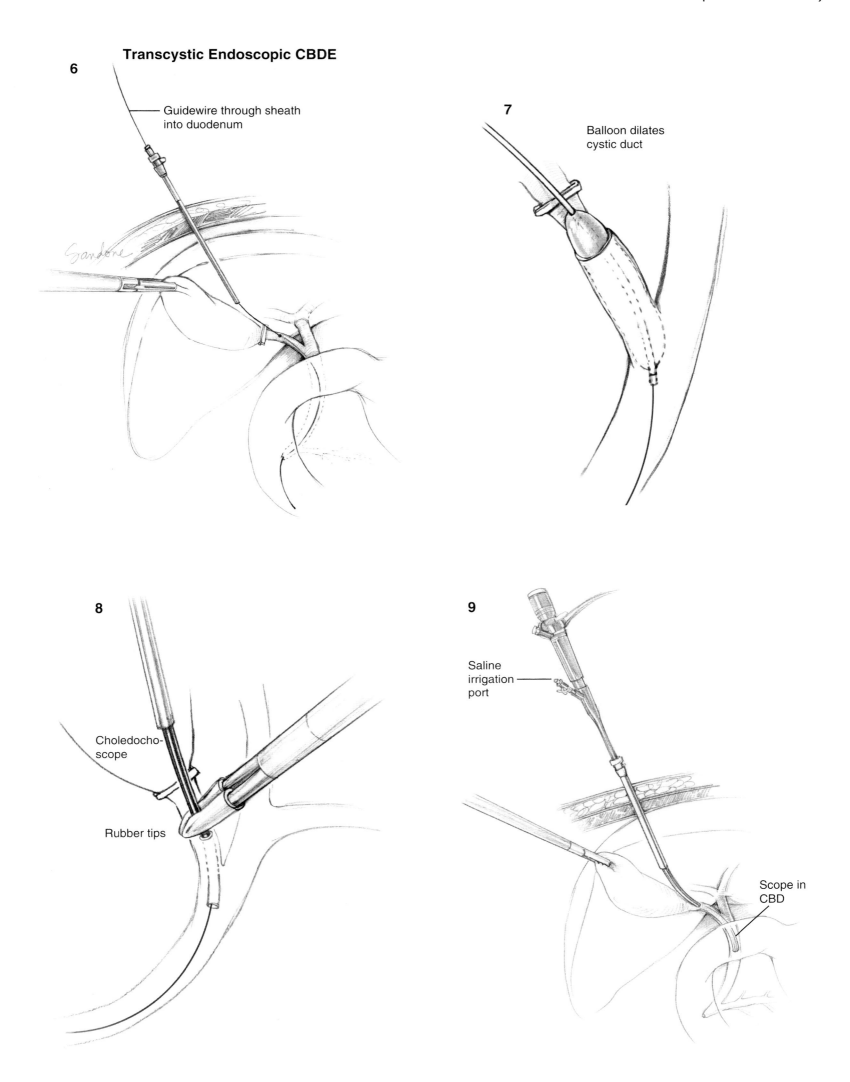

Transcystic Endoscopic CBDE

6

Guidewire through sheath into duodenum

7

Balloon dilates cystic duct

8

Choledocho-scope

Rubber tips

9

Saline irrigation port

Scope in CBD

Laparoscopic Transcystic Endoscopic CBDE Once the stone(s) are visualized in the CBD, a 2.8 French flat wire basket is introduced through the operating channel of the scope. If a Tuohy-Borst "valve" is placed in the operating channel, it is possible to maintain irrigation while basketing is performed. Maintaining irrigation is critical to maintaining vision, which requires that the basket used be smaller in caliber than the size of the operating channel. The tip of the retracted basket sheath is directed immediately past the stone (if possible) and the basket is opened **(FIGURE 10)**. The scope and basket are then retracted slowly, together. The opened basket will usually entrap the CBD stone as the basket is retracted. Once the stone is inside the basket, the basket is closed, and the scope, stone, and basket are removed together, releasing the stone into the peritoneal cavity, where it can be easily retrieved **(FIGURE 11)**. These steps are repeated until the cystic duct is cleared of all stones. Choledochoscopy into the duodenum is then performed if the sphincter of Oddi opens easily with saline irrigation **(FIGURE 12)**. This should not be a "forced entry," as the sphincter may become damaged or edematous after much manipulation. Despite "stone-free" choledochoscopy, a completion cholangiogram should still be performed to create a record that the duct is clear, and to confirm that there are no stones in the common hepatic or intrahepatic ducts.

10

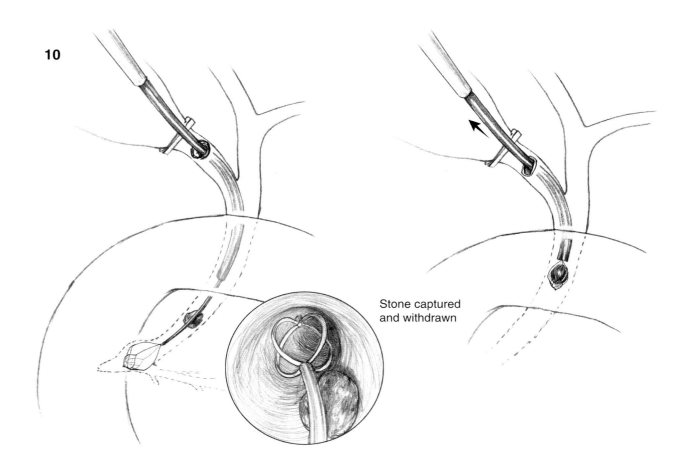

Stone captured
and withdrawn

11

12

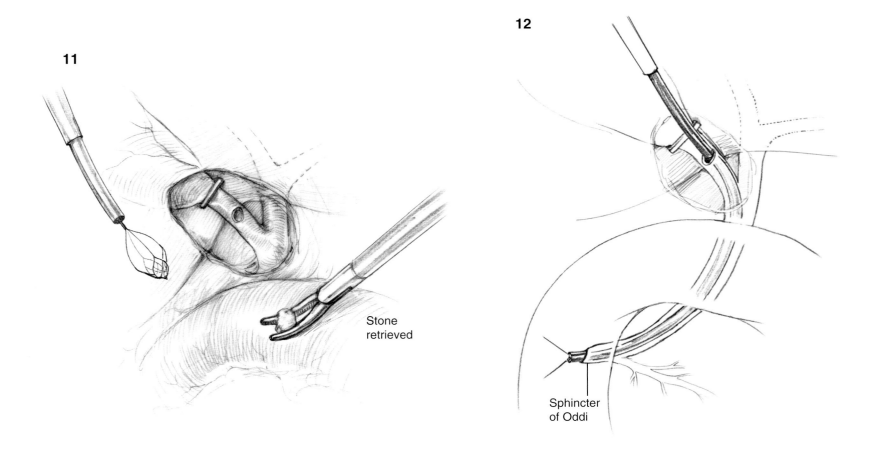

Stone
retrieved

Sphincter
of Oddi

Laparoscopic Choledochotomy and CBDE When stones are lodged in the common hepatic duct or more proximally, it is difficult to use a transcystic route because the oblique entry of the cystic duct into the CBD would require the scope to reverse directions as it entered the CBD. Instead, CHD stones in a dilated biliary system should be addressed with a choledochotomy. If the CBD is small (<6 mm), it may be wise to leave these stones for postoperative retrieval with ERCP. Choledochotomy in a small CBD risks a CBD stricture, even if a stent is left in place. The most common indication for choledochotomy is large stones (>6 mm in longest dimension) in a dilated system. Such stones are unlikely to be successfully retrieved through the cystic duct.

To initiate this procedure, the common bile duct is cleaned off with a fine dissecting hook, near the confluence with the cystic duct, approximately 1 cm above the duodenum. A vertical incision is made in the anterior wall of the CBD with fine, sharp scissors. As a rule of thumb, the incision should be as long as the duct is wide, and a few mm longer than the largest stone. Usually a 1.0- to 1.5-cm choledochotomy will suffice. Bleeding from the choledochotomy is controlled with targeted applications of electrosurgery.

The first step in clearing the duct is irrigation. The simplest method is usually the replacement of the cholangiocatheter into the duct and flushing with large volumes of saline. Next, a Fogarty balloon catheter can be passed in either direction, inflated, and pulled back through the choledochotomy, dislodging more stones (**FIGURE 13**). The Fogarty will often pass into the duodenum, so must be deflated as it is brought through the sphincter of Oddi. Last, a more traditional choledochoscope (5 mm in diameter, used for open CBDE) is introduced into the duct through the right-upper quadrant plastic introducer, described earlier. Stones in the distal CBD are addressed first and cleared with a stone basket as described earlier. The proximal duct

is cleared next (**FIGURE 14**). If stones are truly impacted such that a basket or Fogarty cannot be passed beyond them, they may be broken up with an electrohydraulic lithotripter (a urologic tool) or may be left for subsequent ERCP and sphincterotomy.

At the completion of duct clearance, the cholecystectomy is completed and the gallbladder and all CBD stones are removed from the abdomen. Next, a T-tube is passed through a trocar and sutured into the CBD with interrupted sutures of 4-0 braided absorbable material (**FIGURE 15A**). The duct closure is tested for leaks with pressurized saline injection through the T-tube. When the closure is found to be watertight, a Jackson-Pratt (JP) drain is pulled through the epigastric port and pulled out the most lateral port site, as the trocar is removed. Alternatively, a biliary stent can be placed into the duct before closure (**FIGURE 15B**), or a large duct can be closed primarily (**FIGURE 15C**). With both alternate methods, a JP drain is left in the abdomen adjacent to the closure of the CBD.

POSTOPERATIVE CARE Depending on the complexity and duration of the procedure, the patient may be treated as a laparoscopic cholecystectomy patient with immediate feeding and early discharge (usually postoperative day 1, after duct exploration). If a complicated CBDE is performed with T-tube placement and drainage, ileus resolution may take a day or two longer. JP drains are removed, if the output is not bilious, on postoperative day 1 or 2. If bilious drainage is present, the drain is left until the bile drainage has ceased. The T-tube is usually removed 2 weeks following CBDE. It is customary to perform T-tube cholangiography (with antibiotic prophylaxis) before removing the T tube. If the cholangiogram demonstrates a filling defect, the T-tube tract is dilated and a percutaneous fluoroscopic or choledochoscopic exploration is performed to remove and/or crush the residual stone(s). ■

Choledochotomy and CBDE

13

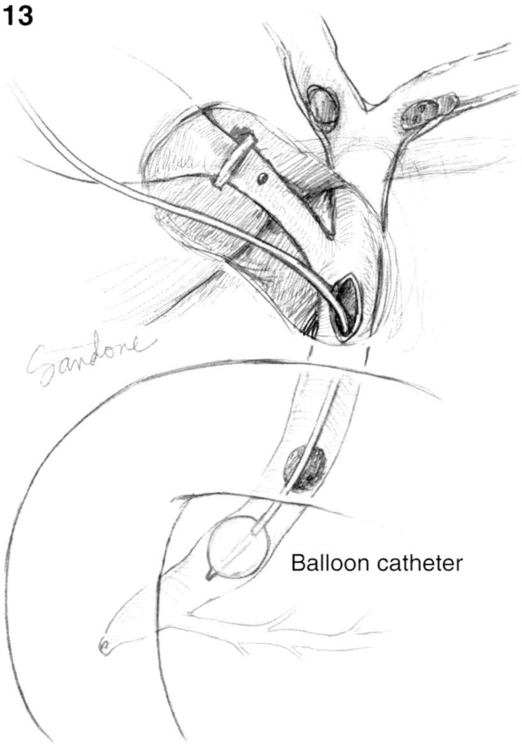

Balloon catheter

14

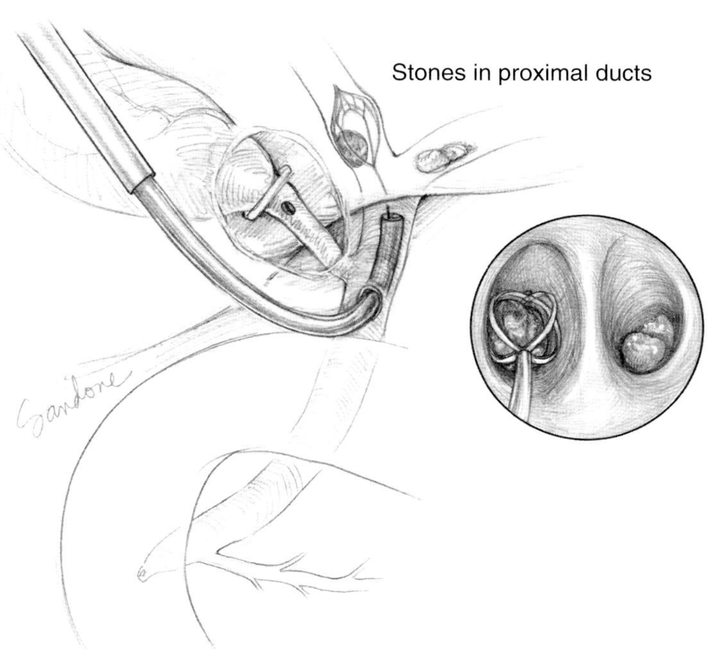

Stones in proximal ducts

15a

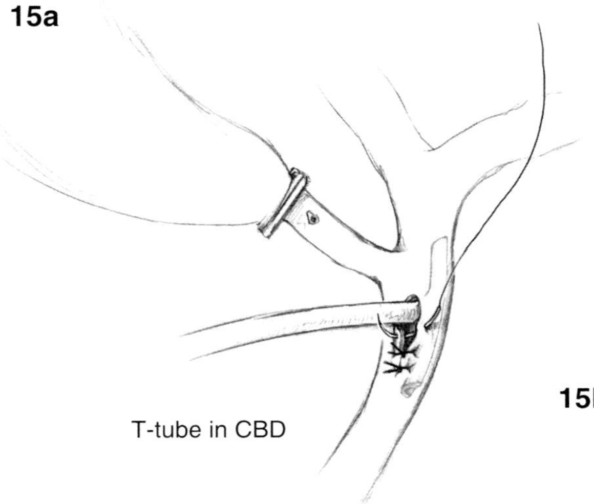

T-tube in CBD

15b

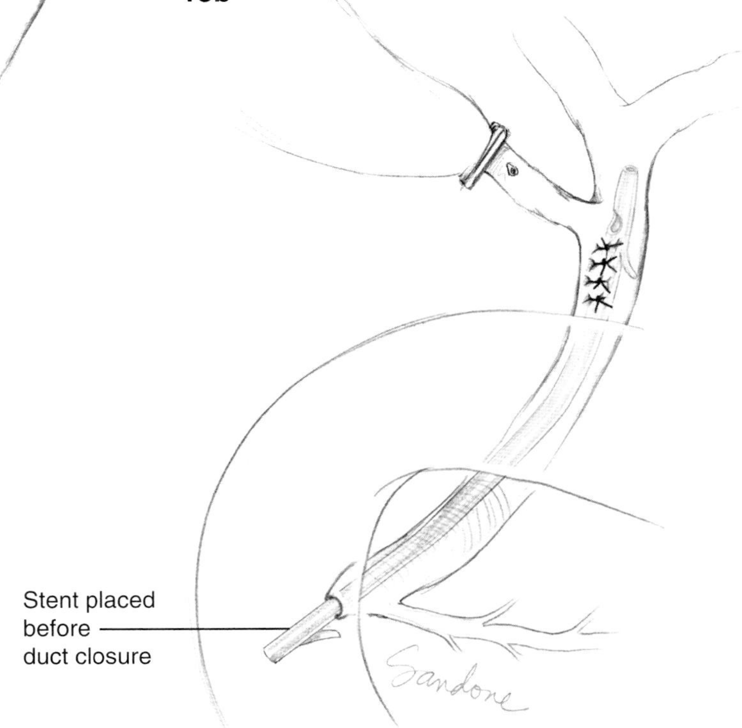

Stent placed before duct closure

15c

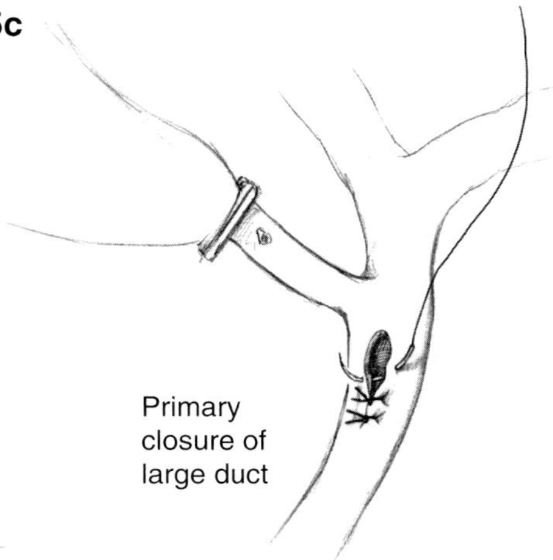

Primary closure of large duct

RADIOFREQUENCY ABLATION OF LIVER TUMORS

INDICATIONS Radiofrequency ablation (RFA) of liver tumors can be performed percutaneously, laparoscopically, or through a traditional open incision. The most common indication for RFA is unresectable primary or metastatic hepatic cancer. RFA can also be applied to a potentially resectable hepatic neoplasm in a patient with a prohibitive operative risk secondary to severe medical comorbidities or compromised hepatocellular reserve (cirrhosis). The role of RFA in non-neuroendocrine neoplasms with extrahepatic metastases is unclear. RFA can provide effective symptomatic palliation for unresectable functional neuroendocrine neoplasms.

RFA is currently considered a form of hepatic directed palliative therapy. Heat produced during RFA induces local tissue destruction by inducing coagulative necrosis. The effectiveness of RFA is limited by the size and the location of the lesion(s). When performed correctly, RFA is effective at destroying hepatic neoplasms up to 5 cm in diameter. Lesions located near a vessel greater than 3 mm in diameter may not be adequately ablated because of a "heat sink" effect in which optimum targeted temperature cannot be achieved due to perivascular heat dissipation. Neoplasms located near the hilar plate must be approached with caution because of the potential for bile duct injury.

PREOPERATIVE PREPARATION Triple-phase contrast-enhanced computed tomography (CT) scan of the abdomen provides critical anatomical information on the number and location of hepatic masses and their relation to major vessels and ductal structures.

Preoperative medical evaluation for cardiopulmonary disease and fitness for surgery are essential. In patients with cirrhosis, laboratory investigation and clinical assessment must be performed to assess the hepatocellular reserve. The model of end-stage liver disease (MELD) score is an objective method to evaluate the hepatic reserve. The MELD score is calculated by measuring serum creatinine, total bilirubin, and the international normalized (coagulation) ratio (INR). The MELD score has been demonstrated to be predictive of perioperative mortality in patients undergoing abdominal and hepatic surgery.

Patients with a metastatic "functional" neuroendocrine neoplasm should have their symptoms appropriately controlled preoperatively, usually with octreotide. Adequate hydration, preoperative antibiotic, and deep venous thrombosis (DVT) prophylaxis are all indicated. Essential equipment includes 30- and 45-degree laparoscopes, a 10-mm flexible laparoscopic ultrasound probe, an ultrasonic dissector, a 10-mm clip applier, and a laparoscopic radiofrequency ablation system with a 5-cm array electrosurgical probe.

ANESTHESIA General anesthesia with endotracheal intubation and complete neuromuscular blockade is required for this operation.

OPERATIVE PREPARATION A dose of prophylactic IV antibiotic is administered per routine. A Foley catheter and nasogastric tube are placed after the induction of anesthesia. The upper abdomen of the patient is shaved from the nipple line to the pubis if necessary. The abdomen is sterilely prepped and draped.

PATIENT POSITION Laparoscopic RFA of a hepatic mass is performed with the patient in the supine position. The upper and lower extremities are well padded and secured to avoid pressure on tissues during extremes of positioning. The surgeon stands on the right and the assistant stands on the left of the patient (**FIGURE 1**).

TROCAR INSERTION Laparoscopic RFA is performed with a two-trocar technique (**FIGURE 2**). The exact location of the trocar placement depends on the body habitus of the patient and the exact location of the hepatic lesion. Typically a 12-mm camera port is placed in the supraumbilical area. After placement of the camera, a thorough abdominal inspection and survey is performed to rule out metastatic disease. A second 12-mm trocar is inserted in the right side of the abdomen based on the location of the hepatic lesion. An additional trocar may be inserted if mobilization of the right hepatic lobe is necessary for complete visualization by ultrasound. Occasionally the falciform ligament must be divided to allow adequate visualization of the left lateral segments of the liver.

DETAILS OF PROCEDURE The basic principles of laparoscopic RFA of a liver tumor are:

a. Accurate placement of the RFA probe requires accurate ultrasound guidance.

b. *Ablation should include a 1-cm margin of surrounding normal tissue. A 3-cm neoplasm requires an ablation area of 5 cm. A 5-cm neoplasm requires an ablation area of 7 cm.*

c. An ablation area of less than 5 cm be performed with a single insertion of the RFA probe. For an ablation area of larger than 5 cm, a staged ablation with multiple insertions of the RFA probe is needed.

d. A preablation strategy for staged insertion of the RFA probe is needed for an ablation area larger than 5 cm.

e. For multiple lesions, the deeper lesion should be ablated first before ablating the more superficial lesion. This technique will avoid obscuring the details of the deeper lesion.

f. Lesions within 1–2 cm of a major bile duct or the hilar plate should be approached with caution.

Laparoscopic Ultrasound Laparoscopic ultrasound is a critical and essential part of this procedure. There are three important steps in examination with ultrasound.

1. *Ultrasound examination of the liver parenchyma.* A systematic examination of the entire liver with the flexible laparoscopic ultrasound probe allows identification of known and additional hepatic neoplasms (**FIGURE 3**). This can be performed by following each hepatic vein from the suprahepatic inferior vena cava (IVC). Starting from the most superior aspect of segment 4a near the suprahepatic IVC, the probe is moved toward the falciform ligament and the umbilical fissure. This allows examination of left lateral sector (segments 2 and 3) and left medial sector (segments 4a and 4b). The maneuver is then repeated to follow the course of the middle hepatic vein, which is from the IVC to the medial border of the gallbladder. This will allow repeat examination of the left medial sector (segments 4a and 4b) and the right anterior sector (segments 8 and 5). Finally, the right hepatic vein course is followed, and this allows examination of right posterior sector (segments 7 and 6). It may be necessary to alter the setting of the ultrasound to allow optimum visualization of both superficial and deeper hepatic lesions.

2. *Ultrasound examination of the hepatic lesions.* Each hepatic lesion is examined from several views to assess its relationship with the blood vessels and bile duct.

3. *Ultrasound examination of the porta hepatis.* With the operating table tilted into reverse Trendelenburg position, the porta hepatis can be examined by the ultrasound. The presence of a larger portal lymph node is not uncommon, but those that are large and round or with heterogeneity may have metastatic disease.

Tissue Diagnosis For a patient who did not have a prior tissue diagnosis, a core biopsy of the hepatic lesions (with ultrasound guidance for deeper lesions) is performed using a spring-loaded biopsy gun.

RFA Ablation for Lesions Less Than 3 cm (5-cm Ablation Zone) The current RFA technology can allow single insertion of the RFA probe for a neoplasm of less than 3 cm in its greatest dimension to get a 5-cm ablation area.

The hepatic lesion is localized by the ultrasound. The RFA needle is passed percutaneously into the liver parenchyma, preferably in the same plane as the ultrasound probe. The RFA needle is advanced to the edge of the neoplasm and then slowly advanced centrally so that the tip of the RFA needle is 1 cm from the center of the intended ablation area. A biplanar view is needed to confirm this central placement. The array is then deployed to the 2-cm mark (**FIGURES 4 AND 5**), and the ablation begins until the temperature reaches 90–100°C (this usually takes about 3 minutes). The deployment is advanced to the 3-cm mark and ablation continues until the temperature reaches 90–100°C. The prongs are sequentially advanced at 1-cm intervals until they reaches the 5-cm mark (**FIGURE 6**). During each advancement, the array temperature must reach 90–100°C. In general, the duration of the last two ablations should be at least 7 minutes at 90–100°C. Aggressive ablation is vital for this form of therapy.

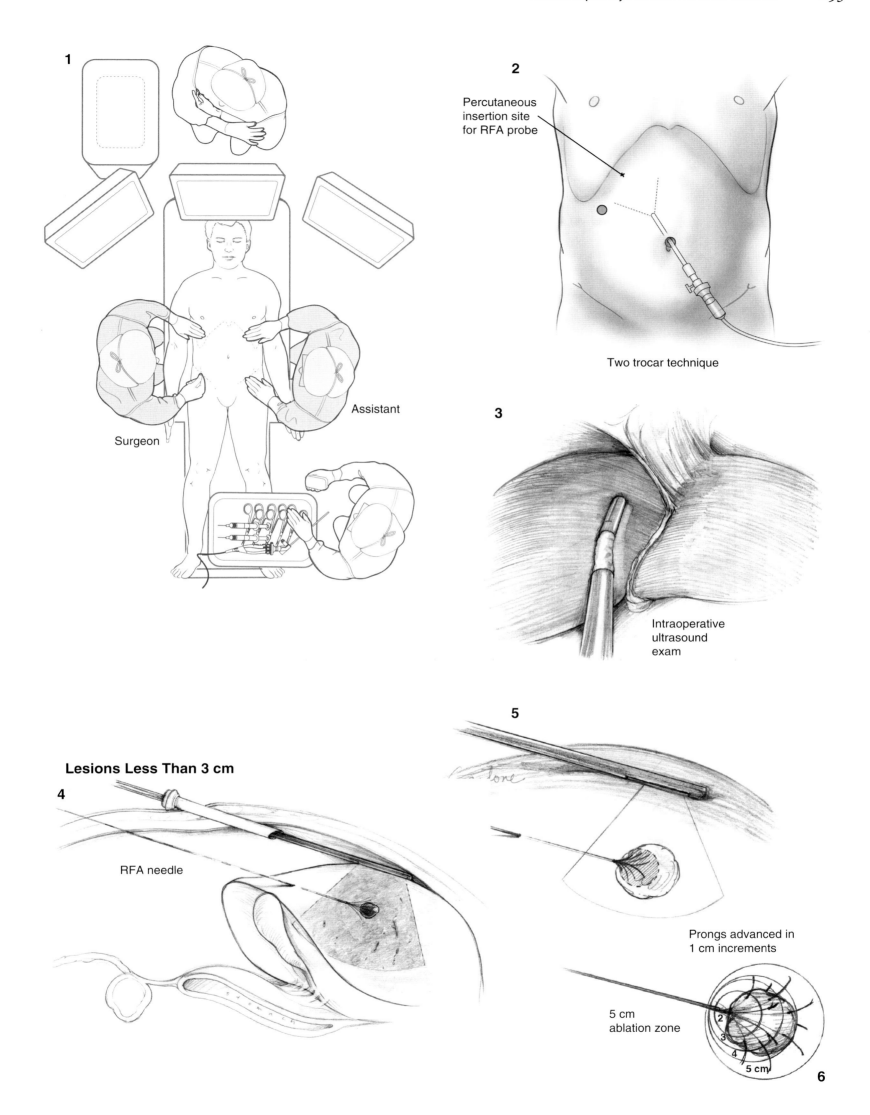

1

Surgeon

Assistant

2

Percutaneous
insertion site
for RFA probe

Two trocar technique

3

Intraoperative
ultrasound
exam

Lesions Less Than 3 cm

4

RFA needle

5

6

Prongs advanced in
1 cm increments

5 cm
ablation zone

5 cm

RFA Planning and Ablation for Lesions Greater Than 3 cm (Greater Than a 5-cm Ablation Zone) A 1-cm ablation of surrounding normal tissue is needed (**FIGURE 7**). Therefore, for a neoplasm larger than 3 cm, staged multiple insertions of the RFA probe are needed to allow an overlapping ablation zone larger than 5 cm. A pre-ablation strategy is needed, because after each ablation the border of the neoplasm is obscured, making ultrasound reimaging of the lesion inaccurate.

The way to plan for a staged deployment is to imagine that the spherical tumor is within a square box. This box should include the tumor and 1 cm of surrounding normal tissue. The location of the imaginary box is measured from the site where the RFA probe enters the hepatic surface. Six spherical ablation sites are staged, correlating to the six sides of the box. Each RFA probe insertion can coagulate a spherical zone of up to 5 cm. Sequential overlapping ablations will allow both the center and the periphery of the tumor to be fully ablated (**FIGURE 8**).

The array is first placed at the posterior interface between the neoplasm and the normal liver parenchyma. The array is deployed and confirmed by biplanar view on the ultrasound. The same sequential advancement of the prongs is used as for neoplasms less than 3 cm, resulting in a 5-cm ablated area. The needle is then retracted and repositioned anteriorly at a 2-cm interval, and the anterior zone is ablated. Four subsequent ablations are done in a clockwise direction at 12, 3, 6, 9 o'clock positions about 2 to 3 cm apart (**FIGURE 9**). Occasionally, an additional (seventh) ablation in the center of the neoplasm may be needed if the neoplasm is large. These will provide a good overlapping ablation, with 1 cm of surrounding normal liver tissue ablated.

It is also important to be familiar with the RF generator, especially in doing overlapping ablation. Within a recently ablated area, the array will sense high temperature. It is important to switch off sensing of this array so that the generator will continue to produce adequate temperature to other arrays.

Needle Tract Ablation To avoid neoplastic cell seeding and to ensure hemostasis, the needle tracts are cauterized while withdrawing the RFA needle under ultrasound visualization (**FIGURE 9**). After inspection for bleeding, the pneumoperitoneum is released and the trocar is removed under direct vision.

POSTOPERATIVE CARE Laparoscopic RFA is well tolerated by most patients. Patients with large-volume RFA may have more postoperative discomfort and low-grade fever. In general, patients can be cared for on the regular surgical floor unless otherwise indicated. The nasogastric tube can be removed the same day, and sips of liquid can be initiated as tolerated. Patients are encouraged to ambulate and use respiratory spirometry as early as possible to prevent DVT and atelectasis.

The overall perioperative mortality should be less than 0.5%, and morbidity less than 5%. The patients usually stay in the hospital for 1 or 2 days. A post-RFA CT scan with IV contrast is obtained to serve as a baseline before discharge. Follow-up CT scans at 3-month intervals are essential to detect recurrent or new lesions that typically occur within the first 18 months after RFA. ■

7   Lesions Greater Than 3 cm

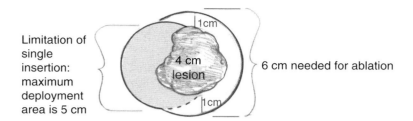

Limitation of single insertion: maximum deployment area is 5 cm

6 cm needed for ablation

8 Visualization of the spherical tumor within a square box

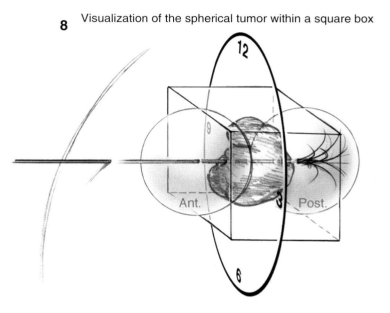

Multiple insertions of the RFA probe

9

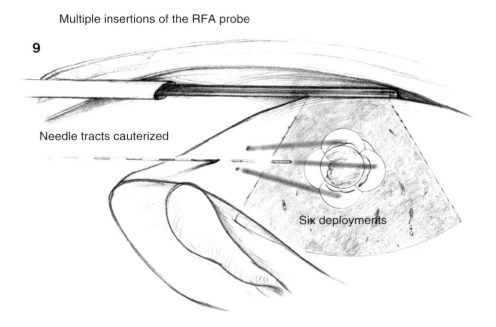

Needle tracts cauterized

Six deployments

INDICATIONS Laparoscopic liver resection is usually performed to remove a cyst or a tumor. It is recommended that initial experience in liver resection be gained with small peripheral lesions, hepatic cysts, liver biopsies, and the use of radiofrequency ablation. Facility with laparoscopic ultrasonography is imperative. As technical expertise grows, most resections that can be performed using open techniques can be approached laparoscopically. Many patients with liver masses are cirrhotic; therefore, evaluation for portal hypertension and careful patient selection is required. For cancers, oncologic principles must be maintained.

PREOPERATIVE PREPARATION Tumors are preoperatively studied to establish resectability using triphasic abdominal and pelvic computed tomography (CT) scans or contrast-enhanced magnetic resonance imaging (MRI). The boundaries of the tumor are established with respect to Couinaud segments to develop an operative strategy. If intraoperative localization of the lesion is to be performed using ultrasound, a preoperative ultrasound should be obtained to ensure that the lesion is visible sonographically.

Laparoscopic liver resections are challenging cases dependent on complex equipment. Rapid performance of certain tasks may be required. Therefore it is recommended that a dedicated operative team be present throughout the case, a team knowledgeable in all aspects of the surgery and the equipment.

Patients should be evaluated with appropriate cardiovascular and pulmonary screening to identify individuals with excessive surgical risk. At minimum, two units of packed red blood cells are typed and cross-matched in preparation for the surgery.

ANESTHESIA General anesthesia with endotracheal intubation is required for laparoscopic liver surgery. Complete neuromuscular blockade is necessary. Intravenous antibiotics with broad coverage (including *Enterococcus*) are given prior to skin incision. To minimize the risk of deep vein thrombosis, compression stockings and sequential compression devices must be in place and working before the induction of anesthesia. The systolic blood pressure should be maintained at 90 to 120 mm Hg. A central line should be placed to enable monitoring and adjustment of the central venous pressure to between 3 and 5 mm Hg to minimize bleeding from hepatic veins.

POSITIONING AND OPERATIVE PREPARATION The patient is placed in the supine position to permit safe induction of anesthesia and line placement. An operating table that allows the surgeon to stand in between the patient's legs is often advantageous (**FIGURE 1**). Adequate access for rapid large-volume resuscitation is assured with at least two large-bore (≤18 gauge) infusion lines. An orogastric tube and a Foley catheter are placed after induction. If the tumor is in the posterior right lobe, the patient may be placed in the left lateral decubitus (right side up) position; otherwise, the supine, split-leg position is maintained. The entire abdomen of the patient, from the nipples to the pubis, is shaved and sterilely prepped. An open hepatic surgery setup with vascular clamps and suctioning equipment should be in the room, open, and ready for use if urgently needed. Endoscopic Satinsky clamps and intracorporeal bulldogs must be available in case of bleeding. Tissue sealants or other hemostatic agents should be available.

During the conduct of the operation, a 30-degree angled scope provides the most versatile image. Because few field changes are necessary, a pneumatic camera holder can be used to provide a stable image. The table can be maintained in a level position or in reverse Trendelenburg position to allow gravity to retract the viscera downward. If air embolism is suspected, the patient should be placed in steep reverse Trendelenburg position with the right side up to trap air in the right ventricle, where it can be evacuated with a central line.

PORT PLACEMENT For patients with portal hypertension, great care must be taken to avoid injury to a patent umbilical vein. If present, a recanalized umbilical vein is usually evident on preoperative CT, MRI, or ultrasound studies. This structure can be avoided by placing ports inferior to the umbilicus or, if superiorly, lateral to the linea alba. In cirrhotic patients care must also be taken to avoid injuring an enlarged spleen.

Hand-assisted surgery is used by many surgeons. It helps optimize exposure, allows for tactile feedback, and provides a means for hemostatic pressure on the liver or vascular structures. In addition, the hand can be used to apply counterpressure on the liver while stapling to minimize the risk of tearing intrahepatic structures. The hand port can be placed in the midline, or laterally, on either side of the abdomen (typically to the right). Depending on its position, a hand-port incision can be extended to produce a full midline or subcostal incision if open surgery is required. In addition, the hand port provides a site for removal of resected tissue. Alternatively, liver tissue can be removed through a Pfannenstiel incision. The downsides of the hand port are that the hand can get in the way and that it requires a 6- to 8-cm incision.

The general principle of port placement requires the maintenance of adequate distance (ideally greater than 8 cm) between ports to allow for optimal triangulation and minimal instrument interference. For accurate positioning, secondary ports should be placed after insufflation. Subcostal ports should be placed at least 2 to 4 cm inferior to the costal margin to allow for unencumbered passage of staplers under the ribs. Subcostal ports placed in an arc (as allowed) facilitate conversion to an open subcostal incision if required. Retractor ports should not be placed too far posterolaterally, as leverage will be lost. Articulating, fan, or sheathed liver retractors can be used and affixed to the table using a retractor system.

RIGHT LOBE LESIONS There are two common approaches: (1) the traditional approach, with full inflow and outflow control, and (2) treating right lobe resection as a large "wedge" resection, with minimal vascular dissection. In the traditional approach to a right hepatic lobectomy, which is based on segmental anatomy, the inflow and outflow vessels are divided prior to dividing the lobe. As such, the resection is performed at the border between the right and left lobes (a line made clear by ischemic demarcation). Recently, a simpler, alternative approach has been developed where the lobectomy is treated as a large wedge resection and the hepatic vessels are dealt with intraparenchymally as they are encountered. The traditional approach has the advantage of having secure vascular control of the lobe during the parenchymal division, but risks bleeding or damage to hilar and retrohepatic structures during their dissection.

Port Placement

Hand Assisted The operation begins with the incision for the hand port. By placing the hand port first, the abdomen is entered under direct visualization, minimizing potential injury to the viscera and allowing for lysis of adhesions. The hand port incision is typically placed in the right upper quadrant (RUQ) or in the midline. In the RUQ, it is typically centered on the right midclavicular line to the right of the midline and superior to the umbilicus. If placed superolaterally, it can be oriented obliquely like a standard subcostal incision. The RUQ position is preferred because it allows for greater mobility of the hand with minimal interference with instruments and the camera. In addition, it allows for work in the far lateral RUQ without extreme dorsiflexion of the wrist. Alternatively, the hand port can be placed to the left of the midline for insertion of the right hand. This strategy will leave the left hand for primary instrument handling, which some surgeons find less desirable.

After the hand port device is in place, a 12-mm trocar is inserted through the hand port for insufflation and visualization of the abdomen. Once insufflated to 15 mm Hg, a 10-mm 30-degree scope is placed for direct visualization of subsequent port placement (**FIGURE 2**). The hand can also be used for tactile guidance during primary port placement by acting as a barrier to protect the underlying viscera.

With the hand port placed laterally in the RUQ, two 12-mm ports and one 5-mm retractor/working port are placed. Initially, the two midline 12-mm ports are placed: a camera port is placed through the umbilicus (or periumbilically) and a working port is placed 6 to 10 cm inferior to the xiphoid process, just right of the falciform ligament. Last, a 12-mm retractor/working port is placed subcostally in the left upper quadrant, in the midclavicular line. Additional 12-mm and 5-mm ports are placed as needed. The primary surgeon stands between the patient's legs with the left hand inserted through the hand port. The assistant is on the patient's left (**FIGURE 3**).

Totally Laparoscopic The operation is begun with insufflation of the abdomen to 15 mm Hg using a Veress needle or the Hasson technique. A 12-mm umbilical (or periumbilical) port is placed. In cirrhotic patients, direct cannulation of the umbilicus should be avoided. Three working ports are placed in a transverse arc across the upper abdomen. This includes a 12-mm right subcostal working port placed in the right midclavicular line, a 12-mm working port placed in the midline just to the right of the falciform ligament 8 to 10 cm inferior to the xiphoid process, and a 12-mm left subcostal working/retraction port placed in the left midclavicular line. The primary surgeon stands between the patient's legs. The assistant is on the patient's left (**FIGURE 4**).

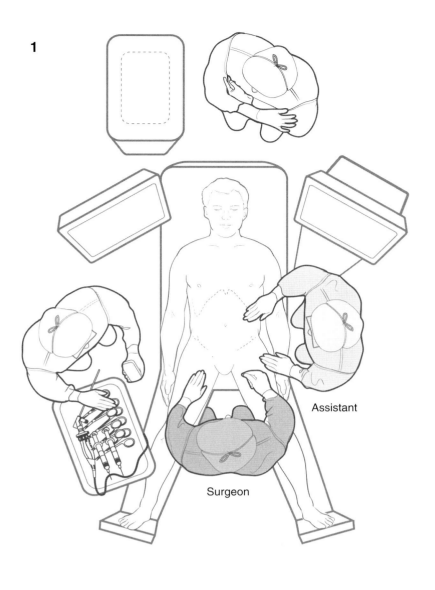

1

Assistant

Surgeon

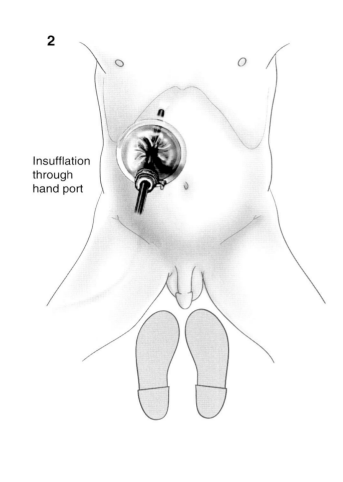

2

Insufflation
through
hand port

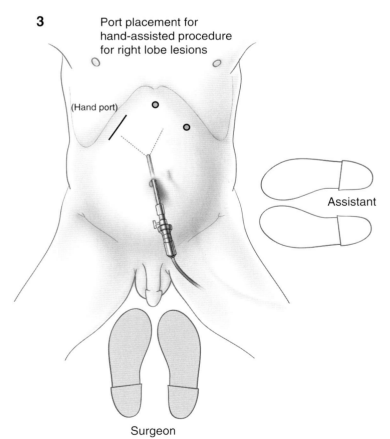

3 Port placement for
hand-assisted procedure
for right lobe lesions

(Hand port)

Assistant

Surgeon

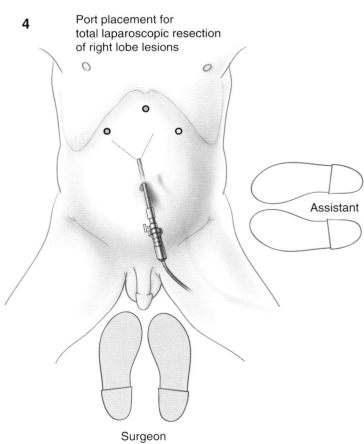

4 Port placement for
total laparoscopic resection
of right lobe lesions

Assistant

Surgeon

DETAILS OF THE PROCEDURE

Vascular Control After an abdominal survey, a meticulous ultrasonic evaluation of the liver is performed. Ultrasound is used to define the boundaries of the lesion in question, to rule out additional hepatic lesions, and to establish the locations of the major portal pedicles and hepatic veins. The falciform ligament is divided and the round ligament (with its umbilical vein) is stapled with a vascular load of the endoscopic stapler (**FIGURE 5**). The gastrohepatic ligament is divided to provide access to the lesser sac. Care must be taken to avoid injury to a possible replaced or accessory left hepatic artery. The remnant of the round ligament can be grasped by the assistant to elevate the liver during exposure of the porta hepatis (**FIGURE 6**). Once isolated, the porta hepatis is encircled with an umbilical tape, a feeding tube, or a vessel loop (**FIGURE 7**). At this point a Pringle maneuver can be performed if necessary. This can be accomplished laparoscopically using the Rummel tourniquet technique on an umbilical tape or a vessel loop (**FIGURE 8**). An endo-Satinsky clamp or endo-bulldogs can also be used for the Pringle maneuver.

Right Lobe Lesion
5   (Right Lobectomy)

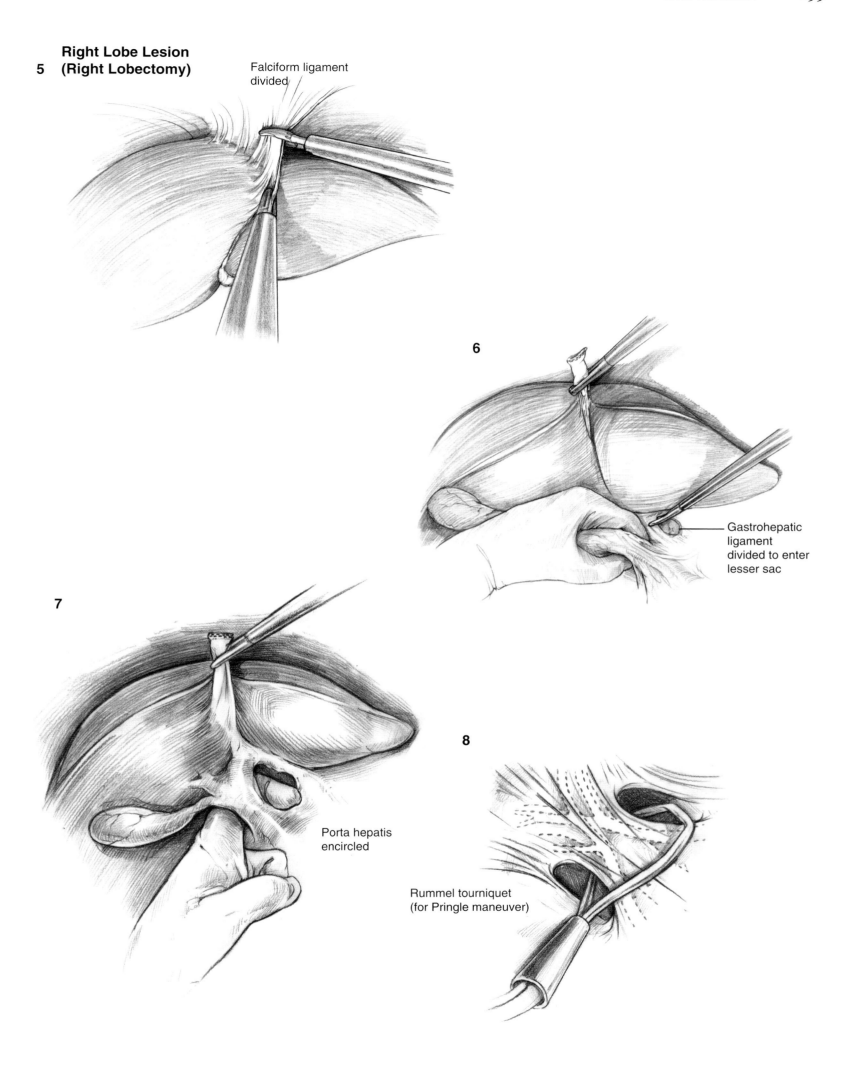

Falciform ligament
divided

6

Gastrohepatic
ligament
divided to enter
lesser sac

7

Porta hepatis
encircled

8

Rummel tourniquet
(for Pringle maneuver)

Vascular Control The lateral right lobe is mobilized by dividing the right triangular ligament (**FIGURE 9**). The vena cava is exposed by carefully dissecting the bare area of the liver off the diaphragm.

For the traditional approach to the right hepatectomy, a cholecystectomy is first performed. For the large wedge resection approach, it may not be needed. A cholangiogram can delineate ductal anatomy (**FIGURE 10A**). The right hepatic duct can be ligated and divided at this time. Next, the right hepatic artery is exposed (a process often made easier by a previous division of the right bile duct) and is divided using clips, ties, or a vascular Endo GIA stapler. The right portal vein is freed (from a lateral approach), ligated, and divided, preferably using the endoscopic stapler with a vascular load. Vascular stapler. Care must be taken to not tear caudate portal vein branches (**FIGURE 10B**).

There are three possible approaches to control of the right hepatic vein. In the traditional inferolateral approach, the vein is visualized superiorly and from the right as it enters the inferior vena cava. To expose the vein after the liver is mobilized from the right, the caval ligament is divided, and the short hepatic veins are ligated and divided.

The second approach is intraparenchymal division of the vein as it is encountered during the parenchymal dissection (see Figures 15 and 16). The benefit of this approach is that the risk of injuring the vein while freeing it in the extrahepatic space is eliminated, and it is safer with respect to the integrity of the middle and left hepatic veins. This is the approach employed in the "large wedge resection" technique, where there is minimal dissection.

Tunnel Technique A third approach is the tunnel technique. In this approach, the right hepatic vein is exposed inferiorly, from beneath the liver, by creating a tunnel along the vena cava. Dissecting from inferior to superior along the inferior vena cava, the short hepatic veins are divided between clips, taken with an ultrasonic dissector, or using a bladed bipolar cautery (a stapler may be needed for a large accessory right hepatic vein) (**FIGURE 11**). The development of this retrohepatic tunnel eventually exposes the right hepatic vein at its insertion and allows the vein to be stapled with an endoscopic stapler with a vascular load. (**FIGURE 12**). The disadvantage of this technique is that there is risk of having inadequate exposure if a venous injury should occur.

9

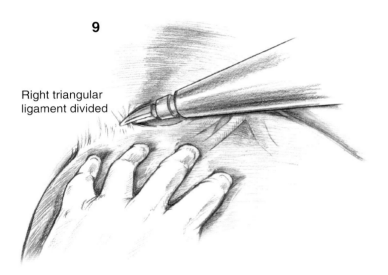

Right triangular ligament divided

10a

10b

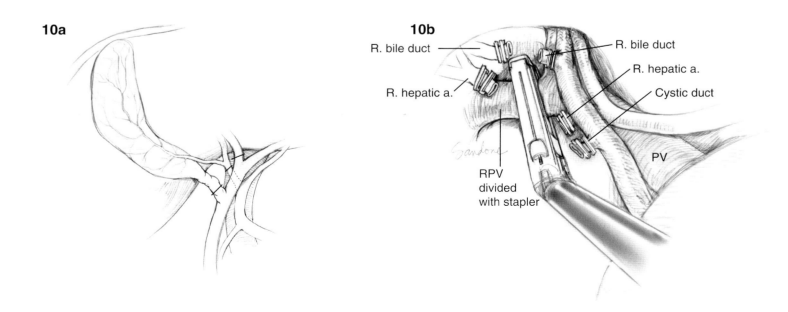

R. bile duct

R. hepatic a.

R. bile duct

R. hepatic a.

Cystic duct

PV

RPV divided with stapler

Tunnel Technique

11

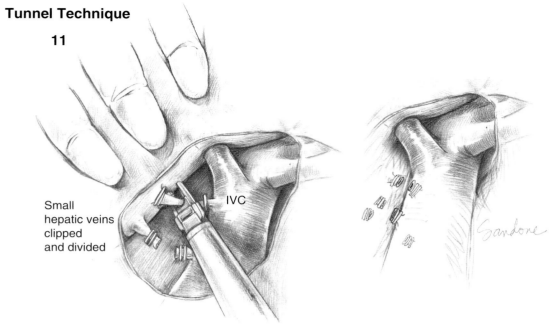

Small
hepatic veins
clipped
and divided

IVC

12

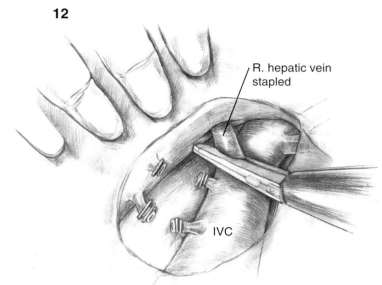

R. hepatic vein
stapled

IVC

Parenchymal Dissection

General Principles If the hand-assisted approach is used, the hand can be used to apply gentle hemostatic pressure during dissection (a significant advantage). An endo-Satinsky clamp and endo-bulldog clamps should be available to aid with hemostasis. If necessary, a Pringle maneuver may be employed to reduce bleeding. If persistent oozing occurs, intraabdominal pressure can be increased (up to 20 mm Hg) to help decrease blood loss.

If the vena cava has been freed with the tunnel technique, an umbilical tape or a drain can be placed beneath the hepatic resection plane for upward traction away from the vena cava. After the lateral attachments of the right lobe have been divided the lobe is mobile and the dissection plane can be moved into optimal position with respect to the ports and the camera.

If pre-resection vascular inflow control has been obtained, the line of demarcation is marked using standard cautery or an argon beam coagulator. For the large wedge resection approach, ultrasound is used to establish the perimeter of the intended resection. This boundary is marked with the cautery. A wide margin is maintained for malignant tumors (at least 1 cm) (**FIGURE 13**).

Dissection Technique Glisson capsule is incised, as is 2 to 3 cm of superficial hepatic parenchyma, using electrocautery, an ultrasonic dissector, or saline-enhanced cautery (**FIGURE 14**). The superficial parenchyma is generally devoid of major structures. Transection of the deeper parenchyma, which contains major hepatic veins and portal triads, can be accomplished in two ways: (1) after the superficial dissection, repeated gross firings of the endoscopic stapler through the tissue can be used to divide the parenchyma. This is referred to as the "gross stapling technique". Alternatively, a more controlled resection can be performed by careful, layered dissection with explicit visualization and dissection of the portal pedicles and hepatic veins as they are encountered; this is referred to as the "visualized dissection technique."

For the "gross stapling technique," the parenchymal division is performed entirely by repeatedly inserting and firing the stapler across the hepatic tissue without identifying particular structures. The stapler must be inserted gently to avoid injury to portal pedicles and hepatic veins. The stapler crushes the parenchyma as it staples and divides hepatic structures. A shorter segment of tissue is incised than is stapled, decreasing the risk of bleeding from incompletely stapled blood vessels. A variety of stapler sizes can be employed; however, the articulating 60-mm stapler with medium-small loads is preferred**.** Instead of directly inserting the thin blade of the stapler into the parenchyma, a tract for the stapler can be created by preinserting a blunt instrument. The hand can be of great assistance in guiding the stapler and in providing gentle countertraction to the liver to minimize stapler-induced shear forces. Greater care is required when stapling across cirrhotic or steatotic livers.

For the "visualized dissection technique," after the superficial layer of the liver is transected, a combination of approaches is used to divide the remaining parenchyma, portal pedicles, and hepatic veins. Several instruments are available for dissection, including standard cautery, saline-enhanced radiofrequency cautery, water jet dissection, radiofrequency dissection, or ultrasonic dissection. Smaller pedicles and veins (<5 mm) can be divided using the ultrasonic dissector or bladed bipolar cautery device. Larger bile ducts may be more prone to leakage if not carefully sealed. Clips can be used, but should be employed with caution as they may interfere with stapling and can be easily dislodged. For larger portal pedicles and hepatic veins, a 30-mm endoscopic stapler with vascular load is used. Similarly, the middle hepatic vein tributaries (V5 and V8), which cross Cantle line from segments 5 and 8, are divided with the vascular stapler (**FIGURE 15**). The right lobectomy dissection is usually carried to the immediate right of the middle hepatic vein. The hand can provide great assistance in maintaining gentle counterpressure on the liver while placing the stapler to avoid tearing of delicate structures.

Typically, the right hepatic vein is ligated and divided as it is encountered at the end of the parenchymal dissection using an endoscopic stapler with vascular load; however, as discussed previously, delaying this step avoids the risks associated with dissecting out the vein (**FIGURE 16**).

13

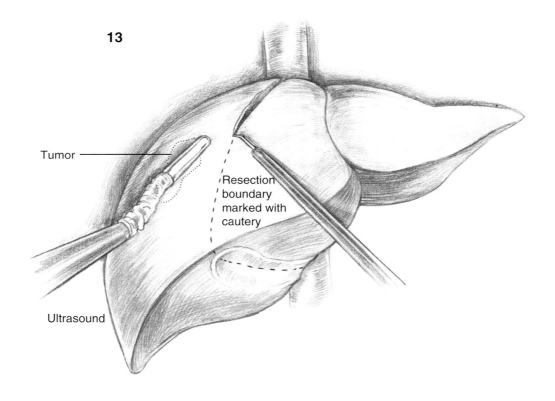

Tumor

Resection boundary marked with cautery

Ultrasound

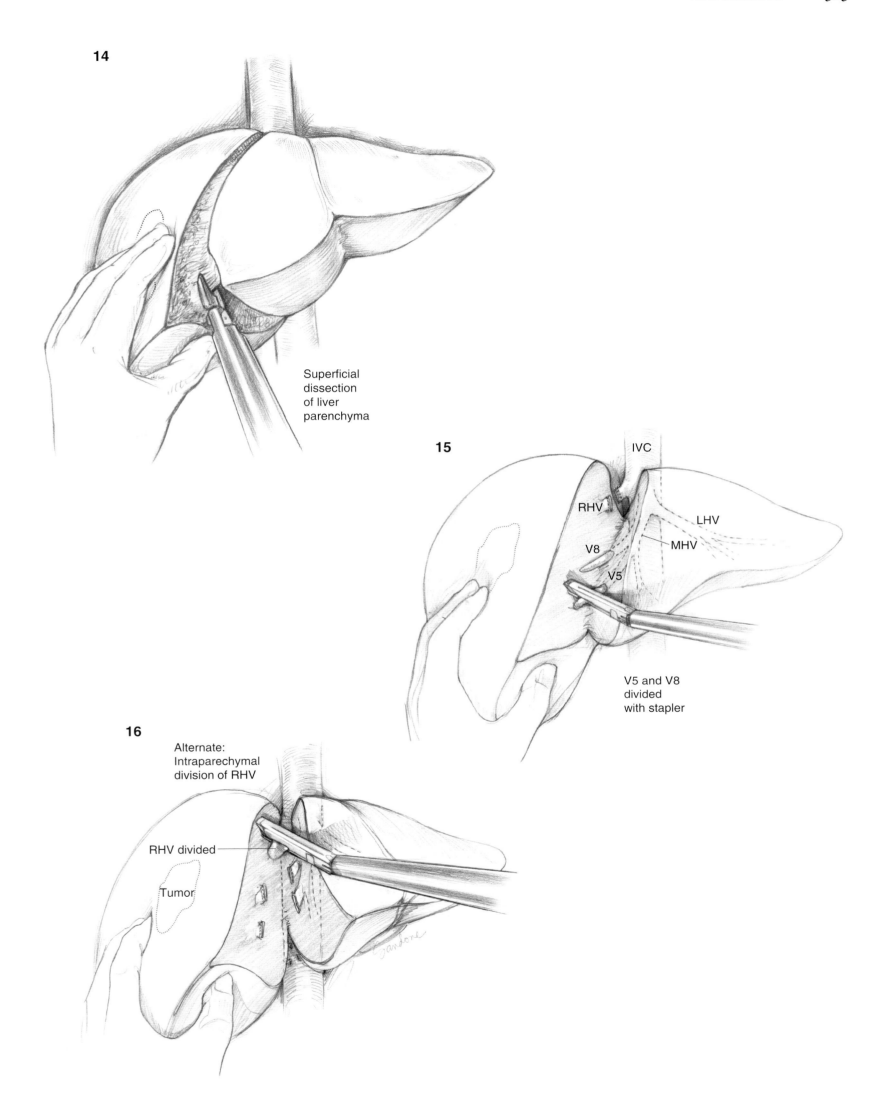

14

Superficial
dissection
of liver
parenchyma

15

IVC

RHV

LHV

V8

MHV

V5

V5 and V8
divided
with stapler

16

Alternate:
Intraparechymal
division of RHV

RHV divided

Tumor

Hemostasis and Biliostasis Significant parenchymal bleeding is controlled by employing several, often complementary, techniques. If hand assisted, the hand can be used to provide direct pressure. A temporary Pringle maneuver may be applied. One should not be reluctant to open (or convert to hand assisted) if the situation demands it for vascular control or for oncologic integrity. Standard cautery, bipolar cautery, or saline-assisted cautery can be used for smaller vessels. Hemostatic sealants, in combination with manual compression, can successfully control small bleeders (**FIGURE 17**). These modalities can be augmented by sheets of hemostatic material (with or without thrombin). The argon beam can be very useful for hemostasis, but it will not achieve biliostasis. Care must be taken to avoid insufflation of argon gas into a defect in a major hepatic vein as it may produce a gas embolism. For bleeding from medium sized vessels (up to 7 mm): clips, standard or bladed bipolar cautery, or the articulating vascular stapler can be useful. For larger vessels, the stapler is most effective. An 0-silk suture that is either clipped or tied at the distal end to allow fast application, can be used to rapidly suture-ligate bleeders. In addition, intraabdominal pressure can be temporally increased to 18 to 20 mm Hg to decrease bleeding while hemostasis is attained.

Biliostasis can also be attained by multiple techniques with variable success. Human fibrin biomatrix tissue sealants or synthetic products can coat the open surface of the liver. Areas of bile leakage can be cauterized, treated with saline-enhanced radiofrequency energy, clipped, or sutured. A drain should be placed routinely through a 5-mm port site and removed after biliostasis is assured.

Specimen Recovery The hand or an endo-bag is used to retrieve the resected specimen (**FIGURE 18**). For pure laparoscopic cases, a Pfannenstiel incision may be needed for liver tumor extraction.

Closure Once hemostasis is secured, intraabdominal pressure is reduced to 5 mm Hg for 5 minutes to expose previously compressed venous bleeders and bile leaks. The hand-port incision is closed with simple interrupted or running 1-0 suture. Before the 12-mm ports are removed, the camera can be reinserted to inspect the incision and trocar sites during removal. The gas is vented. Trocar sites larger than 10 mm are closed if at the level of the umbilicus or below.

Skin incisions are closed with absorbable subcuticular sutures. Long-acting subcutaneous local anesthesia can be applied.

LEFT LOBE LESIONS
General Principles As most of the principles and techniques described for the right side can be applied to left hepatic lobectomies, this description is limited to significant differences. Once the lesser sac is opened, the porta hepatis can be encircled with an umbilical tape or a vessel loop for a Pringle maneuver. A traditional resection can be performed with dissection, ligation, and division of the left hepatic artery and left portal vein prior to parenchymal dissection. As with the right lobe procedure, care must be taken not to accidentally tear caudate branches during dissection of the left portal vein. Typically, to avoid risk of injury to the hepatic veins, the left (and middle) hepatic vein is divided at the end of the parenchymal dissection.

The caudate lobe also can be resected laparoscopically. To accomplish this, first the left lateral segment is mobilized by dividing the left vena caval ligament. Then, the caudate caval branches are divided. The caudate is then further mobilized. Finally, after the portal branches are ligated and divided, the parenchyma is transected.

In this section a nonanatomic left lateral segmentectomy is illustrated.

Port Placement
Hand Assisted For left lateral segmentectomy, the hand-port incision can be placed in the midline or laterally to the right. If placed in the midline, the incision runs vertically beginning at the inferior aspect of the umbilicus. If placed laterally, it is located to the right of the midline and superior to the umbilicus, typically centered on the right midclavicular line. It can also be placed more superiorly and oriented obliquely like a subcostal incision. The lateral location is preferred, as it allows for greater mobility of the hand without requiring extreme dorsiflexion of the wrist. Alternatively, some surgeons place the hand port to the left of the midline and insert the right hand, which allows for unencumbered leftward retraction of the liver, but leaves the left hand for primary instrument handling. If open access to the porta hepatis and the parenchyma is needed, the hand port incision can also be placed superiorly in the midline.

Three ports are placed. First, a 12-mm camera port is positioned a few centimeters to the right of the umbilicus. Second, a 12-mm working port is placed several centimeters to the left of the falciform ligament in the upper midline, 6 to 10 cm inferior to the xiphoid. A 5-mm retractor port is placed in the subcostal left midclavicular line. The primary surgeon stands between the patient's split legs or to the right of the patient. The left hand is inserted through the hand port, and the primary surgeon controls the liver with this hand. The assistant stands to the right of the patient or, for some teams, to the patient's left (**FIGURE 19**).

Totally Laparoscopic The camera port is placed 2 to 4 cm to the right of the umbilicus. For the left lobectomy, 3 working/retractor ports are placed in an arc across the upper abdomen. From right to left, a 12-mm working port is placed in the subcostal right midclavicular line, another 12-mm working port is placed in the upper midline (6–10 cm below the xiphoid process), and a third 12-mm working port is placed in the subcostal left midclavicular line. The primary surgeon stands between the patient's legs or to the right of the, patient and the assistant stands to the patient's right (**FIGURE 20**).

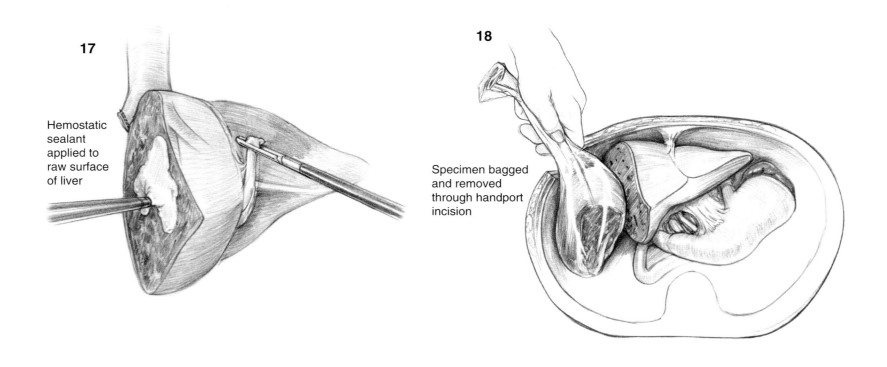

17 Hemostatic sealant applied to raw surface of liver

18 Specimen bagged and removed through handport incision

Left Lobe Lesion (Nonanatomic resection)

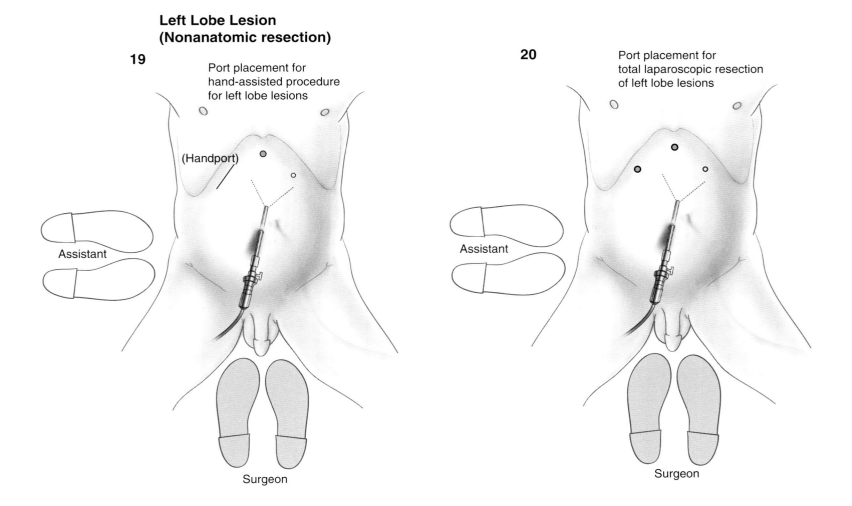

19 Port placement for hand-assisted procedure for left lobe lesions

(Handport)

Assistant

Surgeon

20 Port placement for total laparoscopic resection of left lobe lesions

Assistant

Surgeon

Details of the Procedure The falciform ligament is divided and the round ligament (with its umbilical vein) is stapled and used as a handle. The left lobe is mobilized by dividing the left triangular ligament. The gastrohepatic ligament is divided, as is a possible replaced, or accessory, left hepatic artery if present. Similar to the right lobectomy, the procedure can be approached as a large wedge resection without explicit inflow control, especially for the left lateral segmentectomy.

Using the parenchymal dissection techniques described earlier, small peripheral lesions are often amenable to wedge resection without establishing explicit inflow and outflow control. For a nonanatomic lateral segmentectomy, Glisson capsule is incised (**FIGURE 21**). Next, the superficial parenchymal layers are divided with the Harmonic scalpel (or other device) (**FIGURE 22**). The deep parenchyma, along with the larger portal pedicles and veins, are then divided using a stapler (**FIGURE 23**). After division, the raw surface may be sealed with fibrin glue (**FIGURE 24**).

POSTOPERATIVE CARE The orogastric tube is removed after extubation. Patient-controlled analgesia (PCA) is used postoperatively. For the first 12 hours postoperatively, supplemental analgesia may be needed if the patient cannot maintain adequate pain control using the PCA method. For major resections, patients may have difficulty metabolizing opiates and therefore may not tolerate standard doses of opiates. In this setting, careful dosing must be employed to avoid overdose. Ketorolac is a useful adjunct to opioid analgesia and may be administered. Nausea is treated aggressively. The Foley catheter is removed on postoperative day 1, and ambulation is encouraged. The hemoglobin and hematocrit are checked on postoperative day 1. Liver tests, including coagulation studies, and phosphorus levels are checked daily. The patient may begin on clear liquids on post op day 1 or 2 once the risk of ongoing bleeding has been eliminated. Subsequently, diet is advanced as tolerated. Early resumption of the activities of daily living is encouraged. Patients are counseled to avoid heavy lifting for at least 6 weeks. ■

21

Resection boundary
marked with cautery
under ultrasound guidance

Tumor

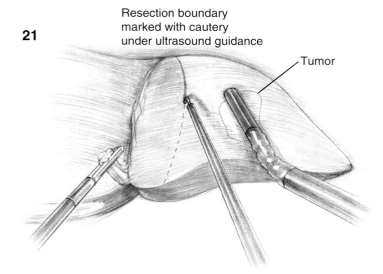

22

Tumor

Superficial
dissection
of liver
parenchyma

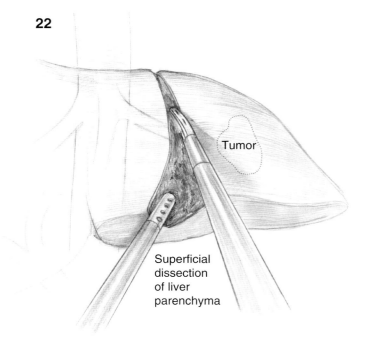

23

Tumor

Deep parenchyma
and vessels divided
using stapler

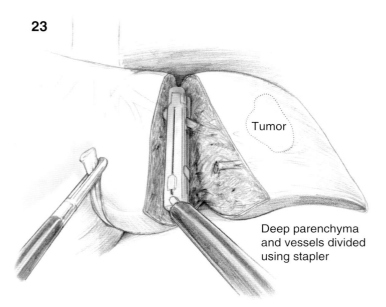

24

Hemostatic
sealant
applied to
raw surface
of liver

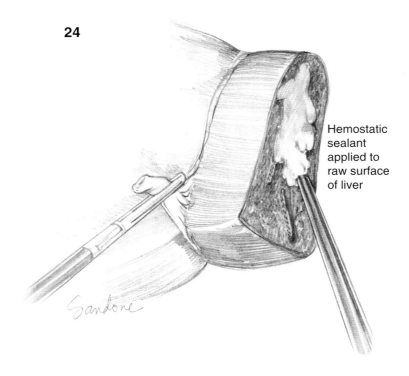

MANAGEMENT OF SIMPLE HEPATIC CYSTS

INDICATIONS Nonparasitic liver cysts are a frequently encountered entity for most surgeons. Although these are rarely large enough to warrant operation, most cases that require surgical intervention can be managed safely and effectively using standard laparoscopic techniques. These lesions are typically discovered incidentally on abdominal imaging performed for other indications. On occasion, symptoms related to stretch of the liver capsule can lead to complaints of epigastric or right upper quadrant pain. Other symptoms that might prompt workup and discovery of these lesions are related to compression of adjacent organs, particularly the stomach. Patients may complain of early satiety, bloating, or upper abdominal fullness. Hepatic cysts may become secondarily infected, but should be differentiated from hepatic abscess. Pain symptoms, especially if abrupt in onset, might indicate hemorrhage into the cyst cavity and require careful patient monitoring. Women are far more likely to present with symptomatic liver cysts. Most solitary, simple cysts can be managed conservatively; operative intervention is indicated for large (>8 cm) cysts with symptoms attributable to the hepatic cyst.

The differential diagnosis for solitary hepatic cysts includes solitary bile duct cyst, ciliated hepatic foregut cyst, hepatobiliary cystadenoma, cystadenocarcinoma, peribiliary cysts, mesothelial cyst, pancreatic pseudocyst, endometrial cyst, and metastatic carcinoma with cystic features. In the setting of a simple hepatic cyst, solitary bile duct cyst and hepatobiliary cystadenoma remain most likely. The vast majority of these lesions are benign; however, surgeons treating these patients must always send resected cyst wall for histologic evaluation to rule out malignant features. Cystadenocarcinoma is a potential risk, especially in the very large and long-standing cyst, or if there has been hemorrhage into the cyst cavity. If cystadenocarcinoma is identified on final pathologic analysis, formal, anatomic hepatic resection should be performed. The presence of septations on imaging is the best noninvasive method for differentiation of simple cysts from these other entities, unless multiple confluent cysts are present wherein adjacent cyst walls can mimic septations.

Echinococcal cysts and cysts in the setting of autosomal dominant polycystic liver disease (ADPLD) are unique clinical problems that require specific interventions beyond the scope of this chapter. It should be noted that the echinococcal cyst has unique imaging characteristics (septations and calcifications) that help differentiate it from simple cysts. Additionally, these patients should all have serum echinococcal titers sent. Extreme care must be taken in the operative management of these cysts, as anaphylaxis can result from cyst rupture into the peritoneal cavity. Cystic disease in ADPLD is typically associated with polycystic kidney disease. These lesions are best managed by combination cyst marsupialization and resection for symptoms. Liver transplantation may be the only therapeutic option in some of these patients.

ANESTHESIA General anesthesia with endotracheal intubation is required for laparoscopic liver surgery. Complete neuromuscular blockade is necessary. Intravenous antibiotics with broad coverage (including *Enterococcus*)

are given prior to skin incision. To minimize the risk of deep vein thrombosis, compression stockings and sequential compression devices must be in place and working before the induction of anesthesia.

Positioning and Port Placement The procedure is performed with the patient in supine position. The surgeon stands on the patient's left and the assistant stands to the right (**FIGURE 1**).

Port location for the laparoscopic approach to hepatic cysts is predicated on cyst location. For lesions located in the left liver, the camera can be placed similar to that for Nissen fundoplication, with triangulation of working ports centered around the camera port. Two 5-mm ports and one 11- or 12-mm port may be all that are required, though additional 5-mm ports can be placed as needed (**FIGURE 2**).

DETAILS OF THE PROCEDURE Whenever possible, cyst marsupialization must be performed, rather than fenestration. This means excising as much of the cyst wall on the capsule (or nonparenchymal) side of the liver as possible (**FIGURE 3**). Simply fenestrating the cyst wall ensures a high likelihood of cyst reepithelialization and recurrence. The cyst cavity should be thoroughly ablated whenever possible. Many authors advocate sclerosing the cavity, usually with concentrated ethanol solutions when an open approach is used. This cannot be accomplished laparoscopically; instead, fulguration with the argon beam coagulator is recommended. Again, the cyst wall must be sent for pathologic evaluation and complete anatomic resection performed at a later date if positive for malignancy.

Initial Approach: Mobilization and Drainage The degree of liver mobilization required depends on the location of the lesion both from a right/left perspective and whether the lesion has a substantial (>50% cyst wall) intrahepatic component. For cysts on the inferior edge of the liver, minimal mobilization is typically all that is required. For very large cysts and those positioned in difficult locations, portions of the left or right triangular ligament must be divided. Taking down the falciform/round ligament may serve a twofold purpose. First, it enables better visualization for work around the anteromedial portion of the left lobe. Second, the round ligament serves as an excellent handle with which to move the liver in the laparoscopic environment. When using this maneuver, the distal round ligament should be divided as near the abdominal wall peritoneum as possible to avoid a large remnant hanging down and obscuring the field.

Often the cyst may be adherent to neighboring organs. These adhesions can typically be taken down with gentle blunt dissection, and this may be done either before or after cyst decompression. The simple cyst should be decompressed with a long laparoscopic needle, such as that typically used to decompress a tense gallbladder. Several hundred milliliters of fluid may be aspirated to render the cavity dry. An alternate technique involves puncturing the cyst wall and advancing a suction/irrigator into the cyst, though there is greater chance for peritoneal leakage with this technique (**FIGURE 4**).

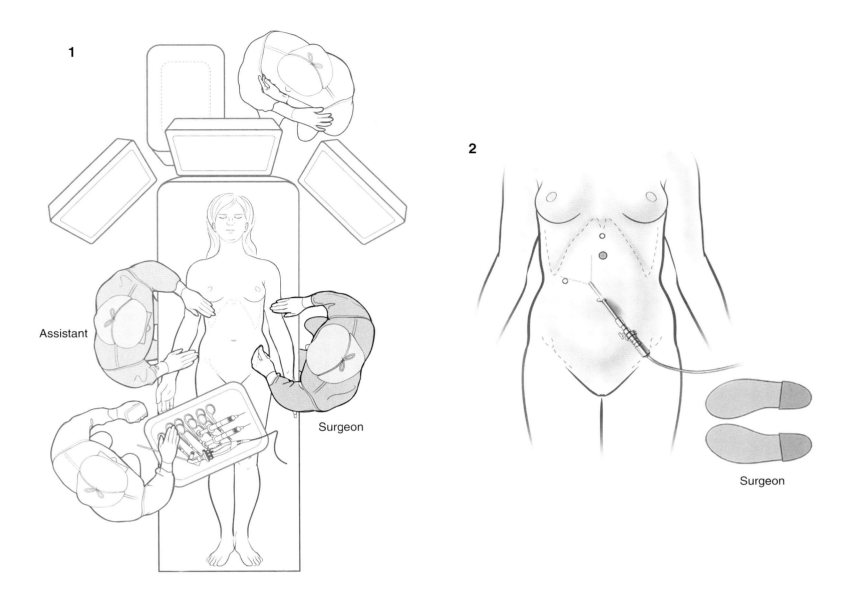

1

Assistant

Surgeon

2

Surgeon

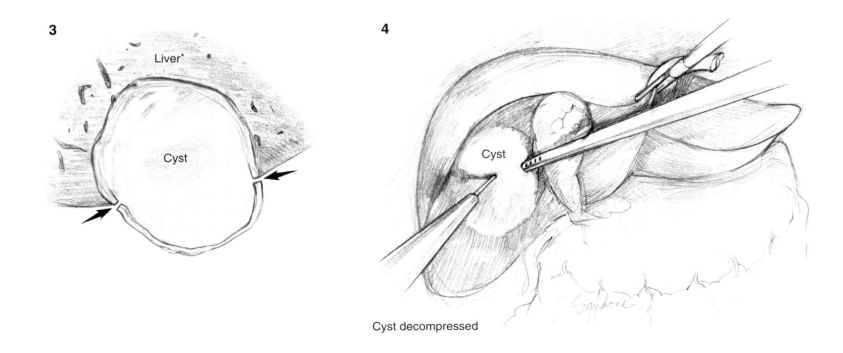

3

Liver

Cyst

4

Cyst

Cyst decompressed

Marsupialization of Cyst Wall Once the cyst has been decompressed, the wall is resected. It is important to resect as much of the wall as possible on the capsular side, right up to the parenchyma. Ultrasonic shears work well in this setting, with countertraction placed on the cyst wall with a grasper in the surgeon's nondominant hand (**FIGURE 5**). Other cutting/ coagulation devices can also be used, including monopolar endoshears or the LigaSure device (Covidien). If the cyst has a dominant intrahepatic component, some parenchymal transection may be required for adequate cyst unroofing. If this is the case, the use of an endoscopic linear stapler is recommended. This technique controls vessels and bile ducts encountered during significant parenchymal transection. As much of the cyst wall as can be resected safely is placed into a specimen bag and sent to pathology for permanent staining. If there is a high index of suspicion for malignancy, an intraoperative frozen section should be performed.

Managing the Cavity Ablating the cyst cavity is important to prevent leakage from the cyst wall and ascites formation. Typically, fulguration with an electrosurgical hook is a reliable technique (**FIGURE 6**). The cavity must be closely inspected for the presence of bile leakage in the setting of a biliary-based cyst or if a biliary radical has been disrupted during cyst wall excision. The presence of bile-stained or dark fluid in the aspirate will indicate the former. If a leak is identified, it should be managed by suture ligation with absorbable monofilament suture or clipping. Close inspection is also required to identify and biopsy any cyst wall irregularities.

An alternative strategy for controlling the cavity is to pack a pedicled omental flap into the defect. The flap is tacked to the liver capsule and the back wall of the cyst cavity with several interrupted absorbable sutures (**FIGURE 7**).

POSTOPERATIVE CARE Most patients require a short, 1- to 2-day hospitalization following laparoscopic management of hepatic cysts. A postoperative closed suction drain is not necessary. Follow-up can be routinely accomplished with ultrasound. If adequate cyst wall resection was performed, the likelihood of recurrence is low. ■

5

Cyst wall resected

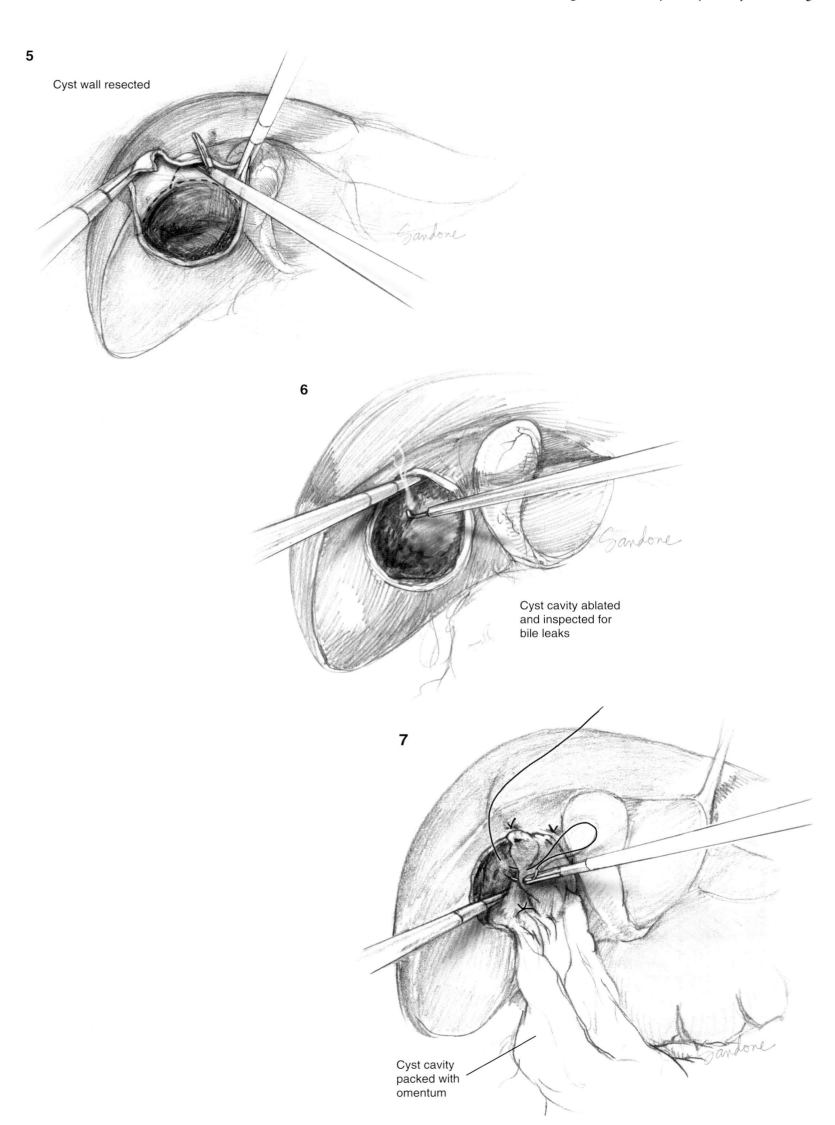

6

Cyst cavity ablated
and inspected for
bile leaks

7

Cyst cavity
packed with
omentum

INTRAGASTRIC SURGERY

INDICATIONS Intragastric surgery may be performed for the local resection of small submucosal tumors such as leiomyomas, as well as for control of bleeding in areas out of reach of a standard upper endoscope (or when upper endoscopy has failed). Intragastric surgery can also be used to create a communication between a pancreatic pseudocyst and the stomach (laparoscopic intragastric cyst-gastrostomy). The indications for each of these procedures are quite different.

Leiomyoma, Lipoma, and Other Small Gastric Tumors The indication for an intragastric approach to a submucosal tumor generally requires that the tumor be sufficiently small that a "shelling out" will not risk the chance of incomplete resection and tumor recurrence. Thus, this approach should only be used for lipomas or leiomyomas, and not GI stromal tumors. Generally leiomyomas are 1 cm or less in diameter and possess smooth muscle cells that are not c-Kit positive by fine-needle aspirate.

Early gastric cancers have generally been approached with endoscopic mucosal resection (EMR) using a flexible endoscope. However, intragastric surgery may be used if experience with EMR is limited but the lesion would otherwise be amenable to a local approach (confined to the mucosa by endoscopic ultrasonography [EUS], and <1.0 cm in diameter).

Pancreatic Pseudocyst Drainage Another indication for intragastric surgery is for drainage of a pancreatic pseudocyst. Although most pancreatic pseudocysts are asymptomatic and/or resolve spontaneously, large cysts may persist and cause symptoms of postprandial pain or gastric outlet obstruction. When a computed tomography (CT) scan shows a mature pseudocyst clearly adherent to the posterior gastric wall, laparoscopic intragastric cystogastrostomy may be indicated.

Intragastric Bleeding Most intragastric bleeding lesions (except gastric varices) can be controlled with endoscopic injection of epinephrin. Occasionally a lesion develops that cannot be adequately controlled with a flexible endoscope, especially those near the gastroesophageal (GE) junction, such as a Mallory-Weiss tear or a Dieulafoy lesion. These lesions may be approached with intragastric surgery for direct suture ligation of the bleeding site.

ANESTHESIA General anesthesia is a requirement. Intravenous antibiotics are administered.

POSITION For most intragastric surgery, the position used for laparoscopic fundoplication is the best. The patient is supine with the legs abducted on leg boards and the patient is placed in a steep reverse Trendelenburg position. The surgeon stands between the patient's legs (**FIGURE 1**).

OPERATIVE PREPARATION Before trocars are placed, an upper GI endoscopy is usually performed to confirm the location of the lesion and to distend the stomach for placement of the intragastric ports after laparoscopic access has been completed.

INCISION AND EXPOSURE For intragastric surgery, three laparoscopic ports and three intragastric ports are placed. The scope is placed through the umbilcus and the working ports are placed to the left and right, slightly cephalad to the camera. The surgeon's right hand uses a 10-mm port on the patient's left (**FIGURE 2**). Through the 5-mm port on the patient's right, an atraumatic locking grasper (bowel clamp) is placed across the pylorus or proximal jejunum (preferably) to keep the gastric insufflation confined to the stomach and duodenum. If the intragastric inflation is allowed to cause small bowel distension, there will be no working room for the eventual closure of the gastric ports.

The three gastric ports are placed in the epigastrium such that all three ports will enter the midbody of the stomach through the greater curvature (**FIGURE 3**). Five- or 10-mm trocars may be used for intragastric surgery. Generally a single large port (10- or 12-mm) is helpful for the passage of an endoscopic probe, a stapler, a clipper, or a suturing device. It is unnecessary to place a 10-mm trocar for the scope, as the intragastric region is adequately illuminated through a 5-mm scope.

The biggest challenge with intragastric surgery is finding a method for keeping the trocars in the stomach. In the past, trocars with balloons on their ends were designed for intragastric surgery. With low demand, these ports were taken out of production in the United States, but are still available in other countries. T-fasteners such as those used with laparoscopic jejunostomy or gastrostomy may be placed in the stomach and used to hold the stomach wall up so that conventional trocars can be placed in the stomach (**FIGURE 4**). Another method is to place three percutaneous endoscopic gastrostomy (PEG) tubes (28 French) and pass 5-mm trocars down each one of these tubes. This technique has the advantage that PEG-tube access to the stomach may be maintained for feeding or resuturing bleeding gastric lesions should rebleeding occur. The disadvantage of the PEG tube technique is the need to remove the PEG tubes transorally at the completion of the procedure or leave them until the gastrocutaneous tract matures. The technique using standard laparoscopic trocars with a radial dilating system, and T-fasteners to avoid slippage of the intragastric ports is depicted in this chapter.

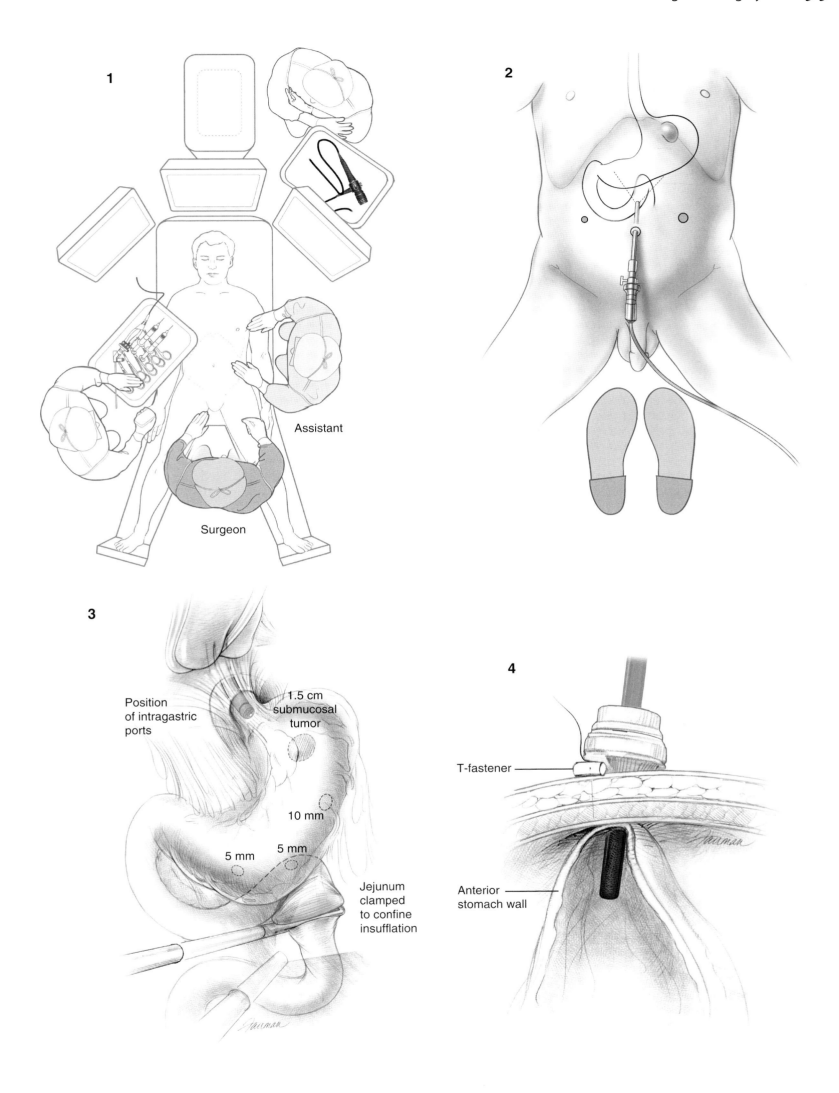

1

Assistant

Surgeon

2

3

Position
of intragastric
ports

1.5 cm
submucosal
tumor

10 mm

5 mm   5 mm

Jejunum
clamped
to confine
insufflation

4

T-fastener

Anterior
stomach wall

DETAILS OF THE PROCEDURE

Leiomyomas, Lipomas, and Early Gastric Cancer Resection of small submucosal tumors can be performed using an atraumatic grasper in the left hand and electrosurgical hook in the right hand. A 0.5- to 1.0-cm cuff of normal tissue around the lesion is marked with electrosurgical "tattooing", and, the submucosal plane is developed with electrosurgical dissection on the left side of the lesion (**FIGURE 5**). Elevating the mucosal flap with the left hand, the surgeon dissects with an electrosurgical hook, under the normal mucosa. The tumor is elevated en bloc with the overlying mucosa, shelling the tumor out of the submucosa with the electrosurgical hook (**FIGURE 6**). The tumor is placed in a specimen bag and either removed transgastrically

or pulled up the esophagus (**FIGURE 7**). Care must be taken not to attempt the removal of lesions of more than 12 to 13 mm in diameter through the esophagus, as the specimen bag may become stuck in the esophagus. The defect in the mucosa is closed with a running absorbable suture (**FIGURE 8**).

A mucosally based early gastric cancer measuring less than 1.0 cm can be removed with a local resection from an intragastric approach by the submucosal injection of saline to elevate it. The resection of the tumor, with scissors or electrosurgical hook, must ensure 1-cm margins circumferentially. The mucosal defect can be closed as described above. Frozen section should ensure that all margins, including the deep (submucosal) margin, are negative for tumor while the patient is still asleep.

Leomyoma, Lipoma, and Gastric Tumor Resection

5

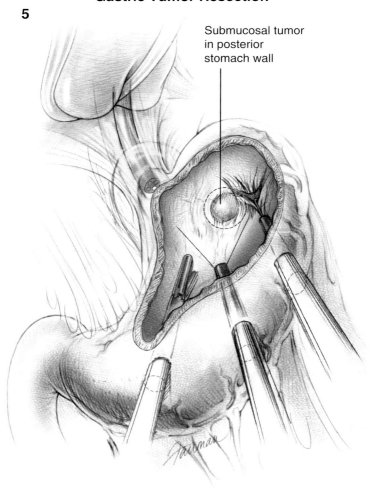

Submucosal tumor in posterior stomach wall

6

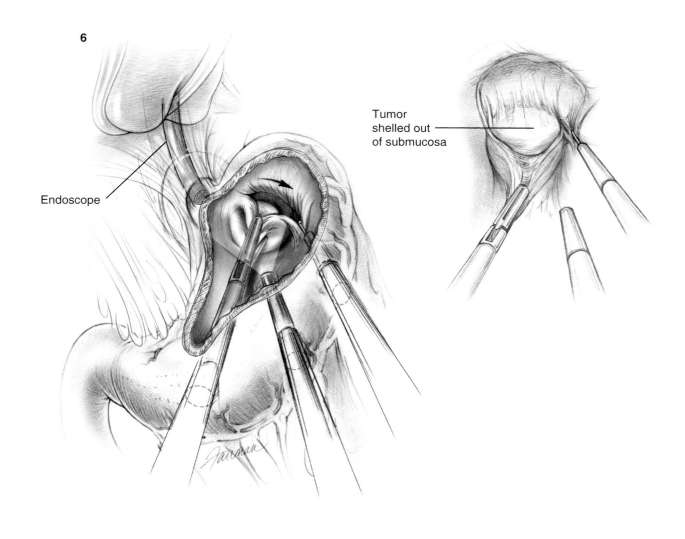

Endoscope

Tumor
shelled out
of submucosa

7

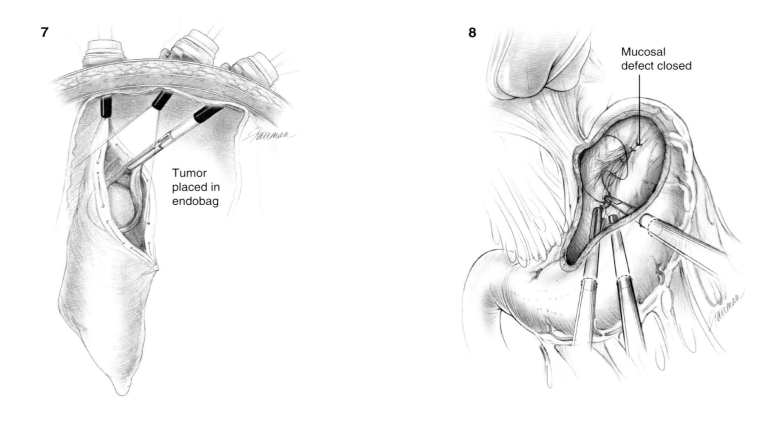

Tumor
placed in
endobag

8

Mucosal
defect closed

Pancreatic Pseudocyst Drainage The operative technique for drainage of a pancreatic pseudocyst is somewhat more complex. The pseudocyst is identified from its large bulge on the posterior wall of the stomach. If EUS has not been performed preoperatively, it is wise to perform intragastric ultrasonography with a laparoscopic ultrasound probe, before draining the pseudocyst, in order to demonstrate tight apposition of the stomach to the pseudocyst wall (**FIGURE 9**). Ultrasound must demonstrate freedom from gastric varices at the proposed site of cystogastrostomy. Gastric varices resulting from splenic vein thrombosis would create massive upper gastrointestinal hemorrhage if incised with an electrosurgical hook or ultrasonic scalpel. A preoperative CT scan can generally rule out the presence of gastric varices, but the surgeon must always be alert to the possibility of vigorous bleeding during this operation.

Three intragastric ports of the same size are placed in the same positions as for leiomyoma excision, described above. Before making a posterior gastrotomy, an aspirating needle is passed into the pseudocyst. The pseudocyst fluid is usually thin and clear or slightly dark, but is rarely cloudy in the absence of infection (**FIGURE 10**). A purulent-looking fluid should alert the surgeon to a pancreatic abscess and the need for external drainage.

A number of techniques have been described for creating the cyst gastrostomy. Although the electrosurgical hook has been the standard instrument to create this opening, ultrasonic shears can also be used with the blade open and the active component opposed to the back wall of the stomach, vibrating its way into the pancreatic pseudocyst. When pseudocyst fluid is seen escaping into the stomach, the jaws of the ultrasonic shears are closed and a larger cyst gastrostomy is made (**FIGURE 11**). It is desirable to take out a button of the posterior stomach so that the cyst wall can be sent for pathology; the opening is left wide enough so that it cannot collapse and reseal quickly. Althernatively, linear openings between the cyst and the stomach can be created using the endoscopic linear stapler. The length of the staple load will depend on the thickness of the stomach and cyst wall. Generally, a medium or thick tissue stapler of 45-mm length is chosen. If the thick tissue load is used, the left upper quadrant gastric cannula will need to be enlarged to 15 mm to admit the larger staple load. If possible, the cyst is opened widely enough that the scope can be placed into the cyst cavity and the cyst cavity can be irrigated.

Intragastric Bleeding For bleeding lesions (Dieulafoy ulcer or Mallory-Weiss tear) one or more figure-of-eight throws of a 2-0 absorbable suture can adequately control most bleeding lesions (**FIGURE 12**).

CLOSURE Upon completion of endogastric surgery, the trocars in the stomach are pulled directly out and the gastrotomies are closed with one or two interrupted sutures of 2-0 nonabsorbable material (**FIGURE 13**). Once all gastrotomies are closed, the stomach is inflated with air while the peritoneum is flooded with saline. Alternatively, the stomach may be filled with blue dye and each closure site tested to make sure there are no leaks. At this point, the clamp is removed from the proximal jejunum and the stomach and duodenum are emptied of gas and air. A nasogastric tube may be placed, if the stomach is unable to be decompressed. The laparoscopic ports are removed from the periumbilical region and the incisions closed.

POSTOPERATIVE CARE Postoperative care depends largely on the indication for the procedure. For an elective gastric resection of a leiomyoma, the patient may be started on liquids the next day and discharged. For more complex lesions such as the drainage of a pancreatic pseudocyst, a multiday hospitalization with a slow resumption of diet may be more appropriate. It is not routine to perform contrast radiographs on these patients before resuming a diet, as the trocar-site gastrotomies are small and not prone to leak. ∎

Pancreatic Pseudocyst Drainage

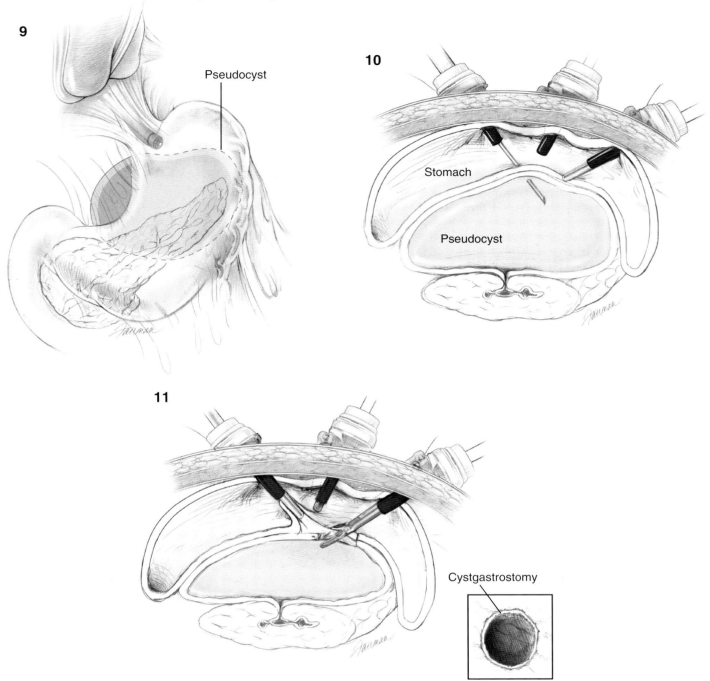

9

Pseudocyst

10

Stomach

Pseudocyst

11

Cystgastrostomy

Intragastric Bleeding

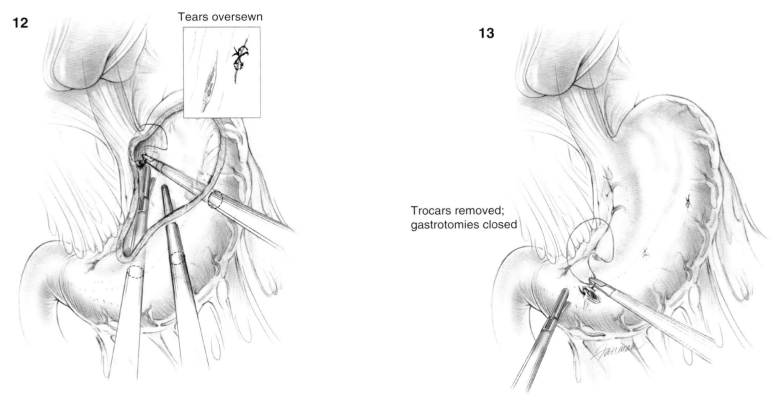

12

Tears oversewn

13

Trocars removed;
gastrotomies closed

PANCREATIC NECROSECTOMY

INDICATIONS Intervention is indicated in patients with infected necrotizing pancreatitis and clinical signs of infection or sepsis. The minimally invasive step-up approach is applicable in nearly all patients and has been shown to be superior to primary open necrosectomy in terms of major morbidity including postprocedural organ failure. The step-up approach consists of percutaneous catheter drainage as a first step followed by video-assisted retroperitoneal debridement (VARD) when needed.

Infection of necrotizing pancreatitis is typically diagnosed a few weeks after onset of acute pancreatitis. It is preferred to postpone any intervention until after 4 weeks following onset of disease, as this reduces postoperative morbidity. During this period, using antibiotics and intensive care, the condition of the patient is allowed to improve and the collections become encapsulated and walled-off. "Walled-off pancreatic necrosis" (WOPN) reduces the risk of bleeding during necrosectomy.

Clinical signs of infection or sepsis are important for determining the need for intervention. Only a small (approximately 5%) subset of patients with infected necrotizing pancreatitis but without signs of sepsis can be treated with antibiotics alone. Computed tomography (CT) depicts bacteria related gas bubbles in only 50% of patients with infected necrotizing pancreatitis. Absence of gas bubbles certainly does not exclude infection. Fine-needle aspiration (FNA) is advised by some surgeons but one should keep in mind that FNA is associated with false-negative test results up to 50%. Sterile necrotizing pancreatitis only rarely requires intervention.

PREOPERATIVE PREPARATION A high-quality contrast-enhanced CT scan is performed to determine the size and position of the collection(s) of infected necrosis and accessibility for percutaneous drains. The CT scan should be viewed with an intent to determine the relationship of the left side of the collection to the left abdominal wall just over Gerota fascia and whether there are any paracolic extensions of the infected collection (**FIGURE 1**). In 95% of patients percutaneous drainage is feasible.

For the VARD procedure, the collection should be within reach of a percutaneous drain placed through the retroperitoneum, which is the case in more than 80% of patients. Typically, this drain is placed over Gerota fascia of the left kidney. Some 30% of patients do not require a VARD procedure and can be successfully treated with one or two 12 to 20 French percutaneous drains. After percutaneous drain placement, drains should be flushed three times daily with 50 mL saline each time to prevent blockage of the drain and to promote lavage of the cavity. The patient should be observed for about 3 days, and if the condition does not improve, a repeat CT is performed to check that the drains are in good position within the collection. If the size of the collection is not significantly improved after 1 to 2 weeks of percutaneous drainage, the next step, VARD, is undertaken.

ANESTHESIA General anesthesia with endotracheal intubation is required. Broad-spectrum antibiotic prophylaxis aimed at intestinal microorganisms is administered.

POSITION The patient is placed in the supine position on a beanbag with the xiphoid over the flex point of the operating table. Before final positioning and draping of the patient, the following landmarks are marked: xiphoid, costal margin, anterior superior iliac spine, and midaxillary line, as well as the planned incision site (**FIGURE 2**). The 4- to 5-cm planned incision site is marked one fingerbreadth below the left costal margin in the midaxillary line. Once the patient is draped, it can be difficult to accurately determine these important landmarks. The left side of the patient is elevated with a roll placed under the left flank, and the left arm is positioned over the patient's head and fixated with proper padding (**FIGURE 3**). The operating table is flexed such that the distance between costal margin and pelvic rim is increased. The entire abdomen of the patient is prepped from nipple to pubis because occasionally laparotomy may be required. Once the patient is draped, the table is rolled 20 degrees to the right. In this way the route of the percutaneous drain from the skin to the retroperitoneal cavity is in the coronal plane. A collection bag may be placed under the incision to collect pus and irrigation fluid.

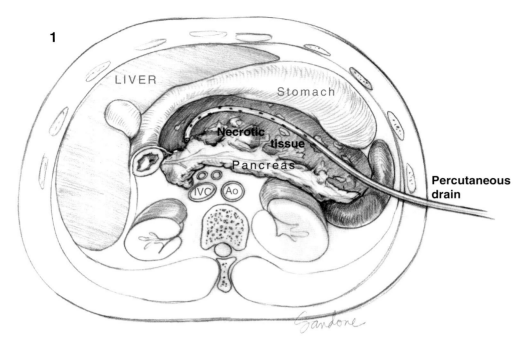

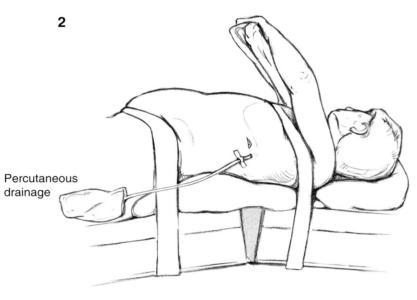

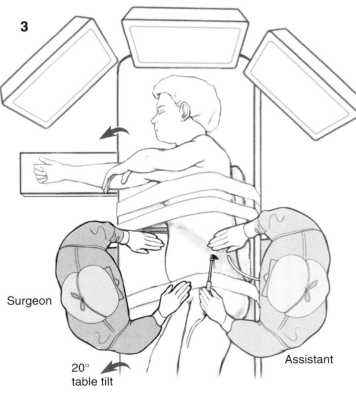

OPERATIVE PREPARATION The preoperative CT scan should be available on a screen in the operating room and reviewed before starting the procedure. Necessary instruments include: 10-mm 0-degree laparoscope, long 10- or 12-mm trocar, long ring forceps, deep Deaver retractors, liberal amounts of warm saline, pulse-lavage system, and two 1-inch Penrose surgical drains. A laparoscopic clip applier is optional but may be helpful in case of bleeding.

DETAILS OF PROCEDURE A 4- to 5-cm left subcostal incision is made as marked in the midaxillary line. The three layers of muscles are divided sequentially. Immediately under the transversus muscle, a thin line indicating the junction of the peritoneum with the retroperitoneum can be visualized. With blunt finger dissection, the drain is identified cranially. The drain is followed along the horizontal plane into the collection with infected necrosis **(FIGURE 4)**. It is important to stay close to the drain in order to avoid the other organs in the near vicinity: the colon (anterior), the spleen (superior), and the kidney (posterior). For the final entrance into the collection, a straight clamp may be applied around the drain, as the wall of the collection is typically firm. Once in the collection, pus will drain spontaneously. Next, a deep Deaver retractor is placed ventrally through the opening, thus enabling a clear view of the infected material near the entrance of the collection.

The first necrotic tissue encountered is removed "blindly" using finger fracture, Yankauer suction, and a ring forceps **(FIGURE 5)**. After a cavity is created, a 10-mm 0-degree laparoscope is placed directly into the collection through an extra-long port in the incision. This port is helpful to prevent impaired vision due to smudging of the camera. The port is placed at the dorsal edge of the incision. The percutaneous drain can be connected to an insufflator and CO_2 gas at 20 mm Hg can be used to help expand the cavity, but this is not essential for all patients. Under laparoscopic vision, further necrosectomy is performed with an instrument placed directly through the incision **(FIGURE 6)**. Without the limitations of a second port, large pieces of necrosis can be removed. It is important to remove only loosely adherent necrosis in order to prevent bleeding from viable pancreatic tissue and nearby vessels such as the splenic artery and vein, which may course through the collection. In case of bleeding, a laparoscopic clip applier may be useful. If this is not feasible and the bleeding is of arterial origin, packing the collection and transporting the patient to interventional radiology for coil embolization is advised. In case of venous bleeding, packing should

suffice to stop the bleeding, followed by repeat necrosectomy after 24 to 48 hours.

The periodic use of the pulse lavage system throughout the operation is helpful to facilitate hydrodissection of the necrotic tissue. It is not the goal of the procedure to remove all necrosis, but large undrained pockets of necrosis may cause ongoing fever. Paracolic collections can also be drained through the same incision if there is, or has been, a connection with the peripancreatic collection.

At the end of the procedure, the cavity is irrigated using pulsed lavage and 2 to 3 L of warm saline. The percutaneous drain is left in place. Two large Penrose drains are then placed into the collection, with one tip placed at the deepest position, and brought out through the dorsal part of the wound. The fascia is closed above the drains, in three individual layers (transversus, internal oblique, and external oblique abdominis muscles) with individual sutures. Failure to close these layers meticulously will contribute to difficult flank hernias. Drains are attached to the skin, and the skin may be closed or left open to heal by secondary intention. The Penrose drains are brought into a urostomy appliance and connected to a Foley urimeter for use in the postoperative lavage system **(FIGURE 7)**. The necrotic tissue is sent for microbiological assessment.

POSTOPERATIVE CARE Postoperatively, broad-spectrum antibiotics are continued and narrowed based on culture results. They are continued until the patient is afebrile with a normal white blood cell count for 24 hours, and then stopped. Continuous postoperative lavage is started with 4 L saline per 24 hours infused in via the percutaneous drains and collected into the Foley urimeter. The nurses should keep careful records of the total fluid in and out.

Once the condition of the patient has clearly improved and lavage fluids are clear, the lavage is stopped and the drains are placed to gravity drainage. The drain output should be monitored closely and amylase/lipase levels measured if they continue to produce spontaneously, because pancreatic fistulas occur in 25% of patients. Two weeks postoperatively, a CT is performed to check for undrained necrosis/collections. In addition to pancreatic fistula, other well known complications are: (1) postoperative bleeding (10–15%), in which case drains are clamped at the bedside and interventional radiology is performed, and (2) colonic perforation (1–5%), in which case a loop ileostomy or transverse colostomy is performed. ■

4

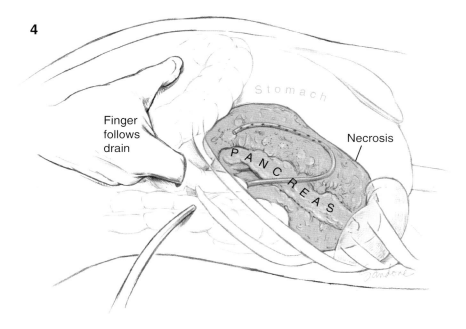

Finger follows drain

Stomach

Necrosis

PANCREAS

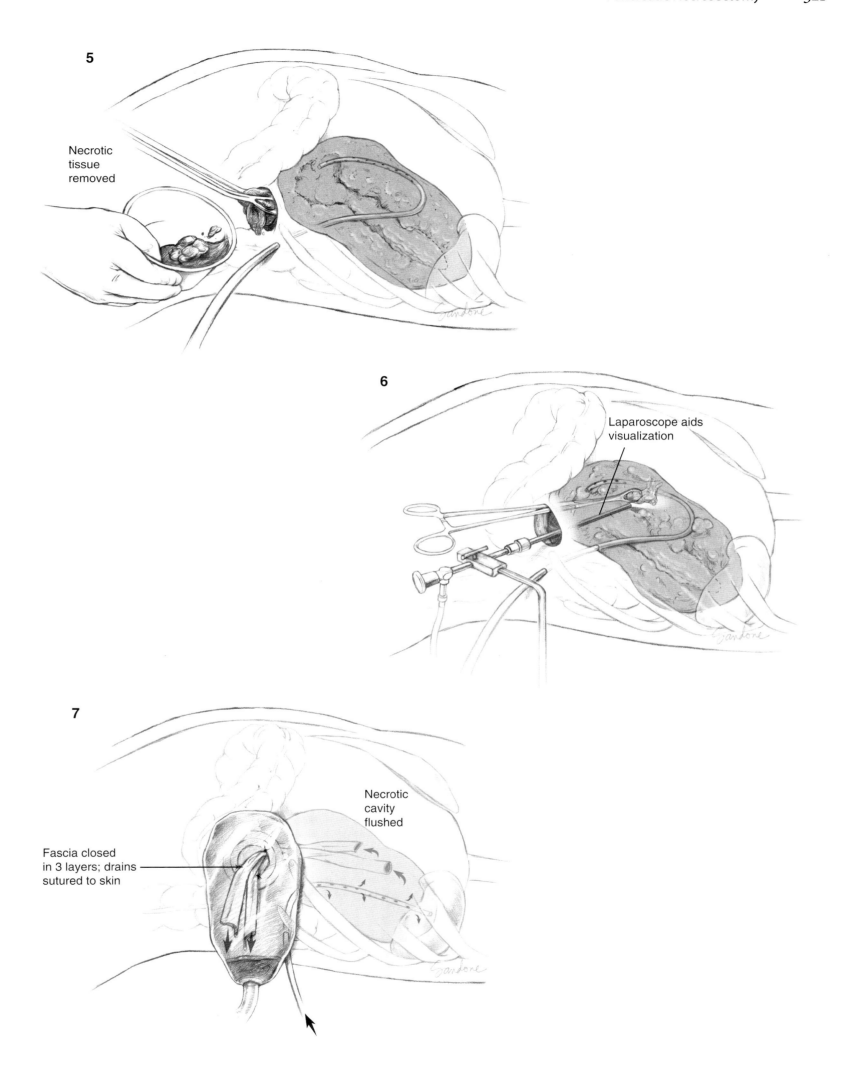

5

Necrotic
tissue
removed

6

Laparoscope aids
visualization

7

Necrotic
cavity
flushed

Fascia closed
in 3 layers; drains
sutured to skin

DISTAL PANCREATECTOMY

INDICATIONS The most common indications for laparoscopic resection of the body and tail of the pancreas are benign neuroendocrine neoplasms, benign cystic neoplasms, symptomatic pancreatic pseudocysts, and pancreatic duct strictures. The role of this procedure for pancreatic malignancy is ill defined, largely because of the lack of clinical data validating its oncologic equivalence to open resection.

PREOPERATIVE INVESTIGATION AND PREPARATION A contrast-enhanced computed tomography (CT) scan using a pancreatic protocol is a necessary assessment tool. This study provides images of the pancreas during the arterial and venous phases. Patients with radiographic abnormalities of the body and tail of the pancreas should undergo endoscopic ultrasound with or without fine-needle aspiration (FNA) and cystic fluid sampling if indicated. In patients with a dilated pancreatic duct, endoscopic retrograde cholangiopancreatography (ERCP) is useful for evaluating the papilla and ductal anatomy in the head of the pancreas.

Preoperative medical evaluation to stratify operative risk is essential. Vaccination against encapsulated bacteria (*Haemophilus influenzae*, *Streptococcus*, *Meningococcus*) is routinely given preoperatively, preferably 7 to 10 days before surgery, as splenectomy is frequently required with distal pancreatectomy. Patients with functional pancreatic neuroendocrine tumors may require preoperative hospitalization to optimize physiologic status. Adequate fluid resuscitation, preoperative antibiotics, and deep venous thrombosis (DVT) prophylaxis are all indicated.

ANESTHESIA General anesthesia with endotracheal intubation and complete neuromuscular blockade is required for this operation.

POSITION Laparoscopic distal pancreatic resection can be performed with the patient in the supine position or in a right semilateral decubitus position. The upper and lower extremities are well padded and secured comfortably. If the patient is in the supine position, the surgeon stands between the patient's legs and the assistant stands to the left of the patient (**FIGURE 1**).

OPERATIVE PREPARATION After the induction of general anesthesia, a Foley catheter and a nasogastric tube are placed. The upper abdomen of the patient from the nipple line to the pubis is shaved with clippers, and the abdomen is sterilely prepped.

OPERATIVE PRINCIPLES Laparoscopic distal pancreatic resection consists of a series of defined steps that include:

1. Lesser sac exposure
2. Splenic flexure and mesocolon mobilization from the spleen and the body of the pancreas
3. Pancreatic mobilization
4. Splenic artery and vein isolation and ligation
5. Pancreatic transection
6. Pancreatic stump management
7. Specimen extraction

There are several technical variations that can be used based on surgeon preference and character of the lesion. Pancreatic mobilization can be performed from lateral to medial or from medial to lateral. In general, the lateral-to-medial approach is easier; however, this does not allow for early control of the splenic artery and vein. Complete splenic mobilization is neither necessary nor desirable unless the spleen is to be removed.

INCISION AND EXPOSURE Pneumoperitoneum is achieved by either the Veress needle technique placed through the umbilicus, or open Hasson technique at the site of the camera port. The laparoscopic distal pancreatic resection is performed via four trocars. The location of these trocars may vary slightly depending on the body habitus of the patient. In general the trocars should be triangulated around the body and tail of the pancreas with a working distance that allows sufficient range of motion. The greatest flexibility can be obtained by using three 12-mm trocars and one 5-mm trocar. A 12-mm trocar is placed in the supraumbilical position to the left of the midline. After placement of this trocar, an angled laparoscope is introduced into the abdomen, and a thorough abdominal inspection is performed. All subsequent trocars are inserted under direct vision after skin infiltration with 0.5% bupivacaine. A 12-mm trocar is placed 8 to 10 cm lateral to the camera port on the patient's left. This trocar will allow passage of the flexible laparoscopic ultrasound probe and the articulated endoscopic staple device. A third 5-mm trocar is placed in the left midclavicular line approximately 10 cm above the camera port. This trocar will allow the assistant to provide suction and retraction. If necessary, this position can be converted into a hand port during the operation. Finally, a fourth 12-mm trocar is placed in the right midclavicular line approximately 5 cm above the camera port. An additional 5-mm subxiphoid trocar can be added for retracting the left lobe of the liver if necessary (**FIGURE 2**).

DETAILS OF THE PROCEDURES

Lesser Sac Exposure The surgeon must be familiar with anatomic relationship of the pancreas and retroperitoneal vascular structures (**FIGURE 3**). To access the lesser sac, the patient is first placed in reverse Trendelenburg position to allow gravity to drop the great omentum and the small bowel from the operating field. If a large left lobe of the liver obscures the stomach, a liver retractor can be placed in the epigastrium and the left lobe retracted (**FIGURE 4**).

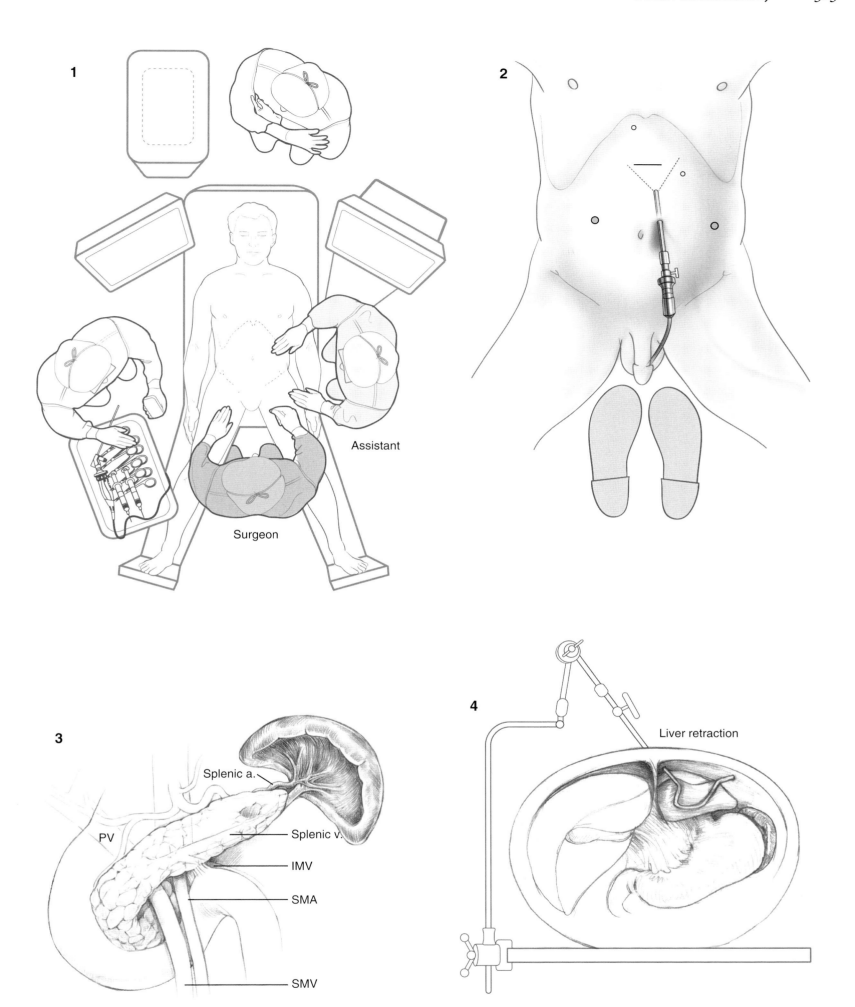

1

Surgeon

Assistant

2

3

Splenic a.

PV

Splenic v.

IMV

SMA

SMV

4

Liver retraction

Lesser Sac Exposure The assistant retracts the stomach in the anterior and cephalad direction. The lesser sac is entered by dividing the greater omentum from the greater curvature of the stomach outside of the right gastroepiploic arcade using an ultrasonic dissector. This dissection can usually be started 5 cm proximal to the pylorus on the greater curve of the stomach (FIGURE 5). Care must be taken to avoid contact with the gastric wall to avoid perforation due to delayed necrosis. Alternatively, the lesser sac can be entered through the avascular plane superior to the transverse colon. However, this approach may leave the greater omentum in the operative field. The mobilization is continued proximally along the greater curvature by dividing all of the short gastric vessels (FIGURE 6). The peritoneal fold between the posterior wall of the stomach and the pancreas is then divided and the lesser sac fully visualized (FIGURE 7). In patients with chronic pancreatitis or a desmoplastic reaction from a pancreatic neuroendocrine tumor, there may be significant adhesions in this retrogastric space. To maintain exposure of the pancreas within the lesser sac, the stomach may be secured to the anterior abdominal wall using percutaneously inserted T-fasteners (FIGURE 8). Although not always needed, this technique improves exposure of the pancreas from its neck to tail.

After exposure of the pancreas is attained, laparoscopic ultrasound will assist in determining the location and morphology of the pancreatic lesion (FIGURE 9). Intraoperative ultrasound can provide useful information regarding the relationship of the lesion to the pancreatic duct and splenic vessels. This may be useful in planning the site of pancreatic transection and the feasibility of splenic preservation.

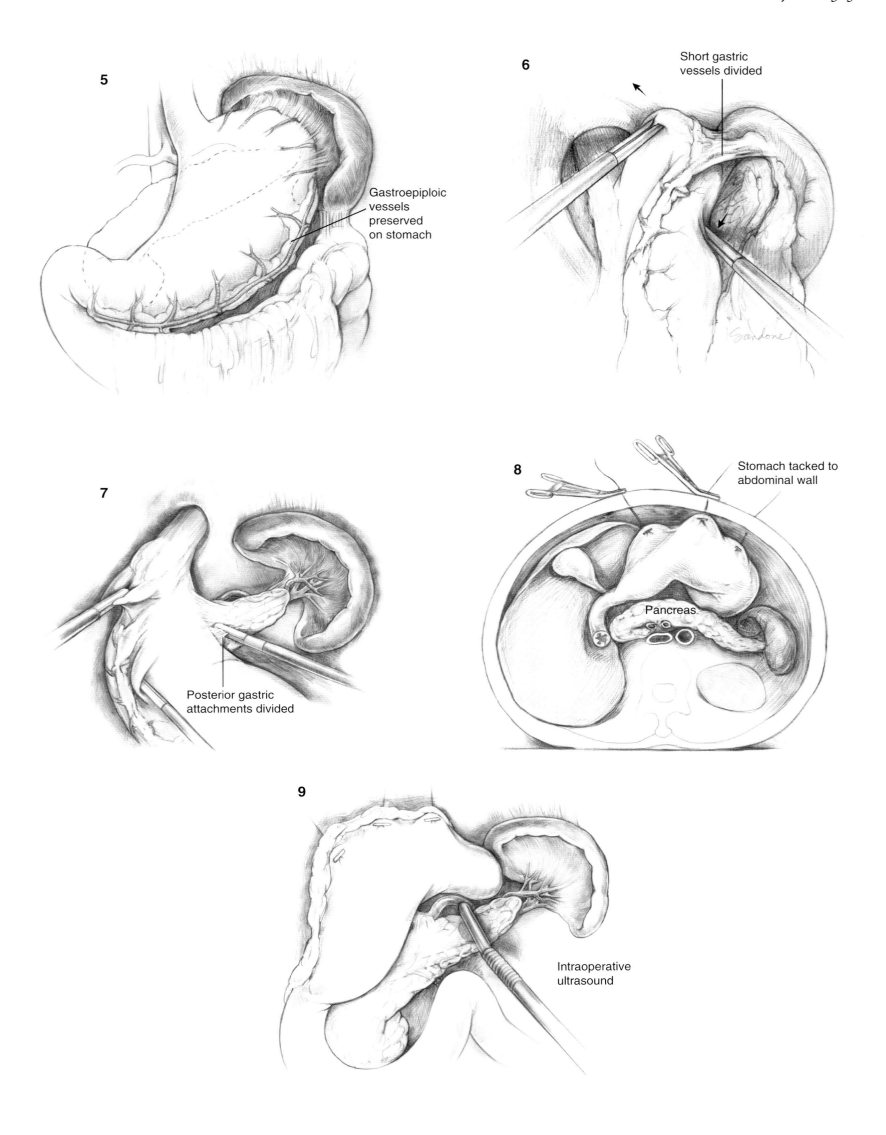

5

Gastroepiploic vessels preserved on stomach

6

Short gastric vessels divided

7

Posterior gastric attachments divided

8

Stomach tacked to abdominal wall

Pancreas

9

Intraoperative ultrasound

Splenic Flexure Mobilization The attachments between the spleen and the colon are divided (FIGURE 10). A large vein is often found in the splenocolic ligament. This vessel may need to be clipped or divided with a laparoscopic energy device. This maneuver will expose the inferior pole of the spleen. Dissection of the ligamentous attachments to the inferior pole of the spleen will allow exposure of the tail of the pancreas. If necessary, the splenic flexure of the colon can be further mobilized to allow greater exposure within the lesser sac. Complete splenic mobilization from its diaphragmatic attachments is intentionally not performed. These attachments will provide lateral retraction to prevent the spleen from entering the operative field during extremes of patient positioning.

Pancreatic Mobilization with Splenectomy Pancreatic mobilization starts within the inferior pancreatic groove and extends laterally. This dissection plane can be difficult to identify in the presence of excessive retroperitoneal fat. Gentle probing will identify the transition point from firm pancreas to loose fatty and alveolar tissue in the inferior pancreatic grove (FIGURE 11). It is sometime easier to have the ultrasonic dissector in the surgeon's left hand, as this direction of dissection is parallel to the inferior border of the pancreas (FIGURE 12). As the lateral dissection continues toward the tail of the pancreas, posterior dissection is simultaneously performed, elevating the splenic vein with the pancreas (FIGURE 13). Loose areolar tissue in this plane can be divided with the ultrasonic dissector. Care must be taken to maintain a horizontal plane of dissection as the retropancreatic space is developed, to avoid injuring retroperitoneal structures such as the kidney. If splenic preservation is to be performed, the splenic vein must be mobilized from its posterior-inferior position along the pancreas. A hand port may facilitate this very tedious dissection, and the hand port site makes a convenient site for specimen retraction at the completion of the resection.

After the inferior and posterior dissection is completed, attention is turned to the superior border of the pancreas. The splenic artery is identified via careful dissection, or direct palpation with the left hand if a hand port has been placed. With the surgeon's thumb in the inferior-posterior space and the index finger on the superior border of the pancreas, loose areolar tissue can be bluntly dissected. The exact location of the splenic artery will be appreciated between surgeon's thumb and index finger (FIGURE 14).

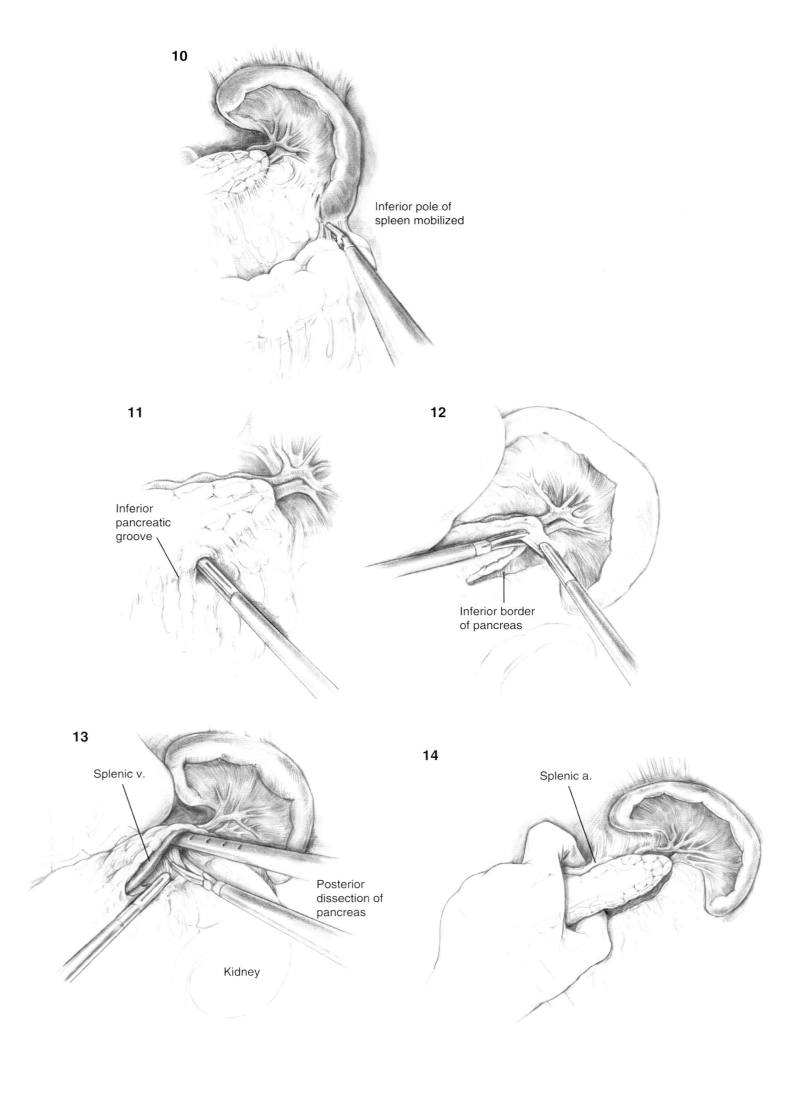

10

Inferior pole of
spleen mobilized

11

Inferior
pancreatic
groove

12

Inferior border
of pancreas

13

Splenic v.

Posterior
dissection of
pancreas

Kidney

14

Splenic a.

Pancreatic Mobilization with Splenectomy The ultrasonic dissector can then be used to dissect the superior border of the pancreas. Small arterial and venous branches must be ligated using the ultrasonic dissector or endoclips (**FIGURE 15**). Once circumferential dissection is achieved, vessels exiting the the tip of the tail of the pancreas originating from the splenic artery and vein can be divided or preserved, depending on whether splenic preservation is to be achieved. Care should be taken to avoid injury to the left adrenal gland, which can be intimately associated with the tail of the pancreas and cause troublesome bleeding that will make further laparoscopic dissection difficult.

There are several structures to consider while mobilizing the medial pancreas. The inferior mesenteric vein (IMV) is often located just lateral to the ligament of Treitz in the retroperitoneum at the midportion of the body of the pancreas. Attempts to save the IMV as it courses superiorly to join the splenic vein should be made to decrease the risk of splenic and portal vein thrombosis. Venous tributaries from the splenic vein will be encountered and should be ligated with the ultrasonic dissector or endoscopic clips.

Pancreatic Transection: Parenchyma, Splenic Artery and Vein If the pancreas is thin, pancreatic transection can be done simultaneously with the splenic artery and vein using an endoscopic stapling device. If the pancreas is thick, the splenic artery, vein, and pancreatic parenchyma should be divided separately. Isolation of the splenic artery can be achieved at the superior border of the pancreas using a laparoscopic right angle and ultrasonic shears. In some instances, the splenic artery is more accessible through the posterior pancreatic dissection plane. At least 1.5 cm of exposed vessel is needed for the application of an articulating endoscopic stapler (vascular load) (**FIGURE 16**). The dissection of the splenic vein is much more challenging because of its thinner wall and numerous branches. Whether or not the spleen and splenic vein are to be preserved, very short venous branches should be divided between endoclips. The ultrasonic shears used in this dissection may be successful, or may leave bleeding side holes in the splenic vein that may be hard to control. If splenic preservation is not to be performed, the splenic vein should be stapled with a vascular load of the endoscopic linear stapler (**FIGURE 17**). Pancreas transection can be performed with the vascular, GI, or thick tissue load of the linear stapler, depending on the thickness of the pancreas at the desired point of resection. Care must be taken to visualize the tip of of the stapler prior to firing to ensure clearance of other surrounding structures, including other branches of the celiac axis (**FIGURE 18**). Gentle and slow firing of the stapler may improve hemostasis and avoid unnecessary traumatic injury to the pancreas.

Pancreatic Stump Management The main pancreatic duct is not routinely identified within the stapled end of the pancreas. The entire end of the gland is oversewn with a running 3-0 Prolene suture (**FIGURE 19**). Alternatively, the stump can be oversewn in a figure-of-eight fashion. Such a closure of the pancreatic stump has not been proven—in randomized trials—to prevent pancreatic fistula.

Irrigation is then performed and the wound bed inspected for hemostasis. If transected, the stapled splenic artery and vein ends are reinspected. The oversewn pancreatic stump is covered with tissue sealant using a laparoscopic delivery system.

15

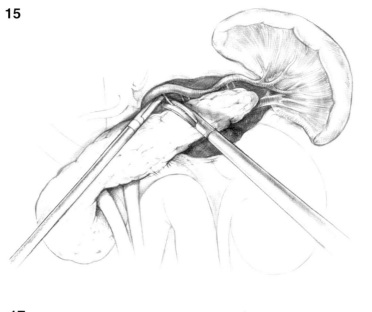

16

Splenic a.
divided

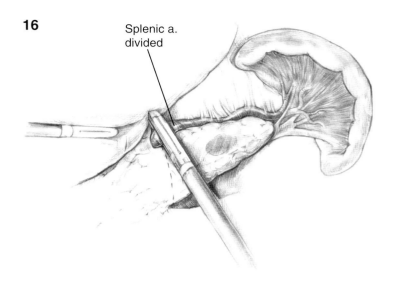

17

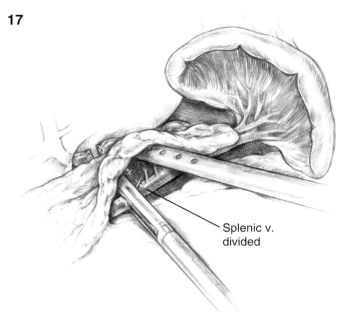

Splenic v.
divided

18

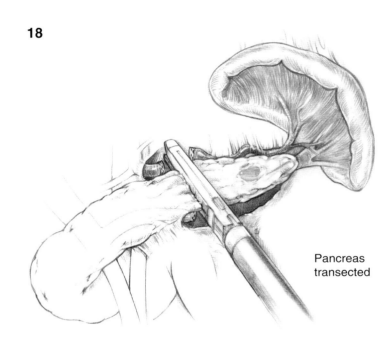

Pancreas
transected

19

Pancreatic
stump oversewn

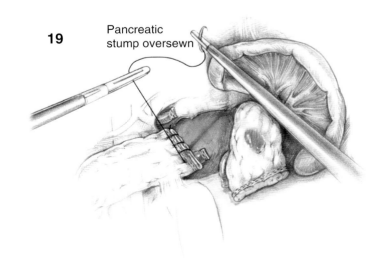

Spleen-Preserving Distal Pancreatic Resection There are two methods of splenic preservation during the laparoscopic distal pancreatic resection. The first preserves the splenic artery and vein, therefore maintaining the inflow and outflow of the spleen. The second method ligates these vessels while preserving the short gastric vessels (not shown). Our preference is to preserve the splenic vein because its ligation carries a higher risk of splenic infarction with subsequent need for splenectomy. The development of gastric varices has also been reported when the splenic artery and vein are divided. If splenic preservation is to be performed, the splenic vein must be mobilized from its posterior-inferior position along the pancreas (**FIGURES 20 AND 21**). A hand port may facilitate this dissection.

Concurrent Splenectomy As previously described, the gastrosplenic, splenocolic, and splenorenal ligaments have been divided to provide exposure of the tail of the pancreas. The splenophrenic ligament is divided to free the spleen completely (**FIGURE 22**).

Specimen Removal The distal pancreas and spleen can be removed from the hand port site if applicable. Alternatively, a large endobag can be inserted via a 12-mm trocar and the skin incision extended to allow extraction (**FIGURE 23**).

Pancreatic Mass Enucleation Neuroendocrine masses such as insulinomas or glucagonomas located within the body or head of the pancreas can often be enucleated. Laparoscopic ultrasound is key to establishing the boundaries of the lesion and its relationship to vascular and ductal structures that may contraindicate enucleation. Enucleation can proceed after the retropancreatic space is established, thus defining the deep margin.

Ultrasonic dissector, cautery, or shears can be used to carefully mobilize the encapsulated specimen. A stitch through the center of the lesion can often provide traction during dissection (**FIGURES 24 AND 25**). After specimen removal, the dissection bed is carefully inspected for hemostasis and ductal leak. Tissue sealant is applied to the pancreatic bed. The specimen is removed using an endobag.

Drain and Closure A closed suction surgical drain is left in the bed of the resected pancreas or adjacent to the site of enucleation, and brought out through the 5-mm trocar site. The pneumoperitoneum is released, and all trocars are removed under direct vision. Fascial incisions greater than 10 mm are closed with large interrupted absorbable sutures.

POSTOPERATIVE CARE The patient can be typically cared for on a surgical ward with intravenous fluids and pain medications. The nasogastric tube can be removed immediately postoperatively, and clear liquids can be initiated as tolerated. Patients are encouraged to ambulate and use incentive spirometry as early as possible to prevent DVT and atelectasis. In the absence of a large wound, perioperative morbidities including wound infections, ileus, and cardiopulmonary compromise remain less than 20%. The overall perioperative mortality is less than 1%.

Pancreatic leak remains as challenging a problem in the laparoscopic approach as in the open. Surgical drain fluid is not routinely sent for analysis unless indicated by high-volume output or persistent intraabdominal irritation manifested most commonly by fever, ileus, or lack of clinical improvement. Most leaks will stop with conservative treatment.

Uncomplicated hospitalizations typically range from 3 to 5 days. ■

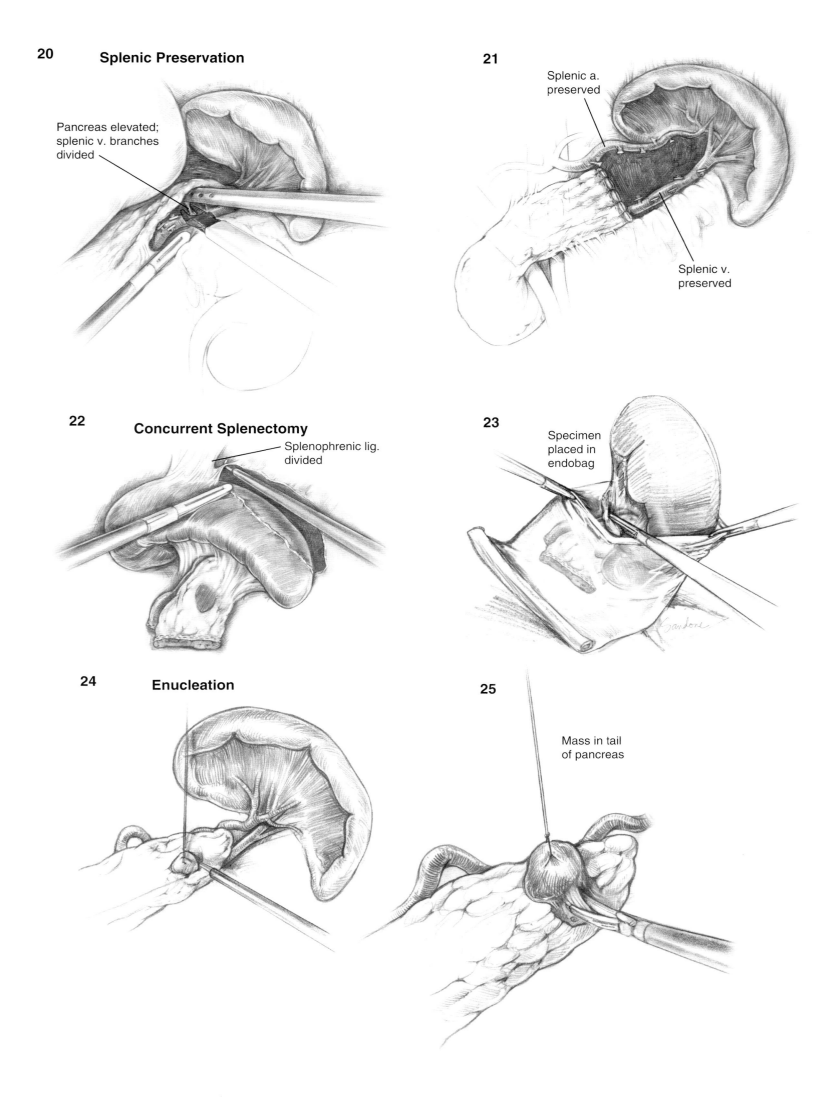

20   **Splenic Preservation**

Pancreas elevated; splenic v. branches divided

21

Splenic a. preserved

Splenic v. preserved

22   **Concurrent Splenectomy**

Splenophrenic lig. divided

23

Specimen placed in endobag

24   **Enucleation**

25

Mass in tail of pancreas

SECTION VII
MINIMALLY INVASIVE ABDOMINAL SURGERY

INDICATIONS Indications for laparoscopic splenectomy are the same as indications for open splenectomy with the following exceptions: acute traumatic hemorrhage is better managed at laparotomy, and extreme splenomegaly prohibiting dissection and removal of the spleen through a small incision is a relative contraindication. The most common indications include hematologic disorders such as idiopathic thrombocytopenic purpura (ITP), which accounts for more than 40% of reported laparoscopic splenectomies. Hereditary spherocytosis, idiopathic autoimmune hemolytic anemia, Felty syndrome, thalassemia, sarcoidosis, sickle cell disease, Gaucher's disease, congenital and acquired hemolytic anemia, thrombotic thrombocytopenic purpura, and AIDS-associated ITP are rare diseases for which splenectomy may be indicated. Laparoscopic splenectomy is also indicated for secondary hypersplenism, splenic artery aneurysm, splenic cyst, and splenic tumor.

PREOPERATIVE PREPARATION Preoperative prophylactic anticoagulation and vaccination against meningococcal, pneumococcal, and *Haemophilus influenzae* type B infections is recommended for all elective splenectomies, unless specifically contraindicated.

For patients with ITP, preoperative imaging such as technetium or indium scanning and postoperative denatured red blood cell scintigraphy may be used to detect accessory spleens. Handheld gamma probe for perioperative examination has shown 100% sensitivity for detection of any accessory spleens.

ANESTHESIA General endotracheal anesthesia with complete neuromuscular blockade is required. A nasogastric or orogastric tube is placed after induction for decompression of the stomach, allowing better access to the operative site. Bilateral sequential compression devices are placed, as is a Foley catheter. Preoperative antibiotics are administered.

POSITION Once asleep, the patient is placed in the right lateral decubitus position with the left side up at approximately 45 degrees (**FIGURE 1**). This position has been called "the leaning spleen." A beanbag or large gel roll is employed to stabilize the patient. All pressure points should be padded and an axillary roll placed. A pillow is placed between the partially flexed knees. The left arm is elevated in a neutral position, and the operating table is flexed to open the operating space between the anterior superior iliac spine and costal margin. Once in the correct position, all air is sucked from the beanbag, and the patient is taped in place with wide cloth tape across the pelvis and across the chest, above the level of the xiphoid. The table is then "airplaned" to the left and right, 30 degrees in either direction, then into steep reverse Trendelenburg to make sure the patient is well secured to the table (**FIGURE 2**).

The patient is shaved from the anterior midline to the posterior midline on the left side between the xiphoid and the pubis, prepped in the same distribution, and draped in a sterile manner. The surgeon and camera operator stand to the patient's right, and the first assistant stands on the patient's left. Monitors are placed at the 10 and 2 o'clock positions.

DETAILS OF THE PROCEDURE With the patient rotated 30 degrees to the left (to nearly flatten the anterior abdominal wall), a Veress needle is placed in the subcostal position in the midclavicular line (Palmer point) and the abdomen insufflated. In patients with splenomegaly, initial access should be in the periumbilical region to avoid iatrogenic splenic injury. Alternatively, initial access through the umbilicus with a Veress needle is preferred by many. The primary trocar, 11 mm in size, is placed halfway between the umbilicus and costal margin, in the midclavicular line (**FIGURE 3**). A 30-degree laparoscope is inserted, and two additional ports are placed under direct visualization. The first is a 12-mm trocar placed at the left anterior axillary line at about the level of the umbilicus for the surgeon's right hand. This will be used for the stapler, later in the operation. This port should be spaced at least 8 cm from the initial trocar to avoid instrument clashing. The second port is a 5-mm trocar placed in the midclavicular line, just below the costal margin, for the surgeon's left hand.

Using sharp or ultrasonic dissection, the left colon is mobilized along the left paracolic gutter to allow visualization of the inferior pole of the spleen and placement of the fourth and final 5-mm port at the posterior axillary line 2 cm below the costal margin (**FIGURE 4**). This will allow retraction of the spleen by the assistant. Once all ports are in position, a systematic exploration of the abdomen for accessory splenic tissue is performed. The patient is then rolled into the lateral position by "airplaning" the table 30 degrees to the right for the next phase of the operation. Some reverse Trendelenburg is usually necessary to allow gravity to retract the omentum, transverse colon, and small bowel inferiorly.

Freeing the spleen from the diaphragm starts at the inferior pole of the spleen, proceeding cephalad, dividing the lateral peritoneal attachments of the spleen with the ultrasonic shears (**FIGURE 5**). The peritoneal reflection at the superior pole of the spleen is left attached to the diaphragm, to hold the spleen in place during hilar dissection. A small vein is often encountered at the inferior pole of the spleen and should be divided with a ultrasonic dissector (**FIGURE 6**). The remnant peritoneum adherent to the spleen is then available for grasping.

1

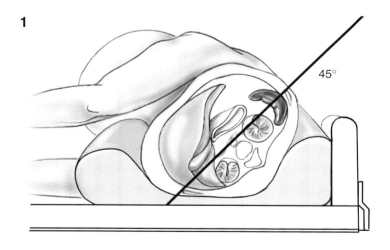

45°

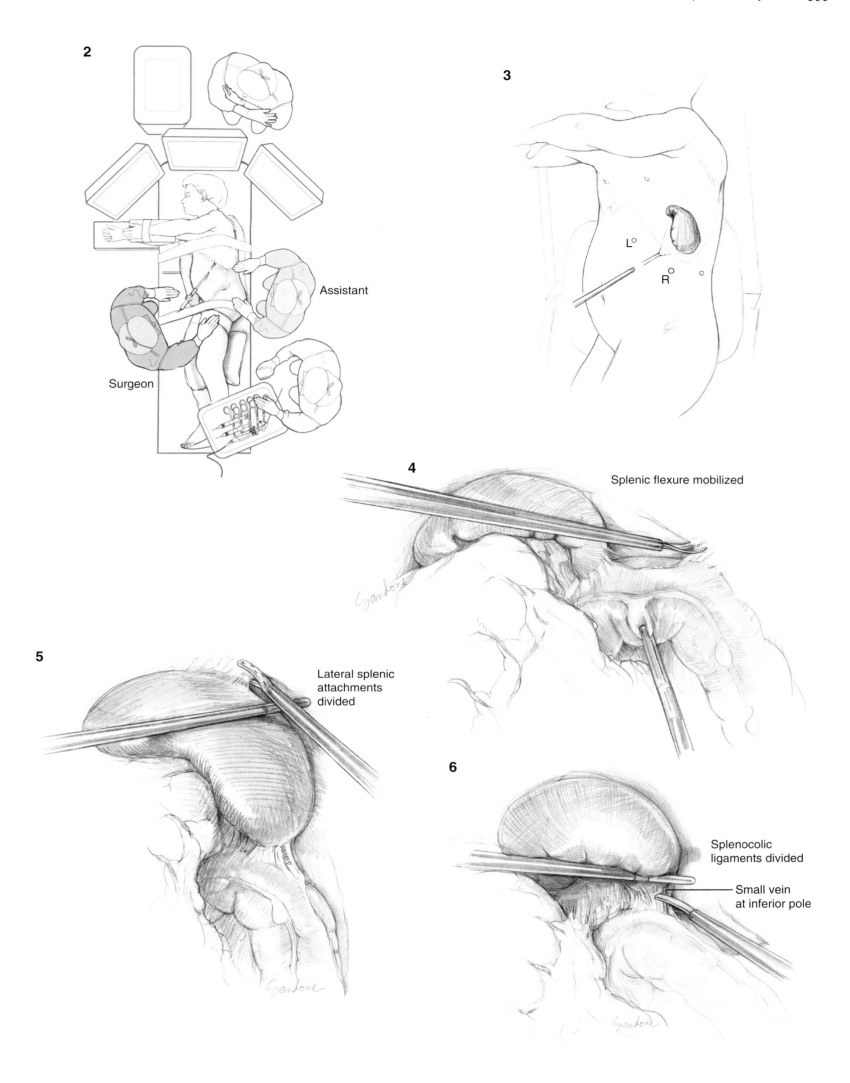

2

Assistant

Surgeon

3

L°

R°

4

Splenic flexure mobilized

5

Lateral splenic
attachments
divided

6

Splenocolic
ligaments divided

Small vein
at inferior pole

DETAILS OF THE PROCEDURE The inferior pole of the spleen is elevated anteriorly by a closed grasper passed through the posterior axillary port by the first assistant, and the table is rotated back to the left to allow access to the gastrosplenic ligament. The short gastrics are divided with ultrasonic shears. Any remaining attachments to the colon are taken down, and the lesser sac is entered (**FIGURE 7**). After freeing all attachments between the stomach and spleen, attention is directed to splenic hilar dissection. It may be desirable to rotate the table to the right again to allow access to the posterior aspects of the hilum.

The splenic hilum is dissected in an inferior-to-superior manner. Because the tail of the pancreas lies in close proximity to the splenic hilum, it is often necessary to divide the splenic artery and vein after their bifurcation. A window is created in the hilum to facilitate identification of the splenic artery and vein (**FIGURE 8**). Small vascular attachments are divided with the ultrasonic dissector or between clips. The splenic artery and vein are dissected circumferentially and divided using a vascular stapler, starting with the inferior branches of artery and vein (**FIGURE 9**) and finishing with the superior branches (**FIGURE 10**). The surgeon's left hand remains free to grasp any bleeding vessel after the division. A "mass stapling" of the artery and vein in a single firing is very acceptable if the window between upper and lower pole vessels is unclear.

The remaining splenophrenic ligament at the superior pole, left earlier in the dissection, is now divided using the ultrasonic dissector. The hilum of the spleen is used as handle to facilitate placement into a large endoscopic bag (**FIGURE 11**). The opening of the bag is brought out of the 10-mm port site, and the spleen is morcellated in the bag (**FIGURE 12**). If the specimen needs to remain intact, the lateral port sites can be connected in a small incision for extraction. All port sites greater than 10 mm are closed using a heavy suture and a suture passer. All skin incisions are closed using an absorbable monofilament suture and skin glue.

POSTOPERATIVE CARE The patient should be admitted for at least 24 hours of observation, and may be advanced as tolerated to a regular diet. Once adequate pain control is achieved by oral analgesia, and no bleeding complications have been identified, the patient may be discharged home with routine postoperative follow-up. ∎

7

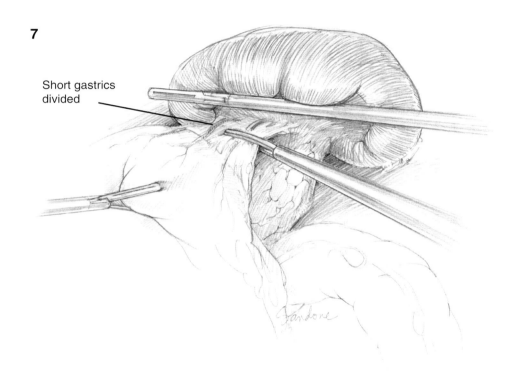

Short gastrics divided

8

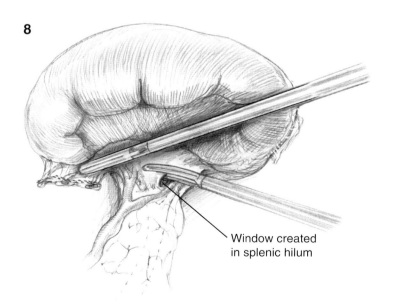

Window created in splenic hilum

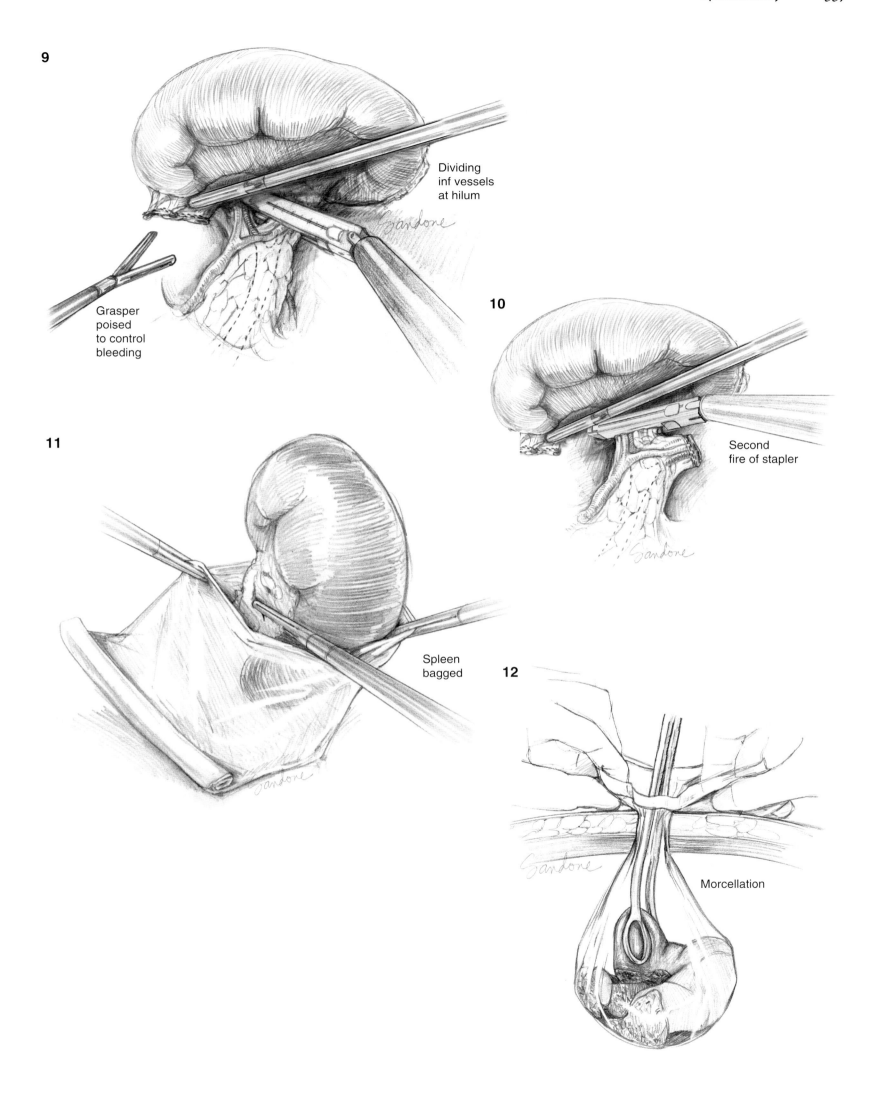

9

Dividing
inf vessels
at hilum

Grasper
poised
to control
bleeding

10

Second
fire of stapler

11

Spleen
bagged

12

Morcellation

CHAPTER 42

ADRENALECTOMY

INDICATIONS Laparoscopic adrenalectomy is indicated for pheochromo-cytomas, and hormonally active adenomas that may secrete aldosterone, glucocorticoids, testosterone, or estrogen. Hormonally inactive lesions >3 cm that demonstrate growth over time on serial imaging studies or tumors >4 cm without evidence of growth are also an indication for laparoscopic adrenalectomy. Functional bilateral adrenal hyperplasia refractory to medical management, primary adrenocortical carcinoma, and solitary metastasis may be treated with laparoscopic adrenalectomy. However, great care should be taken when removing the adrenal metastases from the abdomen in cases of lung or renal cancer, as these are particularly prone to port-site metastasis.

PREOPERATIVE PREPARATION For patients suffering from pheochromocytoma, an alpha blocking agent should be administered for at least 2 weeks prior to adrenalectomy with adequate control of blood pressure. Once adequate blood pressure control is achieved, a beta blocking agent may be added to facilitate heart rate control for pulse rates exceeding 100/min. For patients undergoing adrenalectomy for Cushing disease, a single stress dose of hydrocortisone should be administered intraoperatively, follow by a tapered dose regimen postoperatively.

ANESTHESIA General endotracheal anesthesia with complete neuromuscular blockade is required. An orogastric tube is placed after induction for decompression of the stomach, allowing better access to the operative site. Bilateral sequential compression devices are placed, as is a Foley catheter. Preoperative antibiotics are administered.

POSITION For the left adrenalectomy, the patient is placed on the operating room table in the right lateral decubitus position. This position is stabilized by a beanbag or large gel roll. The arms are supported by armboards in a neutral position. An axillary roll is placed to prevent nerve injury (**FIGURE 1A**). The bed is flexed to widen the angle between the anterior superior iliac spine and the costal margin (**FIGURE 1B**). A kidney rest can be employed to widen this angle if necessary. A pillow is placed between the knees. The patient is secured to the operating table with broad cloth tape, secured at the hips and across the chest. For the right adrenalectomy, this position is mirrored, with the right side of the patient elevated. The patient is shaved from the anterior midline to the posterior flank on the affected side between the xiphoid and the pubis, prepped in the same distribution, and draped in a sterile manner.

DETAILS OF THE PROCEDURE

Left Adrenalectomy A thorough appreciation of the left upper quadrant regional anatomy is particularly important for the left adrenalectomy. Understanding the relationship of the tail of the pancreas, spleen, kidney, and adrenal gland is key to avoiding iatrogenic injury to any of these structures.

Initial port placement occurs with the patient in the decubitus position. A four-trocar technique is typically employed along the costal margin. All trocars should be placed at least 8 cm apart to avoid clashing of instruments during the operation. The abdomen is insufflated by placing a Veress needle in the anterior axillary line two fingerbreadths below the costal margin. After adequate pneumoperitoneum is obtained, a 12-mm port is placed in the same position. A 10-mm, 30-degree laparoscope is inserted through this port for direct visualization of placement of subsequent trocars. An 12-mm port is placed at least 8 cm lateral to the first along the costal margin. A 5-mm port is placed medially along the costal margin 2 cm inferior to the xiphoid. Finally, a 5-mm trocar is placed at the posterior axillary line. Some retroperitoneal dissection is usually necessary, reflecting the left colon off the lateral abdominal wall, before this port can be placed safely (**FIGURE 2**).

Further reflection of the spleen and left colon with the ultrasonic shears or laparoscopic scissors moves the left colon medially, revealing Gerota fascia surrounding the left kidney (**FIGURE 3**). The phrenocolic ligament, splenorenal ligament, and lateral splenic attachments are all incised, to allow medial rotation of the spleen and tail of the pancreas (**FIGURE 4**).

Left Adrenalectomy

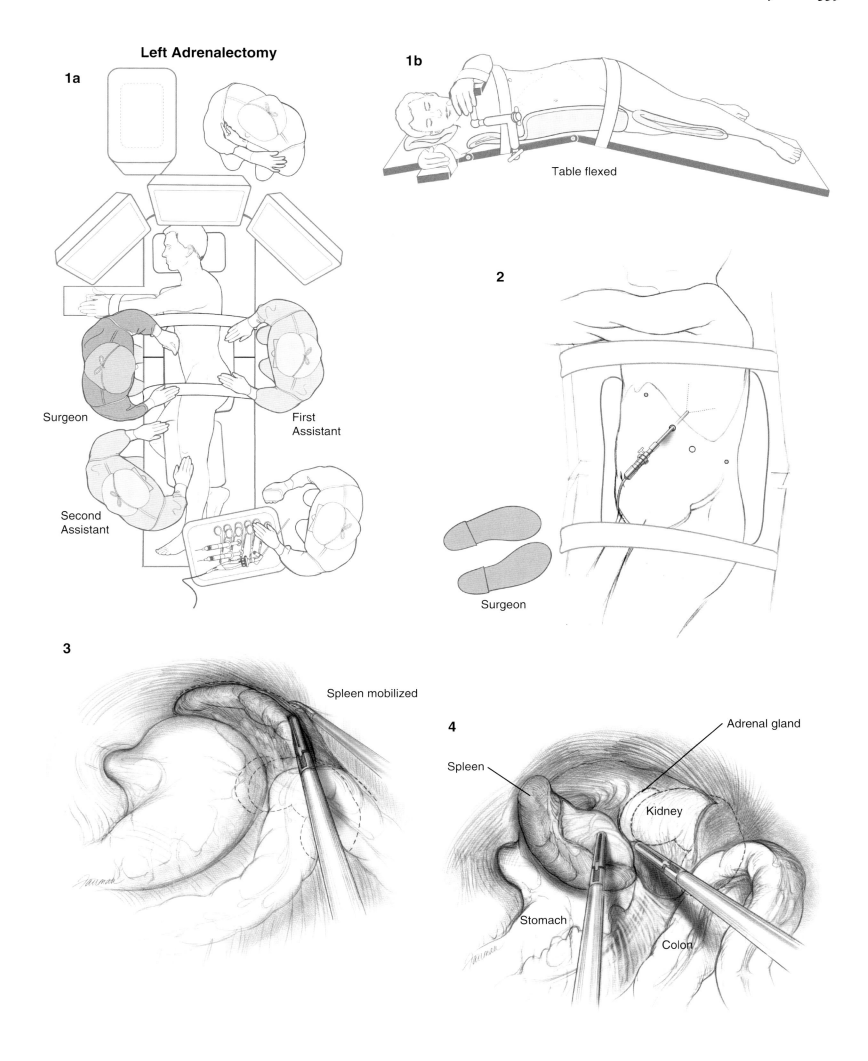

1a

Surgeon

First Assistant

Second Assistant

1b

Table flexed

2

Surgeon

3

Spleen mobilized

4

Spleen

Adrenal gland

Kidney

Stomach

Colon

Left Adrenalectomy The borders of the adrenal gland are often difficult to discern from the surrounding fat; however, careful recognition of the subtle texture change is critical to developing an avascular plane of dissection. The gland is first approached from the inferior medial aspect, where careful dissection will reveal the adrenal vein. In morbidly obese patients, this can be facilitated by identification of the left gonadal vein, which usually inserts immediately opposite the inferior adrenal vein on the left renal vein. The inferior adrenal vein may be joined by an inferior phrenic vein prior to joining the renal vein. The inferior adrenal vein is circumferentially dissected with a right-angle dissector and doubly clipped and divided close to the adrenal gland, leaving a longer stump on the renal vein end (**FIGURE 5**).

The medial aspect of the gland is then carefully elevated and mobilized superiorly. The small arteries supplying the adrenal gland from the diaphragm, aorta, and renal artery are not usually seen or divided specifically. One or two additional adrenal veins may be encountered at the superior medial aspect of the gland. They should be circumferentially dissected and divided between clips or taken with the ultrasonic shears if quite small (**FIGURE 6**). With the gland's blood supply now detached, the ultrasonic dissector can be used to separate it from Gerota fascia inferiorly and peel it superiorly from the underlying psoas muscle, dividing all lateral and superior attachments.

Once the adrenal gland is freed circumferentially, it is placed in an endoscopic catch bag, and removed through the 12-mm subcostal port site (**FIGURE 7**). Fascial defects greater than 10 mm are closed using large absorbable suture in a figure-of-eight fashion, and the skin at all port sites is closed using running subcuticular absorbable monofilament.

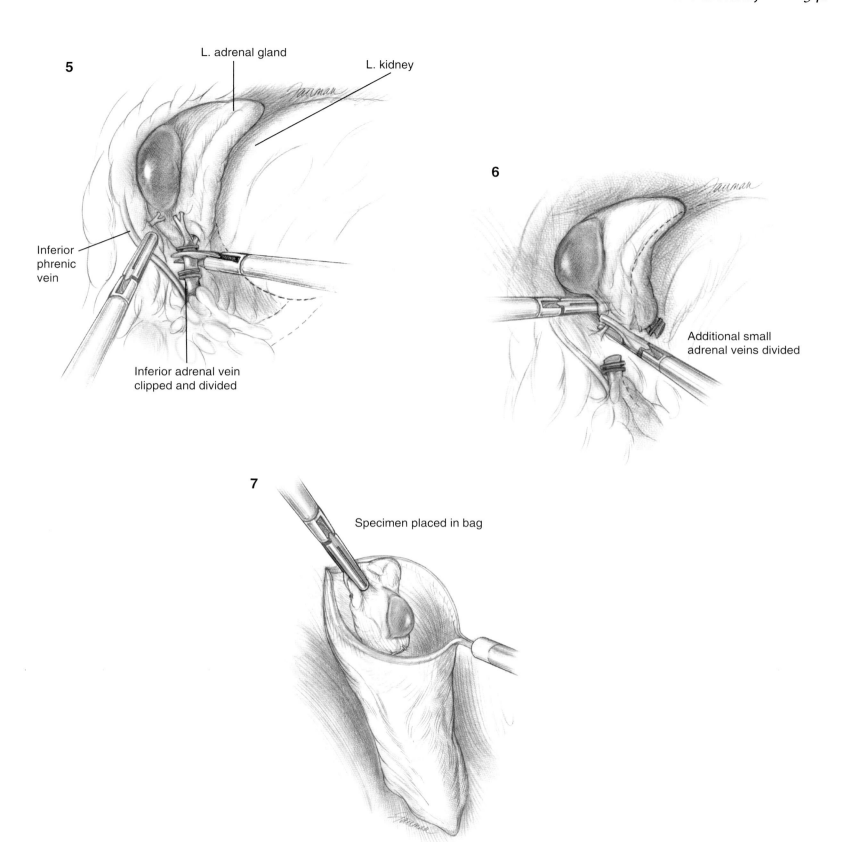

5

L. adrenal gland

L. kidney

Inferior phrenic vein

Inferior adrenal vein clipped and divided

6

Additional small adrenal veins divided

7

Specimen placed in bag

Right Adrenalectomy A thorough appreciation of the right upper quadrant regional anatomy is particularly important for the right adrenalectomy. Understanding the relationship of the porta hepatis, duodenum, inferior vena cava, and adrenal gland is key to avoiding iatrogenic injury to any of these structures.

Initial port placement occurs with the patient in the decubitus position. A four-trocar technique is typically employed along the costal margin. All trocars should be placed at least 8 cm apart to avoid clashing of instruments during the operation. The abdomen is insufflated by placing a Veress needle in the anterior axillary line two fingerbreadths below the costal margin. After adequate pneumoperitoneum is obtained, a 12-mm port is placed in the same position. A 10-mm, 30-degree laparoscope is inserted through this port for direct visualization of placement of subsequent trocars. An 11-mm port is placed at least 8 cm lateral to the first along the costal margin. A third 5-mm port is placed further medially along the costal margin 2 cm inferior to the xiphoid. Finally, a 5-mm port is placed at the posterior axillary line. Some retroperitoneal dissection is usually necessary before this port can be placed safely (**FIGURE 8**).

The right triangular ligament of the liver (peritoneal reflection) is incised, and the right lobe of the liver is retracted superiorly by the assistant from the most medial port (**FIGURE 9**). This step is critical, as adequate mobilization of the liver all the way to the vena cava will be needed to facilitate access to the right adrenal gland. Occasionally it is necessary to mobilize the duodenum and retract it medially with a Kocher maneuver. Typically decompression with an orogastric tube is sufficient to provide the necessary

exposure. The operative field typically lies above the hepatic flexure of the colon, making manipulation of the colon unnecessary. With exposure of the superior aspect of Gerota fascia, the inferior medial aspect of the adrenal gland can be carefully identified. The Harmonic scalpel is used to elevate the inferior medial aspect of the gland separating it from the adjacent inferior vena cava (**FIGURE 10**). The adrenal vein will be encountered as the dissection proceeds medially. This vessel is circumferentially isolated with a right-angle dissector and divided between surgical clips (**FIGURE 11**). The mobilization of the gland proceeds superiorly along its medial border, peeling the gland off of the psoas muscle beneath. Additional veins may be encountered and should be divided between surgical clips or with the ultrasonic shears. The small arteries supplying the right adrenal gland are not often visualized and are divided with the ultrasonic dissector as the mobilization proceeds (**FIGURE 12**). Once the blood supply has been divided, the lateral and superior attachments are freed and the gland is placed in an endoscopic catch bag. The bag is removed through the 12-mm subcostal port site (**FIGURE 13**). Fascial defects greater than 10 mm are closed using large absorbable suture in a figure-of-eight fashion, and the skin at all port sites is closed using running subcuticular absorbable monofilament.

POSTOPERATIVE CARE The patient should be admitted for at least 24 hours of observation and may be advanced as tolerated to a regular diet. Once adequate pain control is achieved by oral analgesia, and no bleeding complications have been identified, the patient may be discharged home with routine postoperative follow-up. ■

8   Right Adrenalectomy

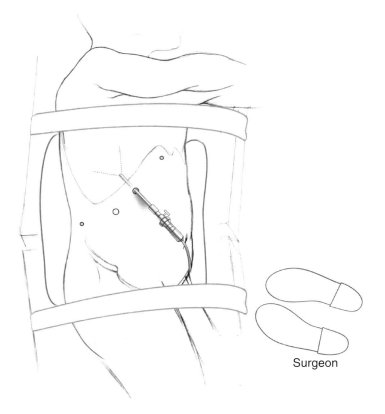

Surgeon

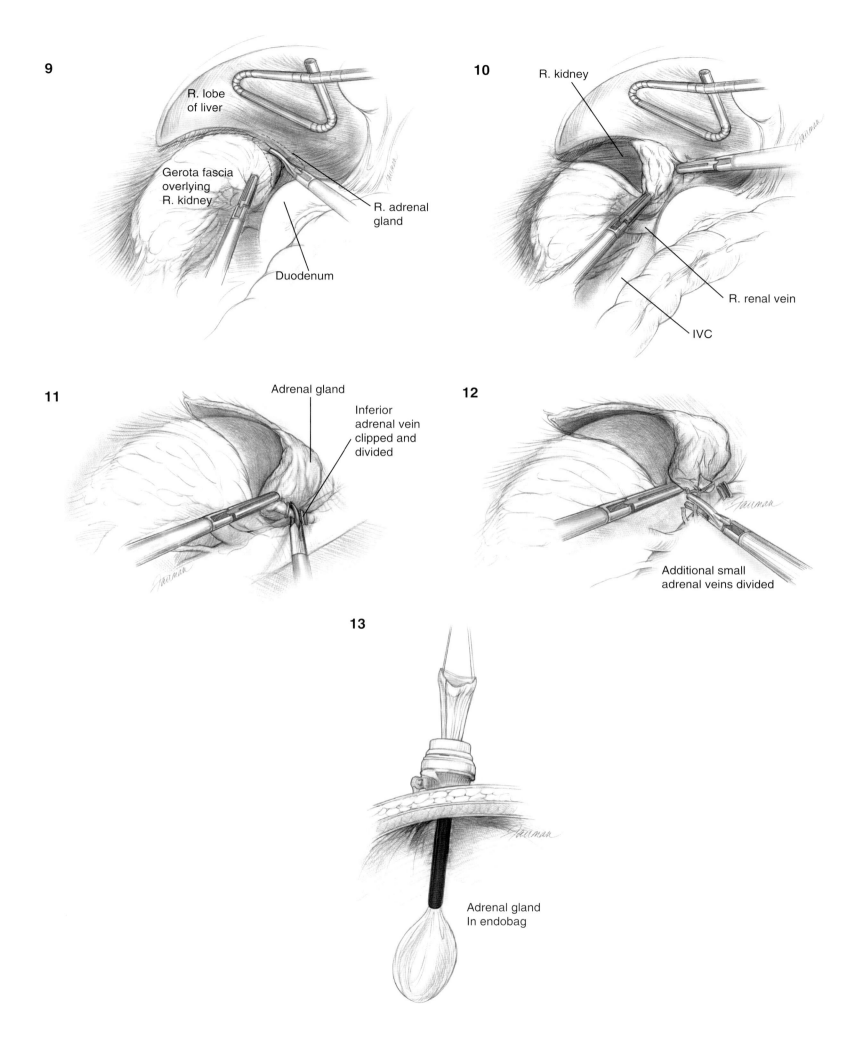

9

R. lobe
of liver

Gerota fascia
overlying
R. kidney

Duodenum

R. adrenal
gland

10

R. kidney

R. renal vein

IVC

11

Adrenal gland

Inferior
adrenal vein
clipped and
divided

12

Additional small
adrenal veins divided

13

Adrenal gland
In endobag

DONOR NEPHRECTOMY

INDICATIONS A donor nephrectomy is indicated for living donor renal transplantation. Potential donors are carefully selected to minimize the risk to the donor and to optimize the success of transplantation.

PREOPERATIVE PREPARATION Before undergoing laparoscopic donor nephrectomy, donor blood type (ABO) and immunologic (HLA) compatibility with the recipient are established. The potential donor's creatinine clearance is measured to assure normal renal function. If needed, the donor is evaluated with appropriate cardiovascular and pulmonary screening. Potential donors with a diagnosis of hypertension must undergo 24-hour ambulatory blood pressure monitoring to more closely examine their blood pressure status. An abdominal and pelvic computed tomography (CT) scan or magnetic resonance imaging (MRI) is obtained to confirm that the donor is anatomically suitable for kidney donation and for preoperative planning. Renal stones are ruled out using either a plain abdominal x-ray or the noncontrast phase of the CT. A contrast CT or MRI ureterogram is obtained to examine the renal collecting system. In selecting the donor kidney, the first order of priority is the well-being of the donor; if a mild abnormality is present, the abnormal kidney is donated. If there are no imperatives regarding the donor, then the best kidney for transplantation is chosen. A kidney with a solitary renal artery is preferred. If both kidneys have a single artery, the left kidney is selected because of its longer renal vein. Two units of packed red blood cells are typed and crossed.

ANESTHESIA General anesthesia with endotracheal intubation is required for the laparoscopic donor nephrectomy. Complete neuromuscular blockade is necessary. Intravenous antibiotics (usually a first-generation cephalosporin, or vancomycin if allergic) are given. The patient is liberally hydrated (2–4 L). Long-acting local anesthesia may be given prior to skin closure. Before emergence from anesthesia, the patient must be protected against postoperative nausea and vomiting with ondansetron, phenergan, or their equivalents. Special attention is given to minimize pain in these volunteers. Postoperative opiates are given, usually via a patient-controlled analgesia (PCA) pump. Supplemental opiates (if the patient gets behind on the PCA) and ketorolac may be given.

POSITIONING AND OPERATIVE PREPARATION To minimize the risk of deep venous thrombosis, sequential compression devices must be in place and working before the induction of anesthesia. The patient is initially placed in the supine position to permit safe induction of anesthesia and line placement. An orogastric tube and a Foley catheter are placed after induction. The patient is aligned such that their iliac crest lies over the flex point in the bed. The patient is then placed in the lateral decubitus position with the nephrectomy side up (**FIGURE 1A**). The bed is flexed to open up the space between the 12th rib and the iliac crest (**FIGURE 1B**). A beanbag (or large gel pads) is used to help secure the patient in the lateral position. Further padding is applied as needed; a large gel pad can be placed between the beanbag and the patient for extra cushioning. The ipsilateral arm is suspended on an arm-shoulder suspension device or on pillows. To protect the structures of the contralateral axilla, an axillary roll is placed. Pillows are placed between the legs (lower leg bent and upper leg straight), and the ankles are padded. The patient is then secured to the bed with tape. The integrity of the positioning can be tested by rolling the table from side to side before prepping and draping. The entire abdomen of the patient from the nipple lines to the pubis is shaved, as needed, with clippers and sterilely prepped (it must be prepared for the possibility that an emergency full-midline incision may be required). As such, a full open surgery setup with vascular clamps and suctioning equipment should be in the room, open, and ready in case of a vascular mishap during the procedure. The bench area for flushing the kidney is also prepared.

LEFT DONOR NEPHRECTOMY

Incision, Placement of Trocars, and Exposure The table is rolled to the left to level the patient for the midline incision. The midline hand-port incision is placed to include the umbilicus. It is made just long enough to easily permit entry of the surgeon's hand (if it is too big, air can escape during the procedure). Typically, two thirds of the incision lies above the umbilicus, and one third lies below the umbilicus. If the patient has an exceptionally long torso or superior kidney, the incision can be oriented more superiorly. A C- or S-shaped incision can be made through the umbilicus to hide some of its length. The fascia is divided and the abdomen entered. If adhesions are present, they are taken down as needed for safe port placement. The hand-port device is placed. An 11-mm trocar is placed through the hand port for insufflation of the abdomen (**FIGURE 2**). Once insufflated to 15 to 18 mm Hg, a 30-degree scope can be inserted for direct visualization of subsequent port placement. The port sites are planned and marked for placement. Two 12-mm ports are placed in the left lower quadrant (LLQ) under direct visualization. One port is placed 4 to 6 cm inferior to the lateral edge of the hand port (approximately 6–10 cm inferior to and 4–6 cm lateral to the umbilicus). The second port is placed approximately 2 cm above and 2–4 cm medial to the medial upper edge of the iliac crest (i.e., the anterior superior iliac spine). The camera is moved to the medial LLQ port. If needed, a 5-mm port can be placed in the lateral left upper quadrant. Different port placement strategies can also be used, such as the placement of the camera port in a superior midline or paramedian position. This strategy provides somewhat easier visualization of the anterior renal hilum, but affords a less clear view of the posterior renal hilum and a less direct line for vascular stapling than the access ports described above.

Details of the Procedure Facing the patient, the surgeon's left hand is inserted through the hand port. The colon is carefully mobilized medially by taking down the colophrenic ligament (which may have a somewhat large vein passing through it) and by opening the white line of Toldt. This can be done sharply, with cautery, or with ultrasonic dissecting shears. Care must be exercised to avoid injury to the colon (**FIGURE 3**). The colonic mesentery is dissected off Gerota fascia (this mesentery can be quite thin, and if it is breached, it should be sutured or clipped closed to reduce the risk of a subsequent internal hernia).

The gonadal vein and the ureter are identified just below the lower pole of the kidney, and a plane between them and the psoas muscle is established. They can be manually dissected as a unit (**FIGURE 4**). Alternatively, the ureter is identified distally (near where it crosses the common iliac artery at the origin of the internal iliac artery), where it can be dissected free and mobilized superiorly. Optimally, to provide maximal periureteral tissue (mesoureter) for maintenance of maximal ureteral blood supply, the gonadal vein is kept with the ureter. It is important to establish the location of the ureter so it will not be injured during mobilization of the kidney.

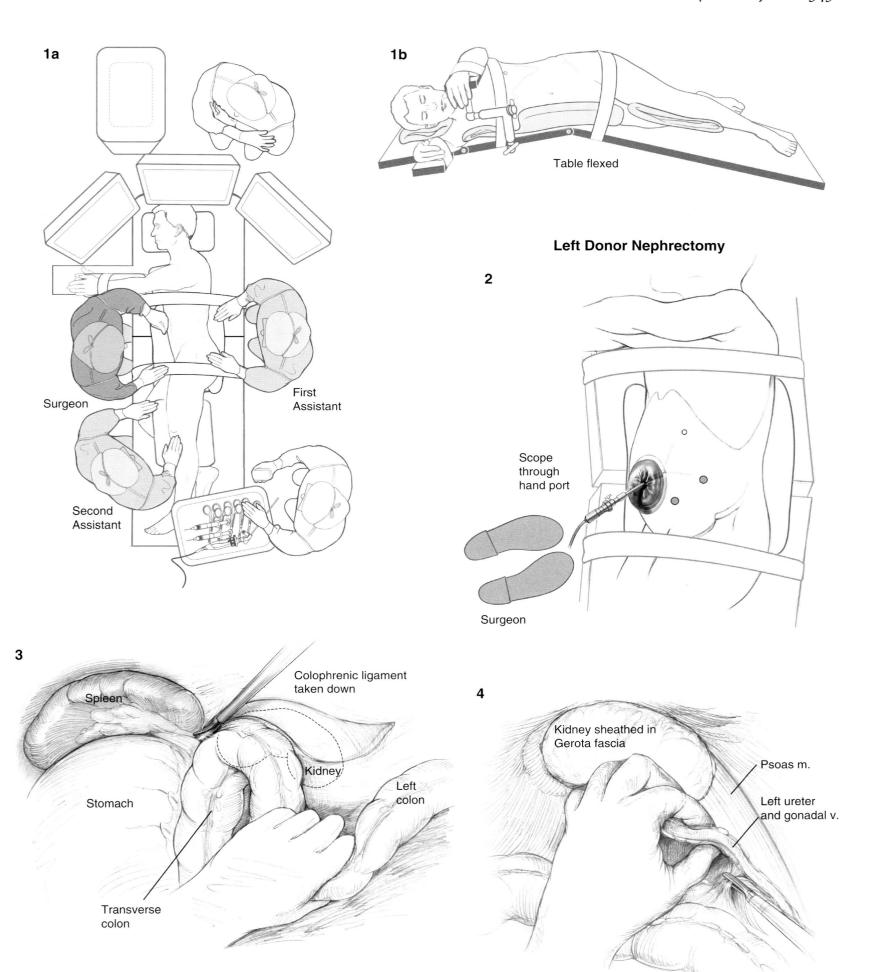

1a

Surgeon

First
Assistant

Second
Assistant

1b

Table flexed

Left Donor Nephrectomy

2

Scope
through
hand port

Surgeon

3

Spleen

Colophrenic ligament
taken down

Kidney

Left
colon

Stomach

Transverse
colon

4

Kidney sheathed in
Gerota fascia

Psoas m.

Left ureter
and gonadal v.

Details of the Procedure   Gerota fascia is entered over the lower pole of the kidney away from the hilum and is dissected superiorly by establishing the plane between it and the renal capsule. The kidney is mobilized by dissecting away Gerota fascia (**FIGURE 5**). This gives maximal exposure for the vascular dissection and, imposes little risk of torsion of the ureter.

The renal vein (which typically lies anterior to the renal artery) is identified and its investing tissue is opened anteriorly along the vein. The left thumb and index finger can be used to assist in this dissection (**FIGURE 6**). This will reveal both the gonadal and the adrenal veins. The gonadal vein is dissected free of its investing tissue, ligated, and divided. There are several ways to ligate and divide the renal vein branches: they can be ligated with bipolar cautery or a Harmonic scalpel, stapled, or clipped. If using clips, care must be taken when clipping the renal vein side to ensure that the clips will not interfere with subsequent stapling of the vein. For difficult, large lumbar veins, greater exposure can be obtained posteriorly by retracting the kidney superomedially. Once the gonadal and lumbar veins are divided, the adrenal vein is likewise divided with the ultrasonic shears or between clips (**FIGURE 7**).

The renal artery usually lies superior and posterior to the renal vein. If it is difficult to identify from an anterior approach, it can be easily found posteriorly by retracting the kidney superolaterally and retracting the fully mobilized renal vein superiorly and anteriorly. The renal artery is freed from its thick plexus of investing neural and lymphatic tissue and separated from the renal vein. This dissection is performed away from the renal hilum to avoid injuring early segmental branches (**FIGURE 8**). Unlike the renal veins, which communicate widely, the segmental renal arteries are noncommunicating end arteries and should be preserved. Small upper pole branches (less than 3 mm in diameter) can be taken without significant consequence, but lower pole arteries must be preserved, as they may provide the principal blood supply to the ureter.

The adrenal gland is dissected off the kidney, staying closer to the gland to avoid upper pole segmental arteries. The kidney is ready for removal.

The ureter is clipped and divided, or stapled where it crosses the common or internal iliac artery origin or deeper (**FIGURE 9**). It is inspected for urine output, which is mandatory for removal of the kidney. If the ureter has been stapled, this step requires the removal of the proximal staple line. Papaverine can be applied topically to the renal vessels to reduce renal vasospasm. Mannitol and furosemide can be given prior to dividing the renal vessels to initiate diuresis before inducing ischemia.

Removal of the Kidney   Once the ureter is divided and the kidney is making urine, it can be removed. Heparin, usually 3000 units (30 units/kg), may be given at this time depending on surgeon preference. The renal artery is divided with a linear stapler using a vascular staple length (**FIGURE 10**). The renal vein is then stapled using the same device and same staple length. The ureter is held and protected by the hand holding the kidney during stapling. The left renal vein is divided distal to the left adrenal and gonadal veins to maximize its length. The kidney is removed through the hand port (**FIGURE 11**) and taken to the back table quickly for flushing with a cold heparinized solution (crystalloid or preservation solution). The vascular bed is inspected for bleeding.

Closure   Once hemostasis is secured, intraabdominal pressure is reduced to 5 mm Hg for 5 minutes to identify previously occult venous bleeding. A single simple stitch can be placed for subsequent closure of the 12-mm port sites. The hand-port incision is closed with simple interrupted 1-0 sutures. Before the 12-mm ports are removed, the camera can be reinserted and the midline closure inspected for problems, such as trapped omentum. The ports are removed. The skin incisions are closed with absorbable subcuticular sutures. Long-acting local anesthesia can be applied subcutaneously.

5

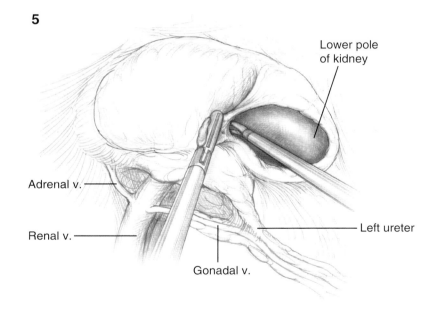

6

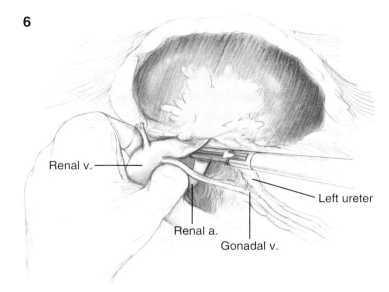

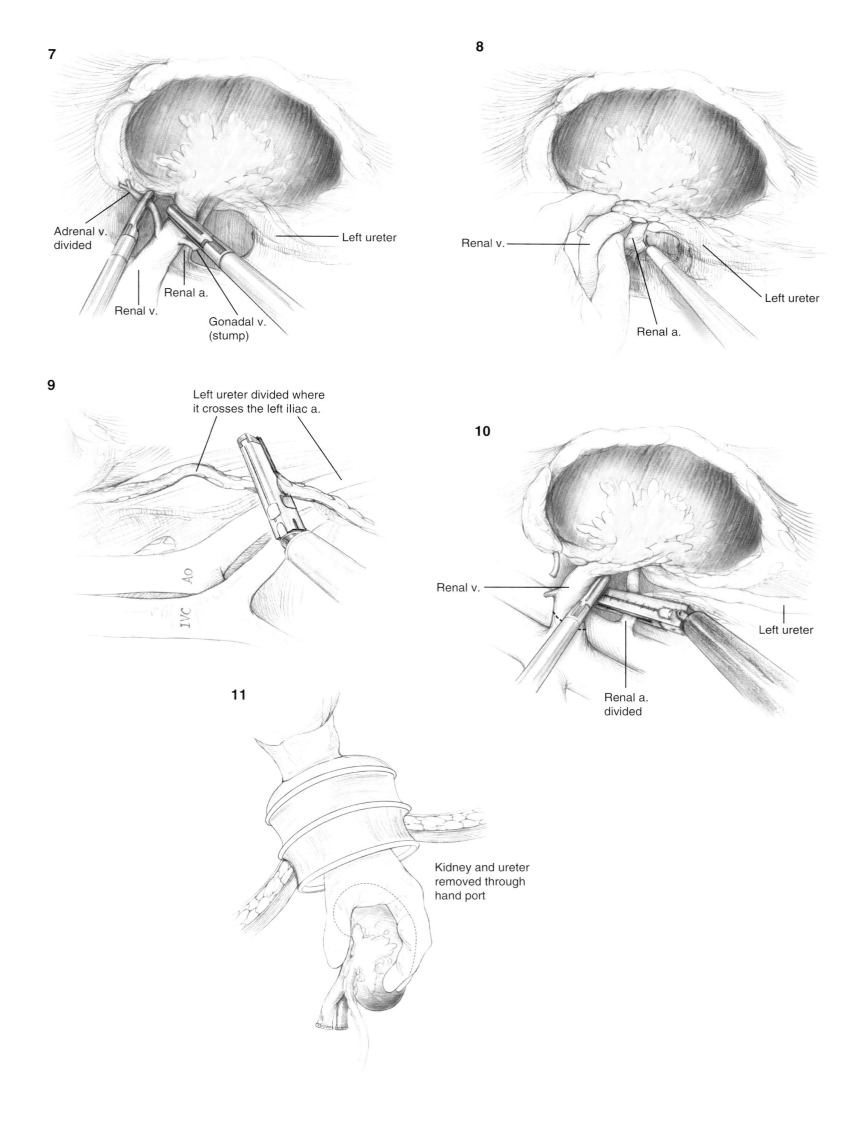

7

Adrenal v. divided

Renal v.

Renal a.

Gonadal v. (stump)

Left ureter

8

Renal v.

Renal a.

Left ureter

9

Left ureter divided where it crosses the left iliac a.

AO

IVC

10

Renal v.

Renal a. divided

Left ureter

11

Kidney and ureter removed through hand port

RIGHT DONOR NEPHRECTOMY

Incision, Placement of Trocars, and Exposure Although the hand port is placed in the same location, laparoscopic port placement for the right kidney differs from that for the left kidney (**FIGURE 12**). The 12-mm camera port is placed 6–8 cm superior to the hand port in the midline (or, for a large patient with a broad abdomen, a few centimeters to the right of the midline). The camera port must be placed to the right of the falciform ligament. A 12-mm working port is placed 2 cm inferior to the costal margin in the midclavicular line. A 5-mm retractor port is placed approximately 2 cm below the xiphoid. This port is for retraction of the liver with a flexible endoretractor.

Details of the Procedure The right colon is mobilized medially, and a Kocher maneuver is performed to expose the inferior vena cava (IVC) (**FIGURE 13**). The anterior tissue investing the vena cava is opened at the level of the right renal vein exposing its origin. Care must be taken to avoid tearing the gonadal vein as it inserts into the IVC just inferior to the right renal vein–IVC junction. The gonadal vein is usually ligated and divided near the vena cava. As in the left nephrectomy, the ureter is identified at the lower pole along with the gonadal vein and dissected off the psoas muscle anterolaterally as a unit to maintain maximal periureteral tissue (meso-ureter). Alternatively, the ureter can be identified in the pelvis and freed superiorly.

Gerota fascia is opened anteriorly, and the kidney is mobilized. This provides maximal exposure for the vascular dissection and, with the ureter in place, imposes little risk of torsion.

The right renal vein, which commonly has small inferior and superior (adrenal) branches, is dissected out anteriorly. The right renal artery is often seen just posterior to the vein. To free the artery, the kidney is retracted anteriorly and dissection conducted from a posterior approach. The renal artery is freed from its investing neural and lymphatic tissue. If there is an early renal artery bifurcation, the lumbar vein, which typically inserts just inferior to the artery, can be in the way. This lumbar vein can be divided to allow for mobilization of the vena cava medially and better exposure of proximal right renal artery. Once the renal vessels are freed, papaverine is applied. Mannitol and furosemide can be given.

The ureter is clipped and divided (or stapled) where it crosses the common iliac artery at the level of the origin of the internal iliac artery. The ureter is inspected for urine output, mandatory for removal of the kidney. The renal artery is divided first, then the right renal vein is divided through the upper medial port (with the camera moved to the more lateral port). It is generally helpful to retract the kidney laterally with the left hand to provide more renal vein length to facilitate stapling (**FIGURE 14**). If this angle is awkward, an extra 12-mm port can be placed inferiorly in the deep right lower quadrant, at or medial to the midclavicular line, to allow for stapling of the renal vein parallel to the vena cava. (The stapler is placed under the hand, which is putting the kidney on stretch laterally.)

THE PURELY LAPAROSCOPIC APPROACH The advantage of the pure laparoscopic approach is the ability to use a lower Pfannenstiel incision for removal of the kidney. At least three ports are needed. For the left nephrectomy, an umbilical port is used for the camera with one lateral port (lateral to the rectus muscle) and one upper midline port (placed half the distance from the xiphoid to the umbilicus). If needed, a hand can be inserted through the Pfannenstiel incision. An endocatch bag (or a hand) is used for removal of the kidney. A similar arrangement can be used for the purely laparoscopic right donor nephrectomy.

POSTOPERATIVE CARE The orogastric tube is removed after extubation. Patient-controlled analgesia (PCA) is used postoperatively. For the first 12 hours postoperatively, supplemental analgesia may be needed if the patient cannot maintain adequate analgesia using the PCA. Ketorolac is a useful adjunct for opioid analgesia and may be administered. Nausea is aggressively treated. The Foley catheter is removed on postoperative day 1, and ambulation is encouraged. The hemoglobin and hematocrit are checked on postoperative day 1. Creatinine can be checked as well. The patient may begin on clear liquids on the day of surgery; diet is advanced as tolerated. To ensure adequate analgesia, patients are typically not discharged until at least postoperative day 2. Comfort level is a primary determinant of the day of discharge for these special patients. Early resumption of the activities of daily living is encouraged. Because there is an abdominal incision, patients are counseled to avoid heavy lifting for at least 6 weeks. ■

12   **Right Donor Nephrectomy**

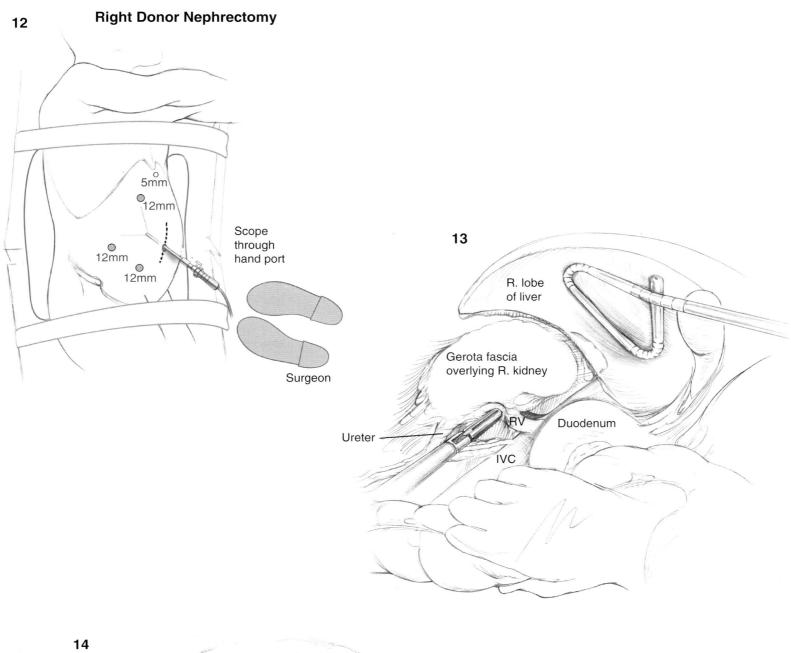

5mm

12mm

12mm

12mm

Scope
through
hand port

Surgeon

13

R. lobe
of liver

Gerota fascia
overlying R. kidney

Ureter

RV

Duodenum

IVC

14

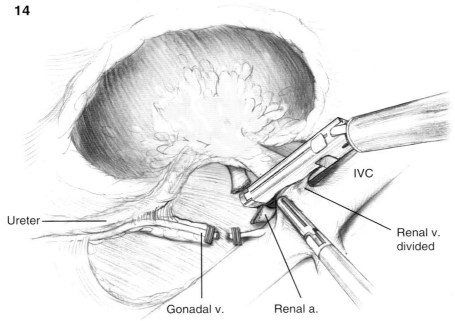

Ureter

IVC

Renal v.
divided

Gonadal v.

Renal a.

SECTION VIII

MINIMALLY INVASIVE HERNIA REPAIR

ABDOMINAL WALL HERNIA REPAIR

INDICATIONS Laparoscopic ventral hernia repair can be considered for all primary abdominal wall hernias and the majority of secondary incisional hernias, including recurrent hernias. The laparoscopic approach has several advantages. First, laparoscopy allows the surgeon to clearly define the edges of the defect from within the peritoneum with the abdominal wall completely relaxed. Second, if pneumoperitoneum can be obtained, the hernia reduced, and adhesions taken down without bowel injury, the surgeon can place a widely underlapping prosthesis that should result in a lower recurrence rate than a traditional open repair. The increased durability of the repair results from tissue ingrowth from the peritoneum to the mesh over a wide surface area rather than from simple defect-edge to mesh-edge suture approximation, which is commonly used for open repair. Finally, postoperative pain and time to recovery are reduced when the mesh is placed laparoscopically.

The main disadvantage of the minimally invasive approach is its technical difficulty. The surgeon must be cautious during laparoscopic hernia reduction and adhesiolysis to avoid bowel injury. As well, the laparoscopic repair may not be ideal for giant incisional hernia, where a large bridging piece of mesh may not provide adequate abdominal wall reconstruction. Under these conditions, component separation techniques, usually performed with an open approach, may be a better option.

PREOPERATIVE PREPARATION Patients with ventral hernias usually complain of mild abdominal pain associated with a noticeable bulge. In the majority of patients, physical examination alone will define the dimensions of the hernia defect. The contents of the hernia, such as omentum or bowel, can also be palpated as they readily reduce from the sac back into the peritoneum. Unless the surgeon cannot determine the presence of a hernia on physical exam, a computed tomography (CT) scan generally adds little to the preoperative planning. If the patient is obese and the hernia shows no evidence of incarceration, significant preoperative weight loss is advisable but often not feasible. The same is true for smoking—smokers are known to have a higher hernia recurrence rate. Smokers should be advised that postoperative coughing may compromise the stability of the repair. The patient should stop all anticoagulants and antiplatelet agents 10 days prior to surgery. The surgeon can consider a bowel prep for larger hernias, although it is not mandatory.

Patients with erythema, skin discoloration, severe pain, very tender hernias, or symptoms consistent with bowel obstruction may have incarcerated bowel and should be emergently or urgently taken to the operating room for open reduction and repair. Experienced laparoscopic surgeons may consider a laparoscopic approach to incarcerated hernias, but open exploration is more appropriate in most cases.

ANESTHESIA General anesthesia with neuromuscular blockade is required for this operation. An intravenous dose of an antistaphylococcal antibiotic should be given 30 minutes prior to skin incision. An orogastric tube decompresses the stomach, and a urinary catheter drains the bladder.

POSITION The patient is supine with both arms tucked. Because the surgeon may need to move from the right to the left side and from superior to inferior as the hernia defect is exposed and the mesh secured circumferentially, an outstretched arm will limit the surgeon's options on that side of the patient. The assistant stands on the same side of the patient so that both surgeon and assistant are facing the same direction. At least two monitors (one on each side of the patient) are recommended (**FIGURE 1**). A plastic adhesive drape can be placed on the patient's abdomen to facilitate marking the borders of the defect and subsequent mesh measurement.

INCISION AND EXPOSURE The initial entry into the peritoneal space must be at least 10 cm from the hernia in order to avoid adhesions and to allow enough room for a 5-cm mesh underlap. The lateral upper quadrants are preferred locations. The open (Hasson) technique or Veress needle entry in the left upper quadrant (Palmer point) is advisable to avoid bowel injury. A 10- to 12-mm port that will eventually accommodate the rolled-up mesh is the ideal first port. Once pneumoperitoneum of 15 mm Hg is obtained safely, the peritoneal cavity is inspected to determine the extent of the adhesions (if any), to define the hernia defect, and to plan further port placement. At least one more 10-mm port on the other side of the defect is usually necessary for circumferential laparoscopic visualization. Two or three 5-mm ports are placed to facilitate dissection with laparoscopic scissors and atraumatic graspers (**FIGURE 2**). The surgeon may need to place additional 10-mm ports or switch out a 5-mm port for a 10-mm port during the procedure. One or two 5-mm ports opposite the operating position are helpful later in the procedure for securing the mesh near the operating ports.

The omentum is the most frequent inhabitant of the hernia sac and can be bluntly teased from the defect under direct vision with atraumatic graspers. A hand pressing externally may facilitate reduction. Careful cauterization of omental adhesions with a curved Maryland grasper will be necessary. If it is determined that small bowel or colon is adherent within the sac, very cautious sharp dissection with minimal cauterization is advised (**FIGURE 3**). The surgeon should not hesitate to move from one side of the patient to the other to approach the adhesions safely. Mature judgment and experience will allow the surgeon to decide if the laparoscopic approach is still feasible.

Once the hernia defect is fully exposed, the surgeon measures the size of the defect and chooses an adequately large prosthesis. A precise measurement is neither possible nor necessary. The pneumoperitoneum is reduced to 7–8 mm Hg, and the dimensions of the defect plus a 5-cm margin are estimated by inserting a local anesthetic needle externally and observing its entrance internally. This maneuver is repeated circumferentially (**FIGURE 4**).

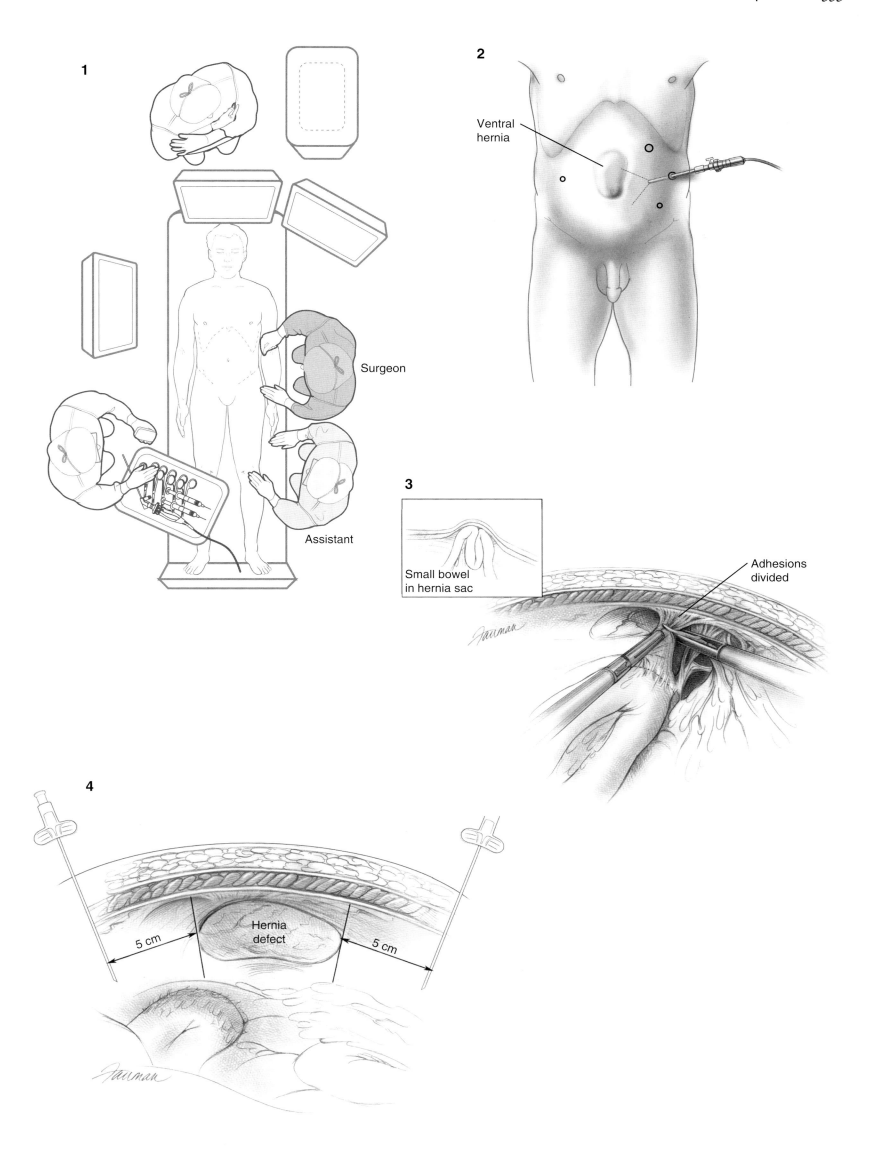

1

Surgeon

Assistant

2

Ventral hernia

3

Small bowel in hernia sac

Adhesions divided

4

5 cm

Hernia defect

5 cm

INCISION AND EXPOSURE If the patient's subcutaneous fat layer is quite thick, this mesh measurement will tend to be an overestimate because the curvature of the skin surface will be larger than the curvature of the peritoneal surface. If an Ioban has been placed, the outline of the fascial defect and 5-cm margin can be marked in concentric circles. This will allow the surgeon to assess the final position of the mesh and plan placement. The prosthesis is chosen and trimmed to the estimated size. At least four tacking sutures of 0 polypropylene are placed at equal intervals 1 cm from the edge of the prosthesis (**FIGURE 5**). The prosthesis is rolled up and placed through the 12-mm port. A single loose suture can be placed through the roll to prevent premature unrolling of the mesh. For large pieces of mesh, it may be necessary to remove the port and place the mesh manually through the port incision. A 15 mm Hg pneumoperitoneum is reobtained.

What follows is often the most tedious part of the operation. The mesh must be laid out over the viscera and the various Prolene tacking sutures disentangled. This process may be simplified if, before the mesh is placed into the abdomen, it is rolled halfway to the middle from two opposite sides. Two of the opposing tacking sutures should be left outside of the mesh roll. After the rolling is complete, a single suture can be placed and loosely tied to hold the complex in place and keep it from unrolling (**FIGURE 5, INSET**). With this technique, only half of the tacking sutures are exposed, and two ends of the mesh are fixed to the peritoneum initially. When ready, the suture holding the roll together can be snipped and the rest of the prosthesis unrolled.

The pneumoperitoneum is again reduced to 7–8 mm Hg and maintained during fixation of the mesh. Two principles guide the surgeon's judgment during mesh fixation. First, a pneumoperitoneum enlarges the surface area of the peritoneum from what it will be once the pneumoperitoneum is released. Thus, by diminishing the pneumoperitoneum during fixation, the surgeon is estimating more accurately the eventual position of the mesh. Second, polypropylene and polyester prostheses contract significantly and unpredictably during tissue ingrowth. The prosthesis should be placed neither taut nor too loose, but some laxity is necessary.

The polypropylene tacking sutures are fixed to the peritoneum by passing a transfascial suturing device through a small stab incision and through the abdominal wall, grasping one arm of the polypropylene suture, and pulling it back through the abdominal wall (**FIGURE 6**). The transfascial suturing

device is then passed back through the same stab incision but through the abdominal wall 1 cm from the first suture passage, and the second suture end is grasped. This process is completed with each of the four preplaced Prolene sutures. A knot is tied in the subcutaneous tissue.

If a very large piece of prosthetic has been placed, additional transfascial sutures may need to be placed. To do this, longer Prolene sutures are fixed to the suture passer, then passed through stab wounds and through the edge of the Prolene prosthesis 3 cm apart, around the circumference of the mesh. With each suture, the free end is left in the abdominal cavity while the suture-passing needle is passed through the same stab wound, but through the fascia and mesh 1 cm from the first puncture. The surgeon places the free end into the jaw of the suture passer; it is withdrawn, and a knot is tied in the subcutaneous fat (**FIGURE 7**). The surgeon may need to revise the locations of the passages to adjust the prosthesis to prevent excessive folds or skewing. A tacking device completes the fixation. These absorbable tacks encircle the hernia 1 cm from the edge of the defect and close the gaps between the tacking sutures (**FIGURE 8**). It is important to avoid placing tacks into the hernia defect, as the tissue may be very thin there, allowing the tacks to penetrate the skin surface.

Before port removal, the omentum is inspected for bleeding and the bowel for previously undetected injury. The pneumoperitoneum is allowed to completely escape, and the ports are all removed. All ports sites are liberally infiltrated with 0.5% bupivacaine mixed 50:50 with 1% lidocaine with epinephrine. The external fascial defects created by the 10- or 12-mm ports are closed in a single fascial layer with the same technique use to fix the mesh. The skin is closed with subcuticular absorbable monofilament suture.

POSTOPERATIVE CARE Patients with smaller hernias and minimal adhesiolysis may be discharged on the day of surgery. Larger hernia repairs necessitate at least an overnight stay for pain control and diet tolerance. Intravenous ketorolac, intravenous or oral narcotics, and antiemetics are ordered. Clear liquids may be started within several hours of surgery and advanced to regular diet as tolerated. Patients are advised to avoid heavy lifting and strenuous activity for 2 to 4 weeks, depending on the size of the hernia. Seromas accumulating in the hernia sac are common and are followed for several weeks or months without aspiration in most cases. ■

5

Prosthetic mesh
trimmed to size
and tacking sutures
placed

1 cm

5 cm

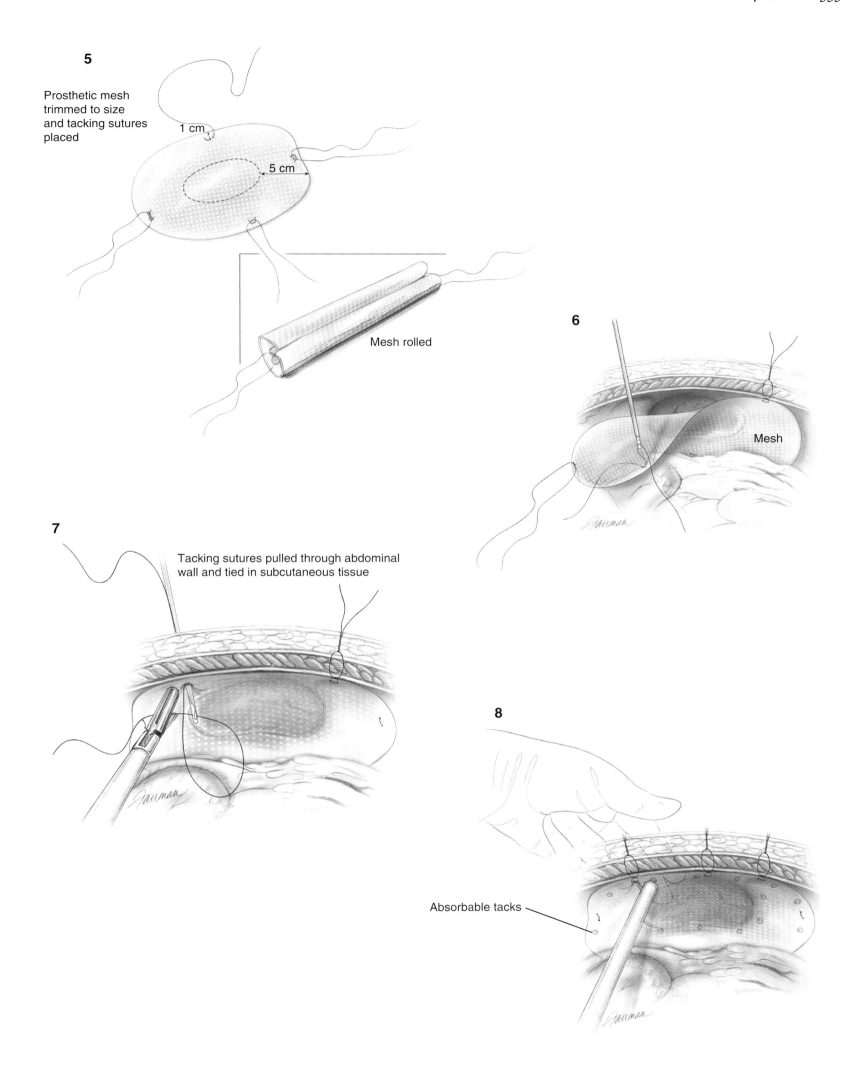

Mesh rolled

6

Mesh

7

Tacking sutures pulled through abdominal
wall and tied in subcutaneous tissue

8

Absorbable tacks

INGUINAL HERNIA REPAIR

INDICATIONS Laparoscopic inguinal hernia repair may be offered to patients who desire a rapid return to full activity, have bilateral inguinal hernias, or have a recurrent hernia where an open anterior approach has failed. The main benefits of laparoscopic repair are a decrease in postoperative pain and an improved time to recovery compared with the open approach. This advantage is particularly beneficial in patients with bilateral hernias because both hernias can be repaired under the same anesthetic without an increase in postoperative pain and disability. The benefit to repairing a recurrent inguinal hernia laparoscopically is that the laparoscopic approach can identify the exact location of the recurrence from the interior of the groin and the defect can be patched without extensive dissection through scarred tissue.

The disadvantages of the laparoscopic approach compared to the open approach are its increased cost and need for general anesthesia. In addition, the laparoscopic procedure is more difficult to learn than open repair, which may result in more complications and early recurrence before the "learning curve" is surpassed. These disadvantages have made laparoscopic inguinal hernia repair less frequently applied than laparoscopic cholecystectomy or laparoscopic appendectomy.

PREOPERATIVE PREPARATION Patients with an inguinal hernia describe the appearance of a groin bulge with minimal or mild groin discomfort. The bulge is usually intermittent in appearance—that is, it generally disappears when the patient is recumbent and reappears when standing. With time the bulge enlarges. Radiographic confirmation is not necessary if the surgeon can see the hernia or palpate it on physical exam. Small inguinal and femoral hernias are not always obvious on physical exam. Groin ultrasound, computed tomography, or magnetic resonance imaging may help confirm the diagnosis, but they are only 80% to 90% sensitive and less specific. An occasional patient may need laparoscopy to diagnose or disprove inguinal hernia. If present, the hernia can be repaired using the intraperitoneal approach.

There are several kinds of inguinal hernia. The laparoscopic approach is appropriate for the three most common types: indirect, direct, and femoral hernia. It is not necessary to differentiate between an indirect and direct inguinal hernia, preoperatively. A femoral hernia will usually be apparent on physical exam, but if not, the laparoscopic approach allows the surgeon to accurately identify the type of hernia and effectively tailor the repair to the pathology. Large and long-standing inguinal hernias, such as scrotal hernias, pantaloon hernias (direct and indirect inguinal hernia combined) and sliding hernias, require more skill to repair with a minimally invasive technique. A painful inguinal hernia that will not reduce opens

the possibility of bowel strangulation and should be explored urgently. The minimally invasive approach is not well suited for this indication except in the most expert surgeons' hands. In this setting an expert may choose to reduce the incarcerated bowel laparoscopically. If it "pinks up," not requiring resection, the surgeon may fix the hernia transperitoneally or "convert" to a preperitoneal approach to fix the hernia.

The patient should stop all anticoagulants and antiplatelet medications 7 days prior to operation. Bowel prep is not necessary. Smokers are known to have a higher recurrence rate for open inguinal hernia repair than nonsmokers but it is unknown if this risk applies to laparoscopic hernia repair as well.

ANESTHESIA General anesthesia with neuromuscular blockade is required for this operation. An intravenous dose of antistaphylococcal antibiotic should be given prior to skin incision. An orogastric tube decompresses the stomach and a urinary catheter drains the bladder. Local anesthetic with 1% lidocaine (including epinephrine) mixed with 0.5% bupivacaine is infiltrated prior to skin incisions.

POSITION The patient is supine with both arms tucked. The monitor is placed over the patient's feet, the surgeon stands contralateral to the hernia to be repaired, and the first assistant stands across the table (**FIGURE 1**).

TOTALLY EXTRAPERITONEAL (TEP) HERNIA REPAIR

Incision and Exposure A 2-cm infraumbilical horizontal incision is made inferior to the umbilicus. Two additional 5-mm ports will be placed later in the suprapubic position and halfway between the pubis and the umbilicus (**FIGURE 2**). The subcutaneous tissue is bluntly retracted to expose the fascia. A 1-cm-wide portion of the midline fascia extending onto the anterior rectus sheath fascia on the side of the hernia should be exposed (**FIGURE 3**). Two Kocher clamps are placed on the fascia—one on the midline, and one on the ipsilateral rectus sheath—and a 1-cm vertical incision is made between the two clamps, thereby exposing fibers of the rectus abdominis muscle. The muscle is retracted laterally to expose the posterior rectus sheath fascia. Using blunt finger dissection, or a blunt pean clamp, the retromuscular space is opened in the midline to allow placement of the dissecting balloon into the space (**FIGURE 4**).

Approximately 30 squeezes of the bulb are adequate to enlarge the retromuscular, preperitoneal space under direct laparoscopic visualization (**FIGURE 5**). The balloon is left inflated for 1 to 2 minutes to allow tamponade of any small bleeding vessels.

1

2   **Totally Extraperitoneal (TEP) Hernia Repair**

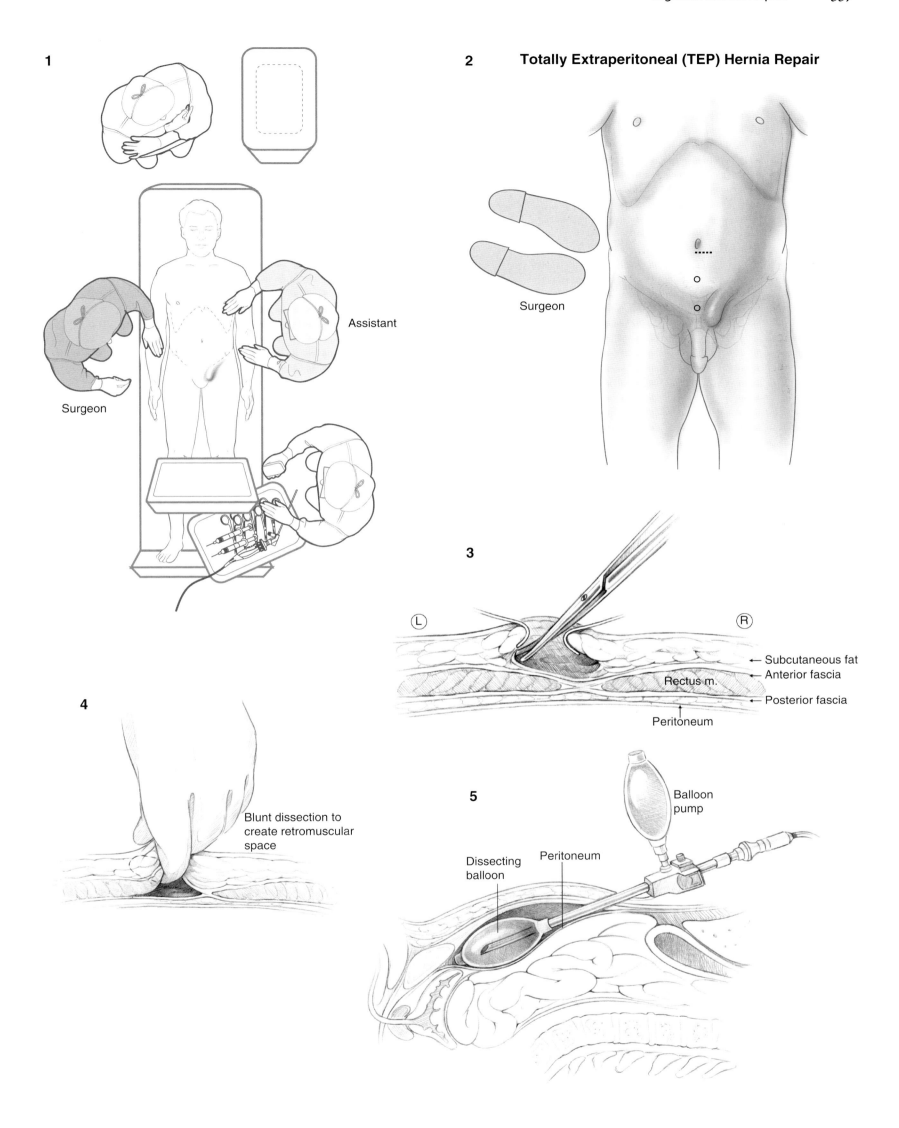

Assistant

Surgeon

Surgeon

3

L   R

← Subcutaneous fat
← Anterior fascia

Rectus m.

← Posterior fascia

Peritoneum

4

Blunt dissection to create retromuscular space

5

Balloon pump

Dissecting balloon   Peritoneum

Incision and Exposure If a specialized dissecting balloon trocar has been used, the large balloon may be removed and replaced with a vertical "structural" balloon that maintains the retromuscular space. Alternatively, a 10- to 12-mm blunt (Hasson) port can be passed into the same space and secured with two transfixing sutures placed through the anterior rectus sheath. The space is insufflated with CO_2 to a pressure of 10 to 15 mm Hg. A 30- or 45-degree laparoscope is passed. At this point, the surgeon should see the midline pubis, the areolar fat of the preperitoneal space, and the inferior epigastric artery and vein. Additionally, the direct, indirect and femoral spaces can be evaluated for herniated contents (**FIGURE 6**). Sometimes it will be necessary to bluntly remove additional extraperitoneal fat to visualize these structures, even after thorough balloon dissection.

The two 5-mm ports are placed in the lower midline after identifying their preperitoneal entry point with the needle of the local anesthetic syringe. The lowest port should be placed no closer than 2 cm from the pubis, and the upper port should split the difference between the umbilical and suprapubic ports (see Figure 2).

Dissection of the Hernia Blunt dissection with blunt-tipped grasping instruments is used to expose the pubis, the iliopubic tract, the medial margin of the femoral vein, the floor of the inguinal canal, and the cord structures. It is rarely necessary to cauterize or cut vessels or tissue during this dissection. Care is taken to avoid injury to the femoral artery and vein, which are covered with fat and lymphatics at the lower, lateral margin of the field. Similarly, bleeding can be minimized by identifying and preserving the inferior epigastric vessels running across the exposed rectus muscle, and obturator vessels that may cross over the iliopubic tract. It is particularly important during dissection and mesh fixation to avoid manipulation or tacking in the area shaded (**FIGURE 7**).

6

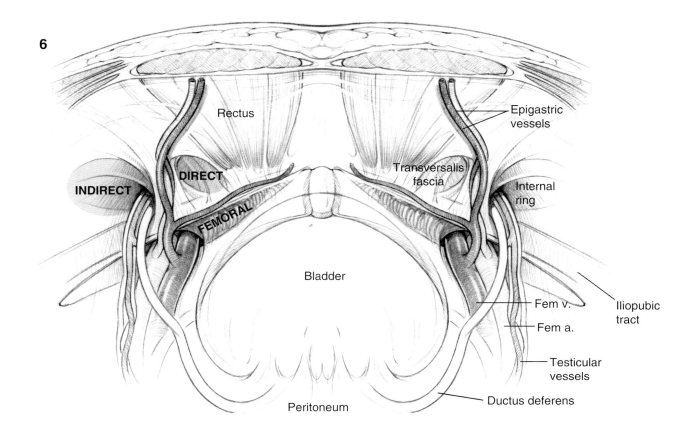

Rectus

Epigastric vessels

DIRECT

INDIRECT

Transversalis fascia

Internal ring

FEMORAL

Bladder

Iliopubic tract

Fem v.

Fem a.

Testicular vessels

Ductus deferens

Peritoneum

7

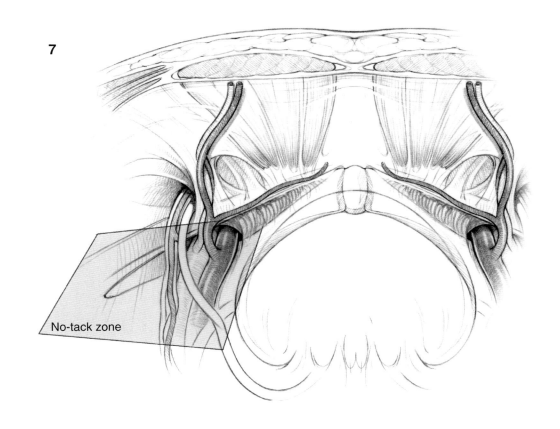

No-tack zone

Dissection of the Hernia At this point it should be anatomically apparent whether the patient has a direct defect through the floor of the inguinal canal or an indirect sac associated with the cord structures. If an indirect sac is present, it is separated from the cord structures bluntly (**FIGURE 8A**). It is possible to completely reduce a small sac into the preperitoneal space, but large sacs, especially those extending into the scrotum, may not be reducible. In this case the sac is ligated with o silk proximally but not distally (**FIGURE 8B**). The sac is then transected with scissors. In the advanced case of a sliding hernia, it may be necessary to open the sac before ligation to ensure that all intraperitoneal structures are protected. The sac is then closed with a purse-string suture. Under these circumstances it is necessary to "vent" the pneumoperitoneum that develops with an additional 5-mm trocar placed into the peritoneal cavity to maintain preperitoneal working room.

If after careful dissection neither a direct or indirect hernia is discovered, it is possible that the hernia is actually femoral and obscured by femoral fat and lymphatics. In this circumstance the preperitoneal approach should be converted to the intraperitoneal approach. The intraperitoneal approach should confirm the location of the expected inguinal or femoral hernia.

At any time during the dissection, if tears are made in the peritoneum that allow the insufflation to enter the peritoneum in enough volume to prevent careful preperitoneal dissection, the tear should be repaired or the operation converted to intraperitoneal hernia repair.

Mesh Repair Once the direct hernia (if present) is reduced, or the indirect sac (if present) is reduced completely or ligated, a piece of mesh that will cover the pubis, the floor of the inguinal canal, the cord structures, and approximately 3 cm lateral to the cord is chosen. The mesh should be contoured to allow passage of the cord. Some surgeons prefer to place a lateral slit in the mesh to allow the cord to enter the center of the mesh (**FIGURE 9**).

The mesh is grasped in the middle and pushed through the umbilical port blindly. The 30-degree scope is replaced and the mesh is manipulated into position. The mesh should cover the defects and a 2-cm margin. If the indirect sac is not ligated, it should be laid proximal to or even tacked to the back of the mesh to prevent it from insinuating under the mesh.

If bilateral repairs are necessary, both sides are dissected before inserting any mesh. Usually two pieces of mesh that overlap in the pubic midline are used.

Tacking the mesh in place is commonly performed, but is not required. If the mesh is not tacked, the size of the mesh should be generous because some slippage of the mesh will occur. Tissue glue or specialized "gripping" mesh products have been used, as well, to help avoid the need for tacking. If a tacker is used, care should be exercised to stay away from the "triangle of pain" and the "triangle of doom," which—when put together—create a tetrahedron (see Figure 7). Tacks in this area risk nerve and vascular injury, which may be disabling. When applying tacks to the abdominal wall, it is critical that the surgeon be able to palpate the end of the tacker through the abdominal wall (**FIGURES 10 AND 11**). The only exception to this are the tacks placed in the pubis and the iliopectineal line (Cooper ligament).

8a

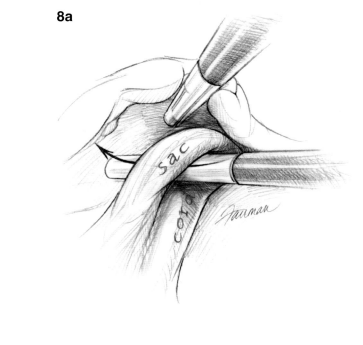

8b

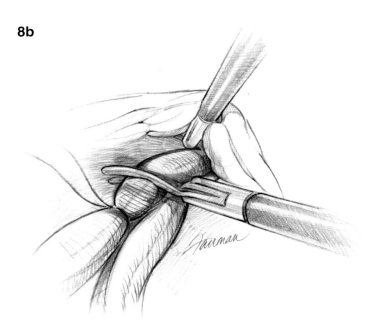

9

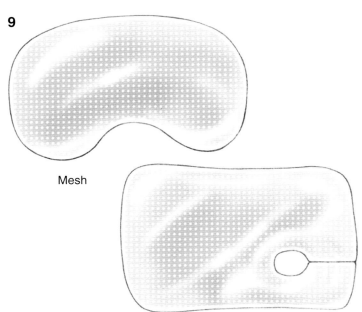

Mesh

10

Tacker palpated
through abdominal wall

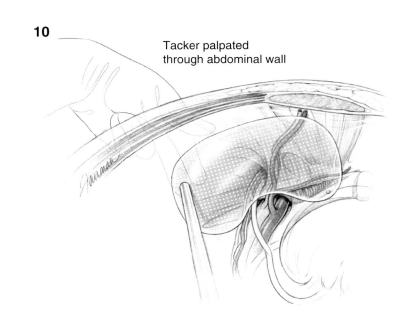

11

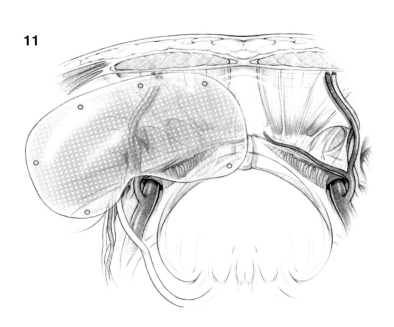

TRANSABDOMINAL PREPERITONEAL (TAPP) HERNIA REPAIR If the intraperitoneal approach is necessary, the trocar positions are spread to allow better "triangulation" than can be achieved with the TEP procedure (**FIGURE 12**). TAPP is most valuable in the case where the preperitoneal space cannot be opened as a result of previous lower midline surgery, when a large tear in the peritoneum is made during TEP, or if the hernia cannot be located preperitoneally.

The floor of the inguinal canal and the cord are exposed through a horizontal peritoneal slit from the midline to a point lateral to the internal inguinal ring (**FIGURE 13**). An indirect sac should be obvious using this approach. Before opening the peritoneum, the indirect sac can be invaginated into the peritoneum bluntly and ligated. The same piece of mesh described above is laid or tacked into place, and the peritoneal slit should be closed with tacks or preferably sutured with absorbable suture (**FIGURE 14**). It is often difficult or impossible to completely close this peritoneum over the mesh. Thus, it may be wise to use a bilayer mesh to help prevent intestinal adhesions when performing this kind of hernia repair. It is this portion of the intraperitoneal approach (TAPP) that is its chief drawback when compared to the completely preperitoneal approach (TEP).

CLOSURE The CO_2 is allowed to escape and the ports are removed. The fascial defect below the umbilicus is repaired with a 0 absorbable suture, either figure-of-eight or two interrupted sutures. Skin incisions are closed with subcuticular absorbable suture and strips. The wounds should be infiltrated again with local anesthetic.

POSTOPERATIVE CARE The patient is discharged home as soon as he/she can urinate. Postoperative urinary retention is uncommon. The patient is counseled to avoid lifting more than 25 pounds for 10 days to 2 weeks, but is allowed to return to work as soon as they feel able depending on their employment. At follow-up, a distal remnant hernia sac may develop a seroma, but rarely is aspiration necessary, as spontaneous resolution is the rule. ■

Transabdominal Preperitoneal (TAPP) Hernia Repair

12

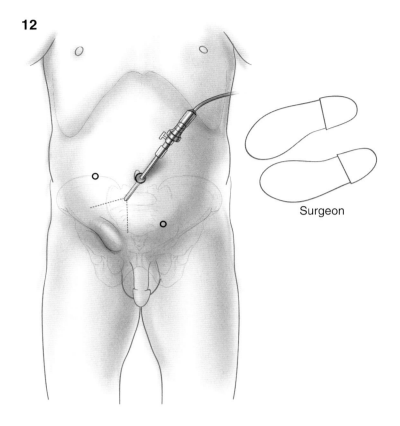

Surgeon

13

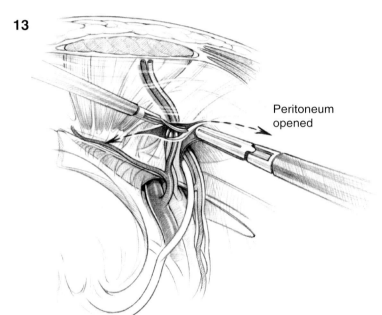

Peritoneum opened

14

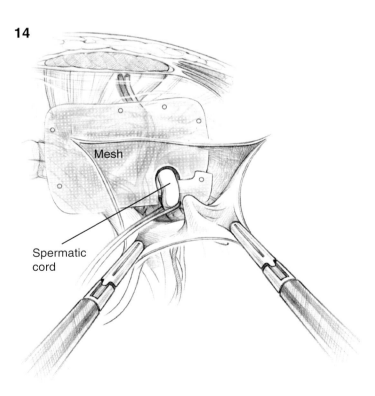

Mesh

Spermatic cord

MINIMALLY INVASIVE COLORECTAL SURGERY

CHAPTER 46

APPENDECTOMY

INDICATIONS Laparoscopic abdominal exploration and appendectomy is indicated when acute appendicitis is suspected. The laparoscopic approach is particularly advantageous in young women, in obese patients, or when the diagnosis is in doubt.

PREOPERATIVE PREPARATION In the majority of cases, the diagnosis is easily established by clinical history and physical examination. Laboratory evaluation such as a complete blood count and urinalysis, may provide supportive data. When warranted, ultrasound or computed tomography (CT) scans may confirm the diagnosis. The patient is given appropriate intravenous antibiotics prior to surgery.

ANESTHESIA General anesthesia with endotracheal intubation is necessary for this operation. Complete neuromuscular blockade is required. If there has been little bleeding during the laparoscopic dissection, ketorolac may be given at procedure completion to diminish postoperative pain.

POSITION The patient is positioned supine with arms tucked at the sides. This allows the surgeon and assistant to move cephalad as required. The surgeon stands on the patient's left side; the assistant stands near the patient's left shoulder. The operative monitor is placed near the patient's hip on the right side (**FIGURE 1**).

OPERATIVE PREPARATION A Foley catheter and orogastric tube are placed after the induction of anesthesia. Decompression of the bladder is of particular importance if a suprapubic port site is used. The abdomen from the nipple lines to the pubis is shaved with clippers after induction of anesthesia, and the abdomen is sterilely prepped in the routine manner.

Depending on the surgeon's preference, the appendectomy may be performed with an endoscopic linear stapler, ultrasonic dissector, or pretied surgical ligature. Generally a 10-mm, 30-degree and a 5-mm, 30-degree laparoscope are made available for dissection and specimen extraction, respectively.

DETAILS OF PROCEDURE

Trocar Position Laparoscopic appendectomy is performed with a three-trocar technique. The size of the trocars depends on the instrumentation. Maximum flexibility is obtained by using one 12-mm trocar and two 5-mm trocars.

Because the abdominal wall is thinnest in the region of the umbilicus, this operation commences with insufflation of the abdomen using the Veress needle technique placed through the umbilicus. Alternatively, initial access is achieved via the Hasson technique at the umbilicus.

A 12-mm port is placed at the umbilicus. A 10-mm 30-degree laparoscope is placed through this trocar and used to guide the placement of additional trocars. A 5-mm port is then placed in the left lower quadrant, keeping lateral to the rectus muscle to avoid injury to the inferior epigastric vessels. The third port is a 5-mm port placed in the midline suprapubic position. Placement of this port is often aided by using a grasper through the left lower quadrant port to place anterior pressure against the supravesicular fat pad that would otherwise be deflected down as the last trocar is placed (**FIGURE 2**).

An alternative port placement to facilitate dissection of a retrocecal appendix uses a 12-mm port at the umbilicus for the camera, a 5-mm port in the right upper quadrant, and a 5-mm port in the left lower quadrant.

Appendectomy The patient is placed in a steep Trendelenburg position with the right side rotated upward to allow the small bowel to slide away from the right lower quadrant. Complete endoscopic inspection of the abdomen and pelvis is performed to confirm the diagnosis. If the appendix appears grossly normal but no other source of pain is found, it may still be reasonable to proceed with the appendectomy. In many cases a fecolith or small focus of inflammation is ultimately documented on the final pathology.

If the appendix is not immediately visible, the antimesenteric taenia coli of the right colon can be traced back to the cecum and ultimately to the base of the appendix. Using the left-hand port, the appendix is elevated anteriorly with an atraumatic grasper or Babcock clamp. If the appendix is significantly inflamed, a pretied surgical ligature can be used to provide secure retraction with less risk of fragmenting the appendix than if it were elevated with a grasper (**FIGURE 3**).

Division of the mesoappendix facilitates exposure of the base of the appendix, ensuring that the appendix is resected in its entirety. The mesoappendix may be divided with cautery and clips or with ultrasonic dissection. An endoscopic stapler may be used to divide the mesoappendix after making a window in the avascular area where the mesoappendix meets the base of the appendix (**FIGURES 4 AND 5**). This may be the most secure method for a very inflamed appendix, as the appendiceal artery may bleed a surprising amount when it is inflamed.

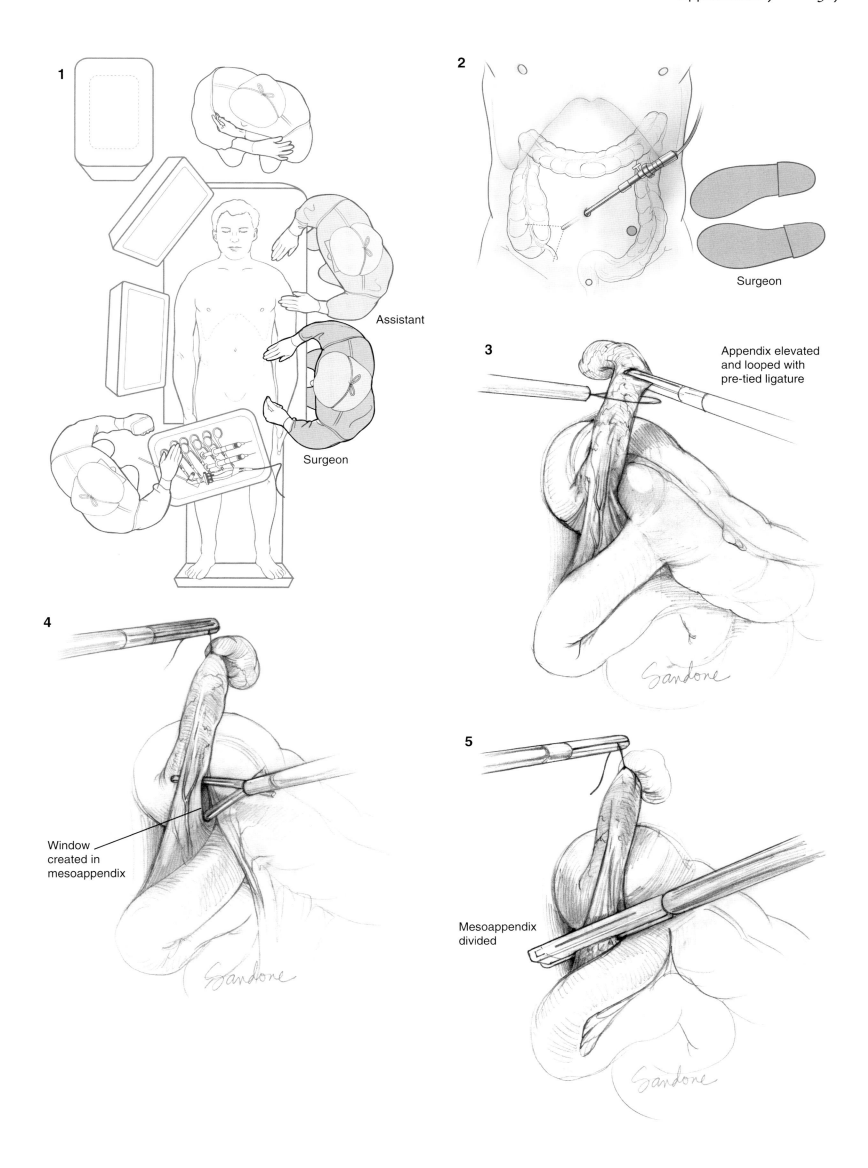

1

Assistant

Surgeon

2

Surgeon

3 Appendix elevated
and looped with
pre-tied ligature

Sandone

4

Window
created in
mesoappendix

Sandone

5

Mesoappendix
divided

Sandone

Appendectomy After division of the mesoappendix, the appendix is divided at its base with a second application of the endoscopic stapler (**FIGURE 6**). In cases where the base of the appendix is inflamed, it may be necessary to incorporate a small portion of the cecum within the staple line. Care should be taken to avoid injury to the ileocecal valve, right ureter, and adjacent small bowel before the stapler is fired.

Alternatively, the appendix may be divided with scissors. The base of the appendix is cleared circumferentially of any adipose or connective tissue. A pretied suture ligature is applied at the base, and a second ligature is placed more distally on the appendix. The appendix is divided sharply between the ligatures (**FIGURE 7**). Care should be taken not to apply excessive electrosurgery to the appendix during its division. Appendiceal stump leaks may occur when excessive coagulation results in tissue sloughing at the point of the proximal ligature.

The appendix may be retrieved by pulling it within the 12-mm port (**FIGURE 8**). The port and appendix are then removed together, thereby avoiding contamination of the abdominal wall. If the appendix is bulky or grossly contaminated, it should be placed in a specimen bag and retrieved through the 12-mm port site (**FIGURE 9**).

Alternative Technique for the Retrocecal or Gangrenous Appendix In the case of an appendix located in the retrocecal position, it is often difficult to start the dissection by finding the tip of the appendix. This may also be true when the tip of the appendix is necrotic or perforated. In these situations, it is easier to begin by isolating the base of the appendix and dividing it with an endoscopic stapler (**FIGURE 10**). This provides visualization of the adjacent mesoappendix, which can then be divided with an endoscopic stapler or ultrasonic shears (**FIGURE 11**). After proximal division, the appendix can be carefully dissected out of the retroperitoneum or "peeled" off the cecum using a combination of blunt and sharp techniques (**FIGURE 12**).

POSTOPERATIVE CARE Pain relief is usually obtained with intravenous ketorolac and judicious use of narcotics. The Foley catheter is removed in the operating room, and the patient transferred to the inpatient ward. Patients should be observed at least overnight to ensure pain control and resumption of a diet. Drains are rarely indicated in acute appendicitis, but may be of value if an abscess cavity is discovered during the dissection. ■

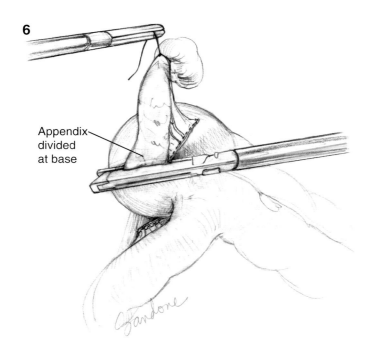

6

Appendix divided at base

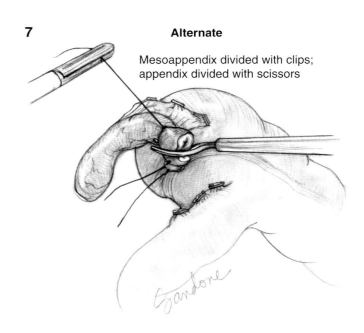

7   Alternate

Mesoappendix divided with clips; appendix divided with scissors

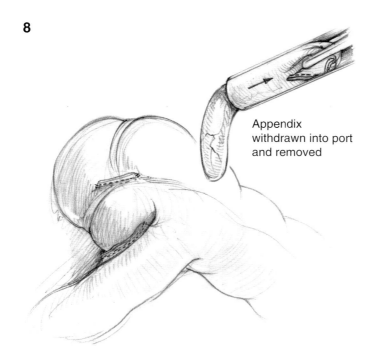

8

Appendix withdrawn into port and removed

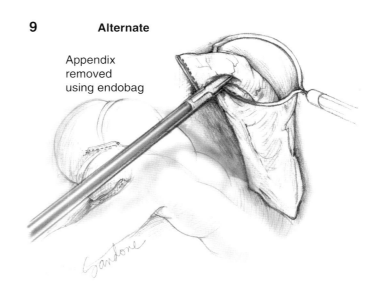

9   Alternate

Appendix removed using endobag

Retrocecal Appendix

10

Base of appendix
divided with stapler

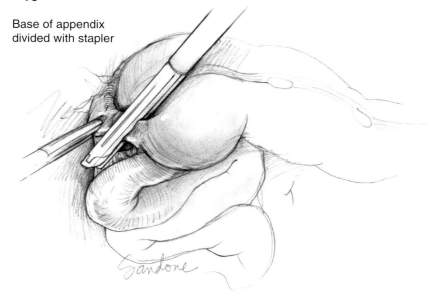

11

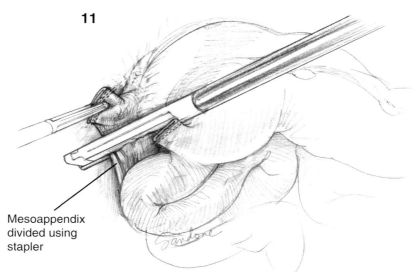

Mesoappendix
divided using
stapler

12   Appendix grasped and dissected toward tip

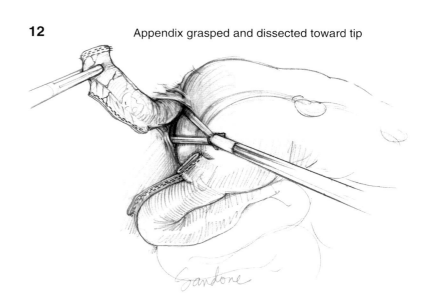

ILEOCECECTOMY AND STRICTUROPLASTY FOR SMALL BOWEL ENTERITIS (CROHN'S DISEASE)

INDICATIONS Although surgical therapy cannot cure Crohn's disease, it can palliate the complications of regional enteritis, including stricture, bleeding, fistula, abscess, or perforation. Bowel preservation is the guiding principle for surgical therapy of Crohn's disease. Only the grossly affected portion of the bowel should be resected. This minimizes the risk of a "short gut" after multiple resections, and reduces the risk of malnutrition. Therefore, if one or more short noninflamed strictures were to cause obstruction, strictureplasty avoids any loss of bowel. This technique can only be done for fibrotic strictures, as this reconstruction will not heal in the setting of acute inflammation. Further, because of a risk of cancer, the stricture should be biopsied prior to any such reconstruction.

PREOPERATIVE EVALUATION When possible the extent of disease should be defined preoperatively with colonoscopy and/or imaging. Imaging techniques include small bowel follow-through, conventional computed tomography (CT), or CT enterography.

Prior to either ileocecectomy or strictureplasty, improvement of nutrition, minimization of steroids, and treatment of anemia are essential. Patients who are severely malnourished, anemic, and on a high dose of steroids and other immunosuppressive agents may not be a candidate for a primary ileocecal anastomosis. Patients on infliximab (Remicade) or other monoclonal antibodies should have elective surgery delayed until 8 weeks have passed following the last dose of medication. Bowel preparation is generally not required. Preoperative steroid doses should be tapered to as low as possible. Ideally, patients should be anabolic prior to elective operation.

Thromboembolism prophylaxis, either pharmacologic or mechanical, is appropriate, particularly in the setting of inflammatory ileocecal disease. Prophylactic antibiotics that cover intestinal flora are given prior to skin incision. After induction of general anesthesia, an orogastric tube and urinary catheter are placed.

POSITIONING A beanbag can be placed under the patient to facilitate positioning. With true ileal or ileocecal disease, simple supine positioning is adequate. If more of the ascending colon is involved and there is a possibility of having to mobilize the hepatic flexure, the patient should be placed into a low lithotomy position with Allen stirrups. Each ankle, knee, and opposite shoulder should be aligned. No pressure should be placed on the peroneal nerves or calves. The angle between the thigh and the plane of the bed should not be more than 10 degrees. Any greater hip flexion will limit the range of motion for instrumentation. Excessive hip extension may lead to an anterior dislocation of the hip.

Each elbow (ulnar nerve) is covered with a gel pad, and both arms are tucked in at the side of the patient. The beanbag is carefully cradled above both shoulders and around the arms to prevent the patient from falling while in extreme Trendelenburg. A gel pad covered by a towel is placed on the upper chest. Tape is placed under the bed, over each shoulder, and across the padded chest to the other side of the bed. Peak airway pressures should be checked to ensure that the tape is not too tight. Security of the patient on the table should be tested using maximal Trendelenburg and left-side-down positioning prior to draping.

The surgeon and camera driver will eventually be on the patient's left. A monitor should be placed at the feet and another monitor should be placed at the patient's right (**FIGURE 1**).

DETAILS OF THE PROCEDURE
Trocar Placement The peritoneal cavity can be accessed with the Veress needle placed through the umbilicus, or with the Hasson technique, through a vertical infraumbilical incision. Pneumoperitoneum to a pressure of 15 mm Hg is established. A 10-mm, 30-degree laparoscope is used to guide placement of two 5-mm ports in the left lateral abdominal wall, just outside the lateral border of the rectus muscle, one above the umbilicus and one below the umbilicus, at least a handbreadth apart (**FIGURE 2A**). Another option is to place a suprapubic trocar 2 cm above the pubis and another trocar in the left lower quadrant, as is done for appendectomy (**FIGURE 2B**).

Ileocecal Mobilization Unlike a right colectomy done for neoplasia, a high ligation of the ileocolic pedicle is not required for inflammatory disease. Furthermore, the mesentery in regional enteritis tends to be thickened and inflamed, and it may not be easily controlled with the available methods for intracorporeal hemostasis. The primary goals of the laparoscopic procedure are twofold: (1) to examine all the intestine to identify all affected bowel, and (2) to mobilize the affected ileocecal region to allow extracorporeal division and anastomosis through a small extraction site at the umbilicus (**FIGURE 3**).

Once all ports have been established, the patient is placed in steep Trendelenburg position. The cecum and appendix are identified and elevated. The inferior side of the ileal mesentery is exposed (**FIGURE 4**). The peritoneum above the iliac vessels is incised, and the cecum is elevated off the retroperitoneum. The retroperitoneal tissues, right gonadal vessels, right ureter, and duodenum posteriorly fall away as the cecum is elevated. The ileal mesentery is dissected until soft, noninflamed tissue is encountered in the mesentery and the ileum itself appears normal, and without fat wrapping. The lateral peritoneal reflection, adjacent to the cecum, is divided with scissors or ultrasonic scalpel, and the cecum is elevated further (**FIGURE 5**). The ascending colon and its associated mesentery are freed until uninflamed bowel is encountered, usually just distal to the cecum. Occasionally, mobilization of the entire right colon and hepatic flexure is required to find suitable bowel for anastomosis.

The adequacy of mobilization is assessed by attempting to retract the cecum past the midline at the level of the umbilicus. Because re-creation of the pneumoperitoneum is difficult after creating the extraction incision (without a hand-port type device), every effort should be made to achieve adequate mobilization of the cecum and terminal ileum before opening the abdomen.

Once adequately mobilized, an extraction incision is made at the umbilicus. Improved cosmesis may be obtained by creating the incision directly through the umbilicus in the midline. The size of the incision depends on the thickness of the ileocecum and its mesentery and can vary between 3 and 7 cm. A wound protector/wound retractor can facilitate exposure at the extraction site.

The diseased bowel is often identified by its indurated, thickened, erythematous appearance with creeping fat. Healthy ileum and ascending colon are identified for anastomosis. The mesentery of the diseased bowel is scored anteriorly with electrosurgery, to connect the planned sites of bowel transection. The mesenteric division can be done with suture ligatures, the LigaSure device, or staplers. The anastomosis should be created with the technique most familiar to the surgeon. A side-to-side stapled anastomosis is described in this chapter.

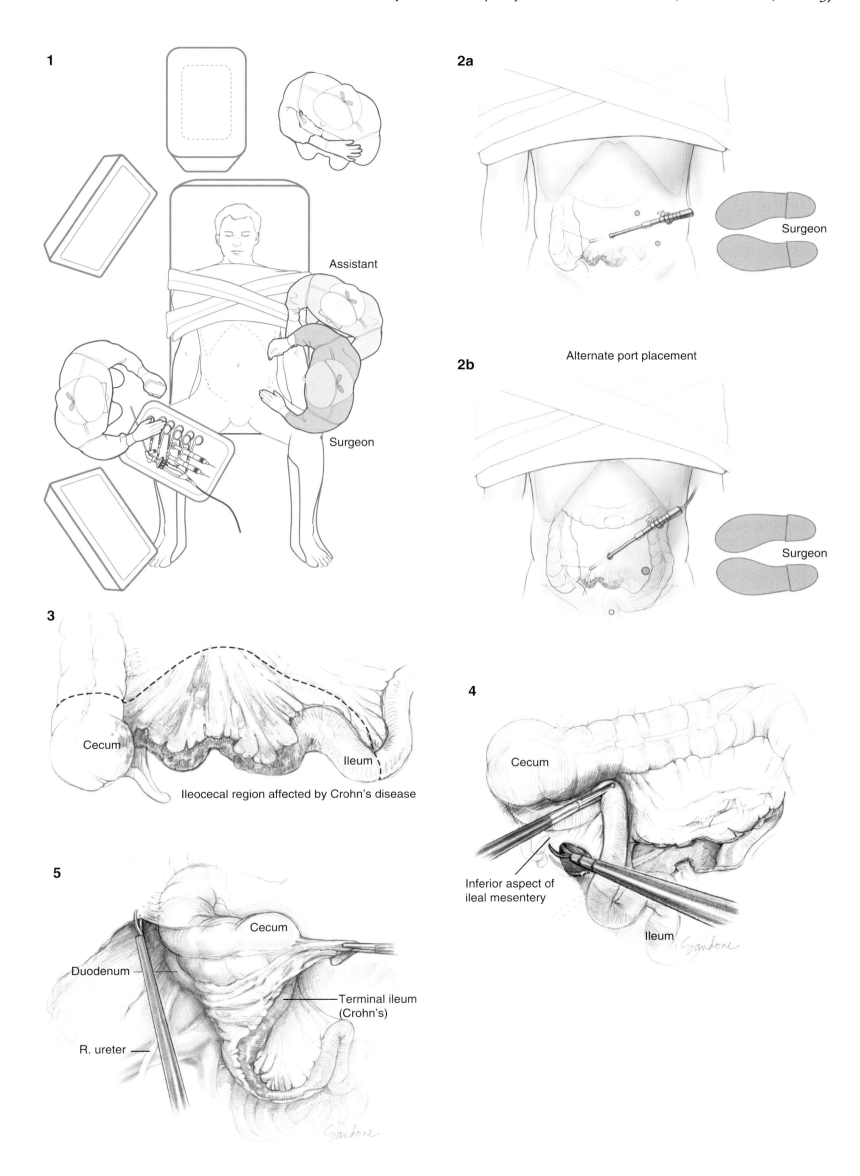

1

Assistant

Surgeon

2a

Surgeon

2b

Alternate port placement

Surgeon

3

Cecum

Ileum

Ileocecal region affected by Crohn's disease

4

Cecum

Inferior aspect of
ileal mesentery

Ileum

5

Cecum

Duodenum

Terminal ileum
(Crohn's)

R. ureter

Side-to-Side Stapled Anastomosis A side-to-side, functional end-to-end, stapled anastomosis can be performed with as few as two firings of a linear stapler. The antimesenteric sides of the ileum and colon are aligned in a side-to-side fashion. Two enterotomies are made on the antimesenteric sides of each limb just inside the proposed resection sites. A side-to-side anastomosis is made with an 80 mm linear stapler (**FIGURE 6**). A second firing of the stapler will complete the anastomosis and resect the specimen at the same time (**FIGURE 7**). The length of the anastomosis should be adequate to prevent obstruction in the event of recurrence of Crohn's disease. Bidigital palpation of the anastomosis is usually possible through the wall of the bowel, to ensure a generous connection between the ileum and colon. If a mesenteric defect is present, it should be closed before the bowel is returned to the peritoneal cavity.

Once the bowel has been returned to the abdomen, the pneumoperitoneum is re-created by closing the incision or the wound protector temporarily, to inspect the mesenteric edges and retroperitoneum for hemostasis. It is also important to make sure that the bowel sits intraabdominally without twists (volvulus) or kinks. Port sites and incisions in excess of 10 mm are closed either directly or with a port-site closure device.

Strictureplasty The setup is the same as is described above, but the surgeon should be prepared to operate from either or both sides of the patient. Three to four 5-mm ports may be needed to complete the operation. An initial inspection with the laparoscope will identify the need for preliminary small bowel dissection and adhesion clearance. Most commonly, the best port placements to accomplish this task will be the same as is described earlier in this chapter for ileocecectomy, but alternative configurations may be chosen once the location of intraabdominal adhesions becomes apparent. The remainder of the small bowel is then examined by running hand over hand with atraumatic graspers, and freed from any significant adhesions. A periumbilical midline extraction incision is then made, and the small bowel damaged by regional enteritis is exteriorized (**FIGURE 8**).

Strictureplasty should not be done for acutely inflamed small bowel. If uncertainty exists as to whether a stricture is obstructing, sterilized marbles (16 mm) or a Foley catheter with the balloon inflated have been used to ensure intestinal patency by placing them intraluminally at the site of the first strictureplasty.

The most frequently performed strictureplasty resembles a Heineke-Mikulicz pyloroplasty. With this technique, a longitudinal incision is made along the stricture (**FIGURE 9**). The stricture is biopsied and sent for frozen section. If a malignancy is detected, a bowel resection with a wide wedge of mesentery must be performed. If the frozen section is benign, the strictureplasty may be performed with one or two layers. If two layers are used, the inner layer is repaired in a transverse fashion with a running 3-0 absorbable monofilament suture. This is followed by an outer layer of interrupted 3-0 braided Lembert sutures of a nonabsorbable suture, such as silk (**FIGURE 10**).

Rarely, the only option available for intestinal obstruction caused by regional enteritis is bypass; however, this is usually due to a fibrotic, shortened mesentery, which would have generally resulted in conversion to an open procedure prior to consideration of any strictureplasty.

CLOSURE Laparoscopic ports are removed under direct vision. The fascia of the umbilical extraction site is closed using long-acting absorbable monofilament suture. The umbilicus is recreated using a dermal suture at the apex of the umbilicus secured to the fascia. The remaining incisions may be closed with sutures or staples.

POSTOPERATIVE CARE No additional antibiotics are needed after the wounds are closed. A nasogastric tube is not routinely left after the operation. Clear liquids are offered the day after the operation, and the diet is advanced as tolerated. The urinary catheter is removed on the morning of the first postoperative day if the patient is not oliguric. Steroids may be rapidly tapered with close attention to symptoms of steroid withdrawal. ∎

6

Extracorporeal, side-to-side
stapled anastomosis

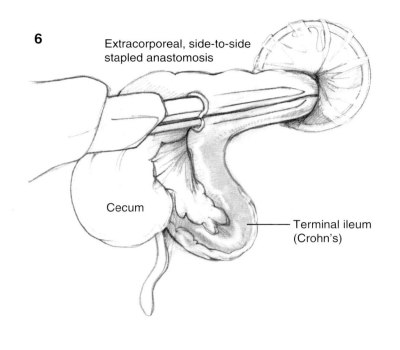

Cecum

Terminal ileum
(Crohn's)

7

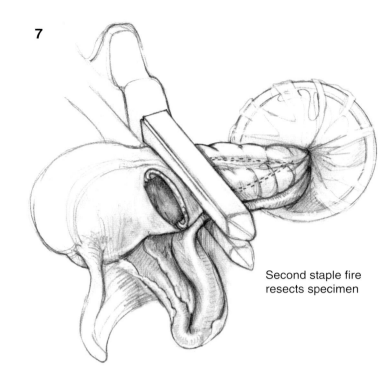

Second staple fire
resects specimen

8   **Stricturoplasty**

Small bowel
exteriorized

Obstructing
stricture

9

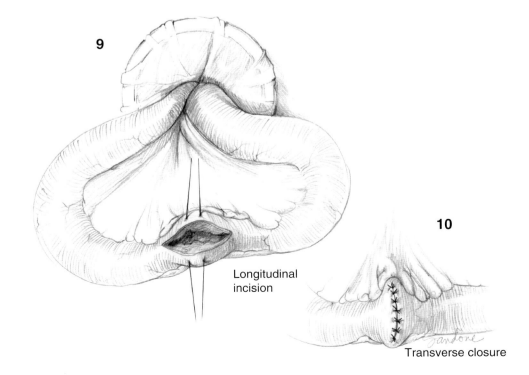

Longitudinal
incision

10

Transverse closure

INDICATIONS Laparoscopic right hemicolectomy is appropriate for pathology in the cecum, ascending colon, or hepatic flexure.

PREOPERATIVE EVALUATION During laparoscopy, loss of tactile sensation makes it harder to find small lesions. Before a laparoscopic procedure, an endoscopist must tattoo the colon just distal to the lesion, so the surgeon can be confident that the lesion will be within the specimen. Further, the colon should be tattooed in each quadrant circumferentially, so that the tattoo may be visualized before the ascending colon mobilization is performed, even if the polyp or small cancer is located in the retroperitoneal portion of the colon.

For malignancies, conventional computed tomography of the abdomen and pelvis with oral and IV contrast is helpful. Although laparoscopy is sensitive for very small surface liver lesions, one cannot effectively palpate the liver.

In most situations, a mechanical and antibiotic bowel preparation is administered preoperatively unless the lesion to be removed is near obstructing.

ANESTHESIA Thromboembolism prophylaxis, either pharmacologic or mechanical, is started prior to induction of general anesthesia. Prophylactic antibiotics that cover intestinal flora are given within 1 hour prior to skin incision. After induction of general anesthesia, an orogastric tube is placed and urinary catheter are placed.

POSITIONING A beanbag under the patient to facilitate positioning. The patient should be placed into a low lithotomy position with Allen stirrups. Each ankle, knee, and opposite shoulder should be aligned. No pressure should be placed on the peroneal nerves or calves. The angle between the thigh and the plane of the bed should be between 0 and 10 degrees. Any more flexion will limit range of motion for the instruments. Any more extension may lead to an anterior dislocation of the hip.

Each elbow (ulnar nerve) is covered with a gel pad, and both arms are carefully adducted. Care must be taken to avoid compromising or kinking the intravenous lines. The beanbag is carefully cradled above both shoulders and around the arms to prevent the patient from falling while in extreme positioning. A gel pad covered by a towel is placed on the upper chest. Tape is placed under the bed, over each shoulder, and across the padded chest to the other side of the bed. Prior to draping, security of the patient on the table should be confirmed using maximal Trendelenburg and left-side-down positioning.

After placement of the trocars, the surgeon and camera driver will both be on the patient's left. The camera driver will be near the patient's left shoulder. Hence, one monitor should be placed at the feet, and another one should be placed at the patient's right (**FIGURE 1**).

INCISION AND EXPOSURE The peritoneal cavity can be accessed with the Veress needle or Hasson technique. Pneumoperitoneum to a pressure of 15 mm Hg is established. A 10-mm, 30-degree laparoscope is used to place two 5-mm trocars in the left lateral abdominal wall, just outside the lateral border of the rectus muscle, at least a handbreadth apart. Another option is to place a suprapubic trocar 2 cm above the pubis and another trocar in the left lower quadrant (**FIGURE 2**).

There are four critical steps for the laparoscopic mobilization of the right colon:

1. High ligation of the ileocolic pedicle and medial dissection of the right colon mesentery from the retroperitoneum.
2. Inferior dissection of the right colon mesentery from the retroperitoneum.
3. Lateral dissection of the right colon mesentery from the retroperitoneum.
4. Superior dissection of the proximal transverse colon away from the greater omentum and the hepatic flexure.

The order in which these steps are performed may vary. In a typical open surgical approach, the lateral dissection is performed first. In a laparoscopic approach, most experts favor the "medial-to-lateral approach," with mobilization in the order listed above. This allows the natural lateral attachments to hold up the colon during the laparoscopic identification of the ileocolic pedicle.

DETAILS OF THE PROCEDURE The patient is placed in steep Trendelenburg position with a left tilt. The cecum and appendix are identified and elevated. The mesentery adjacent to the cecum is lifted up toward the anterior abdominal wall. The bulge of the ileocolic pedicle should be easily identified when anterior retraction creates some tension on the mesentery. There will be a sulcus above and below the ileocolic pedicle. The peritoneum is opened along the sulcus superior to the ileocolic vessels, then inferior to the ileocolic vessels (**FIGURE 3**). Once a window is created, the surgeon's left hand instrument can be placed in this window to lift up as much as possible. The retrocolic plane of dissection can be identified as follows: the small transverse blood vessels lie within the retroperitoneum, while the colon mesentery is a lighter yellow. With the other dissector, the surgeon gently pushes down on the retroperitoneum.

Near the duodenum superiorly, the surgeon either sharply cuts the attachments below the duodenum or brushes the attachments from left to right below the duodenum to isolate the colon from the duodenum. This avoids any contact with or damage to the duodenum.

The next step divides the ileocolic pedicle just inferior to the duodenum. Taking care to avoid the duodenum, a vascular load (2.0 or 2.5 mm) endoscopic stapler or the LigaSure device (illustrated) is used to divide the ileocolic vessels. It is best to keep a free grasper available to grasp the ileocolic pedicle should it bleed (**FIGURE 4**). In case of bleeding, pre-tied endoscopic loop can readily control the stump of the bleeding vessel.

1

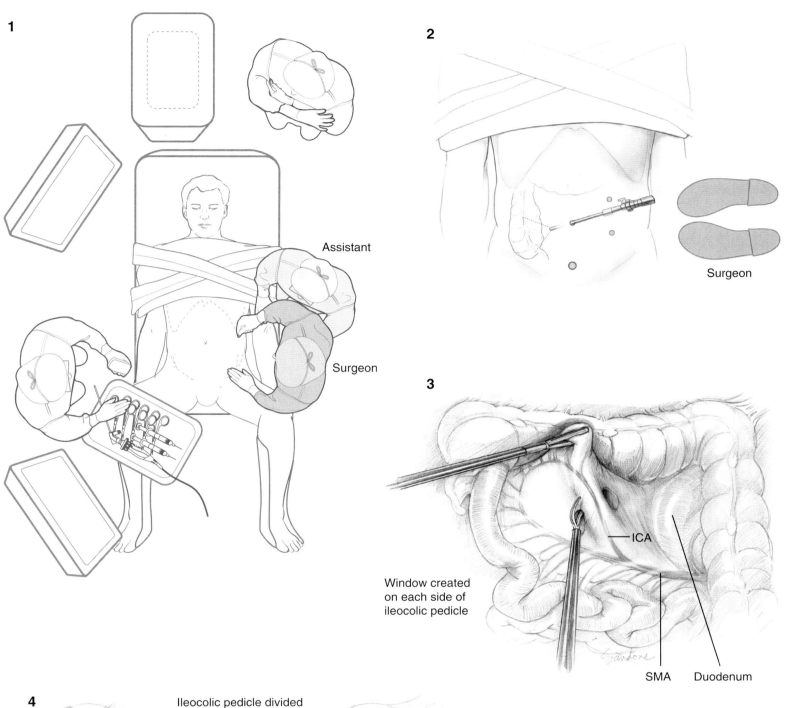

Assistant

Surgeon

2

Surgeon

3

ICA

Window created
on each side of
ileocolic pedicle

SMA   Duodenum

4   Ileocolic pedicle divided

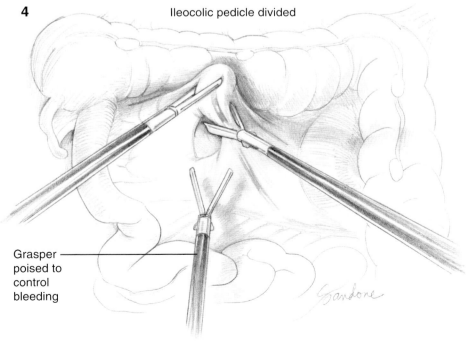

Grasper
poised to
control
bleeding

DETAILS OF THE PROCEDURE Lifting up on the colon mesentery adjacent to the divided ileocolic stump, dissection is continued laterally until the colon is elevated and the lateral peritoneal reflection is reached (**FIGURE 5**).

With the patient in steep Trendelenburg and minimal tilt left, the inferior side of the ileal mesentery is lifted toward the anterior abdominal wall. The small bowel should fall away superiorly. The peritoneum above the iliac vessels is opened (**FIGURE 6**). A grasper is placed under the cut edge and lifted up. By gently pushing down on the retroperitoneum, the cecum and ascending colon mesentery are safely raised away from the right gonadal vessels, the right ureter, and the duodenum, and the prior area of medial dissection is reached (**FIGURE 7**).

With the patient in less Trendelenburg and maximal tilt left, the mesentery is grasped just lateral to the cecum and retracted superomedially. The lateral peritoneal attachments are divided up to the hepatic flexure with scissors or ultrasonic shears (**FIGURE 8**).

With the patient in reverse Trendelenburg and tilt left, the greater omentum is placed up over the liver. The proximal transverse colon is retracted caudally, and the greater omentum is taken off the transverse colon, starting in the middle and working laterally (**FIGURE 9**). The lesser sac is entered. Dissection continues retrograde until the hepatic flexure is reached. Using a grasper, the hepatic flexure is gently pulled medially and inferiorly. The remaining hepatic flexure attachments are divided under direct vision.

The adequacy of mobilization can be determined by three criteria: (1) The proximal transverse colon should be free of the greater omentum to the mid transverse colon, at the level of the umbilical (round) ligament; (2) the hepatic flexure of the colon should be free from the second portion of the duodenum; and (3) the cecum should be able to be reflected past the midline at the level of the umbilicus. Re-creation of the pneumoperitoneum is difficult without a hand-port type device, therefore every effort should be made to achieve adequate mobilization before creating the extraction incision.

5

Medial-to-lateral mobilization of right mesentery

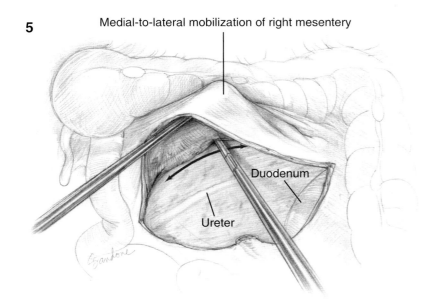

Duodenum

Ureter

6

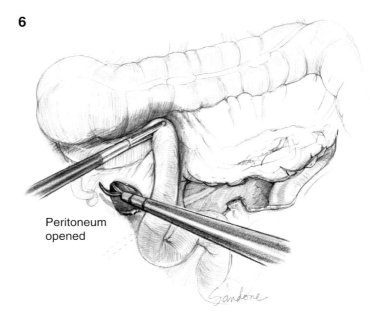

Peritoneum
opened

7

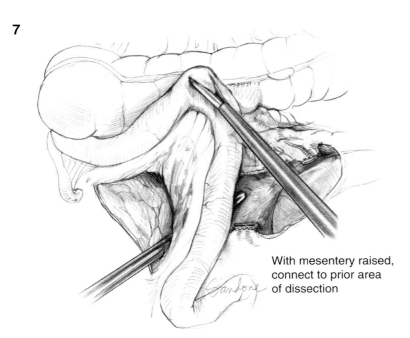

With mesentery raised,
connect to prior area
of dissection

8

Lateral attachments
of right colon divided

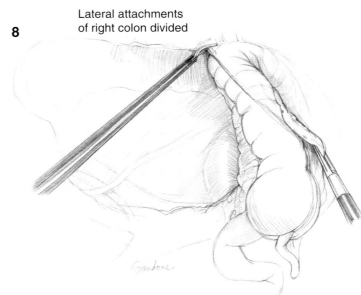

9

Omentum taken off transverse colon

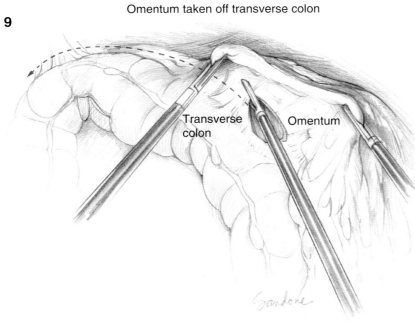

Transverse
colon

Omentum

DETAILS OF THE PROCEDURE Once adequate mobilization is achieved, and before an extraction incision is made, a locking laparoscopic bowel grasper is placed on the ileum just proximal to the ileocecal valve. This grasper is used to pass the specimen medially to the extraction site, after the extraction incision is created and laparoscopic visualization is lost by the collapsing pneumoperitoneum. An extraction incision is made through the umbilicus. The size of the incision depends on the thickness of the ileum, colon, and the mesentery, but should range between 3 and 7 cm. A wound protector can facilitate exposure at the extraction site. Viable ileum and transverse colon are identified for anastomosis, and resection is performed using a surgical stapling device (**FIGURE 10**).

The anastomosis should be performed in the fashion in which the surgeon is most proficient. To perform an anastomosis in a stapled fashion, the antimesenteric sides of the ileum and colon are aligned in a side-to-side fashion. A silk stitch facilitates this alignment and maintains proper retraction later. Two enterotomies are made on the antimesenteric sides of each limb just inside the proposed resection sites. A side-to-side functional end-to-end anastomosis is made with an 80-mm stapler (**FIGURE 11**).

The enterotomies in the now-common lumen can be sutured closed primarily in two layers or stapled. To staple the enterotomy, corner sutures are placed around each anastomotic staple lines and the two interior staple lines are distracted (**FIGURE 12A**). The walls are first aligned with Allis graspers and a TA stapler is then applied to close the defect (**FIGURE 12B**). The length of the anastomosis should be adequate to prevent obstruction in the event of post-operative edema. The last staple line can be oversewn with a running 3-0 braided Lembert suture, and a 3-0 braided "crotch stitch" should be placed to prevent tension on the distal end of the staple line. The bowel is returned to the peritoneal cavity. The mesenteric defect is not routinely closed.

If possible, pneumoperitoneum is recreated by closing off the wound protector/retractor to inspect the resection area for hemostasis and ensure that the ileocolic anastomosis is lying against the right retroperitoneum (**FIGURE 13**). The field is inspected for hemostasis, and all fluid and clot are removed with a suction/irrigator. The ports are removed, and the sites are inspected for bleeding with the laparoscope. The pneumoperitoneum is released.

CLOSURE All ports are removed under direct vision. The fascia of the umbilical extraction site is closed using interrupted figure-of-eight long-acting absorbable monofilament sutures. The umbilicus is re-created using a dermal suture at the apex of the umbilicus secured to the fascia. The remaining incision may be closed with sutures or staples. The port sites may be closed with sutures or dermal adhesive.

POSTOPERATIVE CARE No additional antibiotics are needed after the wounds are closed. A nasogastric tube is not routinely used. Clear liquids are offered the day after the operation, and the diet is advanced as tolerated. The urinary catheter is removed on the morning of the first postoperative day if the patient is not oliguric. ■

10

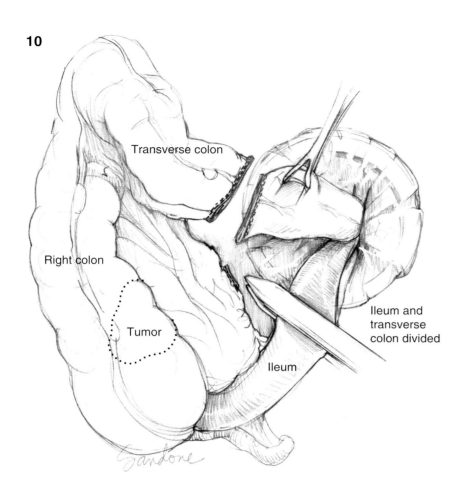

Transverse colon

Right colon

Tumor

Ileum and
transverse
colon divided

Ileum

11

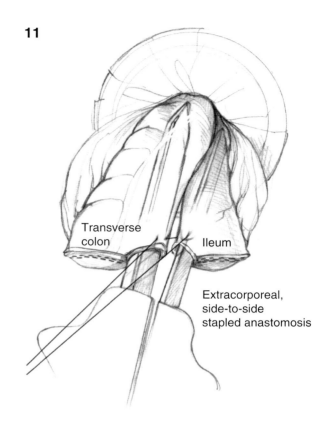

Transverse
colon

Ileum

Extracorporeal,
side-to-side
stapled anastomosis

12a

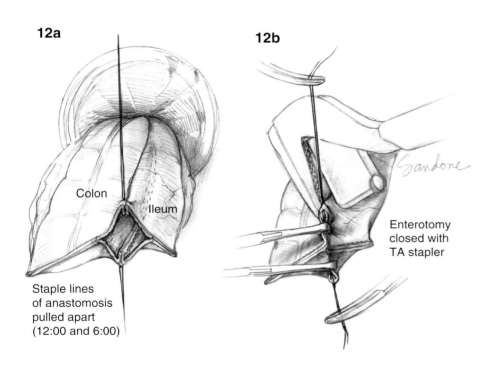

Colon

Ileum

Staple lines
of anastomosis
pulled apart
(12:00 and 6:00)

12b

Enterotomy
closed with
TA stapler

13

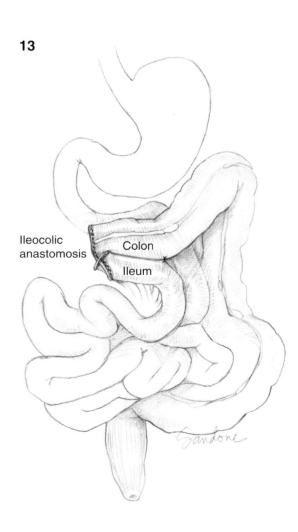

Ileocolic
anastomosis

Colon

Ileum

CHAPTER 49
SIGMOID COLECTOMY

INDICATIONS Diverticular disease, colonic malignancy, endoscopically unresectable polyps, rectal prolapse, and sigmoid volvulus are the most common indications for elective sigmoid colectomy. A primary resection and anastomosis is often considered after one or more episodes of acute sigmoid diverticulitis and is generally performed after resolution of acute inflammation. Laparoscopic surgery for colon cancer is based on the same oncologic principles as open colon cancer surgery. Open surgery may still be recommended for patients with locally advanced large tumors or tumors penetrating adjacent organs or the abdominal wall. Other relative contraindications to laparoscopic colectomy include multiple previous abdominal operations, bleeding disorders, and/or severe cardiopulmonary comorbidity.

PREOPERATIVE EVALUATION AND PREPARATION Preoperative assessment and preparation are the same for laparoscopy and laparotomy. If the lesion is small or resected at the time of colonoscopy, it should be preoperatively tattooed with India ink; additionally, the patient should be prepared for intraoperative colonoscopy. Mechanical bowel preparation, deep venous thrombosis prophylaxis, and oral and intravenous broad-spectrum antibiotics are administered before surgery. Ureteral stents are inserted preoperatively for advanced cancers and advanced diverticular disease where retroperitoneal inflammation or fibrosis is a concern.

OPERATIVE TECHNIQUE The patient is placed in the supine, modified lithotomy position, using Allen stirrups, and secured to the operating table with the arms and legs well padded. Both arms are carefully tucked at the patient's side. The surgeon stands on the right side of the patient, and the first assistant stands on the opposite side. Two video monitors are placed on the patient's left side, one over the shoulder and one over the left leg. An additional monitor is placed over the right shoulder (**FIGURE 1**). Pneumoperitoneum is established using an open Hasson technique. An 11-mm Hasson cannula is inserted through a vertical infraumbilical incision, and pneumoperitoneum is created with CO_2 to a pressure of 15 mm Hg. A 30-degree camera is introduced, and under direct vision, a 12-mm port is placed in the right iliac fossa. A 5-mm port is placed in the right midclavicular line below the costal margin. A fourth trocar is placed in the left lateral abdomen to facilitate splenic flexure mobilization. This port site will be expanded to bring the specimen onto the abdominal wall later in the procedure (**FIGURE 2**).

In obese patients, an additional left-sided port may be used to facilitate exposure (**FIGURE 3**).

The operation begins by incising the white line of Toldt with scissors in a lateral-to-medial approach from the iliac fossa along the left colon to the splenic flexure (**FIGURE 4**). Medial retraction of the sigmoid colon is achieved by using atraumatic graspers and facilitated by a steep Trendelenburg position with a right tilting of the table. After the left colon is mobilized, identification of the left ureter is required. The ureter is identified by following its course from the kidney to the pelvis using the iliac artery pulsation as a landmark. If ureteral catheters are employed, it may be easier to initially identify them by palpation rather than by peristalsis. Mobilization of the descending colon is continued along the white line of Toldt. Full mobilization of the descending colon may provide sufficient length to perform the proximal resection (**FIGURE 5**).

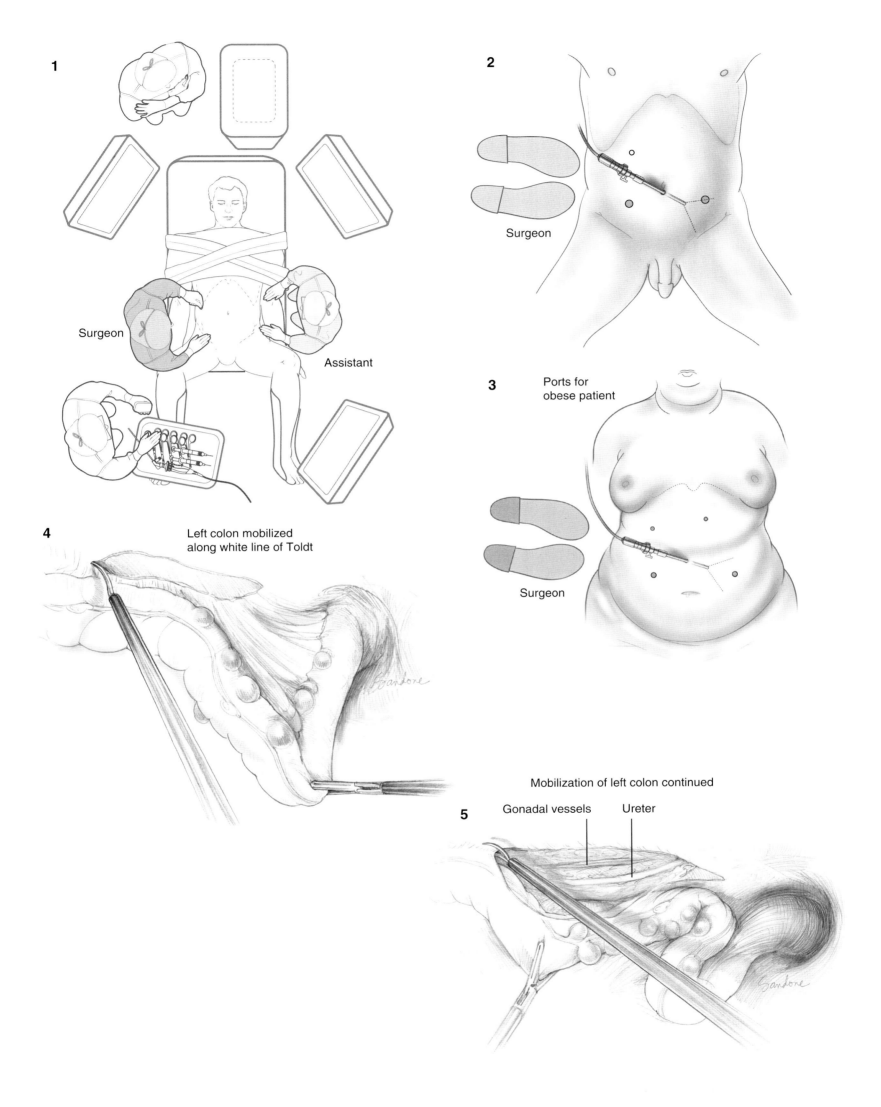

1

Surgeon

Assistant

2

Surgeon

3 Ports for
obese patient

Surgeon

4 Left colon mobilized
along white line of Toldt

Mobilization of left colon continued

5 Gonadal vessels   Ureter

OPERATIVE TECHNIQUE If the left colon is not significantly redundant, it is necessary to mobilize the splenic flexure to provide a tension-free anastomosis. The patient is placed in the reverse Trendelenburg position, and the surgeon stands between the patient's legs. The assistant stands to the patient's right with instruments through the two right abdominal trocars lifting the omentum toward the anterior abdominal wall and retracting the splenic flexure toward the midline (**FIGURE 6**). The splenic flexure is mobilized using an electrosurgical device to continue the lateral peritoneal incision (**FIGURE 7**). The greater omentum is separated from the left transverse colon along the avascular plane. The gastrocolic ligament is divided using the Harmonic scalpel or other tissue sealing device. The extent of the colon resection and the level of vascular ligation depend on the pathology. The proximal level of resection for cancer is the junction between the descending and sigmoid colon. For diverticulosis, the thickened colonic wall is identified and the transection is performed at level of normal colonic wall with no diverticula. The proximal margin may be the descending colon, splenic flexure, or even the transverse colon. The distal level of dissection is the rectosigmoid junction, which is usually located at the level of the sacral promontory, corresponding to the confluence of the teniae and obliteration of the appendices epiploicae.

After lateral mobilization of the left colon, the peritoneum is scored at the root of the mesentery. The mesenteric fat with small vessels is divided using the Harmonic scalpel or other tissue sealing device. The sigmoid branches of the inferior mesenteric artery (IMA) are identified and transected with the LigaSure or a 45-mm vascular linear stapler for diverticular disease (**FIGURE 8**). For sigmoid colon cancer, the IMA is divided close to its origin with a vascular stapler or large clips. If further mobilization is necessary, the inferior mesenteric vein can be treated in an identical manner and the mesentery divided to the base of the middle colic vessels.

At the level of the rectosigmoid junction (sacral promontory), the presacral space is entered by creating a window using the hook cautery (**FIGURE 9**).

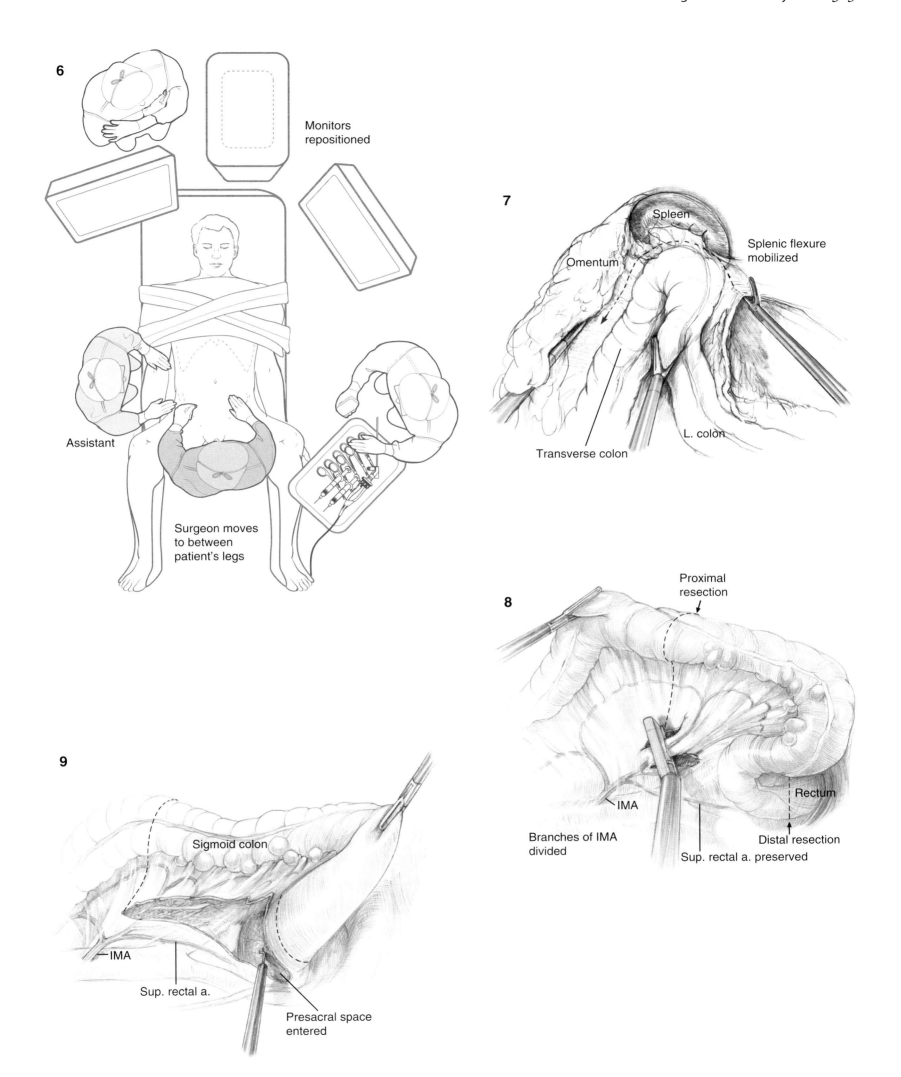

6

Monitors repositioned

Assistant

Surgeon moves to between patient's legs

7

Spleen

Splenic flexure mobilized

Omentum

L. colon

Transverse colon

8

Proximal resection

Rectum

IMA

Branches of IMA divided

Distal resection

Sup. rectal a. preserved

9

Sigmoid colon

IMA

Sup. rectal a.

Presacral space entered

OPERATIVE TECHNIQUE After the upper rectal wall is circumferentially cleared of fat, the bowel is divided with two or three firings of a 45-mm linear stapler (with a blue cartridge, 3.5-mm staple height) (**FIGURE 10**). The rectal stump is assessed for hemostasis and an air-leak test is performed. Our preferred approach is to fill the pelvis with saline and then perform a transanal flexible endoscopic evaluation. The insufflated air tests the staple line integrity while the endoscopy verifies that the chosen level of resection is 15 cm from the dentate line or less. Endoscopy can also verify the absence of any residual sigmoid diverticular disease proximal to the rectal stump. Flexible sigmoidoscopy should be performed before selection of the area for transection, after stapler application, and once more after stapler firing is complete.

The descending–sigmoid colon junction selected for the anastomosis is checked for reach of the distal stapler line to provide a tension-free anastomosis (**FIGURE 11**). A grasper is placed through the left iliac fossa port and used to gently grasp the distal end of the proximal bowel. A transverse incision of 5 cm is made through this port site, and after a plastic wound protector is placed, the bowel is withdrawn (**FIGURE 12**).

The area of the proximal bowel selected for the anastomosis is circumferentially cleared of fat and divided to remove the specimen (**FIGURE 13**). A purse-string suture is applied to the descending colon. The anvil of a circular stapling device (29 or 33 mm) is inserted within the lumen, and the purse-string suture is tied. The mesenteric and serosal fat around the anvil is cleared using electrocautery (**FIGURE 14**).

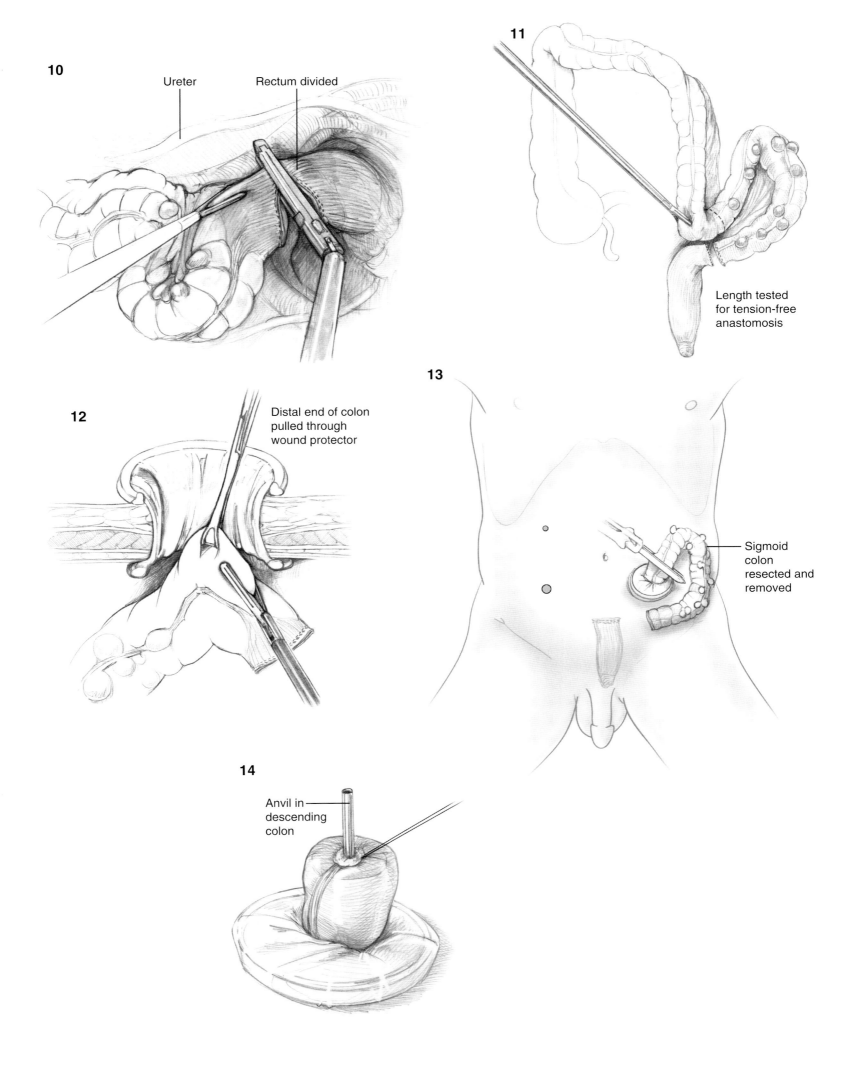

10

Ureter   Rectum divided

11

Length tested
for tension-free
anastomosis

12

Distal end of colon
pulled through
wound protector

13

Sigmoid
colon
resected and
removed

14

Anvil in
descending
colon

OPERATIVE TECHNIQUE The proximal bowel with anvil in place is returned to the abdominal cavity, and the incision is closed. The abdomen is then reinsufflated, irrigated, and meticulously assessed for hemostasis. The circular stapling device is introduced through the rectum and advanced until the staple housing rests flush at the rectal stump and the staple line bisects the end of the device. The circular stapler spike is fully extended so that it pierces the top of the rectal stump through the staple line. The anvil shaft is slid over the spike using a laparoscopic grasping forceps or Babcock, and the stapler is closed (**FIGURES 15 AND 16**). The camera is placed in the right iliac fossa port during closure, and great care is taken to keep the bowel and its mesentery in proper orientation and to avoid inclusion of any extraneous tissue. The stapler is fired, opened, and removed from the rectum; the doughnuts are inspected for completeness.

After the proximal bowel is occluded with a bowel clamp, the pelvis is filled with saline and air is insufflated through the flexible sigmoidoscope to verify a widely patent, circumferentially intact, hemostatic, and airtight anastomosis (**FIGURES 17 AND 18**). The abdomen is inspected for hemostasis and to verify proper orientation of the colon. It should be verified that small bowel is not trapped under the mesentery. The trocars are removed under direct vision, and the port sites are closed.

POSTOPERATIVE CARE No additional antibiotics are needed after the wounds are closed. A nasogastric tube is not routinely used. Clear liquids are offered the day after the operation, and the diet is advanced as tolerated. The urinary catheter is removed on the morning of the first postoperative day if the patient is not oliguric. ■

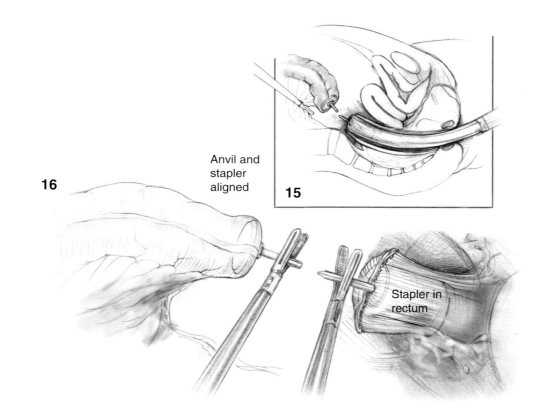

15

Anvil and stapler aligned

Stapler in rectum

16

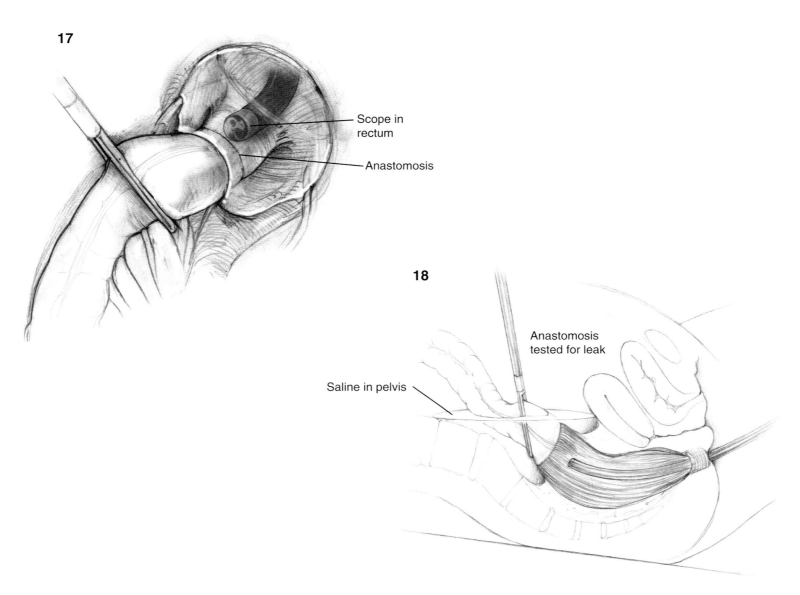

17

Scope in rectum

Anastomosis

18

Anastomosis tested for leak

Saline in pelvis

TOTAL ABDOMINAL COLECTOMY

INDICATIONS Total abdominal colectomy is most commonly performed in the setting of prophylactic cancer prevention (FAP), unidentified bleeding from the lower GI tract, or fulminant ulcerative or *Clostridium difficile*–associated colitis. The stepwise mobilization of the sigmoid colon, cecum, and finally the transverse colon facilitates the greatest control of this large amount of intra-abdominal tissue. Depending on the clinical situation, a hand port can be used to assist in the complete mobilization of the tissue. At the completion of the resection an end ileostomy or ileorectal anastomosis may be performed.

PREOPERATIVE PREPARATION In urgent or emergency circumstances, bowel preparation is not possible and creation of an end ileostomy or ileorectal anastomosis with protective loop ileostomy must be considered at the outset. A Foley catheter is placed in the bladder. An orogastric tube is beneficial to decompress the stomach. The rectum is irrigated with saline and either Betadine or another cytocidal agent. A 34 French mushroom catheter can be left in the rectum to provide intraoperative drainage of the rectal cavity as well as tactile guidance to the anal canal.

ANESTHESIA Thromboembolism prophylaxis, either pharmacologic or mechanical, is started prior to induction of general anesthesia. Prophylactic antibiotics that cover intestinal flora are given within 1 hour prior to skin incision. After induction of general anesthesia, an orogastric tube and urinary catheter are placed. Ureteral stents may be considered in the context of severe intraabdominal inflammation, fibrosis, or retroperitoneal infection.

POSITIONING A beanbag should be placed under the patient to prevent sliding during extremes of positioning. The patient should be placed into a low lithotomy position with Allen stirrups. Each ankle, knee, and opposite shoulder should be aligned. No pressure should be placed on the peroneal nerves or calves. The angle between the thigh and the plane of the bed should be between 0 and 10 degrees. Any more flexion will limit range of motion for the instruments. Any more extension may lead to an anterior dislocation of the hip.

Each elbow (ulnar nerve) is covered with a gel pad, and both arms are carefully tucked at the patient's side. Care must be taken to avoid compromising or kinking the intravenous lines. The beanbag is carefully cradled above both shoulders and around the arms to prevent the patient from falling while in extreme positioning. The air is suctioned from the beanbag so that it retains its shape. A gel pad covered by a towel is placed on the upper chest. Tape is placed under the bed, over each shoulder, and across to the other side of the bed. If the peak airway pressures become elevated, the tape should be loosened. Security of the patient on the table should be confirmed by testing maximal Trendelenburg and left-side-down positioning prior to prepping and draping. The entire abdomen is prepped from nipples to upper thighs, to allow placement of a hand port medially, and placement of the trocars as far laterally as possible.

After placement of the trocars, the surgeon and first assistant will start on the patient's right. The first assistant should stand closest to the patient's right shoulder. One monitor should be placed at the feet, and another one should be placed at the patient's left shoulder. The cautery foot pedal is placed on the patient's right (**FIGURE 1**).

INCISION AND EXPOSURE The peritoneal cavity can be accessed with the Veress needle or Hasson technique. Pneumoperitoneum to a pressure of 15 mmHg is established. A 10-mm, 30-degree laparoscope is placed in the infraumbilical position. Two 5-mm trocars are then placed in the right lateral abdominal wall, just outside the lateral border of the rectus muscle, at least a handbreadth apart. A suprapubic 12-mm trocar is placed 2 cm above the pubis. Two 5-mm trocars are placed in the left lateral abdomen mirroring those on the right (**FIGURE 2**).

There are a number of critical steps for the laparoscopic mobilization of the entire colon. These include mobilization of the left colon, splenic flexure, transverse mesocolon, and right colon; division of the middle colic artery; division of the proximal rectum; and creation of an ileorectal anastomosis or end ileostomy. Accomplishment of these tasks require movement of the surgeon and assistant around the table as needed to optimize instrumentation.

Surgeons vary in their preferences for the order of performing the above steps. In typical general surgery training, residents perform the lateral dissection first. In a laparoscopic approach the "medial-to-lateral approach," is preferred, with mobilization in the order listed. This allows the natural lateral attachments to hold up the colon during the laparoscopic identification of the colonic vascular structures.

DETAILS OF THE OPERATION
Mobilization of the Left Colon and Splenic Flexure The initial steps in the procedure involve placing the patient in steep Trendelenburg and tilting the patient to the right. The surgeon stands on the patient's right side. This allows all the small intestine to fall out of the left lower quadrant and pelvis and into the right upper quadrant. The standard approach to a low anterior resection begins with a medial-to-lateral dissection at the base of the mesentery of the sigmoid colon at the sacral promontory. An incision is made over the sacral promontory behind the superior hemorrhoidal artery as the sigmoid colon is retracted anteriorly and out of the pelvis (**FIGURE 3**). This allows entry into an avascular plane at the sacral promontory. Blunt dissection in a tangential plane over the left iliac artery and vein at the pelvic brim allows identification of the left ureter and the gonadal vessels (**FIGURE 4**). The midline structure first encountered as the dissection moves cephalad is the inferior mesenteric artery (IMA). The thickened dense nerves that arise from the preaortic plexus and extend up on to the IMA can be preserved. The IMA pedicle is carefully dissected, creating a window through which a vascular stapler or energy source can be inserted. Prior to dividing the IMA, care is taken to visualize and protect the ureter and gonadal vessels (**FIGURE 5**).

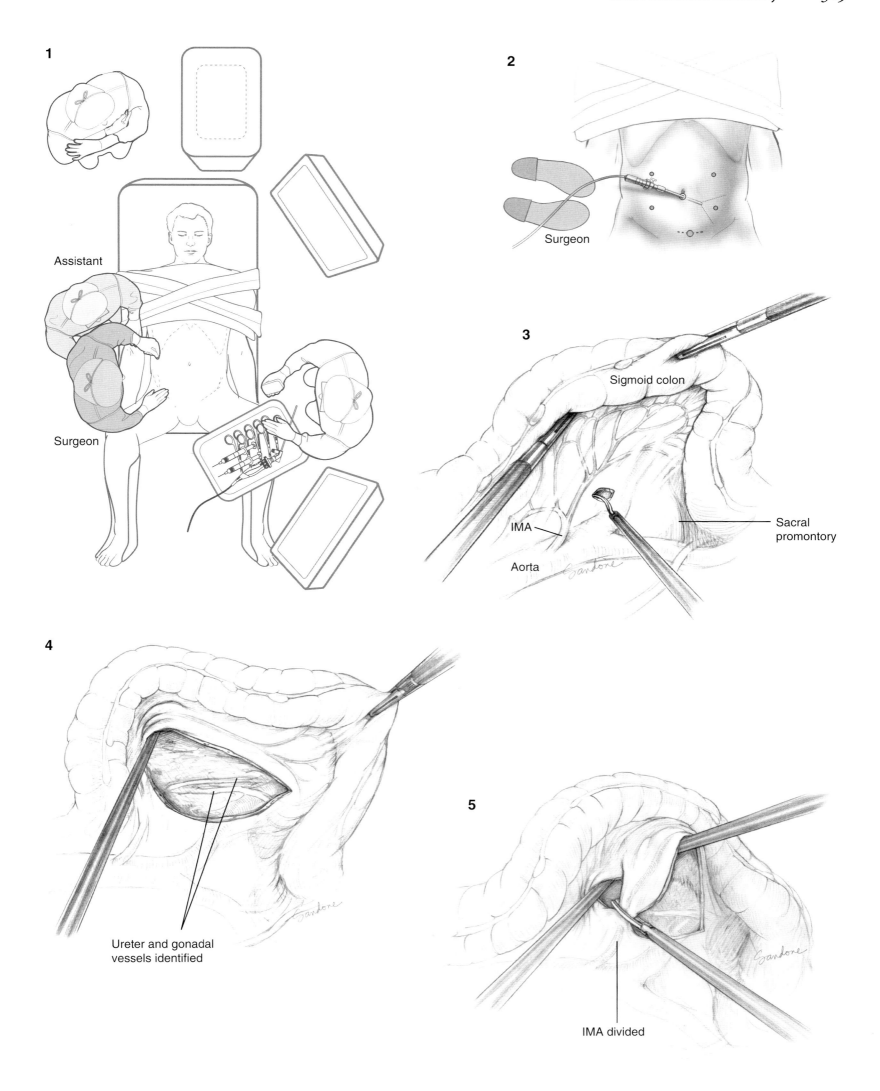

1

Assistant

Surgeon

2

Surgeon

3

Sigmoid colon

IMA

Aorta

Sacral
promontory

4

Ureter and gonadal
vessels identified

5

IMA divided

Mobilization of the Left Colon and Splenic Flexure Once the IMA is divided, the avascular plane behind the IMA is developed cephalad, caudad, and laterally. The next structure encountered in the midline dissection toward the head is the inferior mesenteric vein running at the base of the mesentery of the left colon. The inferior mesenteric vein dives posterior to the third portion of the duodenum at the level of the ligament of Treitz, where the duodenum sweeps out away from the pancreas. Retraction of the inferior mesenteric vein anteriorly toward the abdominal wall allows visualization behind the vein along the undersurface of the pancreas and allows the surgeon to create a window in the base of the mesentery of the left colon at the origin of the inferior mesenteric vein (**FIGURE 6**). The vein is divided with staples or energy sources (**FIGURE 7**).

The avascular plane along the left colon is developed laterally (**FIGURE 8**) and cephalad all the way up and around the splenic flexure. This dissection is continued as far medially as possible to completely free the left colon and its mesentery from the greater omentum and inferior pole of the spleen.

Mobilization of the Transverse Colon The surgeon changes position to stand between the patient's legs to facilitate this maneuver. Monitors are repositioned as needed to optimize viewing (**FIGURE 9**). The surgeon retracts the transverse colon inferiorly with his or her left hand, using an atraumatic grasper through the suprapubic port. The assistant stands to the patient's right with instruments through the two right abdominal ports lifting the omentum toward the anterior abdominal wall and retracting the splenic flexure toward the midline. This exposes the remaining attachments of the splenic flexure (**FIGURE 10**). The mobilization of the splenic flexure is continued with a Harmonic scalpel or LigaSure until the tail of the pancreas is reached. A window into the lesser omental sac allows visualization of the undersurface of the stomach, the anterior surface of the pancreas, and the mesentery of the colon. The flimsy tissue between the transverse colon and the greater omentum is divided until the hepatic flexure is reached (**FIGURE 11**). The hepatic flexure is retracted medially and inferiorly with the surgeon's left hand instrument, and the remaining hepatic flexure attachments are divided under direct vision.

6

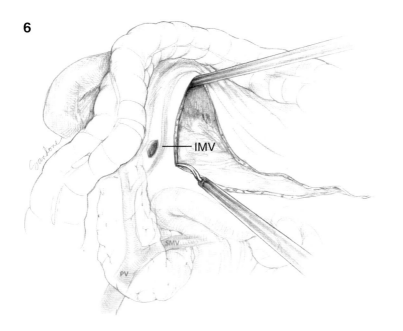

7

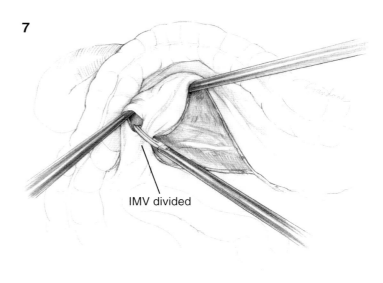

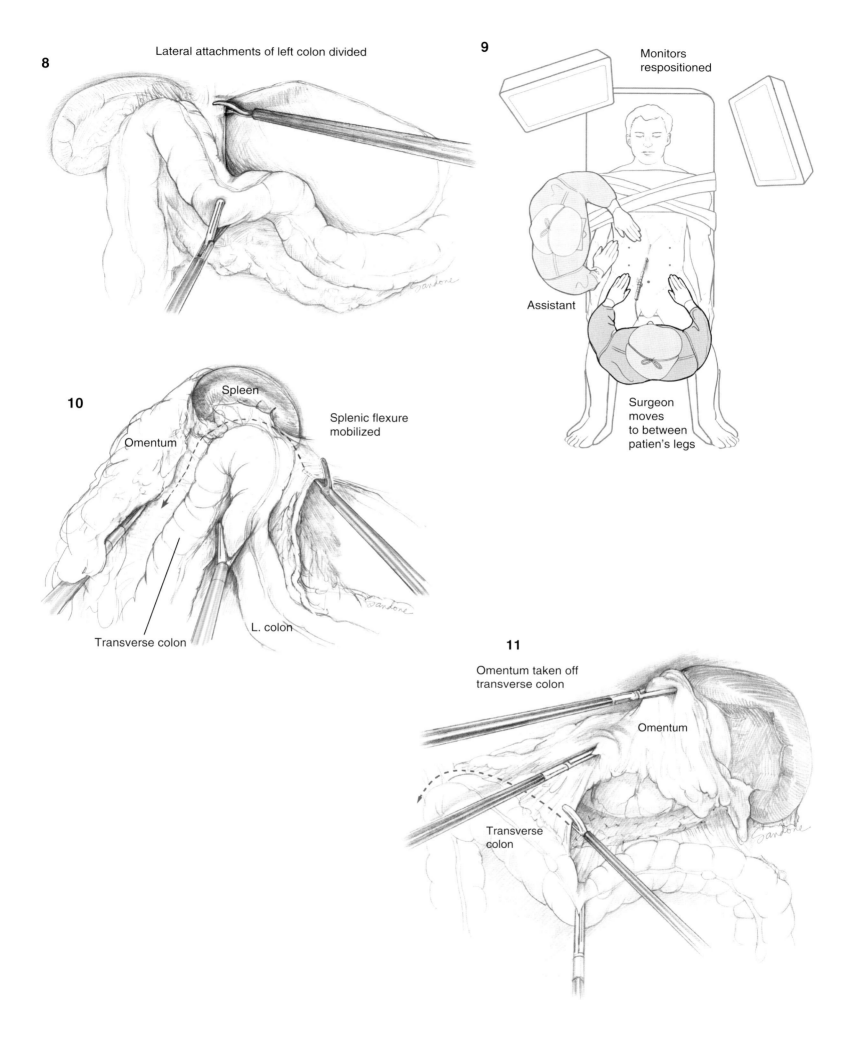

8 Lateral attachments of left colon divided

9 Monitors respositioned

Assistant

Surgeon moves to between patien's legs

10 Spleen

Omentum

Splenic flexure mobilized

Transverse colon

L. colon

11 Omentum taken off transverse colon

Omentum

Transverse colon

Mobilization of the Cecum The surgeon changes position again to stand on the patient's left side. The assistant stands between the patient's legs or to the surgeon's right (FIGURE 12).

The patient is placed in steep Trendelenburg positioning and tilted left. The cecum and appendix are identified and elevated. The mesentery adjacent to the cecum is grasped and lifted toward the anterior abdominal wall. The bulge of the ileocolic pedicle is identified. There will be a sulcus caudal to the ileocolic pedicle. The peritoneum along the sulcus is opened. A window on the cephalad side of the ileocolic pedicle is created by sharply cutting the "bare area" of the mesentery, taking care not to cut too deeply as the duodenum will be close (FIGURE 13).

The ileocolic pedicle is ready for a high ligation. Taking care to avoid the duodenum, a vascular load endoscopic stapler or an energy sealing device is used to divide the pedicle (FIGURE 14). Prior to division of the pedicle, it is prudent to be prepared to control proximal stump. In case of bleeding, a pre-tied ligature can be used to control the stump.

Next, a grasper in the surgeon's left hand is placed under the cut edge of the mesentery and elevated as much as is possible. The plane of dissection can be identified as follows: the small transverse blood vessels lie within the retroperitoneum, while the colon mesentery is a lighter yellow. With the right hand, the plane between the right colon mesentery and retroperitoneum is opened bluntly in a medial-to-lateral fashion until the lateral abdominal wall is reached (FIGURE 15). The attachments from the duodenum to the transverse mesocolon are divided with blunt and thermal dissection (for small bridging vessels).

With the patient in steep Trendelenburg and minimal tilt left, the inferior side of the ileal mesentery is identified and lifted toward the anterior abdominal wall. The small bowel is allowed to fall away into the upper abdomen. The peritoneum is opened above the iliac vessels but below the cecal mesentery (FIGURE 16). A grasper is placed under the cut edge and lifted up. The cecal and ascending colon mesentery is lifted away from the right gonadal vessels, the right ureter, and the duodenum with the right hand as the left hand pushes down on the retroperitoneum, working cephalad until the prior area of medial dissection is reached (FIGURE 17).

12

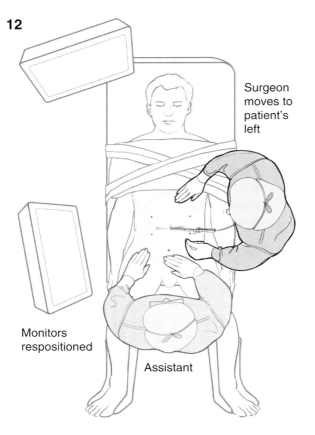

Surgeon moves to patient's left

Monitors respositioned

Assistant

13

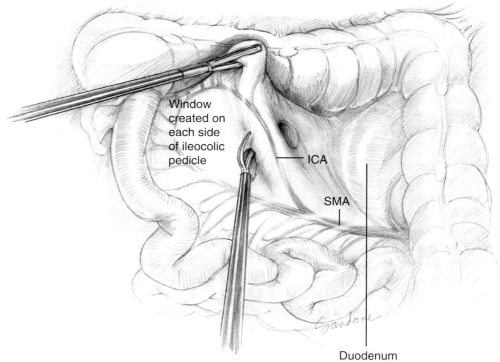

Window created on each side of ileocolic pedicle

ICA

SMA

Duodenum

14

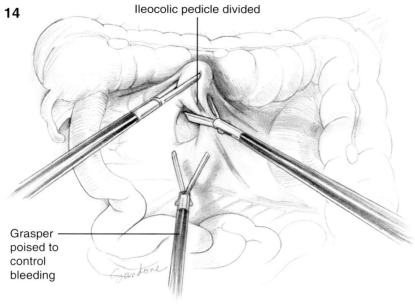

Ileocolic pedicle divided

Grasper poised to control bleeding

15

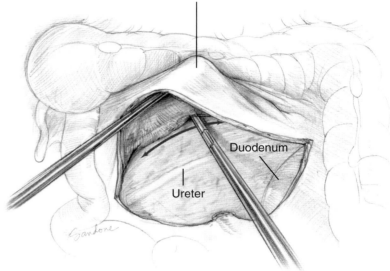

Medial-to-lateral mobilization of right colon mesentery

Duodenum

Ureter

16

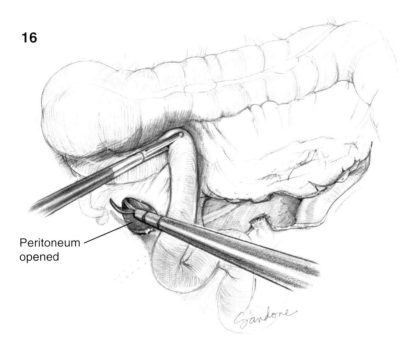

Peritoneum opened

17

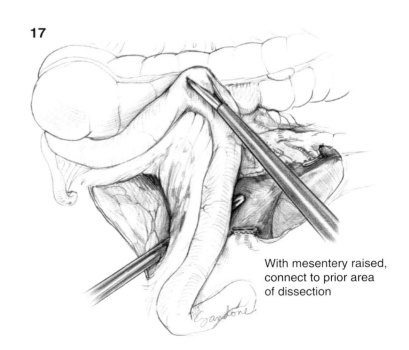

With mesentery raised, connect to prior area of dissection

Mobilization of the Cecum With the patient in less Trendelenburg and maximal tilt left, the lateral peritoneal reflection is grasped just lateral to the cecum and retracted medially. The lateral attachments are divided with scissors or a thermal device until the previously divided hepatic flexure attachments are reached (**FIGURE 18**).

Division of the Middle Colic Vessels This step is optimized by the surgeon moving back to a position between the patient's legs (**FIGURE 19**). Once adequate mobilization of the hepatic and splenic flexure is completed and the omentum is free from the anterior surface of the transverse colon, attention is turned to division of the middle colic vessels. The mesentery is freed from the tail of the pancreas toward the area of transection of the inferior mesenteric vein. Occasionally the arc of Riolan is identified exiting from under the pancreas and entering the mesentery of the left colon. The middle colic vessels are isolated and divided using an energy source or vascular load for the stapler (**FIGURE 20**). The entire colon is now free.

Division of the Proximal Rectum With the left and right colon completely mobilized and the ligation of vessels accomplished, the patient is placed in Trendelenburg position with no lateral tilt. The surgeon moves to the patient's right side. The assistant stands on the left side. The assistant lifts the colon from the retroperitoneum to allow visualization of the posterior rectum. The surgeon uses a 5-mm scissors or hook cautery to dissect in the avascular plane posterior to the rectum beginning at the sacral promontory (**FIGURE 21**). Care is taken to avoid injury to the previously identified ureters.

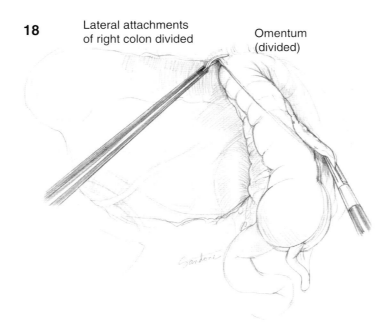

18 Lateral attachments of right colon divided   Omentum (divided)

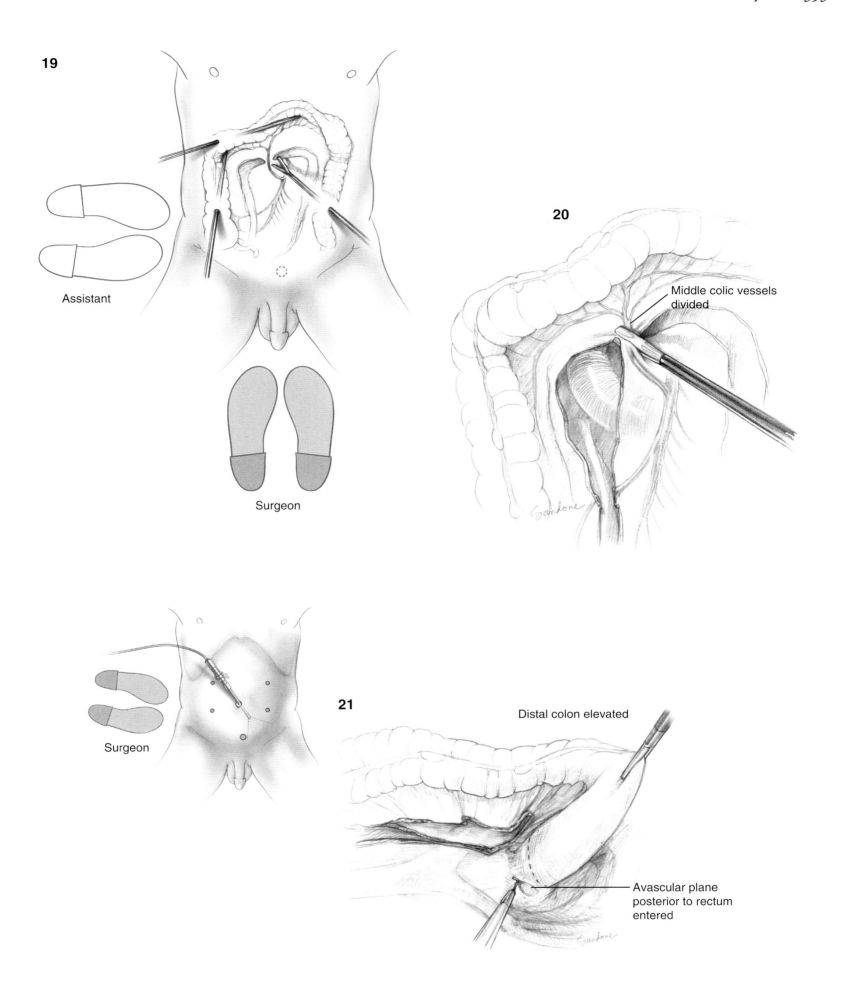

19

Assistant

Surgeon

20

Middle colic vessels
divided

Surgeon

21

Distal colon elevated

Avascular plane
posterior to rectum
entered

Division of the Proximal Rectum The dissection is carried posteriorly in the midline, following the cottony areolar tissue to the level of the rectum just beyond the sacral promontory. The rectum is divided using a roticulating linear stapler (**FIGURE 22**). Multiple firings may be necessary depending on the thickness of the tissue. The mesorectum is divided with additional firings of the stapler or with an energy device. A laparoscopic Babcock clamp is placed on the divided rectum to facilitate extraction (**FIGURE 23**).

Ileorectal Anastomosis In a stable patient without fulminant colitis, an ileorectal anastomosis can be created. To perform an ileorectal anastomosis, an extraction site is made through a low midline suprapubic incision if a hand port was not used previously. A wound protector is recommended. The left colon, transverse colon, and cecum are delivered through the anterior abdominal wall, and the ileum is divided with a linear stapler (**FIGURE 24**).

A purse-string is placed either with a mechanical purse-stringer or by sewing a 0-Prolene around the circumference of the small bowel. The anvil and shaft are secured in the purse-string (**FIGURE 25**). At this point the extraction site can be closed and the anastomosis completed intracorporally or the anastomosis can be performed through the extraction site. The amount of rectal stump and patient body habitus usually dictates this. It may be easy to visualize the anastomosis through the extraction site and reconnect the anvil to the stapler, which is passed up through the anal canal. Alternatively, the anvil and distal ileum may be returned to the abdomen, the wound temporarily closed with towel clips, and pneumoperitoneum reestablished. The anvil and stapling device are connected, closed, and fired under laparoscopic visualization (**FIGURES 26 AND 27**). The doughnuts are inspected for completeness.

22

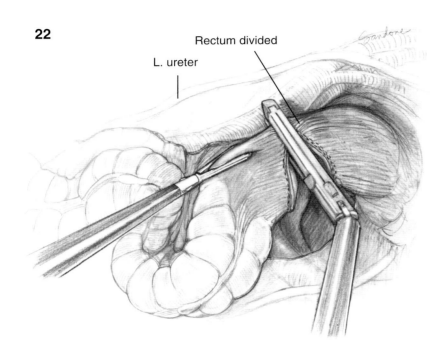

L. ureter

Rectum divided

23

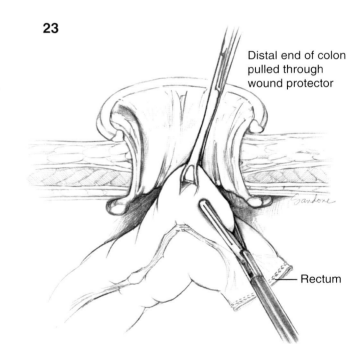

Distal end of colon pulled through wound protector

Rectum

Ileorectal Anastomosis

24

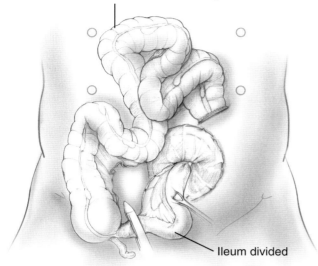

Colon delivered through abdominal wall

Ileum divided

25

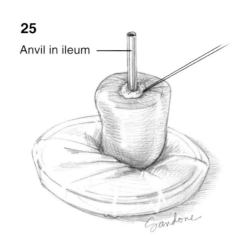

Anvil in ileum

26

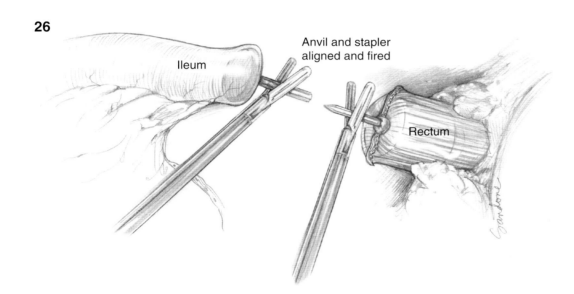

Ileum

Anvil and stapler aligned and fired

Rectum

27

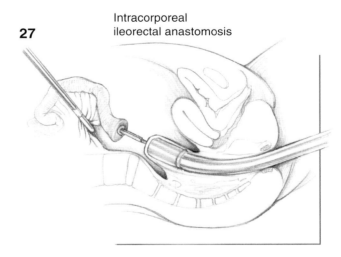

Intracorporeal ileorectal anastomosis

Ileorectal Anastomosis The integrity of the anastomosis should always be tested for leaks by insufflating air through a sigmoidoscope with the proximal bowel occluded and submerged in saline (**FIGURE 28**). If a leak is identified, strong consideration should be given to creation of a diverting loop ileostomy and an attempt made to repair or cover any leak with Lembert sutures. The final anatomy of the ileorectal anastomosis is as shown (**FIGURE 29**).

Alternate: Temporary Diversion Procedure In an unstable patient or one with fulminant colitis, an ileorectal anastomosis should not be performed. An end ileostomy and rectal pouch serve as a temporary diversion procedure. The whole specimen is brought out through the enlarged right lower quadrant trocar site, the ileum is divided, and a Brooke ileostomy is created (**FIGURE 30**). A loop ileostomy (not illustrated) is a third option and may be used to protect an ileorectal anastomosis in a stable patient at high risk for leakage, due to high-dose steroid use or malnutrition.

CLOSURE OF WOUNDS All trocars are removed under direct vision. The fascia of the umbilical extraction site is closed using interrupted figure-of-eight long-acting absorbable monofilament sutures. The umbilicus is recreated using a dermal suture at the apex of the umbilicus secured to the fascia if necessary. The suprapubic extraction site is closed in layers. Port sites greater than 10 mm are closed with interrupted transfascial sutures, and the skin is closed with sutures or dermal adhesive.

POSTOPERATIVE CARE No additional antibiotics are needed after the wounds are closed. A nasogastric tube is not routinely used. Clear liquids are offered the day after the operation, and the diet is advanced as tolerated. The urinary catheter is removed on the morning of the first postoperative day if the patient is not oliguric. ∎

28

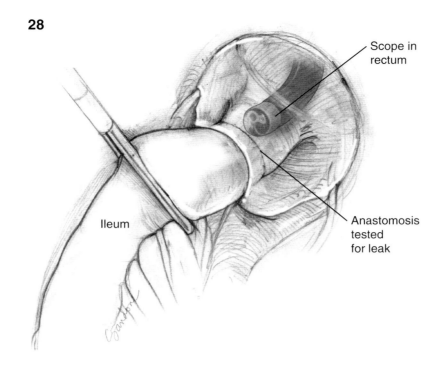

Scope in
rectum

Anastomosis
tested
for leak

Ileum

Ileorectal anastomosis   **Alternate: Temporary diversion**

29   **30**

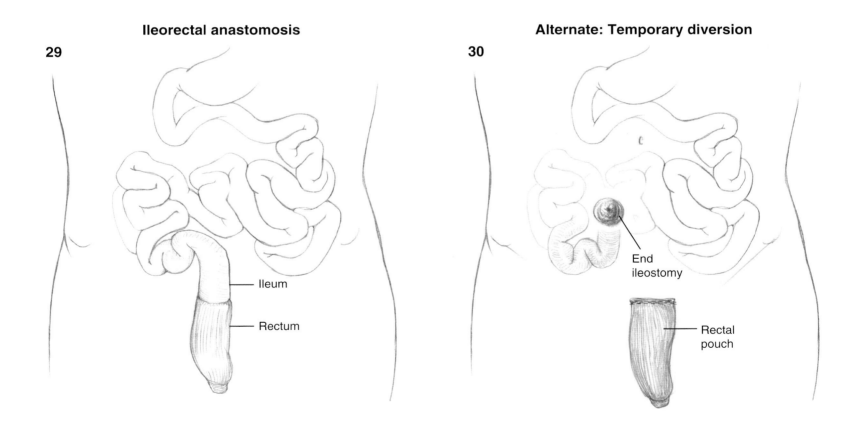

Ileum

Rectum

End
ileostomy

Rectal
pouch

Restorative Proctocolectomy with Ileal J-Pouch Reconstruction

PATIENT SELECTION Patients with either ulcerative colitis or indeterminate colitis are candidates for this procedure after total abdominal colectomy. Though some studies suggest select patients with Crohn's disease may safely undergo this procedure, perianal Crohn's disease and/or fecal incontinence are absolute contraindications.

PREOPERATIVE EVALUATION/PREPARATION Prior to performing a restorative proctocolectomy with ileal J-pouch reconstruction, the patient should have normal nutrition and be marked by enterostomal therapy for possible ileostomy sites. A mechanical/oral antibiotic bowel prep is administered to lessen bowel gas, facilitate bowel manipulation, and reduce the risk of wound infection. Thromboembolism prophylaxis, either pharmacologic or mechanical, is started prior to induction of general anesthesia. Prophylactic antibiotics that cover intestinal flora are given within 1 hour prior to the skin incision. After induction of general anesthesia, an orogastric tube and urinary catheter are placed.

POSITIONING A beanbag should be placed under the patient. The patient should be placed into a low lithotomy position with Allen stirrups. Each ankle, knee, and opposite shoulder should be aligned. No pressure should be placed on the peroneal nerves or calves. The angle between the thigh and the plane of the bed should be between 0 and 10 degrees. Any more flexion will limit range of motion for the instruments. Any more extension may lead to an anterior dislocation of the hip.

Each elbow (ulnar nerve) is covered with a gel pad, and both arms are carefully adducted. Care must be taken to avoid compromising or kinking the intravenous lines.

The beanbag is carefully cradled above both shoulders and around the arms to prevent the patient from falling while in extreme positioning. The air is suctioned from the beanbag so it retains that shape. Tape is placed under the bed, over each shoulder, and across to the other side of the bed. Care is taken to ensure that peak airway pressures are not inappropriately elevated, suggesting that the tape were too tight. Security of the patient on the table should be confirmed using maximal Trendelenburg positioning prior to draping.

DETAILS OF OPERATION

Mobilization of Colon There are a number of critical steps for the laparoscopic mobilization of the entire colon. These include mobilization of the left colon, splenic flexure, transverse mesocolon, and right colon; division of the middle colic artery; division of the proximal rectum; and creation of an ileorectal anastomosis or end ileostomy. The ability to accomplish these tasks requires movement of the surgeon and assistant around the table as needed to optimize instrumentation. Surgeons vary in their preference of the order of performing the listed steps.

Trocar placement and details of left, right, and transverse colon and rectal resections have been described in detail in previous chapters.

After placement of the trocars, the surgeon and first assistant begin the procedure standing on the patient's right side. The first assistant should stand closest to the patient's right shoulder (**FIGURE 1**).

The initial steps in the procedure involve placing the patient in steep Trendelenburg and rotating the patient to the right. This allows all the small intestine to fall out of the left lower quadrant as the left colon is mobilized in a manner similar to the low anterior resection (**FIGURE 2**).

After complete mobilization of the left colon, the surgeon changes position to stand on the patient's left side to facilitate mobilization of the right colon (**FIGURES 3 AND 4**). The assistant stands between the patient's legs or to the surgeon's right. The patient is placed in steep Trendelenburg positioning and tilted left.

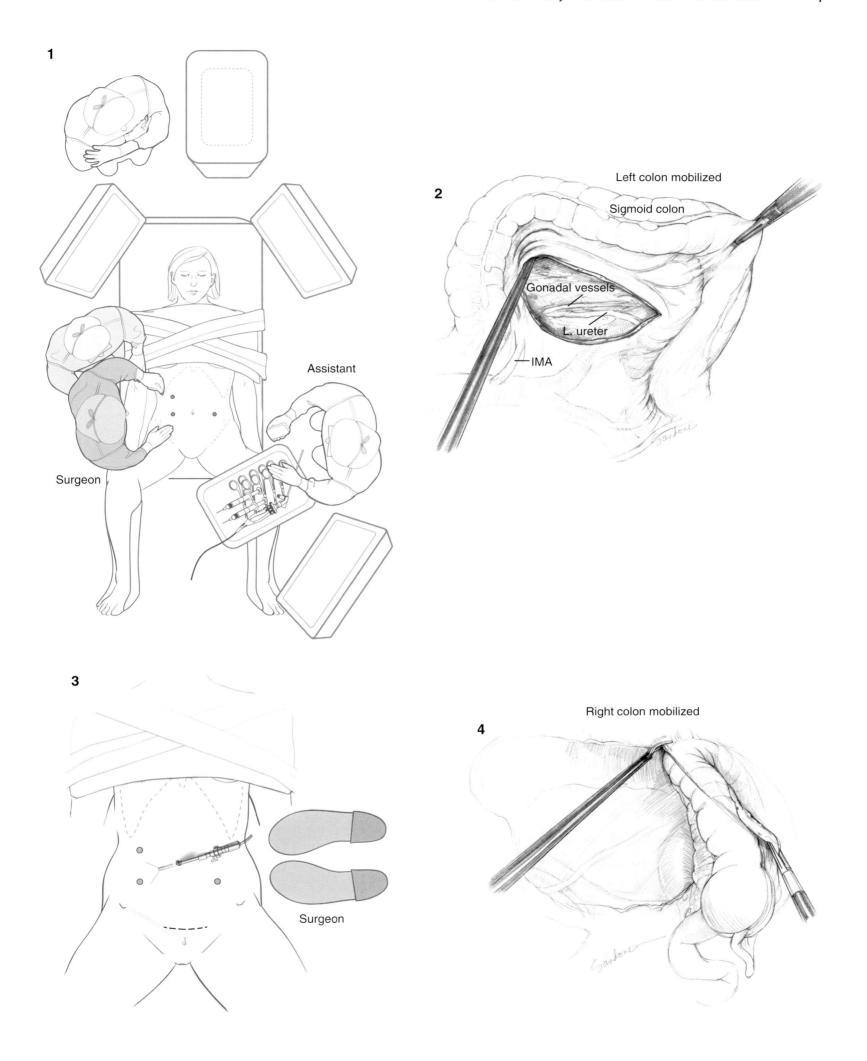

1

Surgeon

Assistant

2

Left colon mobilized

Sigmoid colon

Gonadal vessels

L. ureter

IMA

3

Surgeon

4

Right colon mobilized

Mobilization of Colon The surgeon stands between the patient's legs to facilitate takedown of the transverse colon. Monitors are repositioned as needed to optimize viewing **(FIGURE 5)**. The surgeon retracts the transverse colon inferiorly with their left hand, using an atraumatic grasper through a suprapubic port. The assistant stands to the patient's right with instruments through the two right abdominal trocars, lifting the omentum toward the anterior abdominal wall and retracting the splenic flexure toward the midline. This allows division of the remaining attachments of the splenic flexure. A window into the lesser omental sac allows visualization of the undersurface of the stomach, the anterior surface of the pancreas, and the mesentery of the colon. The flimsy tissue between the transverse colon and the greater omentum is divided until the hepatic flexure is reached **(FIGURE 6)**. These last few steps are described in greater detail in Chapter 50.

To mobilize and divide the rectum, the surgeon stands on the patient's right side **(FIGURE 7)**. The assistant moves to the left side and lifts the colon from the retroperitoneum. The surgeon uses a scissors or hook cautery to dissect in the avascular plane behind the rectum, beginning at the sacral promontory. The dissection is carried posteriorly in the midline following the cottony areolar tissue to the level of the coccyx. Circumferential dissection is completed as described in Chapter 52 to allow elevation of the rectum from the pelvis. A linear stapler is used to divide the rectum **(FIGURE 8)**.

After complete mobilization of the entire colon and division of the rectum distally, the entire specimen is brought out through a suprapubic incision and placed on the abdominal wall.

Creation of the Ileal J-Pouch The antimesenteric terminal ileal fat (ligament of Treves) is dissected away from the ileum. The ileum is divided just proximal to the ileocecal valve using medium thickness staples **(FIGURE 9)**. The cecal mesentery adjacent to the cecum is divided. This divides the cecal branch of the ileocolic pedicle and preserves the ileal branch **(FIGURE 10)**.

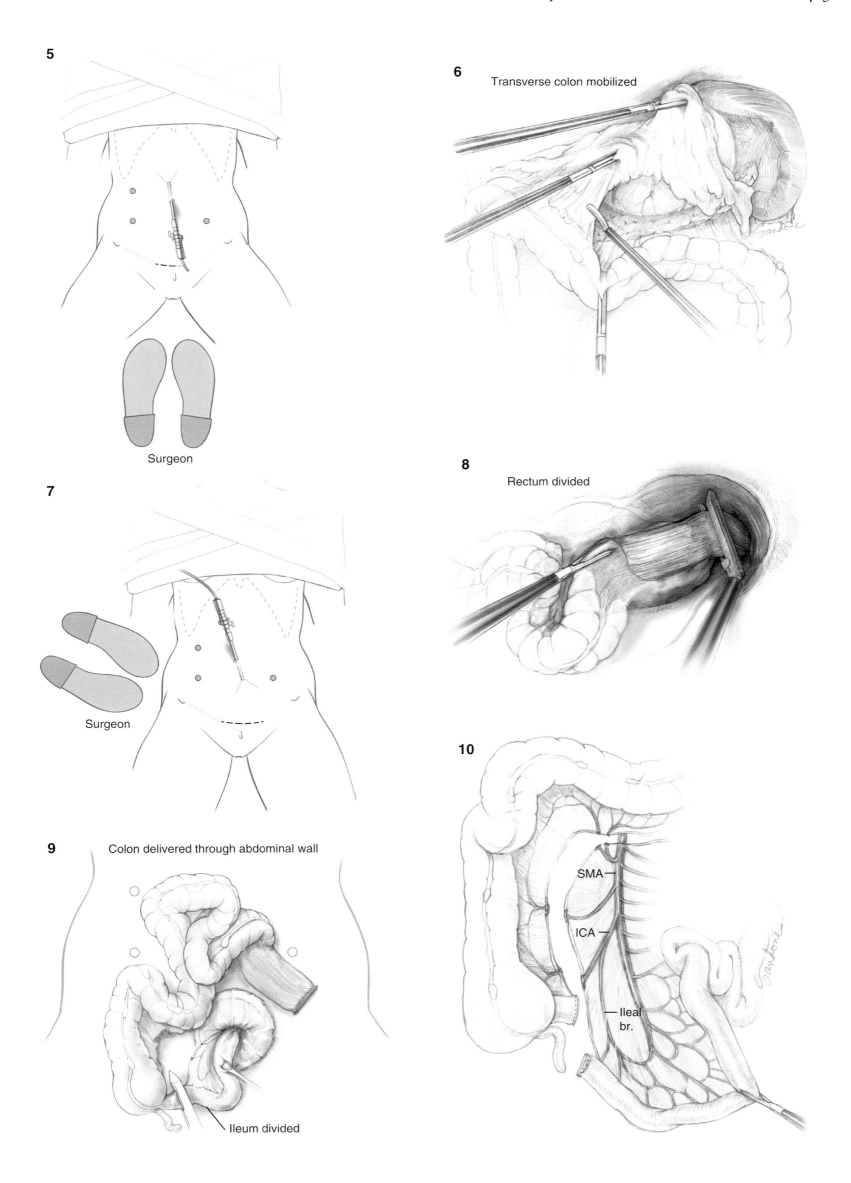

5

Surgeon

6 Transverse colon mobilized

7

Surgeon

8 Rectum divided

9 Colon delivered through abdominal wall

Ileum divided

10

SMA

ICA

Ileal br.

Creation of the Ileal J-Pouch   Under laparoscopy, the portion of the terminal ileum that most easily reaches to the rectal stump is identified. Typically, this is 12 to 25 cm proximal to the end of the ileum **(FIGURE 11)**. If there is difficulty getting the ileum to reach the rectal stump, the following three maneuvers are considered in this order:

1. Adhesions between the ileal mesentery and the duodenum are divided bluntly with the index finger (open), or a blunt grasper (laparoscopic).
2. Without injuring the superior mesenteric artery, small transverse incisions are made in the anterior and posterior peritoneum overlying the superior mesentery artery **(FIGURE 12)**. Each 1-cm transverse incision should give an additional 1 cm in length.
3. If the ileal branch of the ileocolic artery has been preserved, Doppler is used to assess the marginal artery at the proposed apex of the pouch. A vascular clamp is applied to the superior mesenteric artery (SMA) distal to the takeoff of the ileocolic artery. If collateral flow through the ileocolic artery is good, the SMA is divided distal to the ileocolic artery branch (see Figure 12). This final maneuver should provide sufficient length to reach the anal canal.

A 2-cm enterotomy is made at the apex of the pouch. Using two firings of a 100 mm linear stapler, a 12- to 15-cm-long ileal pouch is created **(FIGURES 13 AND 14)**. Extra ileum at the stump end is resected with another firing of the stapler. The tip of the J-pouch (staple line of this ileal stump) is oversewn with interrupted 3-0 Lembert sutures. A "crotch" or apical stitch is placed at the top of the two limbs of the pouch. A 2-0 Prolene purse-string suture is placed into the apex of the ileum at the enterotomy site. The anvil of a 28 or 29 mm circular stapler is inserted into the pouch and the purse-string suture is secured **(FIGURE 15)**.

It is the mesentery of the pouch that limits the reach of the pouch into the pelvis. The mesentery is positioned posterior to the pouch so it travels the shortest distance over the sacral promontory. The anvil and the stapler are mated with the use of laparoscopic graspers, taking care to avoid the bladder in a man or the vagina in a woman. The position is confirmed to ensure there is no tension or twist. After 15 seconds, the circular stapler is fired **(FIGURE 16)**.

The anastomosis is tested for leaks using pouch insufflation and saline. The pelvis is filled with saline. The ileorectal anastomosis is completely submerged. The ileum proximal to the pouch is cross clamped **(FIGURE 17)**. A flexible pouchoscopy is performed. If the pouch distends well and no bubbling is observed, the anastomosis should be sound. A small leak can be repaired with interrupted sutures. A large leak may require a hand-sewn ileorectal anastomosis.

A closed suction drain is placed into the presacral space and brought out through one of the 5-mm trocar sites. A portion of ileum 30 to 40 cm proximal to the pouch is identified and brought up through the right lower quadrant port site, and a diverting loop ileostomy is created **(FIGURE 18)**.

CLOSURE OF WOUNDS   Trocars are removed under direct vision. The fascia of any trocar site larger than 10 mm is closed using interrupted transfascial sutures. The skin incision may be closed with sutures or staples. A stoma appliance is placed.

POSTOPERATIVE CARE   No additional antibiotics are needed after the wounds are closed. A nasogastric tube is not routinely used. Clear liquids are offered the day after the operation, and the diet is advanced as tolerated. The urinary catheter is removed on the morning of the first or second postoperative day if the patient is not oliguric. The presacral drain is removed when the output is serous, usually on the third or fourth postoperative day. ■

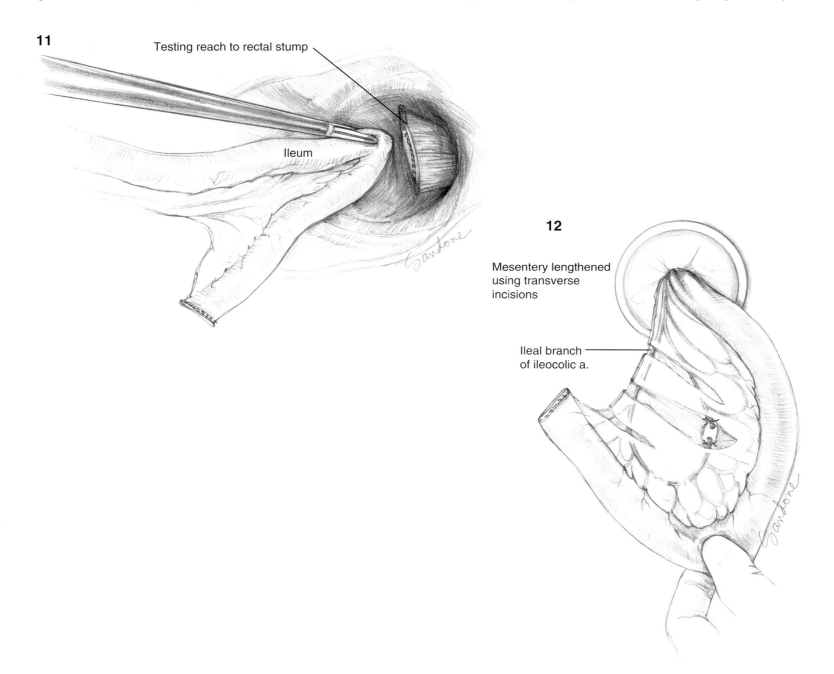

11

Testing reach to rectal stump

Ileum

12

Mesentery lengthened using transverse incisions

Ileal branch of ileocolic a.

13

14

15

Ileal
J pouch
created

Anvil

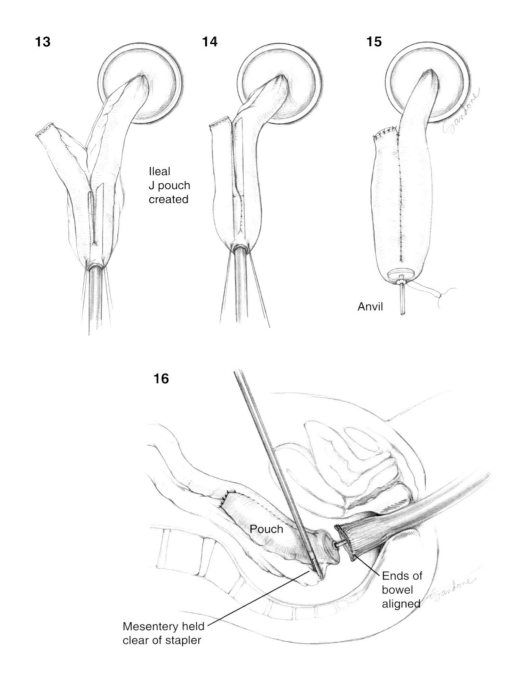

16

Pouch

Ends of
bowel
aligned

Mesentery held
clear of stapler

17

Completed
anastomosis
tested for leaks

Saline level

Pouch

Air through
scope

18

Temporary
diverting
ileostomy

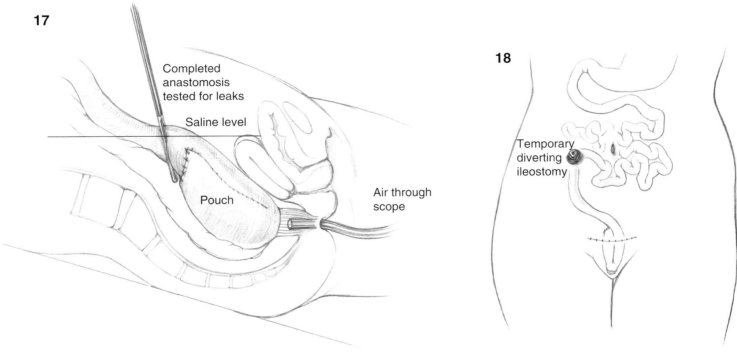

LOW ANTERIOR RESECTION

INDICATIONS Laparoscopic low anterior resection (LAR) is used for removal of rectal cancer and benign diseases with the intent of removing the rectum and restoring the continuity of the bowel with an anastomosis in the pelvis. The LAR has been a standard of care for high and mid rectal cancer for many years and, with certain modifications, is now available to individuals with low rectal cancer. This chapter deals with the routine removal of the rectum and its mesentery and the reconstruction of continuity within the pelvis above the anal canal.

PREOPERATIVE PREPARATION Individuals with rectal cancer, diverticulitis, endometriosis, or other less common tumors will require preoperative imaging with computed tomography (CT) scan or transrectal ultrasound to stage the disease and help plan the procedure. In many instances, patients with rectal cancer will require neoadjuvant chemoradiation, which adds another level of complexity to the procedure and will sometimes influence the surgeon to protect the pelvic anastomosis with a temporary diverting loop ileostomy.

A mechanical and antibiotic bowel preparation is usually recommended. The rectum should be emptied of solid stool and irrigated with some form of cytocidal liquid at the beginning of or during the procedure to wash out any malignant cells if the indication is rectal cancer. This serves the purpose of reducing the number of viable cells within the rectal vault, but it has never been definitively shown to decrease the incidence of local recurrence of rectal cancer.

The patient is maintained on bowel rest after midnight before the operation. Broad-spectrum IV antibiotics with coverage of gram-negative aerobes and anaerobes and gram-positive anaerobes are administered prior to incision. Patients are also given subcutaneous low-molecular-weight heparin preoperatively.

ANESTHESIA General anesthesia with endotracheal intubation is necessary for this operation to provide complete neuromuscular blockade. The patient is supplemented with narcotic analgesia during the anesthetic portion of the procedure to allow a smooth transition to the awakened state. Occasionally, the patient may benefit from an epidural analgesic supplement because of severe chronic obstructive pulmonary disease (COPD). Ketorolac is a reasonable supplement to the narcotic analgesia provided after surgery, if the field is very dry and there is no contraindication to this medication.

POSITION Laparoscopic LAR is performed in the lithotomy position using Allen stirrups to position the patient (**FIGURE 1**). Sequential compression devices are placed on the calves at the time of entering the room before anesthesia induction. A beanbag is very helpful to fix the patient in position because gravity will be used for retraction. The patient will be tilted back and forth from right to left and placed in steep Trendelenburg and even in reverse Trendelenburg positions at times. The beanbag is curled up around the sides and shoulders of the patient, and a tape is placed across the chest to keep the beanbag firmly tucked. A Velcro strap is placed behind the beanbag and attached directly to the table for security. The hip flexion at the Allen stirrups should be less than 10 degrees. The flat angle allows full motion of the instrumentation across the hip flexion and makes all four quadrants available during the operation. Monitors are placed to give view from all three angles of the right side of the patient. The operating surgeon stands on the patient's right side. An assistant stands between the patient's legs or on the left side. The surgeon should always stand opposite the pathology and work with their instruments facing a monitor in line with the pathology and instrumentation.

OPERATIVE PREPARATION A Foley catheter is placed in the bladder. An orogastric tube is beneficial to decompress the stomach. The rectum is irrigated with saline and either Betadine or another cytocidal agent. A 34 French mushroom catheter can be left in the rectum to provide intraoperative drainage of the rectal cavity as well as tactile guidance to the anal canal. After induction of general endotracheal anesthesia, the entire abdomen patient is prepped to allow use of a hand port and placement of the trocars as far laterally as possible.

INCISION AND EXPOSURE Trocar positions are selected based upon body habitus. Generally, the camera port is placed above the umbilicus in the vertical midline, using a 5- or 10-mm trocar to introduce a 30-degree angled laparoscope. 12-mm trocars are placed in the right upper quadrant subcostal area laterally and in the suprapubic midline. The 5-mm trocars are placed in the right lower quadrant and the left lower quadrant. The appropriate placement should be two fingerbreadths below the right costal margin in the anterior axillary line and two fingerbreadths above the anterior superior iliac spine on a line toward the umbilicus. The left trocar should be placed in the left mid lateral position at the level of the umbilicus. The 12-mm trocar in the suprapubic midline should be placed two fingerbreadths above the pubis (**FIGURE 2**). A hand-assisted approach can be achieved through this same incision if the lower edge of the incision is far enough away from the pubis to allow placement of the intraabdominal ring and maintain a pneumoperitoneum with the hand-assist device in place.

The laparoscope is then introduced, and the abdomen should be explored in all quadrants to make sure there are no adhesions that would prevent completion of the procedure or extensive disease that would require an open operation.

DETAILS OF THE PROCEDURE The initial steps in the procedure involve placing the patient in steep Trendelenburg and tilting the patient to the right. This allows all of the small intestine to fall out of the left lower quadrant and out of the pelvis and into the right upper quadrant. The standard approach to a LAR begins with a medial-to-lateral dissection at the base of the mesentery of the sigmoid and left colon at the sacral promontory. An incision is made over the sacral promontory behind the superior hemorrhoidal artery as the sigmoid colon is retracted anteriorly and out of the pelvis (**FIGURE 3**). This allows entry into an avascular plane at the sacral promontory. Blunt dissection in a tangential plane over the left iliac artery and vein at the pelvic brim allows identification of the left ureter and the gonadal vessels (**FIGURE 4**). The midline structure that is first met when proceeding cephalad is the inferior mesenteric artery (IMA). The thickened dense nerves that arise from the preaortic plexus and extend up onto the inferior mesenteric artery can be preserved in benign disease. In malignancy, however, these should be taken with the specimen and the IMA divided within 1 cm of the origin of the vessel. Techniques for dividing these structures include stapling with a vascular staple load of the linear stapler, clips, or energy sources such as bipolar or LigaSure (**FIGURE 5**). Before dividing the IMA, care should be taken to visualize and protect the ureter and gonadal vessels. Once the IMA is divided, the avascular plane behind it is developed cephalad, caudad, and laterally. The lateral dissection extends all the way out to the gutter beyond the colon, until the only structure suspending the colon is the lateral peritoneal reflection (white line of Toldt).

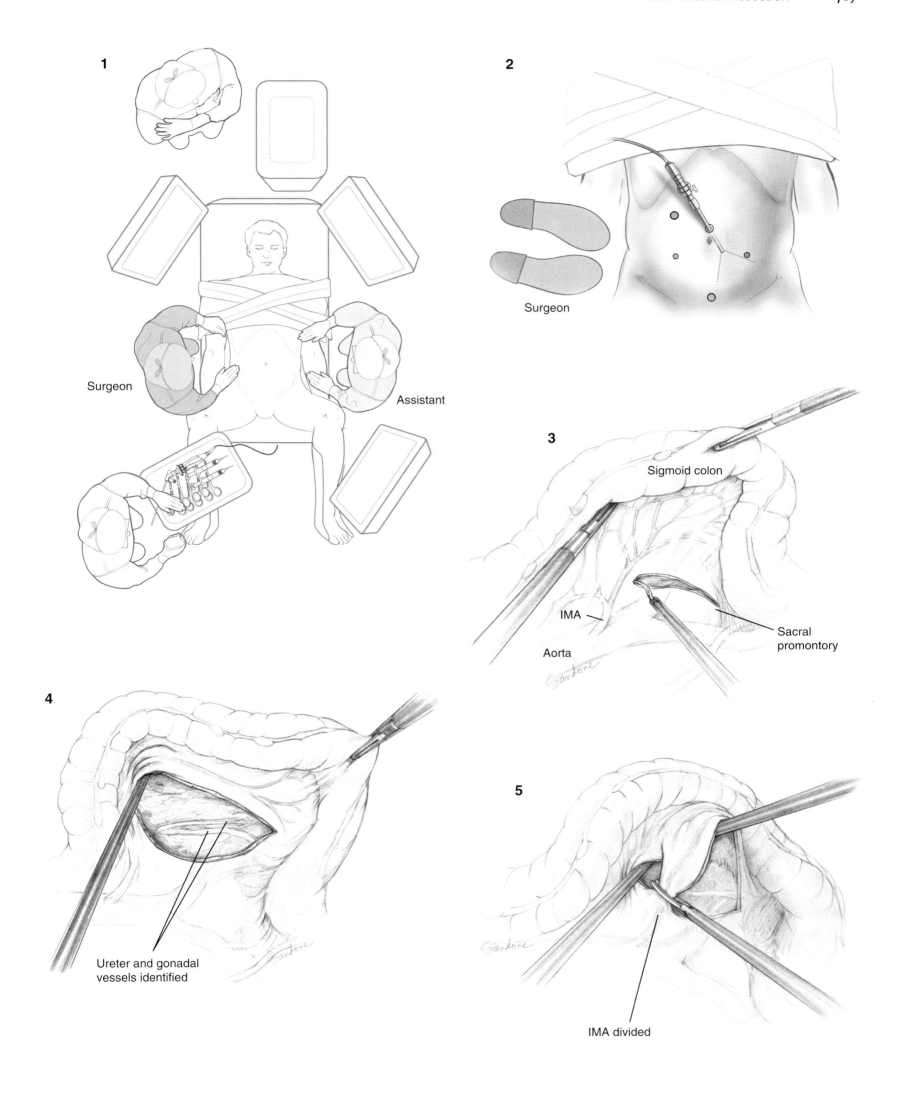

1

Surgeon

Assistant

2

Surgeon

3

Sigmoid colon

IMA

Aorta

Sacral promontory

4

Ureter and gonadal vessels identified

5

IMA divided

DETAILS OF THE PROCEDURE The next structure to be encountered in the midline dissection toward the head is the inferior mesenteric vein running at the base of the mesentery of the left colon (**FIGURE 6**). The inferior mesenteric vein dives behind the third portion of the duodenum at the level of the ligament of Treitz, where the duodenum sweeps out away from the pancreas. Retraction of the inferior mesenteric vein anteriorly toward the abdominal wall allows visualization behind the vein along the undersurface of the pancreas and allows the surgeon to create a window in the base of the mesentery of the left colon at the origin of the inferior mesenteric vein. The vein can then be divided with staples or energy sources as needed (**FIGURE 7**).

The avascular plane laterally and cephalad is developed all the way over the top of the kidney along the tail of the pancreas and out laterally to the sidewall to completely mobilize the left colon and its mesentery from the retroperitoneum.

The next step is to incise the lateral attachments of the colon beginning at the pelvic brim at the sigmoid attachments and all the way up to the splenic flexure. This can be accomplished easily with electrocautery and should move rapidly (**FIGURE 8**).

The mobilization of the splenic flexure has become standard for laparoscopic LAR. It is important to mobilize the colon sufficiently to provide adequate length to reach the pelvis with the patient in reverse Trendelenburg position. The colon is retracted toward the midline. The surgeon stands between the patient's legs with their left hand on the 10-mm instrument through the suprapubic port and the right hand on a scissors or energy source through the left flank trocar (**FIGURE 9**). An assistant stands to the patient's right with instruments through the two trocars lifting the omentum toward the anterior abdominal wall and retracting the splenic flexure toward the midline. This exposes the lateral attachments of the splenic flexure toward the midline (**FIGURE 10**). The peritoneal incision should be continued along the lateral aspect until the tail of the pancreas is reached. A window into the lesser omental sac should be incised to allow visualization of the undersurface of the stomach, the anterior surface of the pancreas, and the mesentery of the colon. The overlying omentum is lifted off of the splenic flexure and is separated off the transverse colon in the avascular plane with electrocautery (**FIGURE 11**).

6

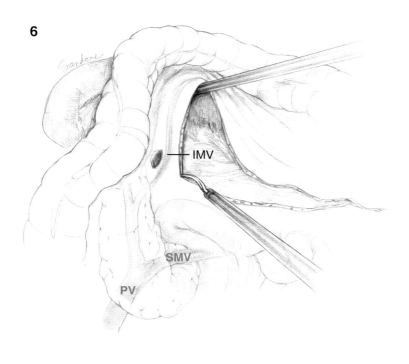

7

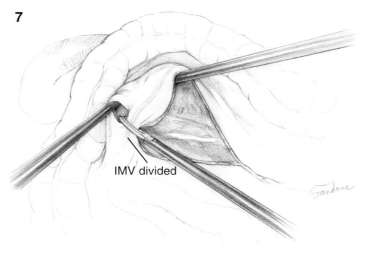

8 Lateral attachments of left colon divided

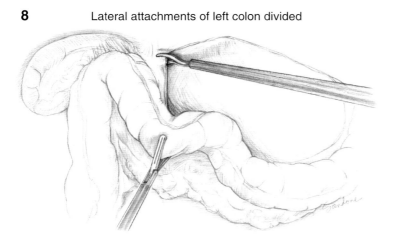

9

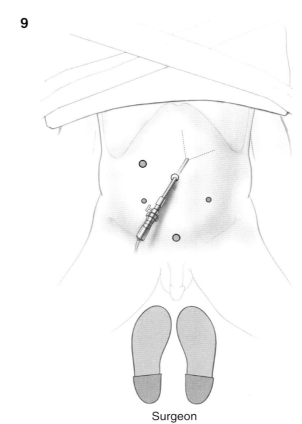

Surgeon

10

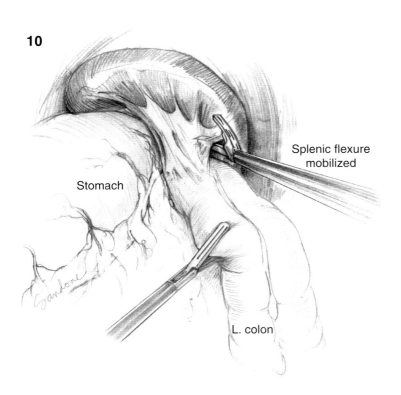

11 Omentum taken off transverse colon

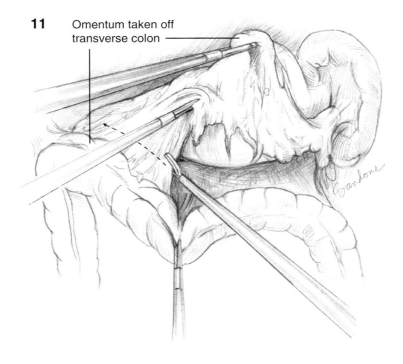

DETAILS OF THE PROCEDURE Once adequate mobilization of the splenic flexure is completed by freeing the omentum from the anterior surface of the transverse colon, the colon mesentery is freed from the tail of the pancreas toward the area of transection of the inferior mesenteric vein. Occasionally the arc of Riolan is identified exiting from under the pancreas and entering the mesentery of the left colon. This leaves the left colon and sigmoid colon vascularized by the left branch of the middle colic artery along the marginal artery of Drummond (**FIGURE 12**). This should allow the left colon to reach the pelvis easily (**FIGURE 13**).

With the left colon completely mobilized and the high ligation of vessels accomplished, the patient is placed back in Trendelenburg position and flat on the table with no left or right tilt. The surgeon moves back to the patient's right side. The assistant moves to the left side. The assistant lifts the colon from the retroperitoneum with an instrument placed behind the cut edge of the mesentery of the sigmoid colon. This can be accomplished with a straight instrument or a curved retractor with flexible tip. The surgeon uses a 5-mm scissors or hook cautery to dissect in the avascular plane behind the rectum beginning at the sacral promontory (**FIGURE 14**).

A mesorectal dissection is completed to remove the rectum intact with its mesorectum. The dissection is carried posteriorly in the midline following the cottony areolar tissue to the level of the coccyx. At this point, a thicker tissue plane is encountered that fixes the back of the rectum to the presacral fascia (**FIGURE 15**). The dissection is then extended laterally along the pelvic sidewall, using a circular motion because of the bowl shape of the pelvis. Straight-line dissection will result in injury of adjacent structures, nerves, and arteries and violate the mesorectal envelope. At the pelvic brim,

the surgeon will find two areas of potential disaster. The ureter runs over the surface of the common iliac artery at the site of bifurcation to the internal iliac and external iliac. Adjacent to the ureter is the splanchnic nerve, which runs along the inner aspect of the pelvic brim from the hypogastric plexus, including parasympathetic and sympathetic nerves that innervate the bladder, prostate, and penis. The nerves at the IMA are sympathetic nerves and, when divided, will result in retrograde ejaculation. Division of the nerves along the pelvic sidewall in the splanchnic nerves will result in impotence and urinary difficulty.

The dissection extends along the peritoneal covering of the mesentery of the rectum along each side of the pelvis. This step will completely release the entire rectum on both sides of the pelvis (**FIGURE 16**).

The final dissection is the anterior aspect of the rectum. Through the left lower quadrant, a retracting clamp is placed behind the anterior peritoneal reflection of the vagina or the prostate and bladder and lifted anteriorly. The 10-mm instrument through the patient's right upper quadrant pulls the rectum downward and cephalad to stretch the attachments at the peritoneal reflection. Scissors are used to incise horizontally behind the peritoneal reflection either anterior or posterior to the Denonvilliers fascia, depending on the indication of the disease (**FIGURE 17**). An anterior rectal cancer requires taking the Denonvilliers fascia and entering the plane adjacent to the seminal vesicles and prostate, putting the nervi erigentes at risk for damage and therefore the patient at risk for impotence. The incision is carried inferiorly in the areolar tissue plane as it continues posterior to the prostate. Some blunt dissection is possible in this area.

12

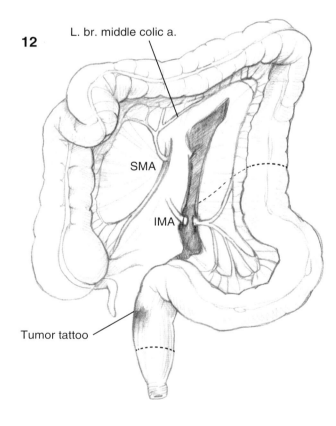

L. br. middle colic a.

SMA

IMA

Tumor tattoo

13

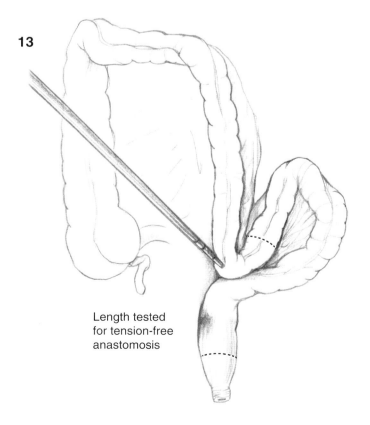

Length tested for tension-free anastomosis

14

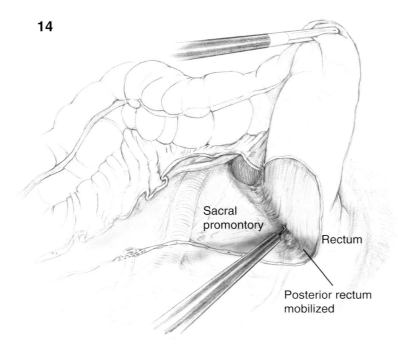

Sacral
promontory

Rectum

Posterior rectum
mobilized

15

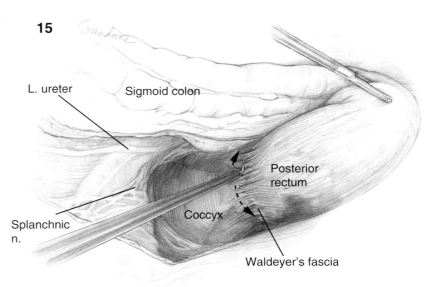

L. ureter   Sigmoid colon

Posterior
rectum

Splanchnic
n.

Coccyx

Waldeyer's fascia

16

Lateral peritoneal attachments divided

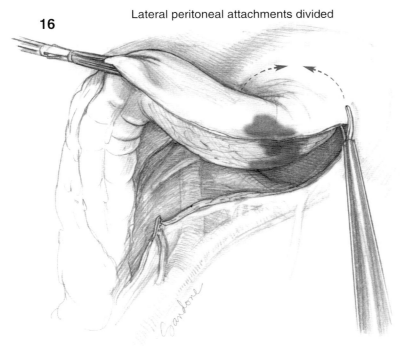

17

Anterior peritoneal
attachments divided

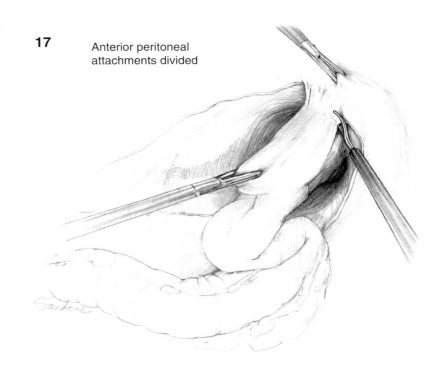

DETAILS OF THE PROCEDURE The final attachments of the rectum are the anterolateral ligaments, which contain the blood supply of the midrectum known as the middle rectal arteries. These anterolateral ligaments are angled from the anterolateral position of the pelvis onto the side of the rectum. They can be divided with electrocautery and the hook cautery tip, as long as the cautery is moved slowly and carefully through the ligaments to obtain hemostasis during the cutting (**FIGURE 18**). Once these anterolateral ligaments have been divided on both sides with gentle curvilinear sweeping strokes, the entire rectum will be completely free from the sidewall of the pelvis and the anterior surface of the sacrum, with the distal rectum heading into the anal canal. The entire mesorectum will have been completely mobilized.

A total mesorectal excision is essential to the local removal of the tumor and its lymphatic drainage. A stapled anastomosis can be constructed by placing a linear stapler or an Endo GIA stapler across the rectum 5 cm below the lowest edge of the tumor (**FIGURE 19**). It is important to have identified the tumor and its position preoperatively, and in some instances it is helpful to have a tattoo of India ink placed at the inferior or distal edge of the tumor to make sure that the tumor site is visible during the operation.

An extraction site can be made either in the left lower quadrant or in the midline suprapubic trocar site. A wound protector is recommended.

The rectum, sigmoid colon, and left colon are delivered through the anterior abdominal wall, and the left colon is divided in the area of the inferior mesenteric vein transection (**FIGURE 20**). The vessels in the mesentery can be divided between o-Vicryl ties, placing clamps across the mesentery through the extraction site.

The purse-string is placed in the left colon at the desired site of transection. It is important to remove all of the sigmoid colon in patients who have undergone neoadjuvant chemoradiation. This will usually result in a purse-string at least in the middle of the left colon or the proximal portion. Testing of adequate length requires that the point of transection pass 4 cm below the pubis when stretched through the extraction site. The point of transection and placement of purse-string is then selected. The purse-string is placed either with a mechanical purse-stringer or by sewing a o-Prolene around the circumference of the bowel. Anvil and shaft should be secured in the purse-string (**FIGURE 21**). The option now exists either to close the extraction site and complete the anastomosis intracorporeally, or to perform the anastomosis through the extraction site. Time usually dictates this, and it is often quicker to use the extraction wound to reconnect the anvil and shaft to the stapler, which is passed up through the anal canal.

18

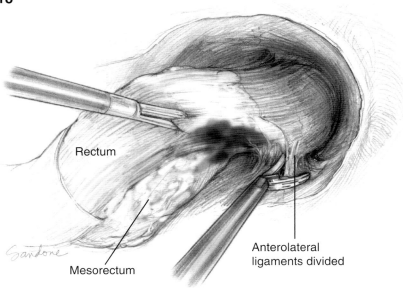

Rectum

Mesorectum

Anterolateral
ligaments divided

19

Rectum divided

Mesorectum   Tattoo

20

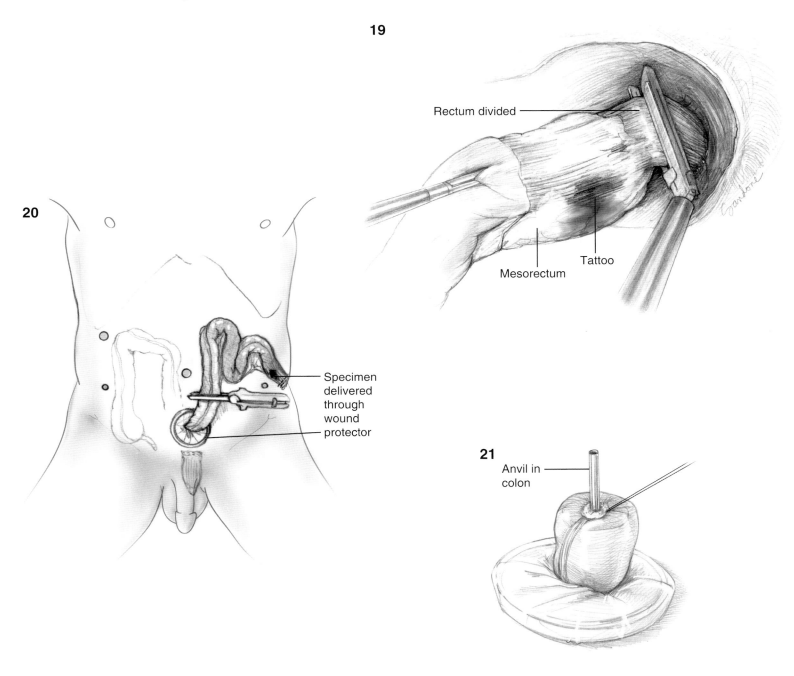

Specimen
delivered
through
wound
protector

21   Anvil in
colon

DETAILS OF THE PROCEDURE The stapling instrument is then reconnected, closed, and fired (**FIGURES 22–24**). The anastomosis should always be checked by insufflating air through the rigid proctoscope with the proximal bowel occluded to allow checking for leakage (**FIGURES 25 AND 26**). If a leak is identified, the anastomosis should be diverted with a loop ileostomy and an attempt made to repair or cover any leak with absorbable Lembert sutures. The decision to place a loop ileostomy for diversion also depends on the use of neoadjuvant chemoradiation.

CLOSURE A Blake drain can be used to drain the pelvis and can be brought out through one of the lower quadrant trocar sites and secured to the skin and hooked to suction bulb drainage. The midline suprapubic extraction site or left lower quadrant extraction site is closed with a running number 1 loop suture. Subcutaneous tissue is irrigated with antibiotics and saline, and the skin is closed with skin staples at all of the sites. Trocar sites larger than 10 mm are generally closed with interrupted transfascial sutures if a cutting trocar was used. Radially expanding trocars only require closure in very thin patients. An attempt should be made to close the supraumbilical site.

POSTOPERATIVE CARE Patients are managed like any bowel resection patients. A nasogastric tube is not necessary unless there was extensive adhesiolysis or other damage to the bowel during the procedure. Patients can be offered ice chips and sips in the first 24 hours. However, they will usually need some form of antinausea medication and will need continued IV fluid therapy for at least 3 or 4 days. The typical bowel function recovery is at 4 to 5 postoperative days. When the patient begins to pass flatus, it is routine to offer them liquid diet and advance rapidly thereafter to a regular diet. Patients who require an ileostomy can be advanced somewhat faster because their ileostomy begins to function much more quickly than the colon would return to function. Patients are encouraged to ambulate at least three times a day after surgery. They are given subcutaneous heparin or low-molecular-weight heparin for deep venous thrombosis (DVT) prevention as indicated by their risk factors. Sequential compression devices are used in the operating room to reduce the risk of DVT. Low anterior resection is a high-risk procedure for development of DVT, and prophylaxis should be maximized with two methods for most of these patients.

A feared complication after a LAR is an anastomotic leak. For this reason, a pelvic drain can be placed for early detection. Drains have not been shown to prevent anastomotic leak. The main reason for using a diverting loop ileostomy in patients who are at extremely high risk for anastomotic leak is to reduce the impact of the leak rather than prevent it. If a contained leak can be identified and drained percutaneously or controlled through an indwelling operatively placed pelvic drain, the patient can be maintained on bowel rest or with diversion until the leak heals and then be returned to normal alimentation. However, a wide separation of the anastomosis with wide contamination of the pelvis and the abdominal cavity requires exploration, diversion, washout, and, usually, takedown of the entire anastomosis and conversion to a permanent stoma. For this reason, it is important to control this problem with a conservative approach if at all possible. ■

22

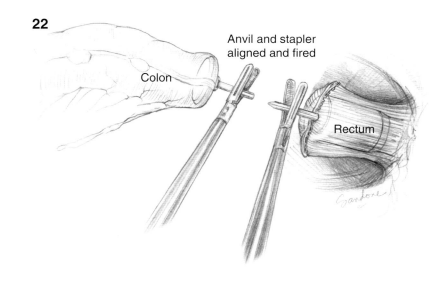

Colon

Anvil and stapler
aligned and fired

Rectum

23

Intracorporeal
colorectal anastomosis

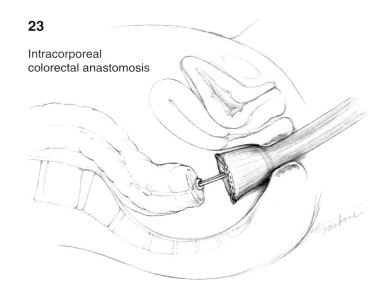

24

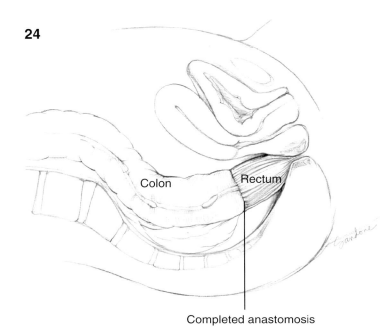

Colon   Rectum

Completed anastomosis

25

Scope in rectum

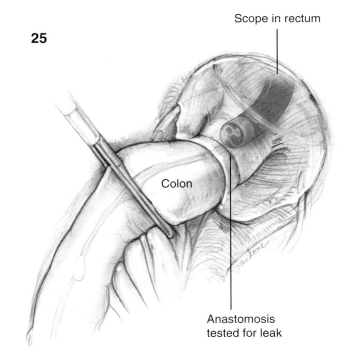

Colon

Anastomosis
tested for leak

26

Saline level

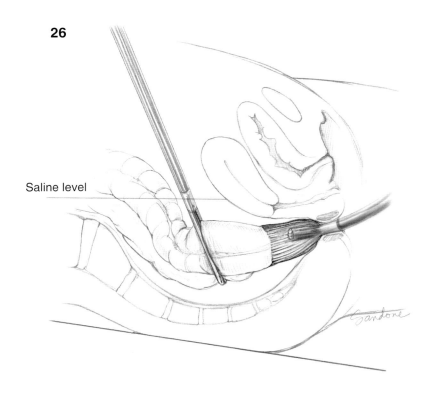

CHAPTER 53

ABDOMINAL PERINEAL RESECTION

INDICATIONS Abdominal perineal resection (APR) of the rectum and sigmoid is used for the removal of rectal cancer that has invaded the anal sphincter mechanism or is too close to the anal canal or too large to perform a sphincter-sparing resection or low anterior resection (LAR) (see Chapter 52). Most patients with rectal cancer who require an APR will also undergo neoadjuvant therapy with chemotherapy and radiation to the pelvis. This causes a special problem with healing in the perineal incision but not with the abdominal portion of the procedure. Preoperative radiation to the pelvis involves the sigmoid colon as well as the rectum, and therefore the sigmoid colon should be removed routinely with the rectum and anus. By definition, a permanent colostomy is the end result of an APR.

PREOPERATIVE PREPARATION The most important aspect of preparing a patient for an APR is consultation with an enterostomal therapist to educate, support, and select the best stoma site for the permanent colostomy. As with a LAR, a mechanical bowel prep and IV antibiotics are usually recommended to reduce pelvic, perineal, and skin infections. The site most at risk for a complication is the perineal wound after closure. The rest of the preoperative measures, including deep venous thrombosis (DVT) prophylaxis, are the same as for LAR.

ANESTHESIA Because the patient will have no large abdominal wound, the risk of postoperative pneumonia and respiratory failure is not generally as great as with open surgery. However, supplemental epidural pain management may be of use due to intense perineal pain. Ketorolac is also useful to reduce the need for parenteral narcotic use (patient-controlled analgesia, PCA).

POSITION The abdominal portion of the procedure is performed with the patient in lithotomy position with sequential devices in place and Allen stirrups. The patient is fixed in position with a beanbag, and both arms are tucked. Thigh flexure is less than 10 degrees, and knee flexure is near 90 degrees (**FIGURE 1**). The perineal portion of the APR can be performed in this position with the surgeon standing between the patient's legs with the table raised to maximum height. Alternatively, the prone flexed position with the hips supported on a roll, rolls under the chest and axillae, and the buttocks taped apart can provide increased access to the pelvis.

For the abdominal portion of the operation, the monitors, surgeon, assistant, and camera operator are placed in the same positions as for a LAR. The table is positioned in steep Trendelenburg and tilted to the right for the majority of the procedure until the rectum is dissected from the pelvis. During the rectal dissection the table is placed in Trendelenburg position.

OPERATIVE PREPARATION A Foley catheter is placed in the bladder. An orogastric tube is beneficial to decompress the stomach. The rectum is irrigated with saline and either Betadine or another cytocidal agent. A 34 French mushroom catheter can be left in the rectum to provide intraoperative drainage of the rectal cavity as well as tactile guidance to the anal canal. After induction of general endotracheal anesthesia, the entire patient abdomen is prepped to allow use of a hand port and placement of the trocars as far laterally as possible.

The colostomy site is marked in the left lower quadrant.

INCISION AND EXPOSURE Trocar positions are determined based on the patient's body habitus. Generally, the camera port is placed above the umbilicus in the vertical midline using either a 5- or an 11-mm trocar to introduce a 30-degree angled laparoscope. The insertion of the umbilical trocar can be accomplished using a Veress needle. Proper positioning is confirmed using the saline drop test and pressure monitoring as the insufflation is continued. If previous operations have been performed or it is felt to be too dangerous to use a Veress needle, open insertion of a 12-mm trocar through this incision is usually possible without greatly enlarging the incision. The operating laparoscope is then introduced, and the abdomen should be explored in all quadrants to make sure there are not adhesions that would prevent completion of the procedure or extensive disease that would require an open operation.

A 12-mm trocar is placed in the right upper quadrant subcostal area laterally and another is placed in the suprapubic midline. The 5-mm trocars are placed in the right lower quadrant and the left lower quadrant. The appropriate placement is two fingerbreadths below the right costal margin in the anterior axillary line and two fingerbreadths above the anterior superior iliac spine on a line toward the umbilicus. The left trocar should be placed in the left midlateral position at the level of umbilicus. The 12-mm trocar in the suprapubic midline should be placed two fingerbreadths above the pubis (**FIGURE 2**). A hand-assisted approach can be achieved through this suprapubic incision if the lower edge of the incision is made far enough away from the pubis to allow placement of the intraabdominal ring and maintain a pneumoperitoneum with the hand-assist device in place. A pneumoperitoneum of 12 to 15 mm Hg is adequate. Higher pressure will cause renal insufficiency and may produce subcutaneous emphysema throughout the body.

The initial steps in the procedure involve placing the patient in steep Trendelenburg and tilting the patient to the right. This allows all the small intestine to fall out of the left lower quadrant and out of the pelvis and to fall into the right upper quadrant. The standard approach to a sigmoid colon resection begins with a medial-to-lateral dissection at the base of the mesentery of the sigmoid and left colon at the sacral promontory. An incision is made over the sacral promontory behind the superior hemorrhoidal artery as the sigmoid colon is retracted anteriorly and out of the pelvis (**FIGURE 3**). This allows entry into an avascular plane at the sacral promontory. Blunt dissection in a tangential plane over the left iliac artery and vein at the pelvic brim allow identification of the left ureter and the gonadal vessels in their normal anatomic positions (**FIGURE 4**). The midline structure that is first encountered is the inferior mesenteric artery (IMA). The thickened dense nerves that arise from the preaortic plexus and extend up onto the IMA can be preserved in benign disease; however, in malignancy, these should be taken with the specimen and the IMA divided within 1 cm of the origin of the vessel (**FIGURE 5**). There are several techniques for dividing the vascular structures including stapling or advanced energy devices. Once the IMA is divided, the avascular plane behind the IMA is developed cephalad, caudad, and laterally. Before dividing the IMA, care should be taken to visualize and protect the ureter and gonadal vessels. The lateral dissection extends all the way out to the gutter beyond the colon, revealing a purple dissection plane when the colon is pulled back toward the midline and the lateral gutter is visualized from above with the laparoscope.

1

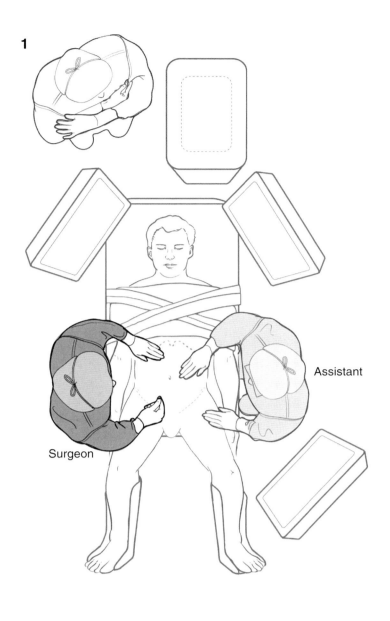

Surgeon

Assistant

2

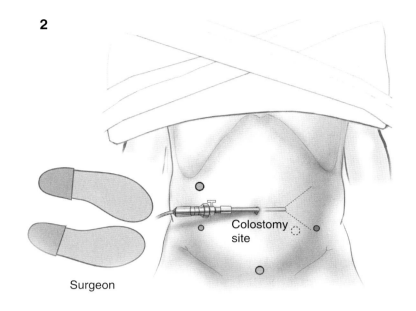

Surgeon

Colostomy
site

3

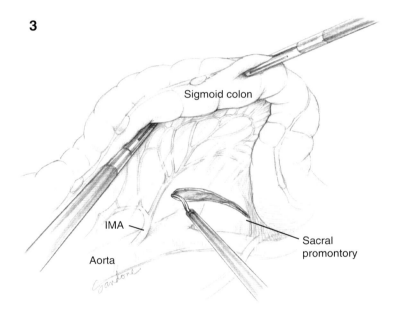

Sigmoid colon

IMA

Aorta

Sacral
promontory

4

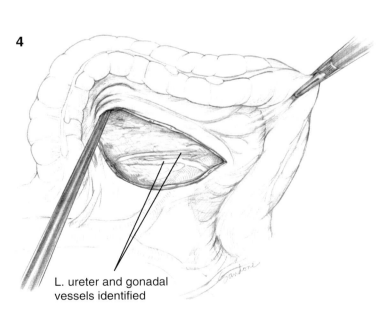

L. ureter and gonadal
vessels identified

5

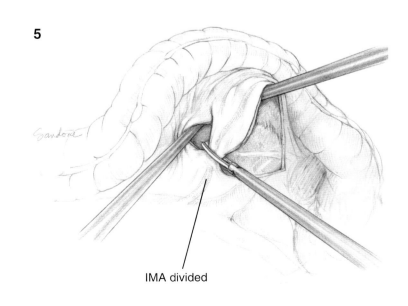

IMA divided

INCISION AND EXPOSURE The next structure encountered in the midline dissection toward the head is the inferior mesenteric vein (IMV) running at the base of the mesentery of the left colon (**FIGURE 6**). The IMV dives behind the third portion of the duodenum at the level of the ligament of Treitz, where the duodenum sweeps out away from the pancreas. Retraction of the IMV anteriorly toward the abdominal wall allows visualization behind the vein along the undersurface of the pancreas and allows the surgeon to create a window in the base of the mesentery of the left colon at the origin of the IMV. The vein is divided with staples or energy sources as needed (**FIGURE 7**).

The avascular plane laterally and cephalad is developed all the way over the top of the kidney along the tail of the pancreas and out laterally to the sidewall to completely mobilize the left colon and its mesentery from the retroperitoneum.

The next step is to incise the lateral attachments of the colon, beginning at the pelvic brim at the sigmoid attachments and continuing all the way up to the splenic flexure. This can be accomplished easily with electrocautery and should move rapidly (**FIGURE 8**). The splenic flexure usually does not need full mobilization. The left colon should reach to the anterior abdominal wall easily even when the pneumoperitoneum is present after dividing the IMA and IMV at their origins and freeing the lateral wall attachments of the left colon (**FIGURE 9**).

With the left colon completely mobilized and the high ligation of vessels accomplished, the patient is placed back in Trendelenburg position and flat on the table with no airplane. The surgeon moves back to the patient's right side. The assistant moves to the left side and lifts the colon from the retroperitoneum with an instrument placed behind the cut edge of the mesentery of the sigmoid colon. This can be accomplished with a straight instrument or a curved retractor with flexible tip. The surgeon uses scissors or hook cautery to dissect in the avascular plane behind the rectum beginning at the sacral promontory (**FIGURE 10**).

A mesorectal dissection is performed. The dissection is carried posteriorly in the midline following the cottony areolar tissue to the level of the coccyx. At this point, a thicker tissue plane is encountered that fixes the back of the rectum to the presacral fascia. This is called the Waldeyer fascia. The dissection is extended laterally along the pelvic sidewall, remembering that this is a circular motion because of the bowl shape of the pelvis. Straight-line dissection will result in injury of adjacent structures, nerves, and arteries and violate the mesorectal envelope. At the pelvic brim, the surgeon will find two areas of potential disaster. The ureter runs over the surface of the common iliac artery at the site of bifurcation to the internal iliac and external iliac. Adjacent to the ureter is the splanchnic nerve, which runs along the inner aspect of the pelvic brim from the hypogastric plexus, including parasympathetic and sympathetic nerves that innervate the bladder, prostate, and penis. Care must be taken to preserve these nerves. The nerves at the IMA are sympathetic nerves, and dividing them will result in retrograde ejaculation. Dividing the nerves along the pelvic sidewall will result in impotence and urinary difficulty (**FIGURE 11**).

6

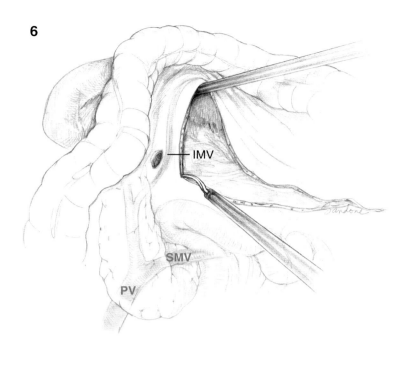

IMV

SMV

PV

7

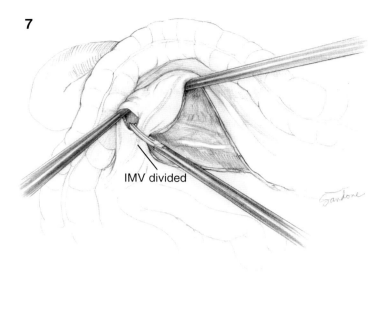

IMV divided

8   Lateral attachments of left colon divided

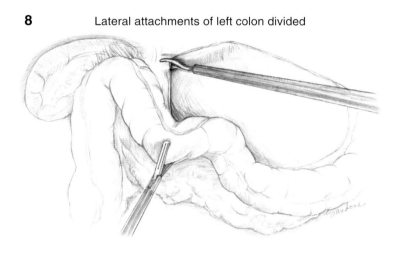

9

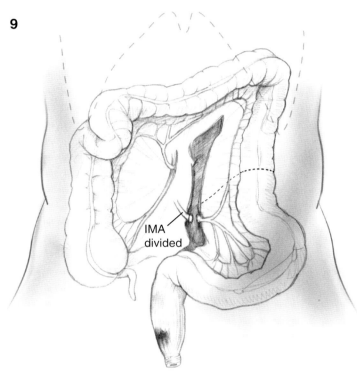

IMA divided

10

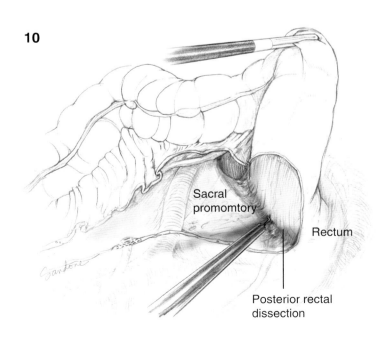

Sacral promomtory

Rectum

Posterior rectal dissection

11

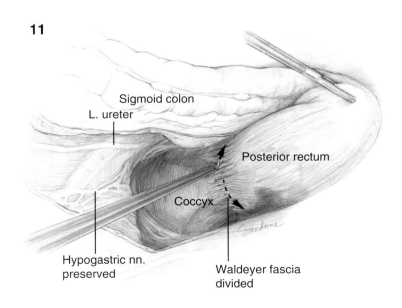

Sigmoid colon

L. ureter

Posterior rectum

Coccyx

Hypogastric nn. preserved

Waldeyer fascia divided

INCISION AND EXPOSURE The dissection then extends along the peritoneal covering of the mesentery of the rectum along each side of the pelvis. This step will release the entire rectum on both sides of the pelvis (**FIGURE 12**).

The final dissection is the anterior aspect of the rectum. Through the left lower quadrant, a retracting clamp is placed behind the anterior peritoneal reflection of the vagina or the prostate and bladder and lifted anteriorly. The 10-mm instrument through the patient's right upper quadrant pulls the rectum downward and cephalad to stretch the attachments at the peritoneal reflection. Hook cautery or scissors is used to incise horizontally behind the peritoneal reflection either anterior or posterior to the Denonvilliers fascia, depending on the indication of the disease. An anterior rectal cancer requires taking the Denonvilliers fascia and entering the plane adjacent to the seminal vesicles and prostate, putting the nervi erigentes at risk for damage and, therefore, the patient at risk for impotence. The incision is carried inferiorly in the areolar tissue plane as it continues posterior to the prostate. Some blunt dissection is possible in this area (**FIGURE 13**).

The final attachments of the rectum are the anterolateral ligaments, which contain the blood supply of the midrectum known as the middle rectal arteries. These anterolateral ligaments are angled from the anterolateral position of the pelvis onto the side of the rectum. They can be divided with ultrasonic dissector or electrocautery as long as the cautery is moved slowly and carefully through the ligaments to obtain hemostasis during the cutting (**FIGURE 14**). Once these anterolateral ligaments have been divided on both sides with gentle curvilinear sweeping strokes, the entire rectum will be completely free from the sidewall of the pelvis and the anterior surface of the sacrum, the remaining attached rectum heads into the anal canal. The entire mesorectum will have been completely removed.

Colostomy Creation Once the entire rectum is mobilized to the pelvic floor, the site for the colostomy is chosen by stretching the left colon to the anterior abdominal wall beneath the marked skin site. There should be no tension. The left colonic mesentery can be divided using vascular staples or energy sources to occlude the mesenteric vessels. The left colon at the descending sigmoid colon junction is divided, at the level of mesenteric vessel ligation, using a linear stapler (**FIGURE 15**). The ostomy is constructed by excising a 3-cm disk of skin and fat and splitting the rectus abdominis fascia and muscle to deliver two fingers into the abdomen. The proximal portion of the divided colon is brought out through the opening without twist or tension (**FIGURE 16**). Once the CO_2 is released, the left colon will reach easily, except in rare circumstances of massive obesity. The staple line is excised, and the colostomy is matured as a flush stoma using absorbable suture placed full-thickness through the colon wall and the skin of the site (**FIGURES 17 AND 18**). An ostomy appliance is placed.

12   Lateral peritoneal attachments divided

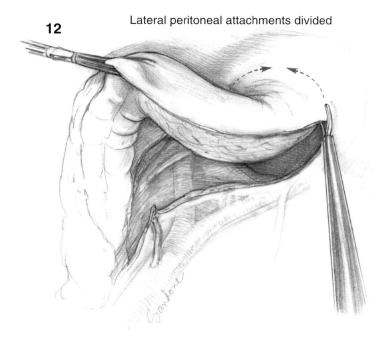

13   Anterior peritoneal attachments divided

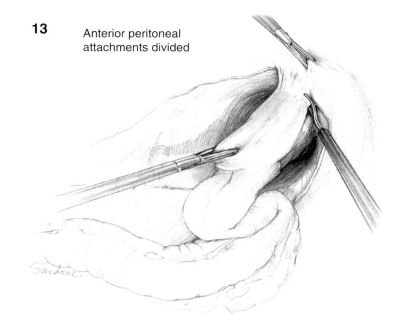

14

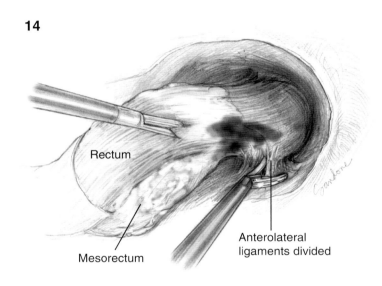

Rectum

Mesorectum

Anterolateral ligaments divided

15   Colon divided

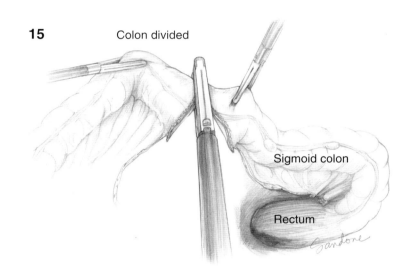

Sigmoid colon

Rectum

16

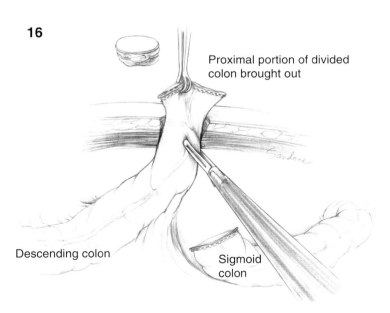

Proximal portion of divided colon brought out

Descending colon

Sigmoid colon

17

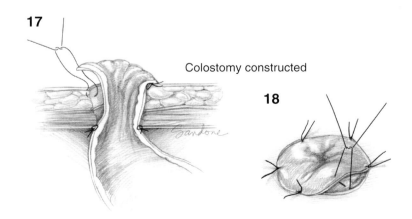

Colostomy constructed

18

Closure of the Abdominal Incisions The abdominal portion of the procedure results in a stoma and five trocar sites, unless a hand-assisted approach has been used. The only trocar site that absolutely must be closed at the fascial level is the supraumbilical port. The skin is closed at all sites with skin glue or staples.

Perineal Incision and Dissection A #1 polypropylene suture is placed at the anal verge to close the anal canal during the dissection.

An incision is made in the skin in the form of an ellipse from the anterior perineal body to the tip of the coccyx, incorporating all of the external sphincter but leaving most of the ischiorectal fossa fat in place (**FIGURE 19**). The pelvis is entered just anterior to the coccyx posteriorly to join the perineal incision to the existing space after the pelvic dissection.

The posterior pelvic floor incision allows placement of the surgeon's or assistant's finger alongside the mobilized rectum on the pelvic side of the levator muscles to act as a guide as a cautery incision is made through the levator plane of muscles on both sides of the pelvic floor, preserving the mesorectal envelope (**FIGURE 20**). A deep blunt perineal rake retractor or skin hooks with elastic attachments can be helpful for this exposure.

This leaves the rectum attached only anteriorly (**FIGURE 21**). The large mass of tissue enveloping the tumor with, hopefully, clear radial margins is delivered through the posterior opening. The anterior dissection is then completed with all aspects of the vagina or prostate exposed and allows for accurate dissection, or resection of attached structures as necessary, to finally remove the sigmoid, rectum, and anus as specimen. This specimen is inked to allow determination of radial margin involvement in the mesorectum or sphincter.

Closure of the Perineal Wound The perineal wound is large and provides a clear view into the pelvis for irrigation, inspection, and proper placement of any suction drain placed during the abdominal portion of the procedure. The technique of finger-guided incision of the pelvic floor muscles leaves a cuff of muscle on each side of the midline that can usually be reapproximated in the midline using large figure-of-eight sutures of heavy absorbable suture (**FIGURE 22**). If a large portion of the muscle has been removed because of tumor position or size, the opening may not be able to be closed primarily. In this circumstance a mesh floor reconstruction using absorbable synthetic mesh or donor-harvested biomaterial may be used to reconstruct the pelvic diaphragm to prevent pelvic floor herniation.

The deep fat of the ischiorectal fossa is then closed in closely situated layers using absorbable horizontal mattress sutures. This obliterates dead space and protects the pelvic floor muscle closure. The skin is left open (**FIGURE 23**). At the conclusion of the APR procedure the patient is left with a closed perineum and a permanent colostomy (**FIGURE 24**).

POSTOPERATIVE CARE Nasogastric decompression is rarely needed. Pain is usually only due to the perineal incision. Colostomy function usually begins rapidly, and early postoperative feeding is appropriate. DVT prophylaxis is appropriate. Patients are encouraged to ambulate or lie flat and to avoid sitting or applying shear forces on the perineal wound closure. The most common complication of this procedure is perineal wound disruption, which results in a morbidity that burdens the patient for many months.

Ostomy care instruction should begin as soon as the patient is coherent and beginning self-care. The stoma will function with the same pretreatment bowel pattern described by the patient at the initial office visit. Some patients prefer to irrigate their colostomy on a daily or every-other-day basis to have some bowel control. This should start only after a month of healing and adjustment. ∎

19

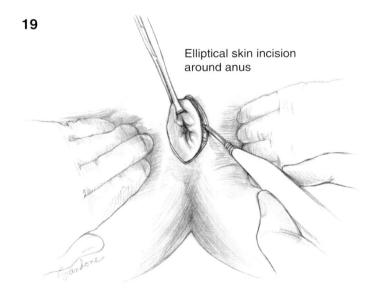

Elliptical skin incision around anus

20

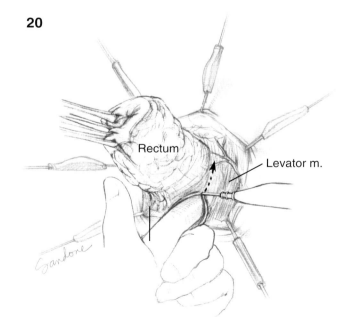

Rectum

Levator m.

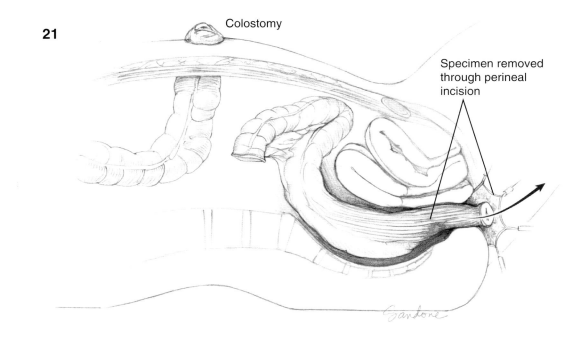

21 Colostomy

Specimen removed through perineal incision

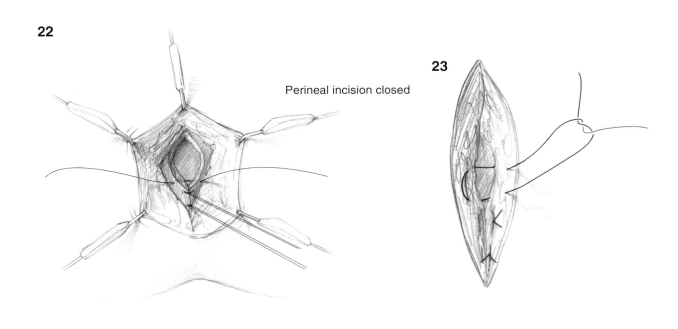

22

Perineal incision closed

23

24

Colostomy

INDICATIONS Laparoscopic colostomy creation is indicated for patients in need of primary fecal diversion. Clinical scenarios include near-obstructing rectal cancers prior to definitive surgery, large sacral decubitus or other wounds at risk of persistent contamination, severe fecal incontinence, or anorectal trauma.

PREOPERATIVE EVALUATION A bowel prep is not required. The patient should be examined in lying, sitting, and standing positions by an enterostomal therapist and be marked for potential ostomy sites. The markings should avoid skin creases, scars, or bony prominences. The patient must be able to see each marking. In obese patients, the upper abdominal wall tends to be thinner and is a better site for ostomies.

ANESTHESIA Thromboembolism prophylaxis, either pharmacologic or mechanical, is started prior to induction of general anesthesia. Prophylactic antibiotics that cover intestinal flora are given within 1 hour prior to skin incision. After induction of general anesthesia, an orogastric tube and urinary catheter are placed.

POSITIONING Some surgeons prefer having a beanbag under the patient. The patient is in a supine position. Each elbow (ulnar nerve) is covered with a gel pad, and both arms are adducted. Care must be taken to avoid compromising or kinking the intravenous lines. The beanbag is cradled above both shoulders and around the arms to prevent the patient from falling while in extreme positioning. The air is suctioned from the beanbag so it retains that shape.

A gel pad covered by a towel is placed on the upper chest. Tape is placed under the bed, over each shoulder, and across to the other side of the bed. If the peak airway pressures become elevated, the tape should be loosened. Security of the patient on the table should be confirmed by testing maximal Trendelenburg and left-side-down positioning prior to prepping and draping. The entire abdomen is prepped from nipples to groin and widely, to allow lateral placement of trocars as needed.

For most of the operation, the surgeon and assistant will both be on the patient's right. The assistant will be near the patient's right shoulder. One monitor should be placed near the feet, and another should be placed near the head on the patient's left. The cautery foot pedal is placed on the patient's right (**FIGURE 1**).

The preoperative markings for ostomy sites are reinforced by scratching the skin with a needle.

DETAILS OF THE PROCEDURE

Trocar Placement The peritoneal cavity can be accessed with a Hasson technique or Veress needle above the umbilicus. Pneumoperitoneum to a pressure of 15 mm Hg is established. With observation through a 30-degree laparoscope, two 5-mm trocars are placed in the right lateral abdominal wall, just outside the lateral border of the rectus muscle, at least a handbreadth apart. A 10- to 12-mm trocar is placed through the future colostomy site (**FIGURE 2**).

Mobilization of the Sigmoid Colon Because there is no need to divide the vascular pedicle, a lateral approach for dissection is used. By gently and medially retracting the sigmoid colon, the lateral attachments can be divided. The left gonadal vessels and left ureter should be identified and preserved (**FIGURE 3**).

Through the future colostomy site (the left lower quadrant trocar site), a locking 10-mm Babcock is used to grasp the sigmoid colon and pull it up to the abdominal wall. It is important to maintain clear orientation of proximal and distal limbs of the colon to avoid maturation of the distal limb as a colostomy. An intracorporeal stitch or endoclip can be placed on the distal limb to mark orientation.

Mobilization of the colon is complete when the bowel easily reaches the proposed ostomy site during full pneumoperitoneum. This should ensure adequate length after desufflation. Otherwise, freeing of the descending colon continues along the white line of Toldt until the length is sufficient.

Creation of the Ostomy Site A plug of skin and fat is excised around the ostomy site. A cruciate incision is made in the anterior rectus fascia. The fibers of the rectus abdominis are spread with a large blunt clamp. While watching with the laparoscopic camera, a vertical incision is made in the posterior fascia. The colon and its mesentery are gently pulled above the fascia (**FIGURE 4**).

Closure of Wounds The pneumoperitoneum is released. Trocars are removed under direct vision. The fascia of any trocar site larger than 10 mm is closed with interrupted 0 braided absorbable sutures. The skin incisions may be closed with sutures or staples.

Maturation of the Ostomy For ease of future takedown, a divided loop colostomy can be created. A linear stapler with a medium thickness cartridge is used to divide the colon. If a distal obstruction is present, a mucous fistula should be created by cutting off the antimesenteric tip of the distal limb and incorporating it into the maturation of the colostomy. The mucous fistula is secured to the skin with interrupted 3-0 braided absorbable sutures. The entire staple line of the proximal limb is cut off (**FIGURE 5**). An interrupted 3-0 braided absorbable suture is placed to join both limbs. The larger proximal limb is matured as usual with interrupted simple 3-0 sutures (**FIGURE 6**). The abdomen wall is cleaned, and a stoma appliance is placed.

POSTOPERATIVE CARE No additional antibiotics are needed after the wounds are closed. A nasogastric tube is not routinely used. Clear liquids are offered the day after the operation, and the diet is advanced as tolerated. The urinary catheter is removed on the morning of the first postoperative day if the patient is not oliguric. The patient will need thorough instruction by the enterostomal therapist prior to discharge. ■

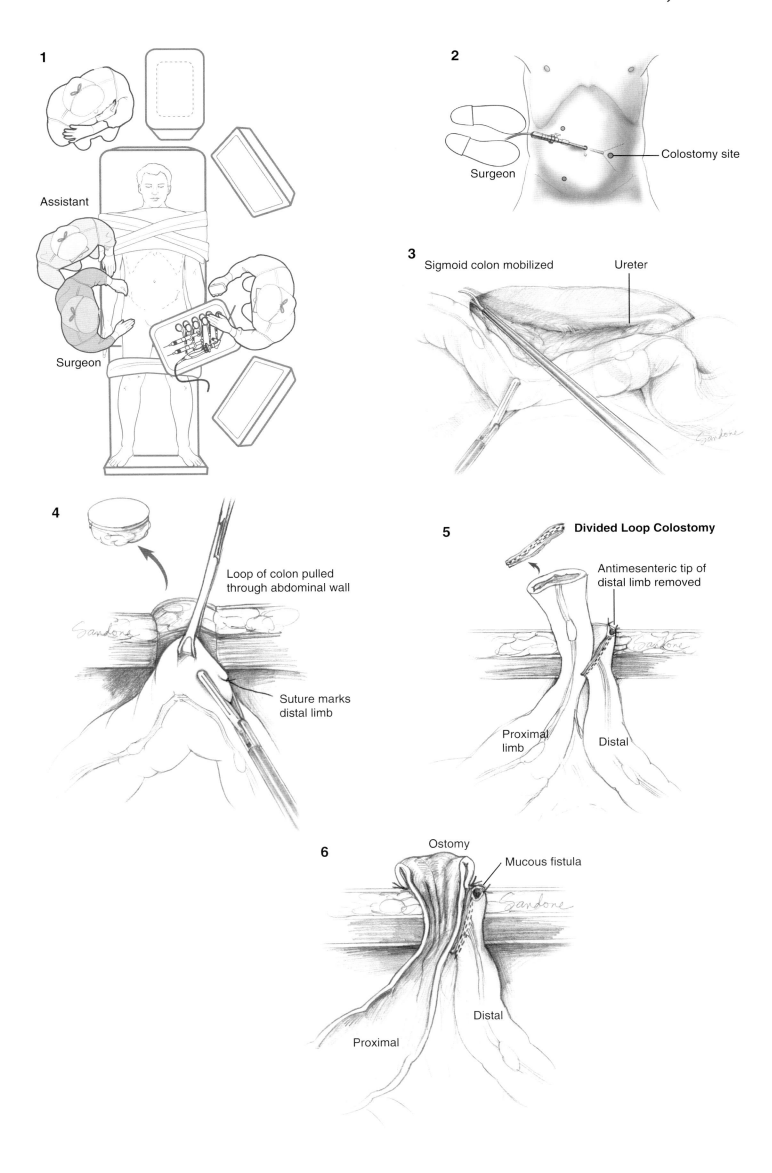

1

Assistant

Surgeon

2

Surgeon

Colostomy site

3

Sigmoid colon mobilized   Ureter

4

Loop of colon pulled through abdominal wall

Suture marks distal limb

5   **Divided Loop Colostomy**

Antimesenteric tip of distal limb removed

Proximal limb   Distal

6

Ostomy

Mucous fistula

Proximal   Distal

CHAPTER 55 | COLOSTOMY TAKEDOWN

PREOPERATIVE EVALUATION Before colostomy takedown, the patient should have a colonoscopy or contrast enema to ensure the absence of pathology in the proximal colon. If pathology were found, that could be treated at the same time as the colostomy takedown.

A mechanical and antibiotic bowel prep is used, as well as irrigations of the rectum through the mucous fistula or through the anus, to ensure that the rectum is cleaned out before colostomy takedown. In addition, with a good bowel prep, the less distended bowel becomes easier to manipulate. Thromboembolism prophylaxis, either pharmacologic or mechanical, is started prior to induction of general anesthesia. Prophylactic antibiotics that cover intestinal flora are given within an hour prior to skin incision. After induction of general anesthesia, an orogastric tube and urinary catheter are placed.

POSITIONING A beanbag is placed under the patient. The patient should be placed into a low lithotomy position with Allen stirrups. Each ankle, knee, and opposite shoulder should be aligned. No pressure should be placed on the peroneal nerves or calves. The angle between the thigh and the plane of the bed should be between 0 and 10 degrees. Any more flexion will limit range of motion for the instruments. Any more extension may lead to an anterior dislocation of the hip.

Each elbow (ulnar nerve) is covered with a gel pad, and both arms are adducted. Care must be taken to avoid compromising or kinking the intravenous lines. The beanbag is cradled above both shoulders and around the arms to prevent the patient from falling while in extreme positioning. Then, the air is suctioned from the beanbag so it retains that shape.

A gel pad covered by a towel is placed on the upper chest. Tape is placed under the bed, over each shoulder, and across to the other side of the bed. If the peak airway pressures become elevated, the tape should be loosened. Security of the patient on the table should be confirmed by testing maximal Trendelenburg and left-side-down positioning prior to prepping and draping. The entire abdomen is prepped from nipples to groin and widely, to allow lateral placement of trocars as needed (**FIGURE 1**).

For most of the operation, the surgeon and the assistant are both on the patient's right with the assistant near the patient's right shoulder. One monitor should be placed near the feet, and another should be placed near the head on the patient's left. The cautery foot pedal is placed on the patient's right.

DETAILS OF THE PROCEDURE Via rigid proctoscopy, any residual mucus is suctioned from the rectal stump. If this step is not performed, the circular stapler may not reach the end of the rectal stump during creation of the anastomosis.

The ostomy is sewn shut with a 2-0 silk suture on a tapered needle. After the standard prep, a folded sponge is placed over the ostomy and secured with a sterile adhesive dressing.

Trocar Placement Because this is reoperative surgery, the peritoneal cavity should be accessed with a Hasson technique above the umbilicus or a Veress needle in the right upper quadrant. Pneumoperitoneum to pressure of 15 mm Hg is established. An 11-mm trocar is placed through or near the umbilicus. Under observation through a 30-degree laparoscope, two 5-mm trocars are placed in the right lateral abdominal wall, just outside the lateral border of the rectus muscle, at least a handbreadth apart. An optional 5-mm suprapubic trocar may be helpful for retraction (**FIGURE 2**).

Identification and Mobilization of the Rectal Stump After a circular stapler sizer is placed through the anus, the rectal stump can be quickly identified (**FIGURE 3**). Adhesions near the end of the rectal stump can be taken down sharply or with an energy source up to the rectosigmoid junction. If any sigmoid colon were remaining, it would need to be resected to the level of the rectosigmoid junction (splaying of the taenia and after the last epiploic fat) with a medium thickness stapler.

Mobilization of the Sigmoid Colon Because there is no need to divide the vascular pedicle, a lateral approach for dissection is used. By gently and medially retracting the colon above the colostomy, the lateral attachments can be carefully divided, if this was not done at the time of colostomy creation (**FIGURE 4**). The freed colon is pulled down toward the rectal stump. If there is any tension or it appears that there will not be enough length, even after the colostomy is released from the abdominal wall, the splenic flexure is taken down (illustrated in Chapter 50).

Takedown of Colostomy from Abdominal Wall The sponge and dressing over the colostomy are removed. Using a knife or cutting cautery, a circumferential skin incision is made 1 mm away from the mucocutaneous junction. Skin hooks with elastic attachments are used to retract the skin edges (**FIGURE 5**). With a combination of sharp and thermal dissection, the colon is dissected away from the subcutaneous tissue and abdominal wall fascia, circumferentially. Once the colostomy is completely free, a wound protector is placed around the ostomy to protect the wound after the colon is reopened.

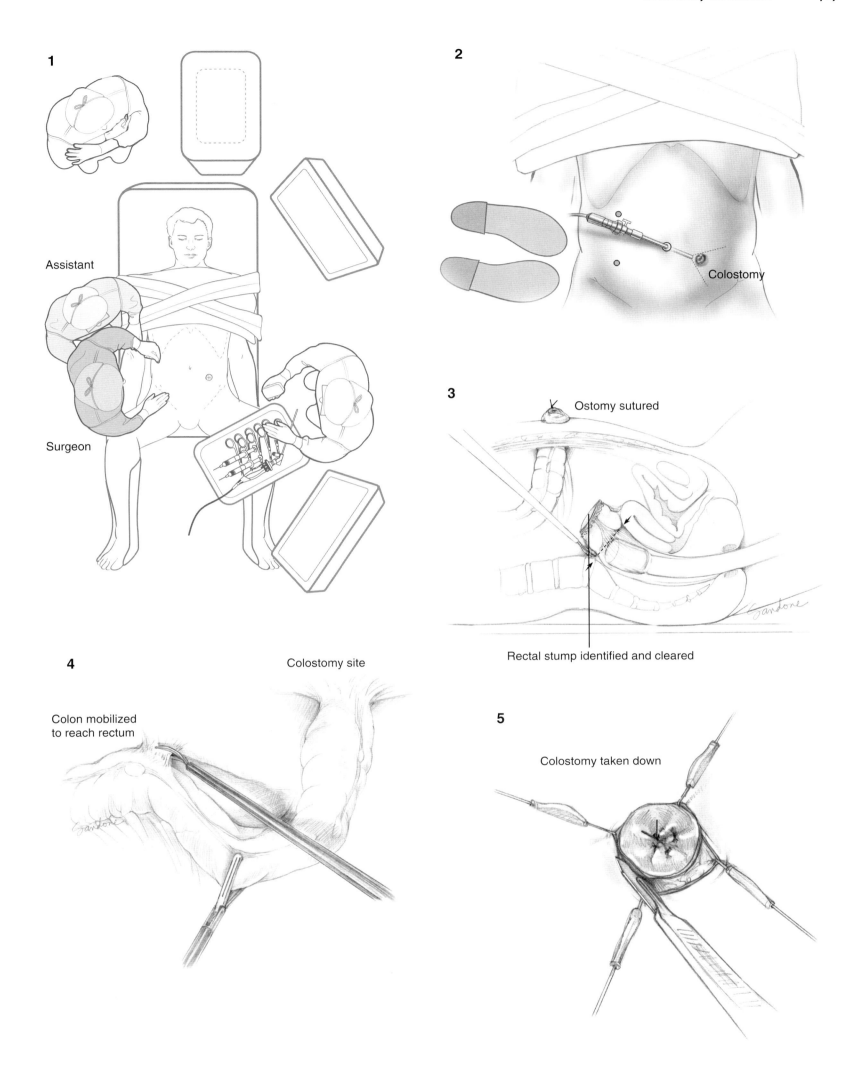

1

Assistant

Surgeon

2

Colostomy

3

Ostomy sutured

Rectal stump identified and cleared

4   Colostomy site

Colon mobilized
to reach rectum

5

Colostomy taken down

Creation of the Anastomosis The silk stitch is removed from the end of the colostomy. A purse-string device is placed in the open end of the colon. The anvil of the 28 or 29 mm circular stapler is placed into the colon, and the purse string is tied down (**FIGURE 6**). The end of the colon and anvil are returned to the abdomen. Pneumoperitoneum is reestablished by twisting the wound protector, towel clipping the skin, or formally closing the fascia with interrupted absorbable sutures.

The circular stapler is passed through the anus and advanced until it is flush with the end of the rectal stump. The spike pierces the rectal stump adjacent to the staple line and is advanced until it is fully deployed. The anvil and the stapler are coupled (**FIGURES 7 AND 8**). Making sure no extraneous tissue gets caught in the new anastomosis and the colon is not twisted, the stapler is closed and fired.

The anastomosis is tested for leaks by filling the pelvis with saline. The colon is occluded above the anastomosis and the rectum is filled with air.

If the colon above the anastomosis distends and there are no bubbles, the anastomosis is fine (**FIGURE 9**). The air and saline are evacuated from the colon and pelvis, respectively.

CLOSURE OF WOUNDS Trocars are removed under direct vision, and the pneumoperitoneum is evacuated. The fascia of any trocar site larger than 10 mm is closed using interrupted absorbable sutures. The skin incisions may be closed with glue, sutures, or staples. The skin of the ostomy site will be left open for twice-daily dressing changes.

POSTOPERATIVE CARE No additional antibiotics are needed after the wounds are closed. A nasogastric tube is not routinely used. Clear liquids are offered the day after the operation, and the diet is advanced as tolerated. The urinary catheter is removed on the morning of the first postoperative day if the patient is not oliguric. ■

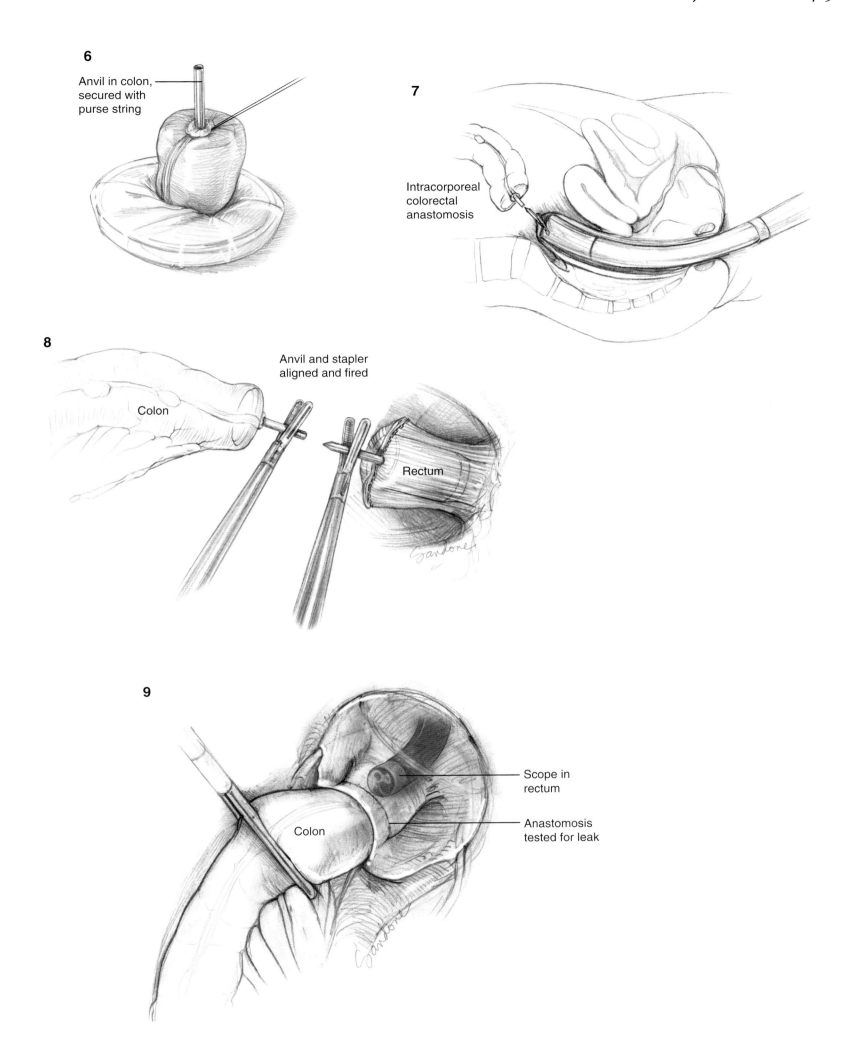

6

Anvil in colon, secured with purse string

7

Intracorporeal colorectal anastomosis

8

Anvil and stapler aligned and fired

Colon

Rectum

9

Colon

Scope in rectum

Anastomosis tested for leak

RECTOPEXY AND POSTERIOR MESH REPAIR FOR RECTAL PROLAPSE

INDICATIONS For full-thickness rectal prolapse, there are several commonly used laparoscopic operations. Laparoscopic sigmoid colectomy and suture rectopexy is ideal for patients with full-thickness prolapse and with moderate to severe constipation (<1 bowel movement every 3 days). For patients without constipation, resection is to be avoided. A simple sutured rectopexy or a posterior mesh repair (modified Wells repair) will suffice. The anterior mesh repair (Ripstein procedure) is not favored, as it tends to lead to postoperative constipation because the rectum is completely surrounded by nondistensible mesh (anteriorly) and sacrum (posteriorly).

PREOPERATIVE EVALUATION When the patient sits on a commode and strains, the rectal prolapse can be confirmed by the surgeon. A rectal prolapse is seen as a series of concentric folds representing the full thickness of the rectum, protruding from the anus (**FIGURES 1 AND 2**). The full-thickness prolapse should be distinguished from prolapsed hemorrhoids. Hemorrhoids do not have concentric folds and may be discernible as a series of three folds on the left lateral aspect of the anus, the right anterior anus, and the right posterior anus (**FIGURES 3 AND 4**). Significant edema may obscure the anatomic definition of the three hemorrhoid columns.

A colonoscopy should be performed before any operative procedure. Should the patient have significant constipation, colonic inertia should be ruled out with a colonic transit study. The patient should undergo a mechanical bowel preparation the day before surgery. On the day of surgery, the patient should have pneumatic sequential compression devices (SCDs) placed on both legs prior to induction of anesthesia. Intravenous prophylactic antibiotic is given within 1 hour before incision.

1

Prolapse

2

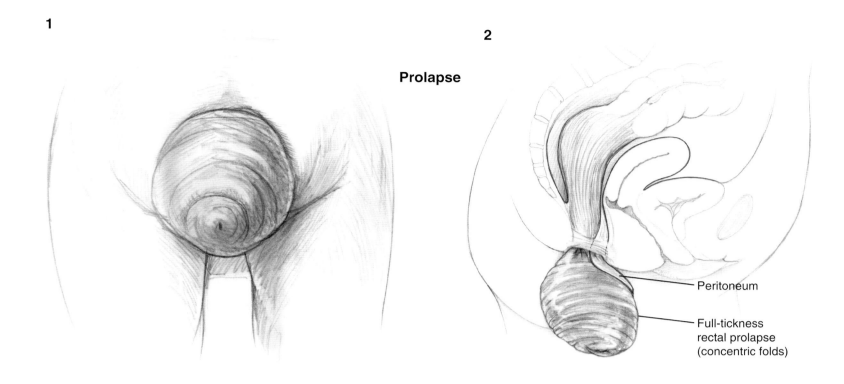

Peritoneum

Full-tickness
rectal prolapse
(concentric folds)

3

Hemorrhoids

4

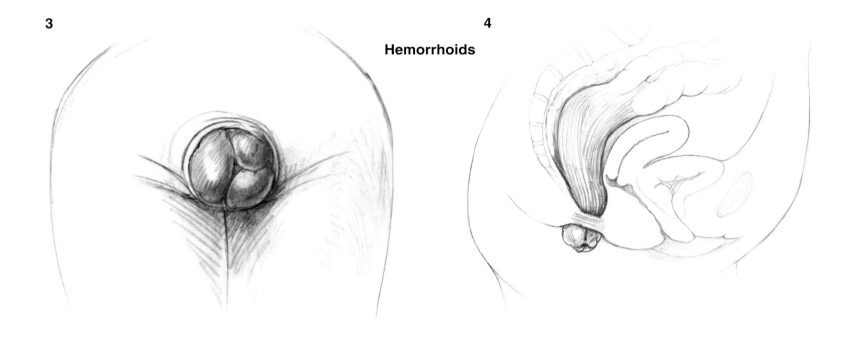

POSITIONING The patient should be placed on a beanbag to facilitate positioning. After induction of general anesthesia, an orogastric tube and Foley catheter are placed. The patient should be moved to a low lithotomy position with Allen stirrups (**FIGURE 5**). There must be free access to the anus. Each ankle, knee, and opposite shoulder should be aligned. No pressure should be placed on the peroneal nerves or calves. The angle between the knee and the plane of the bed should be between 0 and 10 degrees. Any more flexion will limit range of motion for the instruments. Any more extension may lead to an anterior dislocation of the hip.

Each elbow (ulnar nerve) is covered with a gel pad, and both arms are adducted and tucked at the sides of the operating table. Care must be taken to avoid compromising or kinking the intravenous lines. The beanbag is cradled above both shoulders and around the arms to prevent the patient from falling while in extreme positioning. The air is suctioned from the beanbag so it retains that shape. A gel pad covered by a towel is placed on the upper chest. Tape is place under the bed, over each shoulder, and across to the other side of the bed. Peak airway pressures should be monitored for elevation during taping to avoid excessive chest compression. The patient is placed in extreme Trendelenburg and right tilt prior to starting the case to make sure that the patient has been adequately secured. The surgeon and assistant stand on the patient's right. A monitor should be placed at the feet. Another should be placed at the patient's left shoulder.

DETAILS OF THE PROCEDURE

Trocar Placement The abdomen can usually be safely accessed with a Veress needle below the umbilicus. Alternatively, the surgeon may use a Hasson technique. Pneumoperitoneum up to a pressure of 15 mm Hg is established. A 30- or 45-degree laparoscope may be used to place the other trocars under direct vision. After numbing the skin and peritoneum with local anesthetic, a 10-mm trocar is placed in the right lower quadrant 2 cm medial and 2 cm superior to the right anterior superior iliac spine. A third 5-mm trocar is placed one handbreadth superior and a little medial to that last trocar. Finally, a 10-mm suprapubic trocar is placed 2 cm above the pubic symphysis. An optional 5-mm trocar can be placed in the left lower quadrant for an assistant (**FIGURE 6**).

Pelvic Dissection for the Rectopexy The patient is placed into a steep Trendelenburg and tilt right position. The small bowel is pulled out of the pelvis with atraumatic graspers. Typically, the space between the sacrum and mesorectum is quite long. The mesentery of the sigmoid colon is held adjacent to the colon and lifted up to the abdominal wall. The bulging fat overlying the inferior mesenteric artery should become obvious. The peritoneum is scored between the superior rectal artery and the sacral promontory to enter the presacral plane (**FIGURE 7**). The posterior dissection of the rectum is carried inferiorly in this avascular plane until the pelvic floor is reached (**FIGURE 8**).

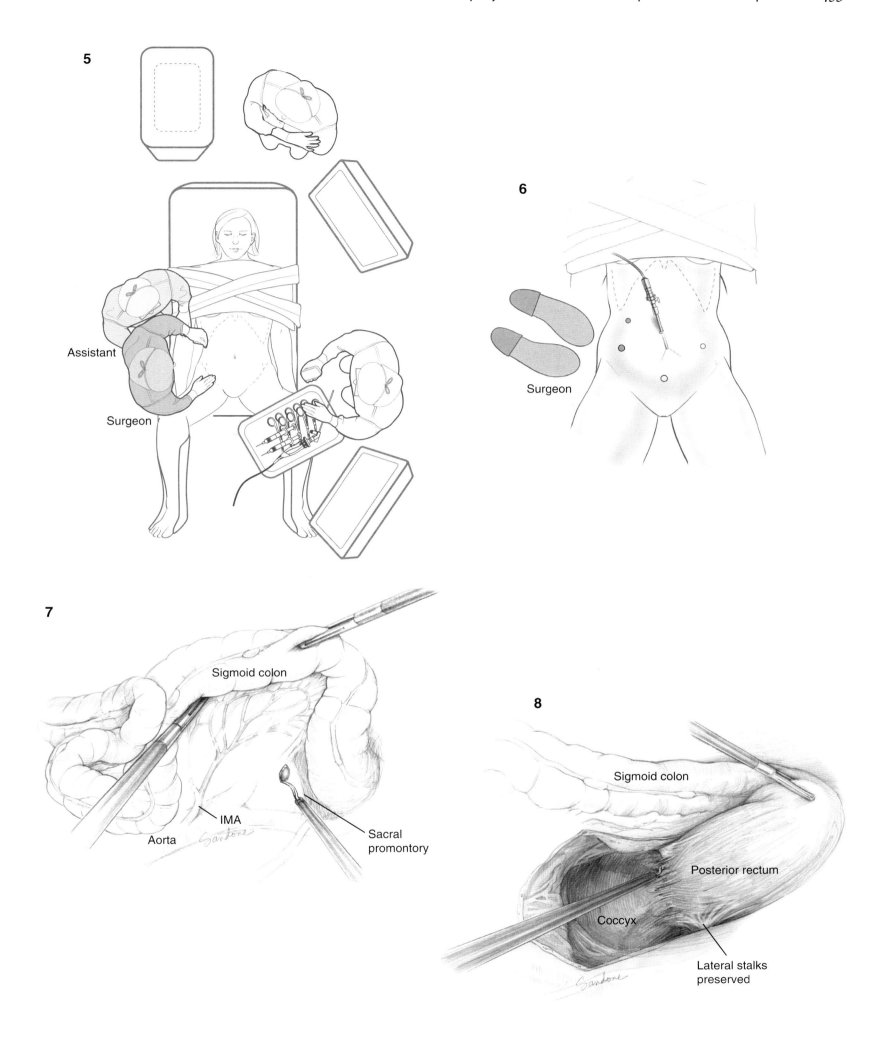

5

6

Assistant

Surgeon

Surgeon

7

Sigmoid colon

IMA

Aorta

Sacral
promontory

8

Sigmoid colon

Posterior rectum

Coccyx

Lateral stalks
preserved

Pelvic Dissection for the Rectopexy Next, the anterior plane is developed between the rectum and the bladder (in men) or the vagina (in women). The peritoneum of the anterior rectal reflection is scored (**FIGURE 9**), and dissection proceeds inferiorly along the rectal wall until the pelvic floor is reached. Once the anterior dissection is completed, two lateral stalks remain (**FIGURE 10**). These stalks must be preserved. Division of the stalks may lead to postoperative constipation. If constipation is not a problem, then either suture or mesh rectopexy is indicated.

If the patient has constipation, a sigmoid colectomy and anastomosis should be performed before rectopexy (see Chapter 49) to reduce the length of the colon. When performing colectomy and rectopexy, synthetic mesh should not be used. If the laparoscopic tacker is to be used for the rectopexy, a 5-mm port is placed through the suprapubic extraction site after sigmoid colon removal, and the fascia is closed around the trocar.

Sutured rectopexy Typically, three sutures of braided nonabsorbable o suture are used to secure the right margin of the rectum to the presacral fascia. The first suture is placed through the lateral stalk and then into the midline fascia just below the sacral promontory in a horizontal mattress fashion (**FIGURE 11**). A single armed suture may be used, but a double-armed suture avoids the need for backhanded suturing. The suture is tied intracorporeally or extracorporeally. The hypogastric nerves and iliac vein are avoided by staying in the midline of the posterior pelvis. The second suture is placed through the right lateral stalk and then through the sacral fascia in the same fashion as the first stitch (**FIGURE 12**).

The third and last stitch is placed between the superior right rectal stalk and the proximal sacral promontory, just to the right of the midline, to avoid the middle sacral artery (**FIGURE 13**). The completion of the rectopexy elevates the rectum higher into the pelvis (**FIGURE 14**).

Mechanical Rectopexy Tacking the rectum to the sacrum is an alternative to suturing. The laparoscopic tacker is placed through the suprapubic port. The right lateral rectal stalk is tacked to the sacral promontory just off the midline to avoid the middle sacral artery, the hypogastric nerve, and the iliac veins. At least three helical tacks should be placed.

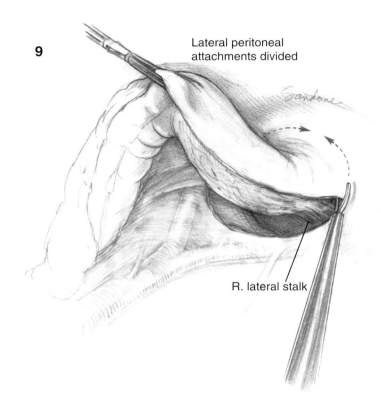

9

Lateral peritoneal
attachments divided

R. lateral stalk

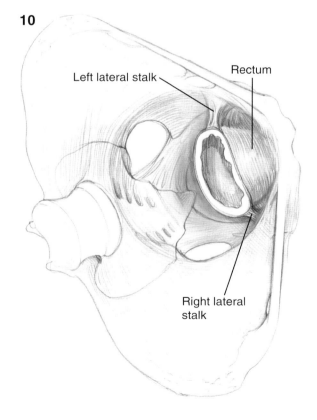

10

Left lateral stalk

Rectum

Right lateral
stalk

11   Sutured Rectopexy

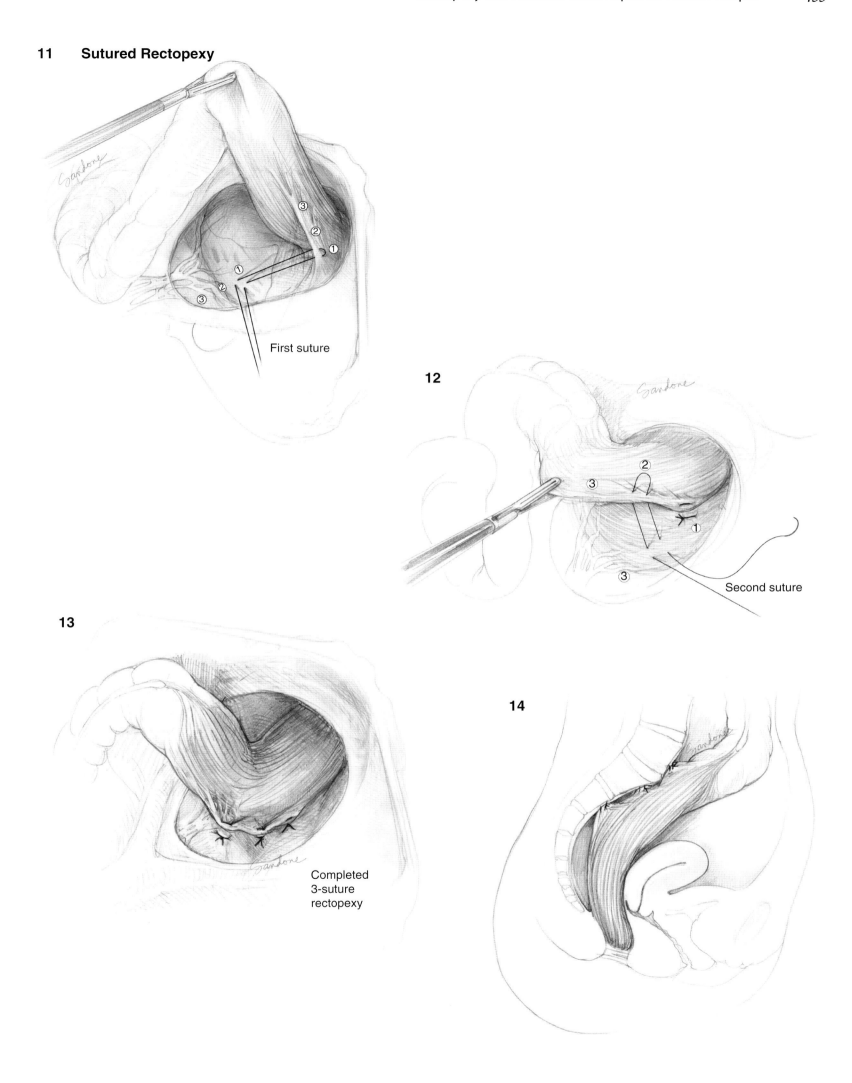

First suture

12

Second suture

13

Completed
3-suture
rectopexy

14

Posterior Mesh Rectopexy If sigmoid colectomy has not been performed, a mesh repair is an attractive option and provides firm fixation of the superior rectum. Some surgeons reserve this procedure for those patients who failed sutured rectopexy. A 3 × 8 cm² polypropylene or similar mesh is rolled up and placed through the right lower quadrant (RLQ) 10-mm trocar. The middle of the mesh is tacked or sewn to the sacral promontory just off the midline **(FIGURE 15)**. Each end of the mesh is sewn to the lateral stalks with two 0 braided nonabsorbable sutures (modified Wells procedure) **(FIGURE 16)**.

Alternatively, the mesh can be sewn directly to the rectum after posterior fixation (Wells procedure). After mobilization of the rectum, 2 to 3 cm of peritoneum on each side of the upper rectum is divided. The ends of the mesh are wrapped around each side of the rectum and sewn to the rectal serosa using interrupted 2-0 polypropylene sutures. Part of the anterior rectum should be free of mesh **(FIGURE 17)**. The peritoneum of the divided lateral stalks can be used to cover the mesh with a running 3-0 braided absorbable suture.

Pelvic Drain A 10 French Jackson-Pratt drain is usually placed through the RLQ 10-mm trocar and positioned in the presacral space, adjacent to the rectopexy.

CLOSURE OF WOUNDS All trocars should be removed under direct vision. The fascia below the 10-mm trocar sites should be closed with 0 braided absorbable sutures. A laparoscopic suture passer may be used to secure the fascia. The wounds should be irrigated. The skin may be closed with a 4-0 absorbable monofilament suture and skin glue.

POSTOPERATIVE CARE No antibiotics are needed after the wounds are closed. A nasogastric tube should not be needed. The patient may have clear liquids the night of surgery. The diet is then advanced as tolerated. Typically, the drain is left for 4 to 5 days. As long as the drainage is not purulent, bilious, feculent, or bloody, it may be removed on postoperative day 4 or 5. ∎

Mesh Rectopexy

15

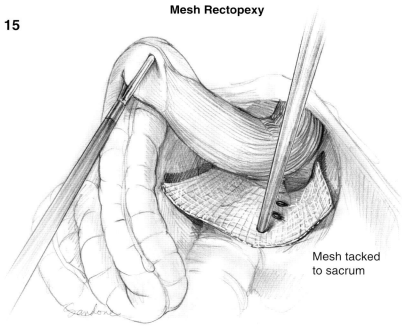

Mesh tacked
to sacrum

16

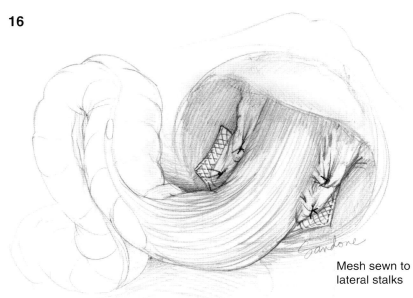

Mesh sewn to
lateral stalks

17

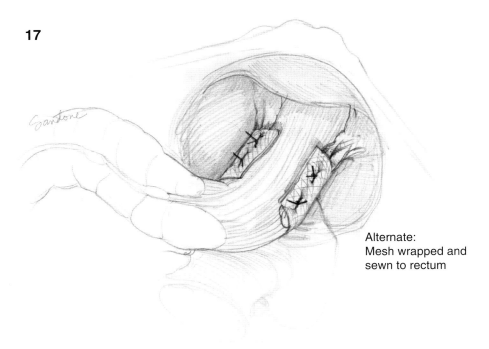

Alternate:
Mesh wrapped and
sewn to rectum

Transanal Endoscopic Microsurgery

INDICATIONS Transanal endoscopic microsurgery (TEM) is a minimally invasive technique for the excision of rectal tumors located between 8 and 18 cm above the anal verge. Lesions located below 8 cm can usually be approached with traditional instruments, whereas exposure using a traditional transanal approach becomes difficult above this point. TEM provides excellent exposure of tumors up to 18 cm from the anal verge. When compared to the techniques of low anterior resection, parasacral approach, or sphincter-splitting approaches, TEM offers greater precision, lower morbidity, and a shorter hospital stay. The technique is not widely established because of the specific instrumentation required, the unusual technical demands of the approach, and the specific patient selection criteria.

The main indication for the TEM procedure is any benign lesion that cannot be removed by the traditional endoscopic snare technique. These consist mainly of lipomas, leiomyomas, tubular or villous adenomas, or carcinoids. Depending on the skill of the surgeon, any size benign lesion can be considered for TEM; however, "optimal" tumor size ranges from 2 cm in diameter to three fourths of the lumen circumference. TEM is also used for the removal of malignant neoplasms in patients with low-risk cancers (T1). In a high-risk operative candidate or as a palliative modality, these criteria can be extended. Careful selection and meticulous operative technique is critical for the outcome when operating with curative intent. A full-thickness resection is recommended to ensure a negative surgical margin. This resection technique also decreases the risk of missing small rectal cancers that may be located deep inside a villous adenoma that might occur if only a mucosectomy is performed.

Lymph-node invasion is the primary factor limiting the effectiveness of local treatment in early rectal cancer. The lymph-node metastasis rate of T1 rectal tumors lies between 0% and 15.4% depending on tumor grade. Cancer recurrence rates after TEM are generally lower than those reported with conventional transanal surgery. The indications for neo-adjuvant or adjuvant radiation chemotherapy following local resection of rectal cancer by TEM remain controversial.

TEM may be also be an alternative for the resection of rectal stenoses within 5 to 15 cm of the dentate line (i.e., inflammatory stenoses after high fistulae or colorectal anastomotic stenoses).

PREOPERATIVE PREPARATION Preoperative assessment of type, stage, and grade of the tumor is crucial to the success of TEM. This generally consists of a clinical examination with rectoscopy and biopsy, endorectal ultrasound, and a sphincter function test. Patients with known benign lesions do not need evaluation by computed tomography (CT). Lesions should be assessed for mobility. Patients with malignant lesions greater than 3 cm or with ulcerated appearance on sigmoidoscopy are at greater risk of penetration through the rectal wall and must be carefully evaluated before TEM is attempted. Patients should also be asked about fecal or urinary incontinence, which may be made worse by a TEM procedure.

Routine mechanical bowel preparation is usually recommended. The rectum should at least be emptied of solid stool and irrigated with some form of cytocidal liquid such as Betadine at the beginning of the procedure or during the procedure to reduce fecal contaminants or malignant cells if

the indication is rectal cancer. The patient receives nothing by mouth after midnight before the operation and is given broad-spectrum IV antibiotics prior to the operation. A Foley catheter is placed.

ANESTHESIA TEM is usually performed under general anesthesia, but epidural or spinal anesthesia is also possible. Neuromuscular blockade is not necessary.

POSITION The position of the patient is dependent on the position of the tumor on the rectal wall. To obtain a constant operating position for the surgeon, the tumor should be located in the inferior part of the operative field. The patient can be placed:

1. in a supine position (posterior tumor)
2. in a prone position (anterior tumor)
3. in a right or left lateral decubitus position (right or left rectal wall tumor) (**FIGURE 1**).

INCISION AND EXPOSURE The instrumentation used in TEM procedures is specific to this technique. An operative rectoscope 40 mm in diameter and 120 or 200 mm in length is typically used. A magnified stereoscopic lens or standard laparoscopic digital camera is affixed to the scope. The end of the rectoscope is beveled downward to provide maximum exposure of the lesion positioned in the inferior aspect of the field.

The surgical instruments used in the TEM procedure are similar to those in laparoscopic surgery; however, the tips are angled 40 degrees to enhance the view of the tumor. Typically two instruments, such as a grasper and coagulation scalpel, suction, or needle holder, are introduced through sealed ports on the rectoscope (**FIGURE 2**). To optimize visualization and access to the entire tumor, the position of the rectoscope must be changed frequently to compensate for the limited operating field and length of the surgical instruments. The use of a bed-mounted supporting arm makes such frequent shifts in perspective possible while still allowing the surgeon to operate with both hands.

The rectoscope is inserted after ample lubrication and gentle dilatation of the rectum is performed. Carbon dioxide is used to insufflated the rectum to 10 mm Hg. Enlargement of the intrarectal space facilitates optimal visualization and resection. To avoid air leakage, the surgical instruments are inserted in the operative rectoscope through a sealed cap. The combined suction-insufflation endosurgical unit is used to ensure a constant, high flow of gas and to evacuate the smoke from coagulation. The high flow is regulated by the pressure and is similar to the high flow used during conventional laparoscopy. The tumor is then well exposed and can be dissected.

Tumor Resection The first step in TEM is a gentle grasping of the tissue near the base of the tumor to apply tension to the mucosa. Coagulation is used to label the region and identify the boundaries of resection. Usually a rim of normal tissue of 5 mm or greater is allowed to ensure complete resection of the lesion (**FIGURE 3**). The mucosa is then incised with electrocautery at a right angle full thickness through the rectal wall and into the perirectal fat tissue (**FIGURE 4**). During this procedure, it is important to retain at least 5 mm of healthy tissue up to the coagulated surface.

1

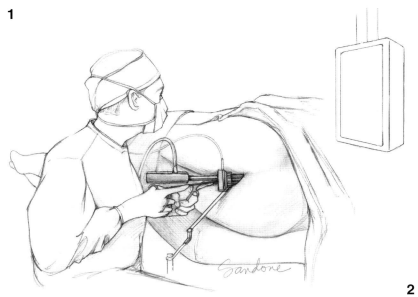

2

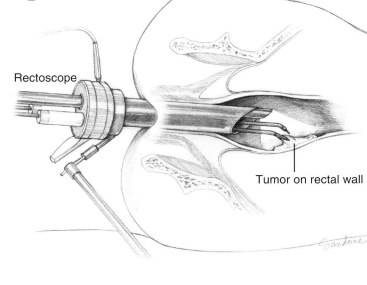

Rectoscope

Tumor on rectal wall

3

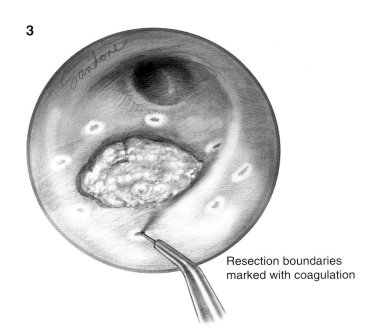

Resection boundaries
marked with coagulation

4

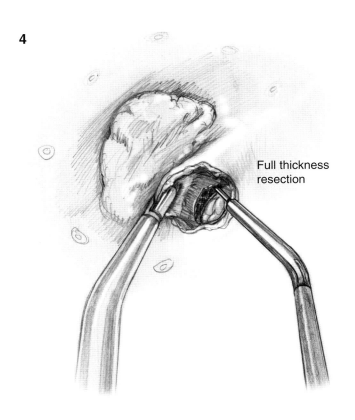

Full thickness
resection

Tumor Resection Coagulation is performed progressively in a right caudal to left cranial direction in the perirectal fat tissue (**FIGURE 5**). Visualized vessels are coagulated. Periodic cleaning of the cautery probe to remove coagulated tissue particles will facilitate dissection and visualization of the target. When vessels are encountered, it is important to perform coagulation before division, as the bleeding vessels may retract into the fat tissue, making further coagulation more difficult. After the lesions is separated from its posterior attachments, the specimen is extracted (**FIGURE 6**). After the tumor is resected, hemostasis becomes easier and the bleeding vessels may be grasped and coagulated at the base. The operative region is washed with a Betadine solution.

Rectal Repair The suture of the mucosa defect should incorporate some perirectal fat tissue to facilitate adequate hemostasis. A transverse closure of the rectal defect is performed with an interrupted or a running suture working from right to the left using a 3-0 absorbable monofilament synthetic polyglycol (**FIGURE 7**). Stitches are passed caudad to cephalad, successively taking the inferior margin and then the superior margin of the resection region. The suture is followed transversely until complete closure

of the rectal wall is achieved. The transverse closure aims to avoid a secondary rectal stenosis. The small operative space makes intracorporeal knot tying difficult, so compressible beads crimped on the suture ends are used to secure the suture ends. Once the continuous running stitch is complete, it is fixed by a bead (**FIGURE 8**).

POSTOPERATIVE CARE Patients are allowed to sit and walk as soon as the anesthesia wears off. A liquid diet is maintained for 48 hours. Initial clinical follow-up occurs 6 weeks postoperatively and final clinical examination, including endorectal sonography, 3 months afterwards. For malignant lesions, serial follow-up, every 3 months during the first year, every 6 months during the second, and yearly thereafter, is necessary to detect recurrence of cancer.

Overall, the rate of local complications associated with transanal resection lies between 4% and 8.3% of cases, while systemic complications range between 14% and 21%. Lethal complications are very rare. Prolonged anal dilatation of 4 cm (due to the operative rectoscope) induces few sphincter function problems. Transitory, grade II incontinence, if it occurs, usually resolves within 3 months. ■

5

Tumor

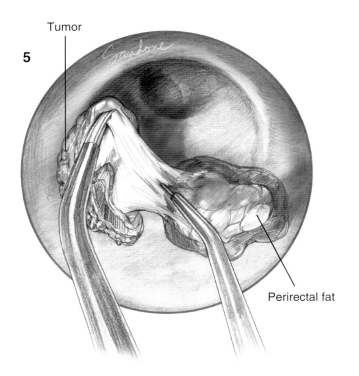

Perirectal fat

6

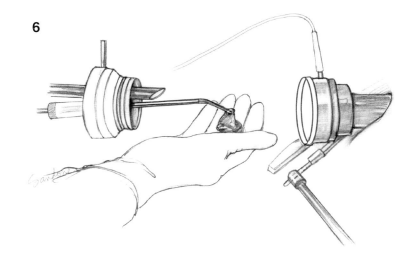

7

Mucosal
defect
closed

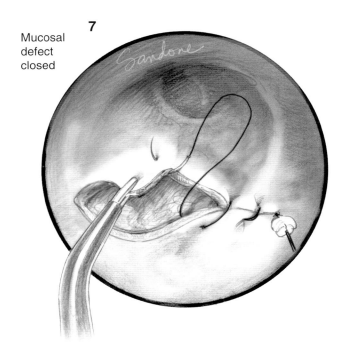

8

Suture
secured
with
beads

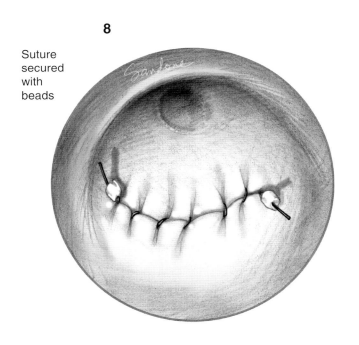

Section X
MINIMALLY INVASIVE PEDIATRIC SURGERY

MINIMALLY INVASIVE PEDIATRIC SURGERY: GENERAL CONSIDERATIONS

BACKGROUND The pediatric surgery community was relatively slow to adopt the techniques of minimally invasive surgery (MIS). This reluctance may have stemmed from several factors. Pediatric surgeons typically utilize small incisions during open procedures and therefore the advantage of the MIS approach was not readily apparent. Additionally, adequate instrumentation for MIS in small children required technologic advances above and beyond the standard tools used in adult MIS. Finally, a poor understanding of pain in the pediatric patient tempered enthusiasm for the minimally invasive approach. Despite the aforementioned barriers, pediatric MIS has seen an exponential upsurge in interest in recent years.

INSTRUMENTATION The equipment used during pediatric MIS is similar to that used in adults but on a smaller scale. Pediatric surgeons commonly use 3- to 5-mm scopes and instruments. These instruments are often shorter than their adult counterparts (**FIGURE 1**). When used, trocars are short and may be disposable or reusable. Smaller trocars (3–4 mm) are usually reusable. Because of the thin abdominal wall in neonates and infants, trocars can often become dislodged with instrument changes during the course of an operation. Thus, trocars are often secured to the abdomen by suture or commercially available adhesive products. A standard insufflator may be used for pediatric MIS with the understanding that settings must be adjusted appropriately. Neonates and infants require low pressure (6–8 mm Hg) and flow rates (3–5 L/min). These settings can be increased with age and as tolerated by each patient's individual physiology.

POSITIONING Positioning may vary depending on the organ or body cavity of interest. Abdominal procedures are typically performed with the patient in the supine position with the arms tucked. However, a modified decubitus position may be used during a splenectomy or adrenalectomy. In the case of infants, positioning the patient transversely on the table can often facilitate easier access to the patient and instrumentation. Similarly, when performing upper abdominal surgery, such as gastric fundoplication, in patients too small to be placed in stirrups, modified lithotomy or "frog-leg" positions can be used to shorten the distance between surgeon and target area for the operation (**FIGURE 2A**). In all cases, in order to maximize the freedom of (anterior-posterior) movement for instruments in lateral port sites, smaller children can be elevated off the table with stacked blankets or towels.

Thoracoscopy is often performed with patients in a lateral decubitus position. Unlike what is typical for adults, prepping the ipsilateral arm into the field may allow for greater flexibility of trocar placement and freedom of instrument movement. As with laparoscopy, neonates and small infants may be positioned transversely on the bed (**FIGURE 2B**). This allows both the surgeon and the anesthesiologist to be close to the patient.

INITIAL ACCESS TECHNIQUES Gaining access to the abdomen or chest is a critical maneuver and requires specific considerations in the pediatric population. A full bladder in a small infant or child can become a significant impediment to initial access and procedures in the lower abdomen. A Foley catheter will decompress the bladder and allow for safe trocar placement. Because of the smaller dimensions of a child's abdomen, many surgeons choose not to use a standard Veress needle for entry but instead enter the abdomen using some form of an open technique. In toddlers and young children, the abdomen can be entered directly through the umbilical ring, which usually remains open during the first few years of life. For this technique, the umbilical skin is elevated using toothed forceps, a vertical incision is made in the umbilicus with a #11 blade, and a fine hemostat is used to enter and dilate the ring to the appropriate size (**FIGURE 3**). In neonates and infants up to about 6 weeks of age, an incisionless entry directly through the umbilicus is possible.

Once an umbilical trocar has been placed in a neonate, it is important to ensure that the umbilical vein has not been inadvertently cannulated. Insufflation directly into the umbilical vein can result in massive air embolus and cardiopulmonary collapse. The surgeon can minimize the risk of this by placing the laparoscope into the trocar to ensure an intraperitoneal position *before* insufflating the abdomen. Additionally, it is important to note that the aortic bifurcation and iliac vessels often lie within 1 to 2 cm of the umbilicus. Therefore, when inserting the umbilical cannula, it should be directed superiorly or laterally to avoid major vascular injury. Directing the cannula inferiorly risks injury to the iliac vessels and bladder. It is important to note that in infants, the bladder is considered an intraabdominal organ.

SECONDARY TROCAR PLACEMENT Efficient and ergonomic trocar placement is an essential component of successful MIS. For abdominal cases, the largest trocar is usually placed at the umbilicus. Additional trocars should be placed in such a fashion as to triangulate the operative region of the abdomen. Because of the small working space, trocars and instruments can quickly become crowded in the pediatric abdomen. Therefore, in addition to the use of standard reusable or disposable trocars, needlescopic instruments can be used. Alternatively, instruments can be passed directly into the cavity of interest through stab incisions without the use of trocars. Needlescopic instruments are essentially a combination trocar and instrument with a 2-mm cross-sectional profile. Needlescopic wounds are small enough to heal with virtually no visible scar. Most pediatric patients have thin abdominal or chest walls and allow for instruments to be passed into the cavity through stab incisions. This is accomplished by creating a small incision directly through skin into the abdomen using a #11 blade.

This technique is best used to introduce instruments that will not be exchanged often during the course of the procedure. The stab incision does not typically require fascial closure. Skin closure is typically accomplished through an absorbable suture placement, Steri-Strip coverage, or surgical glue closure. The benefits of the stab incision technique include smaller incisions, improved cosmesis, and reduced cost.

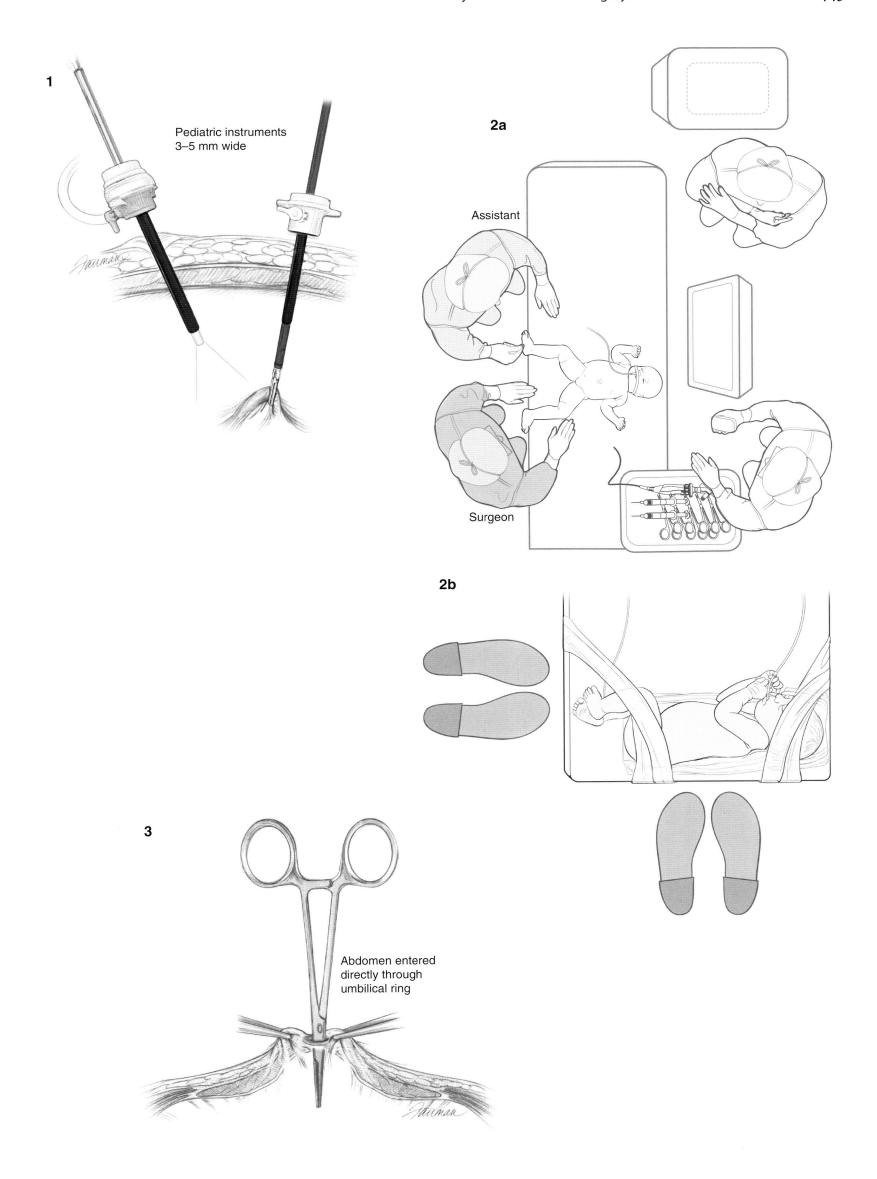

1

Pediatric instruments
3–5 mm wide

2a

Assistant

Surgeon

2b

3

Abdomen entered
directly through
umbilical ring

EXPOSURE TECHNIQUES Because of the small working space in the pediatric abdomen, adequate retraction and exposure are essential components of MIS. Upper abdominal procedures can be facilitated by proper liver retraction. Liver retraction can be accomplished using a variety of techniques. A flexible ring retractor can be passed through a right upper quadrant 3-mm stab incision in order to facilitate liver retraction during a laparoscopic Nissen fundoplication. Liver retraction can also be achieved by passing a transabdominal suture around the falciform ligament, then tying the knot extracoporeally over a buttress (**FIGURE 4A**). When dissecting the porta hepatis, such as in resection of a choledochal cyst, a transabdominal suture can be placed through the fundus of the gallbladder in order to improve exposure (**FIGURE 4B**). The technique of transabdominal suturing is also useful for any procedure that requires suspension of an organ to the anterior abdominal wall. For example, pelvic dissection in girls can be facilitated by temporarily suturing the uterus to the anterior abdominal wall (**FIGURE 4C**).

Creating working space in the pediatric chest is a particularly challenging problem. Single-lung ventilation as performed in adults during thoracoscopic procedures is not always possible, as manufacturers do not produce double-lumen endotracheal tubes for small children and infants. However, effective single-lung ventilation can be achieved through the use of bronchial blockers or contralateral main stem bronchus intubation. Fogarty balloon catheters (sizes 4 and up) can be placed through the endotracheal tube (ETT) and insufflated in the ipsilateral main stem bronchus to act as bronchial blockers. For lobar lung resection, the Fogarty can also be passed through the ETT into the contralateral main stem bronchus and used as a guide over which the ETT can be advanced or pulled back as needed during the procedure to achieve intermittent single-lung ventilation. In this case, intermittent ventilation allows one to test the patency of the airways to the remaining lobes prior to definitive bronchial division of the pathologic lobe. In other cases, simple low pressure (3–4 mm Hg) and low flow (4–6 L/min) CO_2 insufflation can be used to create lung collapse and thus working space for many thoracoscopic procedures.

HEMOSTATIC TECHNIQUES Standard hemostatic techniques and energy devices can by employed during pediatric MIS. Most manufacturers produce a shorter version of their special energy devices. Such devices commonly used in pediatric MIS are Harmonic Scalpel, LigaSure, and Enseal. These devices require the placement of a 5-mm port. For neonates and infants, simple electrocautery applied through 3-mm instruments can be used to divide relatively large vessels such as the short gastrics, cystic artery, and appendiceal artery. Caution should be taken when applying electrocautery in neonates, as collateral heat spread can quickly injure nearby bowel or blood vessels.

As in adults, clips and pre-tied loops of suture can also be used to control bleeding. These commercially available loops have the added benefit of using a 3-mm incision for deployment. Direct pressure of troublesome bleeding in the neonate and infant often results in excellent hemostasis.

UTILITY OF UMBILICAL INCISION The plasticity of the pediatric abdominal wall allows for the umbilical incision to be an extremely versatile tool during MIS. By extending the fascial incision of an umbilical wound a few millimeters in either direction, much of the small bowel or colon can be eviscerated and manipulated. Extracorporeal bowel anastomoses can be readily performed using this approach. By extending the fascial incision cephalad, the pylorus can be delivered through the wound for pyloromyotomy in infants with hypertrophic pyloric stenosis (**FIGURE 5**).

The umbilical incision also provides an excellent portal for specimen extraction. Relatively large tumors, cysts, or specimens can be retrieved from the abdomen by creating a circumferential umbilical skin incision and extending the fascial incision as needed. Large benign cysts can be drained through the umbilical incision by placing a purse-string stitch at the apex of the cyst and passing a suction device into the cyst for decompression. The cyst wall can then be marsupialized or resected laparoscopically. The umbilical incision typically heals well with little to no visible scar.

An appendectomy may be performed through the umbilicus by identifying the appendix, grasping the tip, then externalizing the appendix through the umbilical wound (**FIGURE 6**). The surgeon then performs an extracorporeal ligation of the mesoappendix and transection of the appendix. Given the loose retroperitoneal attachments of the pediatric colon, the entire ascending or descending colon can be readily mobilized using an umbilical incision. The bowel can then be eviscerated through the umbilical wound and an extracorporeal resection and anastomosis can be performed.

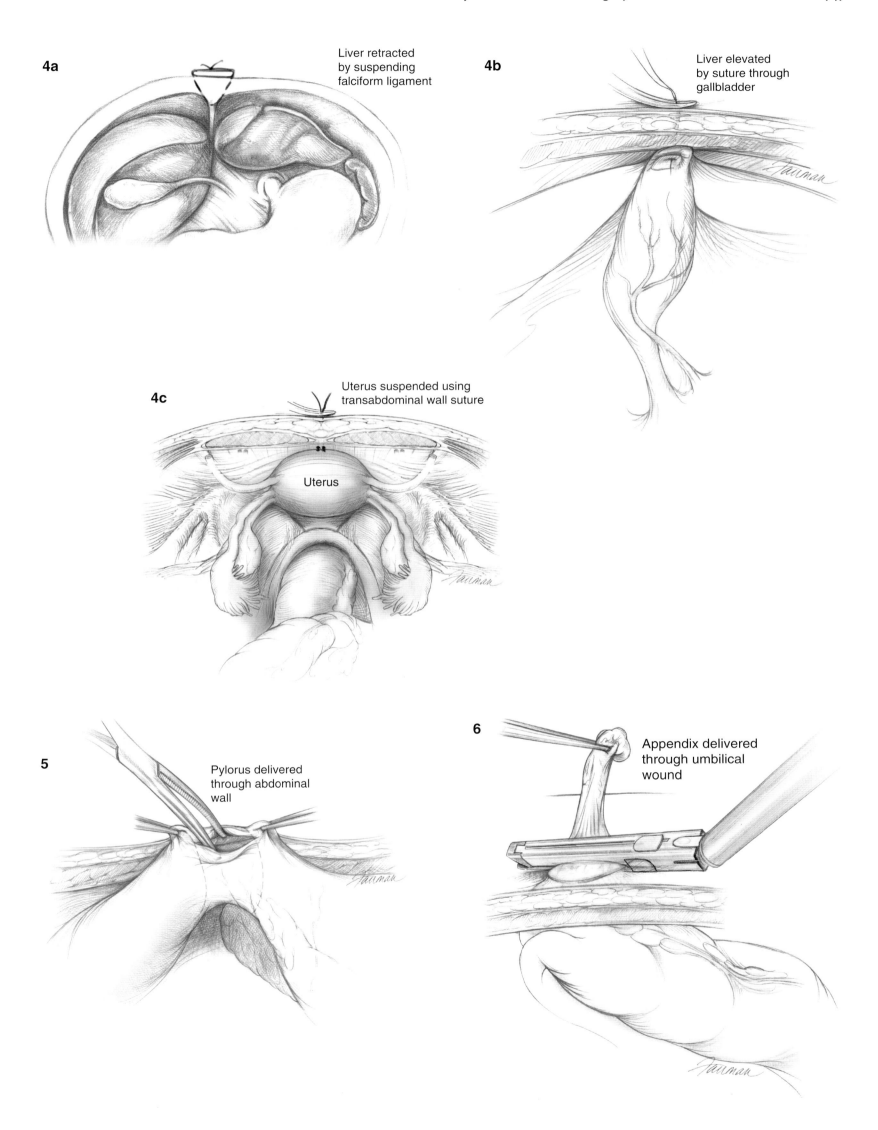

4a

Liver retracted
by suspending
falciform ligament

4b

Liver elevated
by suture through
gallbladder

4c

Uterus suspended using
transabdominal wall suture

Uterus

5

Pylorus delivered
through abdominal
wall

6

Appendix delivered
through umbilical
wound

RESECTION TECHNIQUES Pediatric surgeons often need to resect lesions within the thorax, or hollow and solid viscous organs within the abdomen. In neonates and infants lung parenchyma can be sealed with an advanced energy device. Stapling devices are often too large and cumbersome to use in these small patients. When malignancy is not suspected, specimens can often be retrieved from the chest in piecemeal fashion.

Lesions within the small bowel or colon can be delivered through an umbilical incision for extracorporeal resection (described above). In larger children, intracorporeal resection may be required. For example, a total colectomy can be performed with the use of endoscopic staplers and an advanced energy device (LigaSure, Enseal, Harmonic scalpel). Resection of solid organs such as the spleen, adrenal glands, liver, and ovaries is facilitated using advanced energy devices. Retrieval of these larger organs can be accomplished through cosmetically appealing periumbilical, right lower quadrant, or Pfannenstiel incisions. Transanal retrieval of colon specimens has also been described. In the case of splenectomy, the spleen can be placed intraabdominally within a bag and retrieved in piecemeal fashion through a small umbilical incision. Tumors such as small neuroblastomas or teratomas can also be resected with MIS techniques. The incision required to retrieve the specimen is always smaller than would be required for open resection.

INTRACORPOREAL SUTURING Intracorporeal suturing is an important technique for advanced pediatric MIS procedures. This technique is an essential component of the Nissen fundoplication, thoracoscopic congenital diaphragmatic hernia (CDH) repair, and reconstruction after choledochal cyst resection. The first step of intracorporeal suturing is to pass the needle and suture through the abdominal or chest wall. Because of the radius of the needle, curved needles do not usually pass easily through 3-mm or 5-mm trocars, and, although 12-mm trocars can accommodate most needles, these are used sparingly in pediatric MIS. Therefore, the suture and needle are often passed through stab incisions. The so-called ski needle is a straight needle with a slight curve at the tip. A ski needle can be purchased from a vendor or fashioned by straightening a curved needle. The ski needle has a smaller profile and can usually pass through a 5-mm trocar (**FIGURE 7**). The disadvantage of the ski needle is that it does not work well in small spaces (CDH repair) or when constructing a small anastomosis (hepatojejunostomy).

Knot tying can be performed either extracorporeally or intracorporeally. Extracorporeal knot tying requires a long suture and a knot-pushing device. Intracorporeal knot tying requires greater skill and a larger working space.

Another type of suturing technique can be used to close defects such as inguinal hernias or anterior diaphragmatic hernias (Morgagni hernia). This technique involves making a small skin incision (2 mm) with a #11 blade and passing the needle through the abdominal wall under laparoscopic vision. The surgeon controls the needle extracoporeally and passes the needle around the hernia defect. The needle is driven out through the abdominal wall, but is not completely pulled through all the tissues of the abdominal wall. Once the butt of the needle is in the subcutaneous tissue, it is then driven back toward and through the original small skin incision. Thus a loop of suture is placed around the neck of the hernia defect with both ends of the suture passing through a 2-mm skin incision. The suture is tied down, and the hernia defect is obliterated. The knot buries itself below the level of the skin. This technique is illustrated in Chapter 59.

CLOSURE TECHNIQUES Closure of access sites requires special consideration after pediatric MIS. The fascia of all umbilical access sites should be closed with an absorbable suture. The abdominal wall in children is quite thin, and gaseous distension of the large bowel is common. Thus, great care should be taken when closing access sites in order to prevent occult bowel injury. A thin metal device with a longitudinal indentation such as the grooved director is often used to help guide the needle through the fascia and protect the underlying structures from puncture. This is particularly helpful in thoracoscopic repair of a congenital diaphragmatic hernia where the spleen is at risk just below the repair site (**FIGURE 8**).

In small children with thin abdominal walls, the anterior fascia of 5-mm access sites is often closed as is the skin. In infants and toddlers wearing diapers, no special precautions are typically needed to protect the wounds from urine or fecal contamination. Frequent diaper changes and routine wound care are usually sufficient. ∎

7

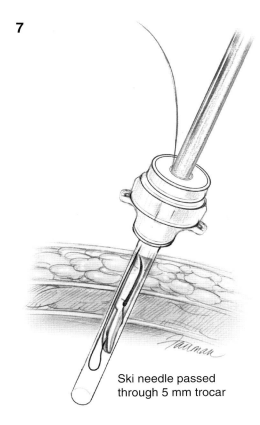

Ski needle passed
through 5 mm trocar

8

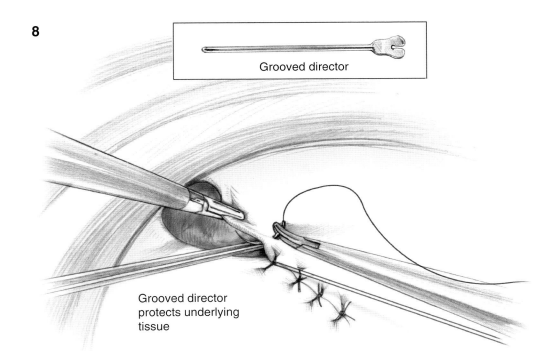

Grooved director

Grooved director
protects underlying
tissue

Pediatric Laparoscopic Inguinal Hernia Repair

BACKGROUND AND INDICATIONS Inguinal hernia repair is the most frequent elective pediatric surgical operation performed by pediatric surgeons. The exact incidence of inguinal hernia in children is not known, but it is somewhere between 1% and 5% and is two to three times more common in premature infants. It is much more common in boys than girls. The diagnosis is almost always made by physical exam, with the palpation of a reducible mass in the inguinal region. In a child the presence of an inguinal hernia is ample indication for surgical repair. If the mass is not reducible, an urgent operation is warranted and the reduction of the bowel is performed as well as inguinal hernia repair.

The essential step in an open surgical repair is performing a high ligation of the patent processus vaginalis (PPV) while maintaining the integrity of the vas deferens and testicular vessels in boys. In girls the round ligament can be divided. Since the advent of minimally invasive techniques, surgeons have devised laparoscopic techniques that accomplish the same goals. The advantages to laparoscopic techniques is that they avoid a groin incision, or make only a very small one. The laparoscopic techniques for inguinal hernia repair differ for boys and girls; both are described here.

ANESTHESIA AND PREOPERATIVE CONSIDERATIONS The patients are consented by their parents for possible bilateral repairs, as it is not infrequent to encounter a contralateral asymptomatic PPV. General anesthesia with endotracheal intubation is necessary for this procedure. Intravenous antibiotics are given at the discretion of the surgeon.

POSITION The patient is draped leaving their umbilicus and groin exposed. The surgeon stands opposite the side of the hernia; the assistant stands opposite the surgeon. Monitors are placed at the feet (**FIGURE 1**).

DETAILS OF PROCEDURE: BOYS A small (3 or 5-mm) laparoscope is placed through the umbilicus after pneumoperitoneum has been established (**FIGURE 2**). Inspection for the presence of PPV is undertaken (**FIGURE 3**). It is sometimes necessary to push from the outside over the inguinal canal to express fluid or air bubbles from the patent process if there is any doubt of its presence. If doubt still remains, then the anatomy can be examined more closely once the instruments are inserted.

A small stab incision is made contralateral to the known hernia in the left or right lateral lower abdomen at the level of the anterior iliac crest. A 3-mm Hunter grasper is inserted. It is helpful if graspers are positioned so that there is a relatively straight approach for the grasper to enter the PPV. If there are bilateral hernias, there is no need to make a second incision and both hernias can be closed with the Maryland grasper from either side.

The external location of the PPV is found by placing the tip of the Maryland grasper at the internal opening of the PPV and palpating the tip through the abdominal wall. Alternatively a needle on a syringe can be used to locate the internal opening under direct visualization (**FIGURE 4**). A small 2-mm skin incision is made over that point.

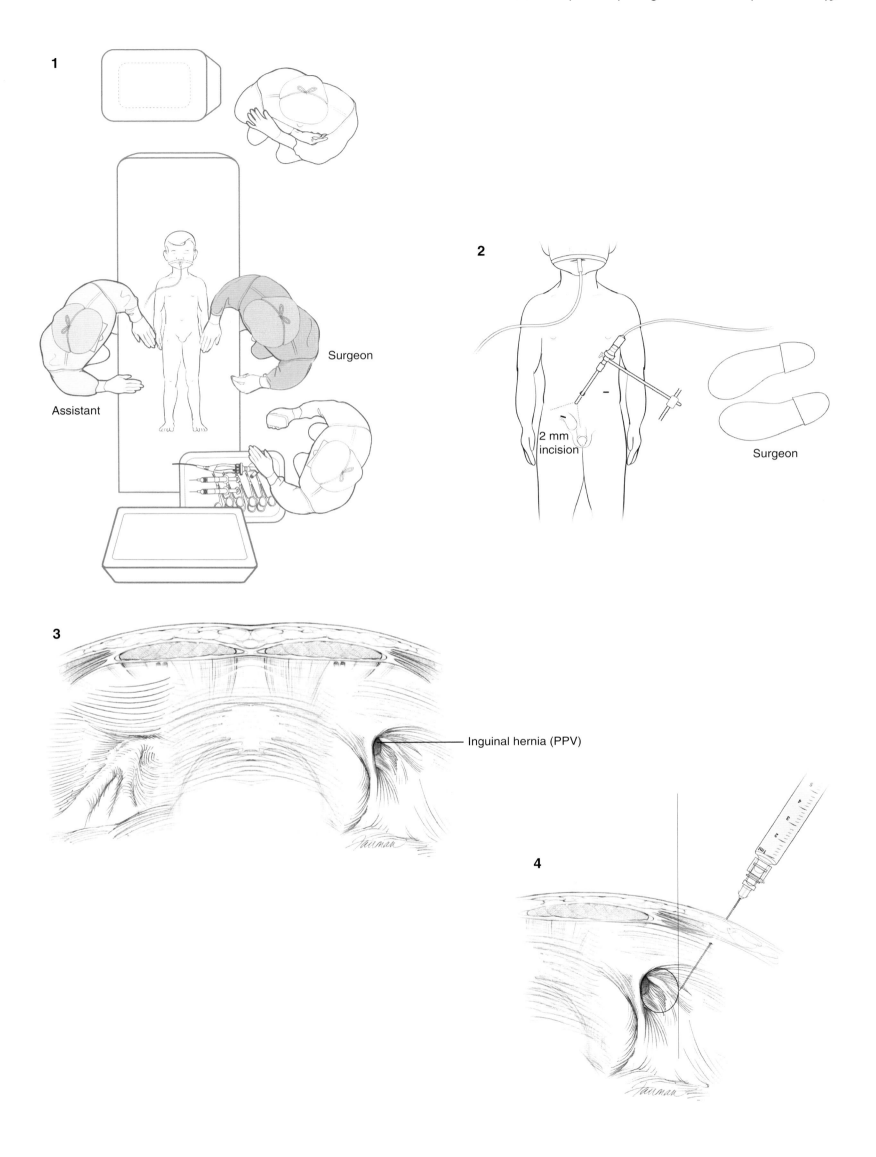

1

Assistant

Surgeon

2

2 mm incision

Surgeon

3

Inguinal hernia (PPV)

4

DETAILS OF PROCEDURE: BOYS Using a 2-0 nonabsorbable-braided suture loaded onto a conventional needle driver, the surgeon inserts the needle in a lateral-to-medial direction to encompass the PPV. The needle is advanced between the femoral vessels and the peritoneum, taking care not to encompass the vessels into the repair (**FIGURE 5A**). With the aid of the Hunter grasper, the needle is directed through the peritoneum, skipped over the vas deferens and spermatic vessels (**FIGURE 5B**), and then reinserted into the peritoneum medial to the vas deferens. The needle is then directed through the peritoneum medial to the vas with the tip partly out of the skin (**FIGURE 5C**). Before leaving the skin, the back of the needle is reinserted medial and anterior to the PPV and directed backward and out of the skin incision near the original point of insertion (**FIGURES 5D–5F**). The suture is tied eliminating the opening to the PPV (**FIGURES 5G AND 5H**). The umbilical incision is closed with an absorbable suture, and the stab wound and groin wound are closed with a single subcuticular stitch. Another perspective on these steps is also shown (**FIGURES 6 AND 7**).

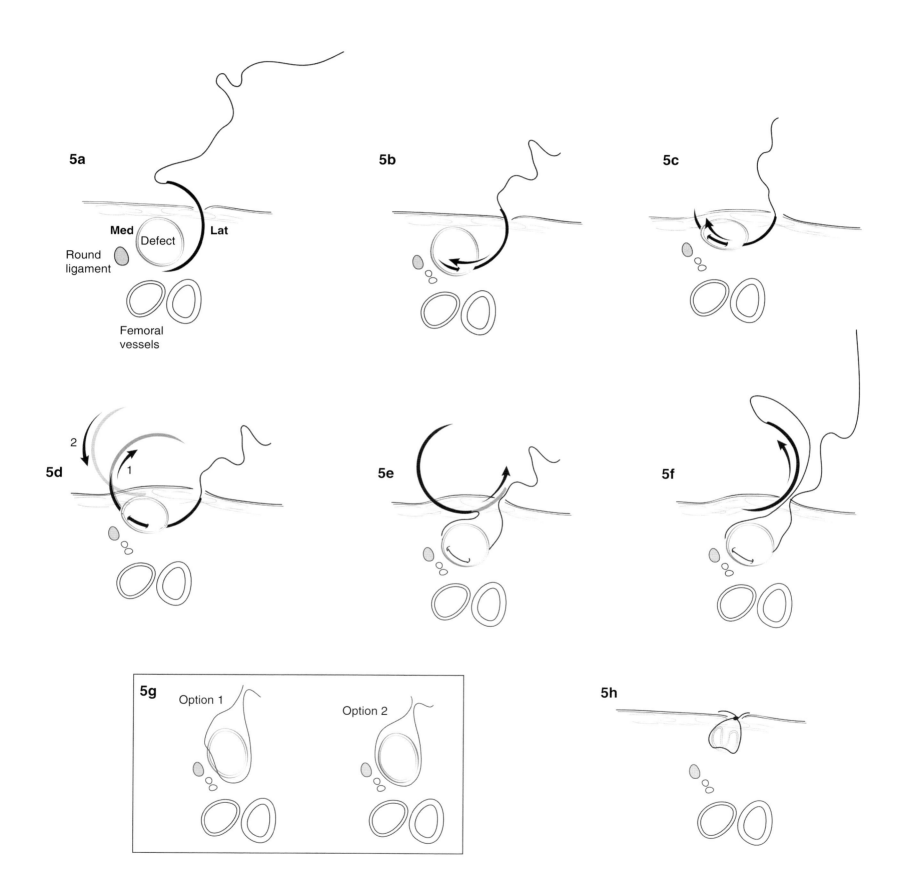

6a

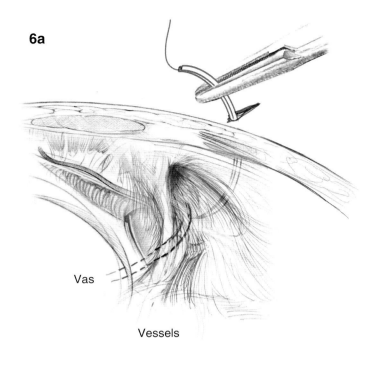

Vas

Vessels

6b

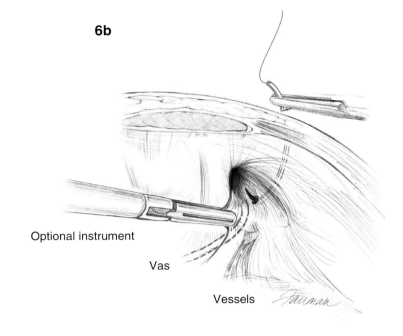

Optional instrument

Vas

Vessels

6c

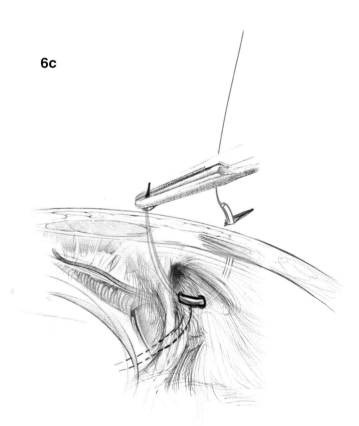

7

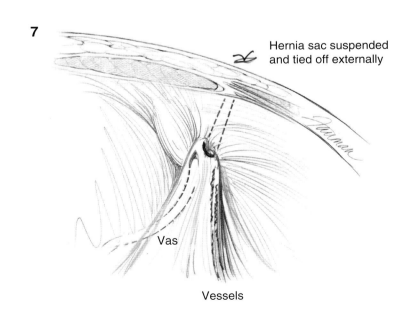

Hernia sac suspended
and tied off externally

Vas

Vessels

DETAILS OF PROCEDURE: GIRLS Similar to laparoscopic hernia repair in boys, two stab wounds that are only large enough to accommodate either 3-mm or 5-mm instruments (depending on patient size) are placed in the bilateral lower quadrants. It is helpful if they are positioned so that there is a relatively straight approach for the grasper to enter the PPV (**FIGURE 8**).

There are two options for closing the PPV in girls. The first technique is similar to that described above for boys (**FIGURE 9A–D**).

Alternatively, an pre-tied ligature of monofilament absorbable suture can be used to ligate the sac internally. It is placed through an incision on the contralateral side of the PPV (**FIGURE 10**). The loop is placed near the opening to the PPV. A Hunter grasper is inserted in the ipsilateral incision and placed down the PPV, through the loop, until it reaches the end of the sac (**FIGURE 11**). The grasper is opened and the sac is grasped and pulled into the abdomen, inverting the sac (**FIGURE 12**).

If the sac is inverted slowly, it will not slip out of the jaws of the grasper. If the fallopian tube is adherent to the sac, the loop is tightened down on the distal part of the sac. The loop serves as a leash for the sac while the fallopian tube is gently dissected off the sac. The suture holding the sac can

be cut short and used as a handle in the abdomen, or it can be left long and brought out either of the stab wounds to facilitate the dissection of structures adherent to the hernia sac. Use of the pre-tied ligature as a handle prevents shredding of the sac that can occur if it is repeatedly grasped during a dissection. If the sac can be completely inverted, it is twisted, and the loop is tightened down at the base of the sac, completing the ligation.

To establish a high ligation of the sac a second loop is placed around the PPV. The sac is grasped and twisted until a high ligation can be established. The inverted sac is cut distal to the second loop and removed (**FIGURE 13**).

The instruments are removed from the abdomen, and the umbilical trocar is removed. The stab wounds are closed with a single 5-0 interrupted subcuticular absorbable suture. The umbilicus is closed with two 2-0 absorbable sutures.

POSTOPERATIVE CONSIDERATIONS Dressings are applied and the patient is awakened. Patients are discharged home with Tylenol for pain relief and are instructed that they can return to normal activities as soon as their discomfort subsides. ∎

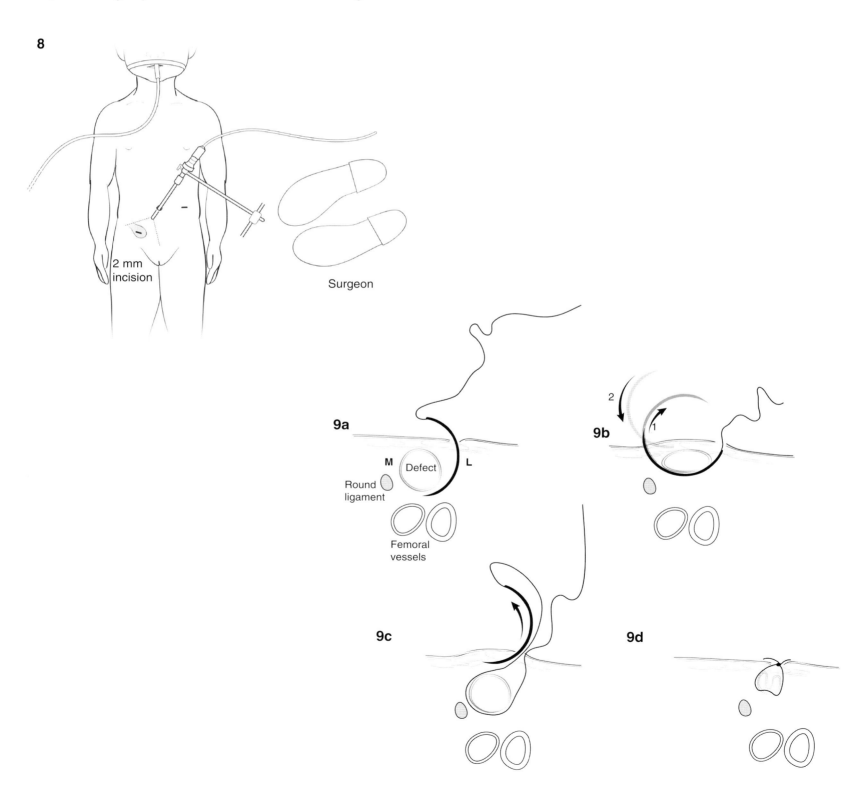

Internal Ligation of the Sac

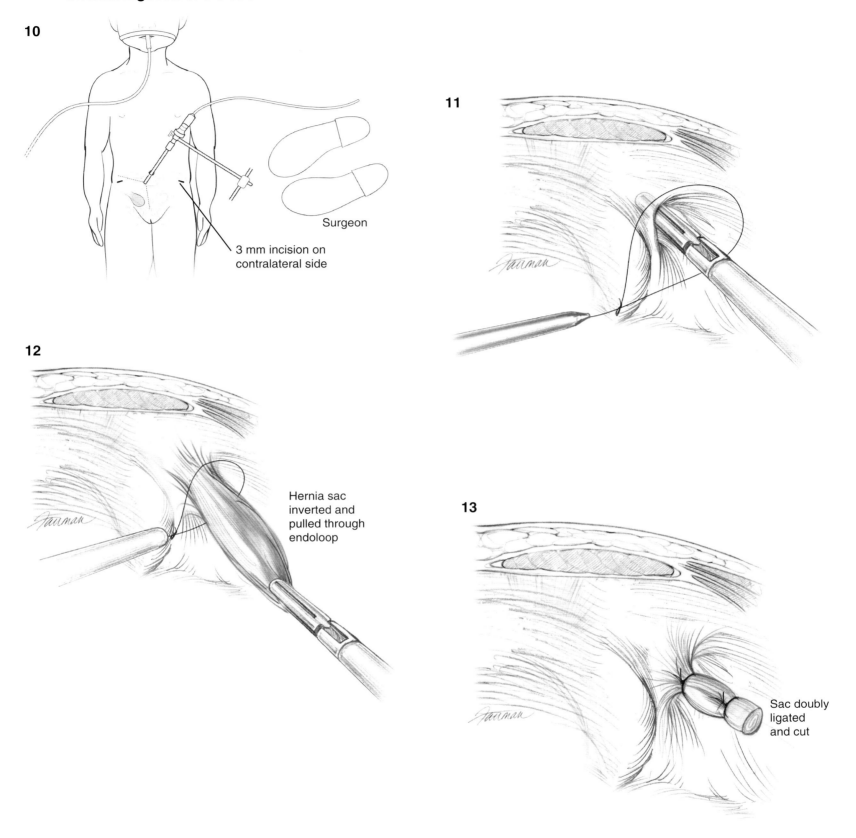

10

Surgeon

3 mm incision on
contralateral side

11

12

Hernia sac
inverted and
pulled through
endoloop

13

Sac doubly
ligated
and cut

PYLOROMYOTOMY FOR PYLORIC STENOSIS

BACKGROUND AND INDICATIONS Pyloric stenosis remains the most frequent surgical cause of vomiting in infancy since its original description more than 100 years ago. The etiology of this disease is still uncertain, but it most commonly presents between 2 and 8 weeks of age and rarely up to 3 months. The typical presentation consists of repeated, nonbilious emesis that can become projectile in nature. The presence of bilious emesis dictates a different workup, as this is almost never pyloric stenosis. Diagnosis is made most frequently with ultrasound. A pylorus that measures greater than 3 mm thick and 17 mm long and does not open to allow the passage of food into the duodenum is diagnostic for pyloric stenosis. Diagnosis can also be made on exam by palpating for the classic "olive" in the right upper quadrant. This can be facilitated by placement of a nasogastric tube and gastric decompression.

Mortality for this disease remained unacceptably high until a muscle-splitting extramucosal pyloromyotomy was perfected and eventually led to an almost 100% survival rate. This technique has since been adapted to a minimally invasive procedure that accomplishes the same operation using smaller incisions.

PREOPERATIVE PREPARATION Once the diagnosis of pyloric stenosis has been established, a careful analysis of the infant's fluid and electrolyte status is important. Electrolyte disturbances, especially hyponatremia, hypokalemia, and hypochloremia in the face of a metabolic alkalosis, are not uncommon and should be corrected prior to surgery. Placement of an IV catheter and administration of normal saline boluses and maintenance fluid should be given until the electrolytes normalize and the infant is making at least 1 mL of urine per hour. The placement of a nasogastric tube is not always necessary during the fluid resuscitation phase, but prior to induction of anesthesia the stomach should be suctioned to help prevent aspiration.

LAPAROSCOPIC TECHNIQUE After the induction of general anesthesia, the infant is positioned across the middle of the OR table with the head turned facing the anesthesiologist. If not already present, an orogastric tube is placed. A large syringe is attached to the tube for later insufflation of the stomach. The infant's legs should be placed frog legged on the table so they do not dangle over the edge (**FIGURE 1**). The infant is prepped and draped and the operators stand at the feet of the infant. A 3-mm trocar can be easily placed through the middle of the umbilicus. Once the trocar has been placed, the abdomen is insufflated to 8 to 10 mm Hg pressure. A 3-mm nontraumatic bowel grasper is placed laterally in the right upper quadrant just below the liver edge. The instrument can be placed directly through the abdominal wall, and a trocar is usually not necessary. A third 3-mm incision is made through the abdominal wall directly over the pylorus (**FIGURE 2**).

Once the instruments are in place, the duodenum is grasped with the bowel grasper. Care must be taken to get a firm grasp on the tissue yet avoid injuring the duodenum by just pinching a little bit of tissue in the graspers. The pylorus is positioned out from under the edge of the liver. The Bovie or pyloromyotomy knife is used to make an incision from the duodenal side of the pylorus to the stomach (**FIGURE 3**). The incision should be no more than 3 mm deep and should not start distal to the pyloric vein of Mayo to avoid a full-thickness incision through the mucosa. Once the incision is made, the Bovie blade is inserted into the incision and the beginning of the "cracking" of the muscle is made by turning the blade back and forth. The goal is to divide the serosa and underlying muscle fibers, while keeping the mucosa intact. The Bovie blade is removed, and either a 3-mm bowel grasper or a laparoscopic pyloric spreader is used to complete the spreading of the muscles (**FIGURE 4**). The myotomy needs to be carried up to the longitudinal muscles of the stomach. The myotomy is considered complete when the two sides of the divided pyloric muscle are able to be moved independently (**FIGURE 5**).

While the duodenum is still grasped, the stomach should be insufflated with air or water to look for a leak from the mucosa. When intact mucosa is confirmed, the instruments are removed, and the abdomen is desufflated through the umbilical trocar.

POSTOPERATIVE CONSIDERATIONS The umbilicus is closed, and the other two incisions can be closed with an absorbable suture or Steri-Strips. The patient is started on a clear liquid diet and advanced as tolerated. ■

1

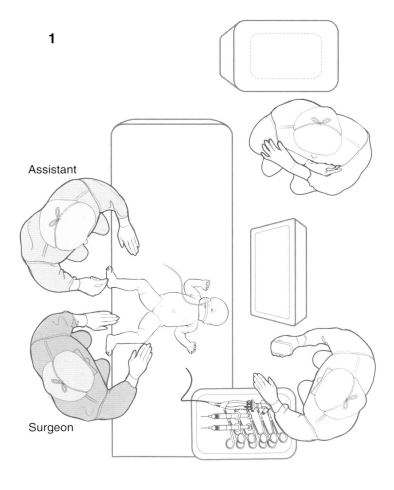

Assistant

Surgeon

2

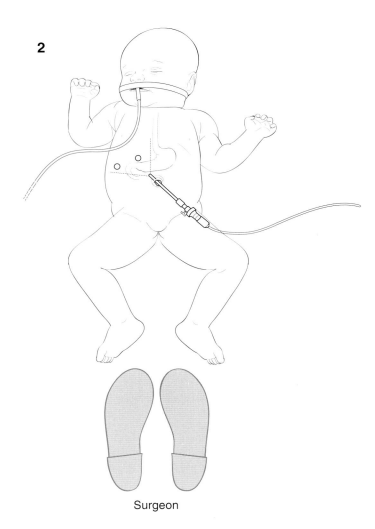

Surgeon

3

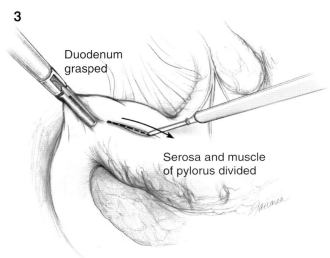

Duodenum grasped

Serosa and muscle of pylorus divided

4

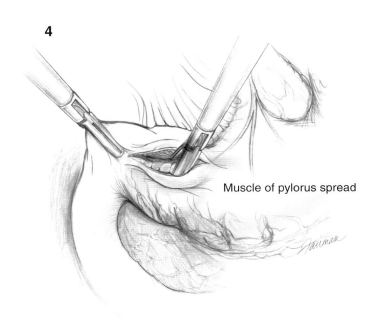

Muscle of pylorus spread

5

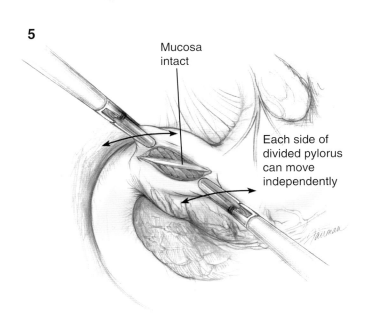

Mucosa intact

Each side of divided pylorus can move independently

Repair of Congenital Diaphragmatic Hernia of Bochdalek

BACKGROUND Posterolateral congenital diaphragmatic hernia (CDH), also known as hernia of Bochdalek, occurs in approximately 1 in 4000 live births. A defect in the diaphragm allows abdominal organs, typically the intestines and stomach, to protrude into the thorax (**FIGURE 1**). The causative factors have yet to be elucidated. Children with this anomaly have variable degrees of both macroscopic and microscopic pulmonary hypoplasia as well as pulmonary arteriolar muscular thickening. The pulmonary hypertension and resultant shunt physiology are the most significant contributors to the life-threatening physiologic compromise that is seen initially in the majority of these patients.

A variety of methodologies including "gentle" ventilation strategies, delayed operative intervention, and extracorporeal life support have increased overall survival from 60% to greater than 80% at some centers. This improved survival has increased the likelihood that surgical repair of the diaphragmatic defect will be needed.

The thoracoscopic approach to CDH has several advantages over the traditional open transabdominal or transthoracic approaches. In addition to the obvious cosmetic benefits, there is decreased intraabdominal adhesion formation and thus a potential for decreased incidence of small bowel obstruction (seen in up to 18%–20% of patients who have undergone open transabdominal CDH repair). Additionally, minimally invasive techniques avoid significant thoracotomy-related complications including secondary scoliosis, shoulder girdle weakness, and chest-wall asymmetry.

INDICATIONS The following criteria are used to determine if the thoracoscopic approach is feasible:

1. Absence of lethal chromosomal or cardiac abnormalities
2. Stable ventilatory status as defined by pre-ductal SaO_2 >90% on less than 0.5 FiO_2, and mean airway pressures ≤15 mm Hg on a nonoscillating ventilator
3. Lack of significant metabolic disturbances by blood gas analysis
4. Minimal or no need for vasoactive drips
5. Echocardiographic evidence of pulmonary pressures in the mild suprasystemic range or lower.

Early postnatal physiologic instability or use of extracorporeal membrane oxygenation (ECMO) in the preoperative period are not seen as contraindications, provided that the patient fulfills the above criteria prior to operative intervention. No specific preoperative anatomic or radiologic criteria are useful in determining the feasibility of the thoracoscopic approach.

PREPARATION A complete discussion of the preoperative care of these children is beyond the scope of this chapter. Once the child has stabilized sufficiently to otherwise be considered for operative repair, nursing staff is asked to reposition the child in the decubitus position for a minimum of 2 hours to mimic operating room positioning and confirm the child's ability to tolerate dependency on the contralateral lung.

ANESTHESIA The risk of precipitous pulmonary hypertension defines much of the intraoperative management. Single-lung ventilation is not needed and may result in greater hypoxemia and increased risk of pulmonary hypertension. Oxygen saturations in the preductal and postductal positions are monitored as indicators of both overall oxygenation and degree of shunt.

Given the heterogeneous physiology of these infants, the choice of monitoring adjuncts such as arterial and central venous lines, specific anesthetic medications and alternatives, crystalloid versus blood product administration, and other diagnostic and therapeutic options are evaluated in each individual's context. Essential principles include maintenance of stable oxygenation, permissive hypercapnia with reasonably consistent end-tidal CO_2 and arterial PCO_2, adequate cardiac preload, minimization of the use of myocardial depressant drugs, and preservation of normal body temperature.

The child is administered a single dose of a first-generation cephalosporin or equivalent antibiotic. Bladder and gastric drainage are important adjuncts.

POSITIONING Once anesthesia is induced, the child is positioned transversely at the end of the bed. The trunk and extremities are elevated on a 5-cm thickness of towels, and the head is extended and rotated away from the side of the defect and supported with a gel or foam doughnut. The cautery pad is placed on the contralateral lower back or thigh. The ipsilateral chest is rotated forward approximately 60 degrees to expose the area of the tip of the 12th rib back to at least the posterior axillary line. This position is maintained using gel rolls. A small cloth roll is used for support of the dependent axilla. The skin is prepped in the standard fashion and draped, allowing access to the upper abdomen (including the umbilicus), ipsilateral chest, neck, shoulder, arm, back, and sternum. Ideally, there are no monitoring devices or lines in the upper extremity on the side of the defect.

The monitor is positioned at the feet of the patient. The surgeon and assistant stand at the child's head and side respectively. The scrub nurse and instruments are positioned between surgeon and assistant (**FIGURE 2**). As working space for the scrub nurse is limited, it may be helpful to position a Mayo stand near the drapes overlying the patient's feet onto which the most frequently used instruments can be placed.

ACCESS After the infiltration of 0.25% bupivacaine in the 2nd or 3rd intercostal space at the midclavicular line, a 3-mm cannula is placed using an open technique with a blunt trocar. The chest is insufflated to 3 cm H_2O pressure at a flow rate of 3 to 5 L/min. Using a 70-degree scope, additional 3-mm trocars are placed under direct vision in a low, parasternal position and in the 5th intercostal space in the midaxillary line. A fourth port in the 7th or 8th intercostal space in the posterior axillary line is placed if necessary (**FIGURE 3**).

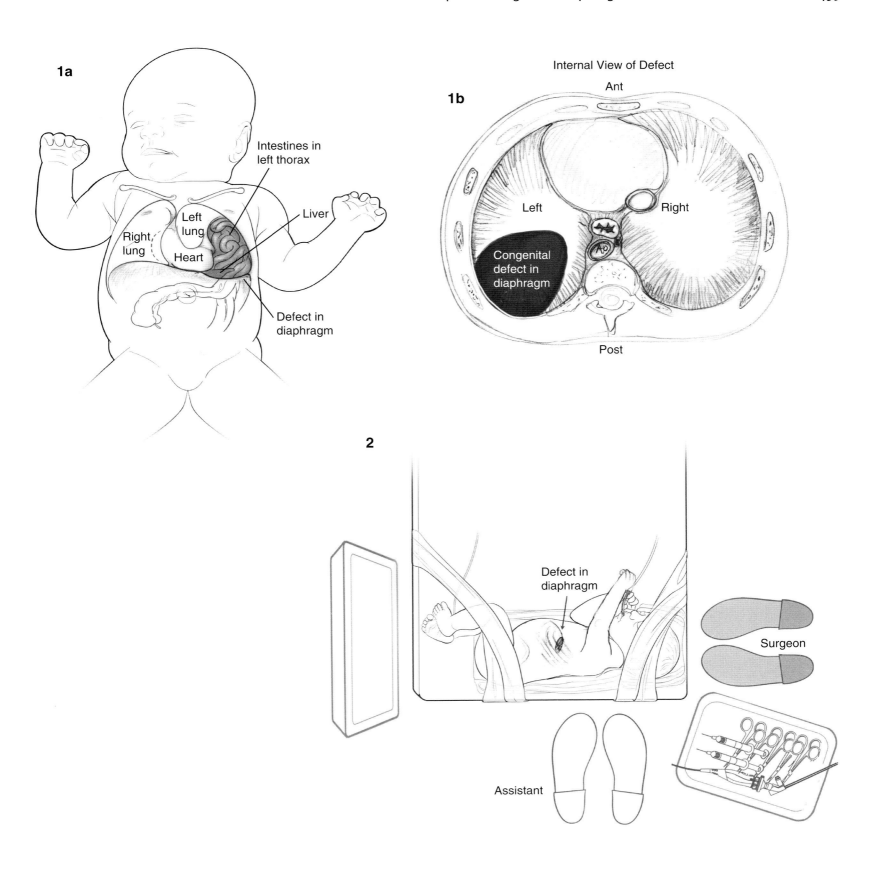

1a

Intestines in
left thorax

Left
lung

Liver

Right
lung

Heart

Defect in
diaphragm

Internal View of Defect

1b

Ant

Left

Right

Congenital
defect in
diaphragm

Post

2

Defect in
diaphragm

Surgeon

Assistant

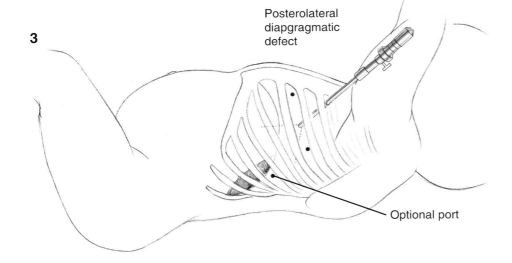

3

Posterolateral
diapgragmatic
defect

Optional port

PROCEDURE The patient is positioned in the reverse Trendelenburg position to facilitate reduction of the abdominal viscera. Using 3-mm Hunter-style graspers placed through the parasternal and mid-axillary trocars, the bowel is gently pushed into the abdomen through the diaphragmatic defect (**FIGURE 4**). As neonatal bowel and mesentery are thin and fragile, gentle and sustained pressure applied across a broad surface area is the safest and most effective technique for reduction. In children with adequate abdominal domain, the viscera will reduce easily and stay within the abdomen, without insufflation. If the viscera will not reduce easily or will not stay reduced, a lack of abdominal domain should be suspected. In this case consideration should be given for a small subcostal abdominal incision to facilitate placement of a temporary preformed abdominal silo. This allows expansion of the abdominal cavity and gradual reduction of viscera over time.

Reduction and maintenance of herniated solid viscera such as liver, spleen, or kidney into the abdomen can be facilitated by the use of a 3-mm coiled retractor (**FIGURE 5**). Special care is taken when reduction of these solid organs is required, as they are easily injured, and this can result in significant hemorrhage.

Once the entire diaphragmatic defect is visualized, the surgeon must determine whether it is amenable to primary repair or will require a prosthetic patch. With the camera in the uppermost trocar and a coiled retractor holding the abdominal viscera below the diaphragm, the anterior diaphragm is grasped with the right-hand device near the widest portion of the defect, and the posterior diaphragm is grasped with the left-hand instrument. If the two sides can be apposed, primary repair should be possible (**FIGURE 6**). If not, the posterior rim may, in some instances, be mobilized. This is accomplished by grasping the posterior rim with the left hand instrument and carrying out sharp or blunt dissection between the diaphragmatic edge and the ipsilateral retroperitoneal organs (**FIGURE 7**). The maneuver to test apposition of the anterior and posterior edges is repeated. If this remains impossible, a prosthetic patch or plug will likely be necessary.

Primary Repair The low, parasternal trocar is removed to facilitate introduction of suture through the orifice. A 2-o Teflon-coated braided polyester suture on a small, curved needle is used with or without felt pledgets. A grooved director instrument can be used to protect underlying tissues and facilitate guidance of the needle. The medial corner of the defect is closed first with an interrupted suture tied extracorporeally. The previous suture is left uncut and secured outside of the patient to facilitate retraction and to flatten the diaphragm medially prior to placement of the following stitch (**FIGURE 8**).

4

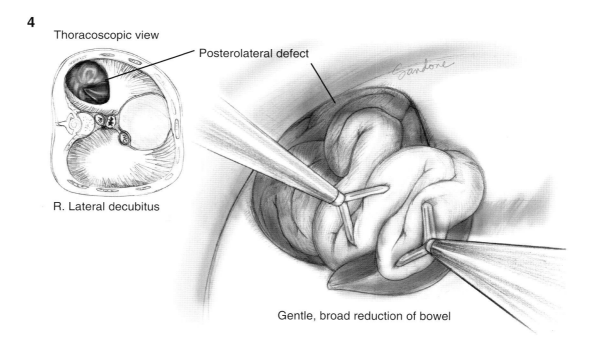

Thoracoscopic view

Posterolateral defect

R. Lateral decubitus

Gentle, broad reduction of bowel

5

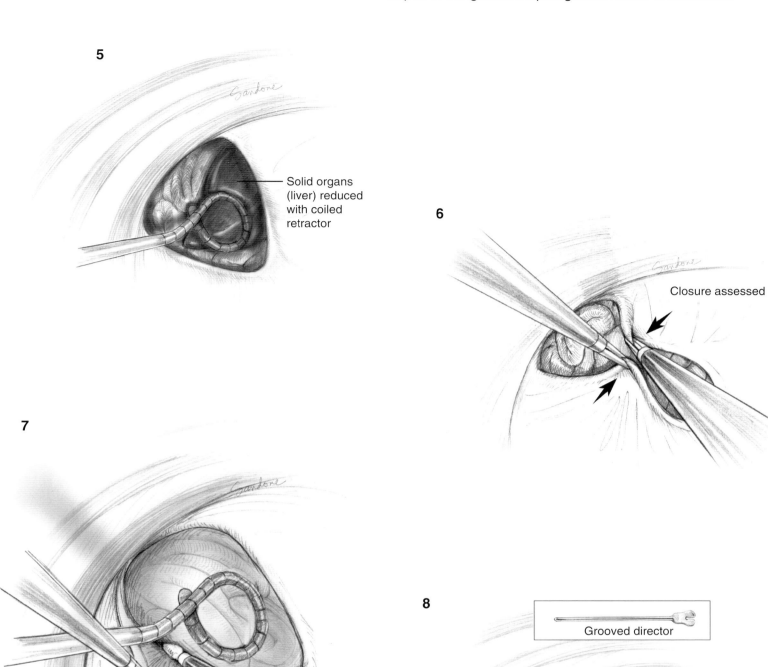

Solid organs
(liver) reduced
with coiled
retractor

6

Closure assessed

7

Posterior rim of defect
mobilized

8

Grooved director

Grooved director
protects
underlying tissue

Primary Repair The diaphragm is closed incrementally with interrupted sutures until the lateral sulcus is reached. At this juncture, there is often little rim of posterior diaphragm, the open space is very small, and the angle to achieve intracorporeal suturing is extraordinarily challenging. Moreover, it can be difficult to see the intraabdominal viscera, leading to increased risk of bowel injury. There are two different means to address this depending on the size of the residual defect. The first uses externally placed sutures and the other uses a prosthetic plug.

If the residual defect is small (angle of remaining defect <90 degrees), it can be repaired with sutures passed directly into the area of the orifice via a small counterincision at the skin correlating with the level of the internal diaphragmatic defect (**FIGURE 9**). This is accomplished by using a needle to define the appropriate location to make an incision. A 2-mm skin incision is made at the indicated point, and the suture is passed into the chest and through the anterior diaphragmatic rim while protecting the abdominal organs. A suture-passing device is then passed through the same skin incision, but enters the chest and brings the suture through the posterior portion of the defect and out the body wall. The suture is tied externally, approximating the defect to the body-wall fascia. Additional sutures are placed until the defect is completely closed (**FIGURE 9**).

Prosthetic Repair When a defect is too large to close primarily (angle of defect >90 degrees), a prosthetic bridge is required (**FIGURE 10**). Very large defects, such as those seen with diaphragmatic agenesis, are closed using dual sided mesh. The defect size is estimated by comparing the length of instrument required to traverse it from medial to lateral as well as in an anterior-to-posterior dimension. The patch is sized, rolled tightly, introduced through the midaxillary trocar incision, and unfurled. It is sewn in place using the identical suture and technique described above, including using externally introduced sutures in the lateral sulcus (**FIGURE 11**).

More commonly the defect is 4 cm or less, and in this case a premade inguinal hernia plug is used. The midaxillary trocar site is enlarged slightly to accommodate the size of the plug. The plug is then inserted apex-first into the chest and, in the same orientation, into the residual diaphragmatic defect. The plug is secured at four to six positions with sutures until it does not appear to move or dislodge with negative intrathoracic pressure created by suctioning within the free space of the chest (**FIGURE 12**). Because fewer sutures are needed for fixation, the use of a prosthetic plug has greatly reduced operative time when compared to a patch technique in cases where the defect is not amenable to complete primary closure.

CLOSURE All trocar sites are closed at the fascial level. Postoperative pneumothorax may occur because of minor abrasions to the lung that were incurred during diaphragmatic repair. Therefore, a 10 French chest tube is placed via the midaxillary trocar incision and visualized thoracoscopically to lie in an anterior position. The skin sites are closed to be airtight, and routine postoperative dressings are placed.

POSTOPERATIVE CARE Routine care is undertaken once the patient returns to the neonatal intensive care unit. A chest x-ray is obtained to establish a radiographic baseline after repair and to confirm proper endotracheal and chest tube positioning. Sedation is typically provided while the infant is mechanically ventilated. For analgesia, patients are placed on acetaminophen 15 mg/kg around the clock for the first 48 hours, and IV narcotics are administered as needed.

Ventilator weaning is accomplished based on the patient's physiology. The thoracostomy tube is removed once any air leak resolves, which is typically within the first 48 hours. Enteral feeding is commenced once any postoperative ileus has resolved and is given via nasogastric tube if the patient remains ventilated for an extended period. ■

9

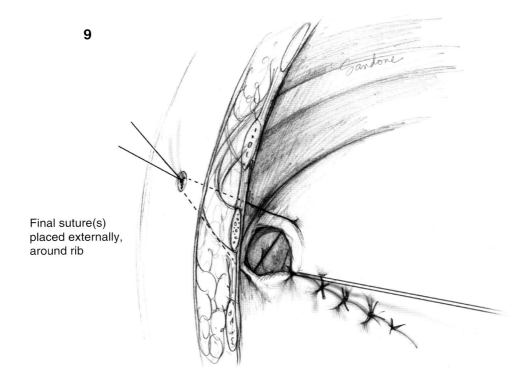

Final suture(s) placed externally, around rib

10

Angle of closure evaluated

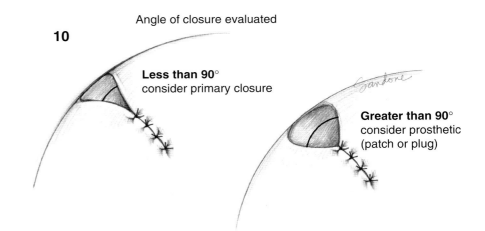

Less than 90° consider primary closure

Greater than 90° consider prosthetic (patch or plug)

Angle greater than 90° requires a patch or plug

11   **12**

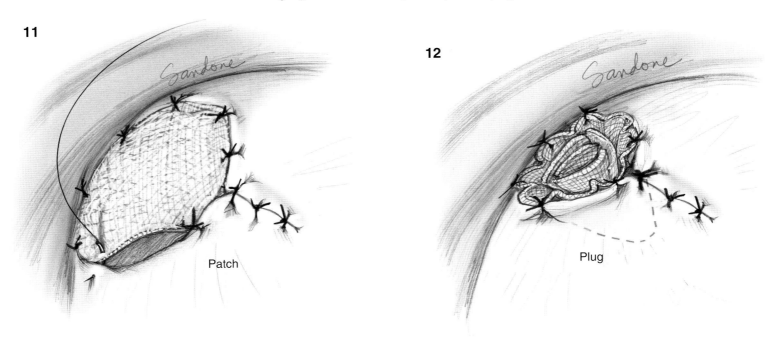

Patch   Plug

ENDORECTAL PULL-THROUGH FOR HIRSCHSPRUNG DISEASE

INDICATIONS Minimally invasive correction of Hirschsprung disease (congenital megacolon) may be employed in nearly all affected children. Approximately 80% of children afflicted with Hirschsprung disease will have aganglionosis confined to the rectum and rectosigmoid. The principles of operation for Hirschsprung disease are to remove the aganglionic section of the rectum and sigmoid and to perform a coloanal anastomosis in a portion of the colon with biopsy-proven ganglion cells present. In order to define the point of resection and pull-through, biopsies must be obtained. Often a clear transition from spastic, narrow distal bowel to the often thickened, dilated colon can be visualized (**FIGURE 1**).

Five percent of patients will have longer segment disease, especially when associated with a syndrome (Down—10%, congenital central hypoventilation, or Von Wardenburg) or a strong family history (5%). Hirschsprung disease is four times more common in boys than in girls. Over 80% of Hirschsprung patients will present with failure to pass meconium in the first 24 hours of life, whereas the remainder may have enterocolitis or varying degrees of chronic constipation. A small percentage will escape detection early in life and may reach adolescence or adulthood and present to adult general surgeons.

Although the vast majority of children may be candidates for corrective operation using MIS techniques, there are a few relative contraindications including active enterocolitis, chronic and severe colonic dilatation, and extension of aganglionosis beyond the terminal ileum.

In many cases, pull-through procedures may be completed by a transanal method alone. Circumstances where laparoscopic assistance is beneficial include transition zones that are unclear or are proximal to the sigmoid colon, difficult transanal mobilization, or concern for bleeding from mesenteric vessels.

PREPARATION Though the majority of children with this disorder have no associated significant anatomic or physiologic derangements, a complete history and physical is required to determine the coincidence of Down syndrome and its associates, neural cristopathies, and family history of Hirschsprung disease or lifelong constipation. Special attention should be paid to the child's nutritional state, degree of abdominal distension, and signs or symptoms of enterocolitis.

In general, mechanical bowel preparation is not required in neonates. However, older children may have a significant amount of stool stored within the colon that must be washed out by both antegrade and retrograde means. A complete blood count with or without a type and cross are obtained to ensure adequate red cell mass. Urinalysis may be needed if symptoms are evident, as urinary stasis and infection may coexist in a child with chronic megarectum. Single-agent preoperative antibiotics such as a second-generation cephalosporin should be administered. In the operating room after the induction of anesthesia, the surgeon should perform rectal irrigations until the effluent is clear prior to initiation of the operation.

ANESTHESIA General anesthesia is the most common approach to this disorder, though regional techniques such as single-shot caudal injection can be used. If the technique used is entirely transanal, it may be unnecessary to employ chemical paralytic agents. However, to perform laparoscopy, a deep plane of general anesthesia and paralysis is generally needed. Standard monitoring methods are employed unless additional devices are indicated for comorbidity. An upper-body radiant warmer may be employed. Gastric decompression may be needed intraoperatively but is generally not required postoperatively. In neonates, it is desirable to have the lower torso and extremities free of any attachments, including intravenous catheters and monitoring devices. An indwelling bladder catheter is placed once the child is positioned.

POSITION Patient positioning is dependent on patient age and habitus. The vast majority of Hirshsprung disease is addressed operatively prior to the age of 6 months. After the successful induction of anesthesia and the performance of a final rectal irrigation, the child is positioned supine at the end of the bed away from the anesthesiologist. The endoscopic control tower is placed cephalad to the patient's left shoulder with the monitors facing the perineum. The right-handed surgeon stands at the patient's right shoulder and the assistant on the opposite side (**FIGURE 2**). The cautery pad is placed high on the posterior thorax. The lower body is cleaned circumferentially, towels are placed at the level of the breast nipples, and an extremity drape is pulled over the legs and torso. The legs are wrapped to prevent heat loss, and the wrapping is secured to the drape on the anterior chest.

OPERATIVE PROCEDURE

Laparoscopic Mobilization The umbilicus is cannulated using a 3-mm trocar. CO_2 insufflation is initiated with pressures of 8 to 15 cm H_2O, determined by the child's age, size, and tolerance. Additional trocars are placed in the left upper quadrant and the right lower quadrant (**FIGURE 3**). If a vessel sealing device is to be used, at least one trocar will need to be 5-mm diameter. The 30- and 45-degree scopes are essential for this procedure.

In order to define the point of resection and pull-through, biopsies must be obtained. If a clear transition from spastic, narrow distal bowel to the often thickened, dilated colon is visualized, partial-thickness biopsies are obtained from at least one area above and below the transition area using a laparoscopic shears without the application of energy. It is important to perform the proximal biopsy at least 2 to 3 cm above the end of the transition zone to avoid areas of hypoganglionosis. Additional frozen-section biopsies are obtained more proximally, as needed, until normal ganglia are present and neural hypertrophy is not present (**FIGURE 4**).

1

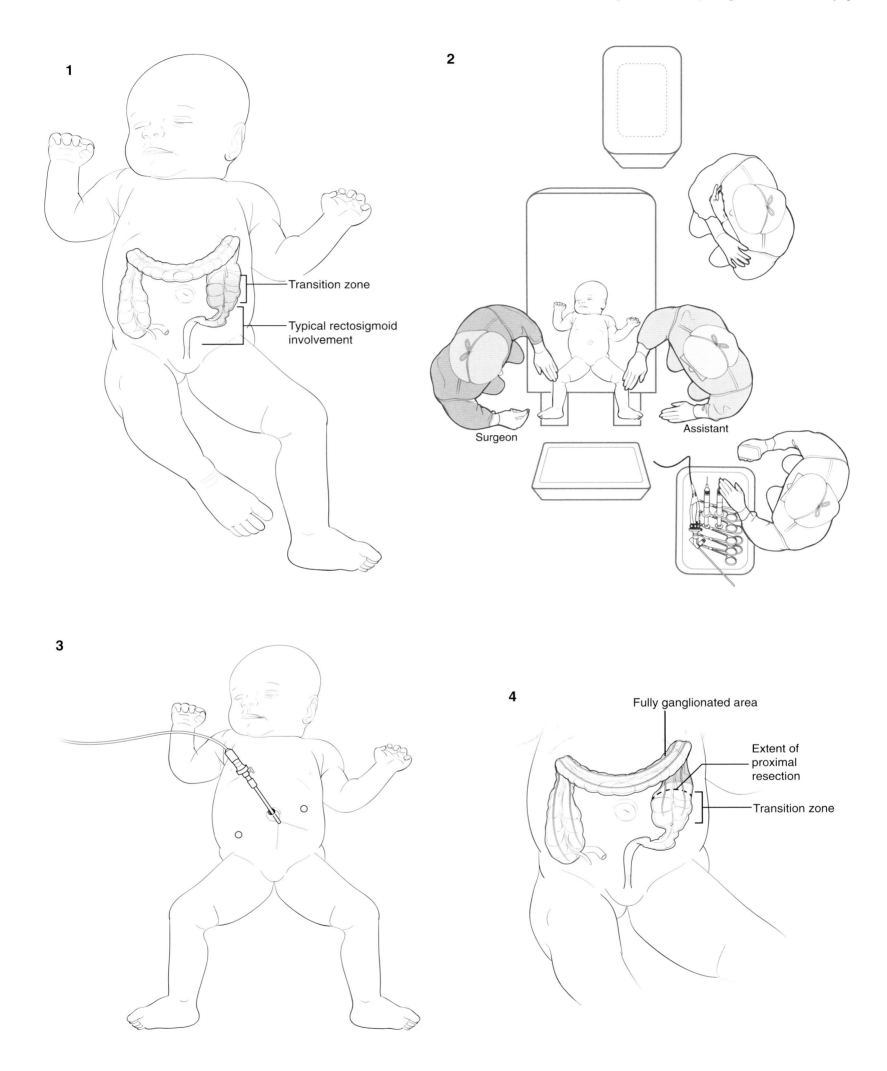

Transition zone

Typical rectosigmoid involvement

2

Surgeon

Assistant

3

4

Fully ganglionated area

Extent of proximal resection

Transition zone

Laparoscopic Mobilization The descending colon is grasped and retracted medially until the white line of Toldt can be visualized and divided. The dissection is carried caudad, with care taken to identify and preserve the gonadal vessels and the ureter (**FIGURE 5**). The extent of proximal dissection is determined by the colonic mobility. In the majority of cases it is not necessary to divide the splenic flexure attachments.

In the event that a transition zone is not apparent, serial biopsies should be performed in the same manner described above at 5- to 8-cm intervals until normal bowel is defined. The blood supply to the distal bowel is divided using either hook cautery (neonates) or a vessel sealing device. As the pelvic brim and more distal blood supply are approached, dissection should be confined to the mesentery nearest the bowel wall to avoid injury to pelvic nerves. The dissection is continued distally into the pelvis, where it will be later met by the upper extent of the transanal dissection. The trocars are removed and the incisions closed at fascial and skin levels.

Transanal Dissection Sterile towels are placed under the perineum to support the pelvis and catch any effluent from the rectum. The surgeon and assistant may sit or stand facing the perineum (**FIGURE 6**). A headlamp is recommended.

Traction sutures are placed at the anal verge and immediately caudad to the dentate line in a radial fashion to cause prolapse of the anal mucosa. At a distance of 0.5 to 1.0 cm cephalad to the dentate line, the mucosa is marked with cautery circumferentially (**FIGURES 7A AND 7B**). Epinephrine in saline 1:100,000 is injected submucosally cephalad to the cautery line to facilitate hemostasis. While applying downward traction, a submucosal flap is created circumferentially, beginning at the previously mentioned mark and progressing cephalad using cautery (**FIGURE 8**). Gradual traction on the mucosa will deliver it from the anal canal. Perforating vessels are cauterized as the muscular layers of the rectum are separated circumferentially. Dissection is carried cephalad until the mucosa "rolls out" easily and circular smooth muscle of the rectosigmoid is noted. Care must be taken to remain in the submucosal plane so as not to injure the sphincter mechanism and to achieve complete mucosal extirpation. Once adequate mucosa has been delivered, an umbilical tape may be used to ligate the rectum to stop any continued leakage and to provide better traction.

Traction sutures are placed through the muscular layer at the 3 and 9 o'clock positions. At a small distance beyond the muscular sutures, a full-thickness, circumferential incision is made in the rectosigmoid muscle (see Figure 8).

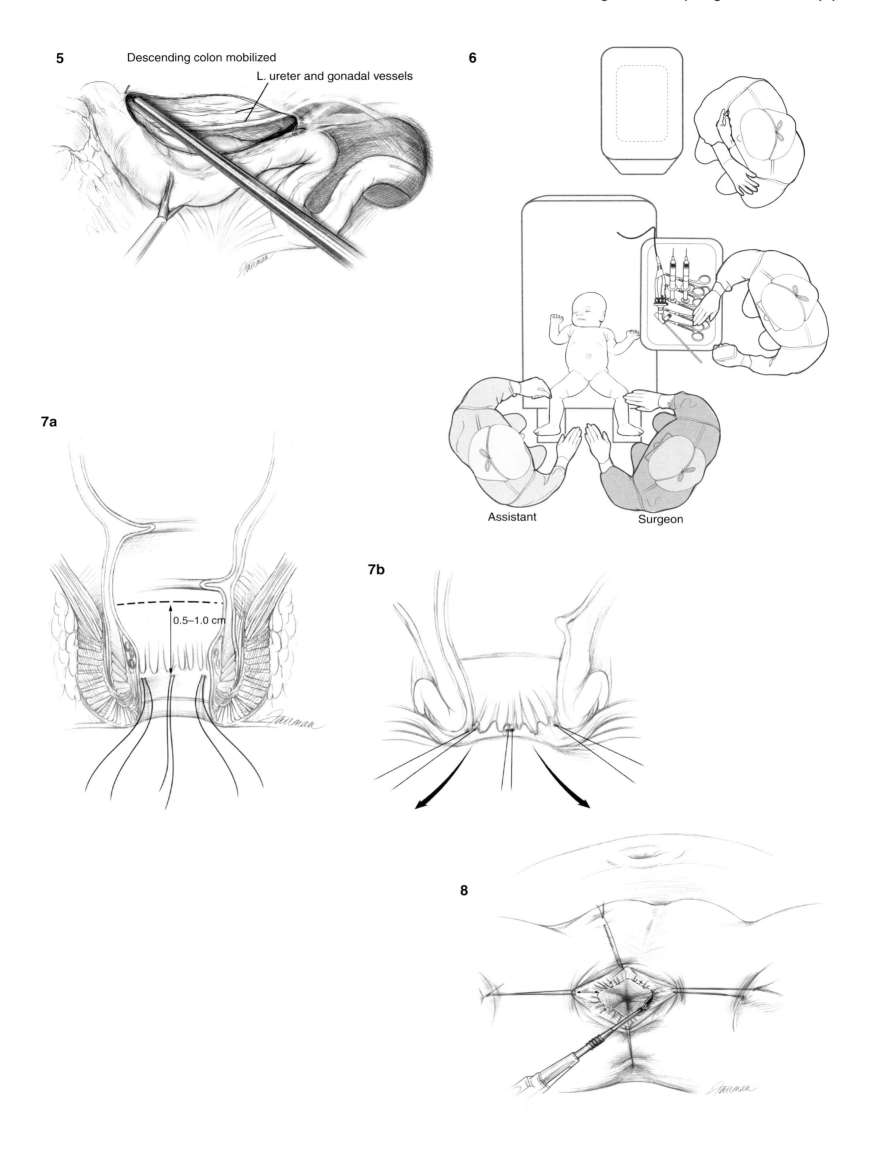

5 Descending colon mobilized

L. ureter and gonadal vessels

6

Assistant   Surgeon

7a

0.5–1.0 cm

7b

8

Transanal Dissection   Further traction on the umbilical tape will begin to deliver full-thickness rectosigmoid (**FIGURE 9**). A marking stitch is placed in the anterior wall of the pull-through segment to maintain orientation. Mesorectal vessels are divided close to the serosal edge to avoid injury to pelvic structures, including the nerve plexus, vas deferens, seminal vesicles, and ureters.

Mobilization by this method continues cephalad until the transition zone is visible or the surgeon wishes to obtain intraoperative frozen-section biopsy to define the location of normally ganglionated bowel without neural hypertrophy (**FIGURE 10**).

Once the appropriate point is defined by biopsy, the pull-through segment is opened across the anterior 50% of the colon (**FIGURE 11**). A rigid dilator is passed into the cephalad bowel to ensure that it has not been inadvertently twisted. Using a 4-0 absorbable suture on a fine needle, the pull-through segment is transfixed to the anorectum at the site of the original cautery entry at the 12, 3, and 9 o'clock positions with partial thickness of rectal muscle and mucosa followed by full thickness of the pull-through bowel (**FIGURE 12**). These stitches are left untied and clamped until the surface area between each is approximated.

It is not necessary to secure the pulled-through bowel to the retroperitoneum. The surgeon should ensure that the pull-through bowel is not twisted prior to initiating the anastomosis.

The anterior portion of the anastomosis is completed in an interrupted fashion with care taken to avoid creating any gaps that predispose to a leak. The posterior portion of the bowel is divided and the specimen sent for pathologic examination to confirm the presence of normal ganglion cells and the absence of neural hypertrophy. The midline posterior of the pull-through bowel is transfixed to the 6 o'clock position of the rectum in the same fashion as above. The remaining gaps are closed with interrupted, absorbable

sutures, and the corner stitches are tied (**FIGURE 13**). The anastomosis is once again inspected, and if no problems are encountered, the external traction sutures are removed and the anorectum returned to its anatomic position.

POSTOPERATIVE CARE   In general, pain is managed with oral acetaminophen and/or codeine. Parenteral narcotics are used judiciously and require monitoring for apnea, bradycardia, and hypoxemia. All individuals involved in the care of the child should be informed that, during the first 2 weeks, no one should perform digital rectal examination, suppository placement, rectal temperature, or other interrogation of the anus other than under controlled circumstances such as in the operating room. Oral feedings may be initiated as soon as postoperative day one and are advanced depending on the child's bowel function. Fever, abdominal pain, or prolonged ileus may prompt investigation for anastomotic leak, obstruction, or injury to intraabdominal gastrointestinal structures. The combined incidence of these complications should be less than 1%.

A high percentage of coloanal anastomoses in infants will narrow sufficiently to require serial dilation. In infants, daily dilations are initiated in the office beginning with an 8- or 9-mm rigid dilator. Every 2 weeks the dilator is exchanged for the next larger size until the anus can admit a 14-mm dilator. Digital rectal exam is performed every 4 weeks until dilations cease. Rarely, surgical revision or strictureplasty is needed.

Long term outcomes are determined by the length of aganglionosis, associated anomalies, and the quality of anal sphincter function. In addition, children remain at risk for potentially life-threatening enterocolitis for up to 2 years after surgery. Patients should be followed intermittently until continence is assured. Many will require physician-directed bowel programs, treatments for anal sphincter hypertonicity, and occasional antegrade enema systems. ∎

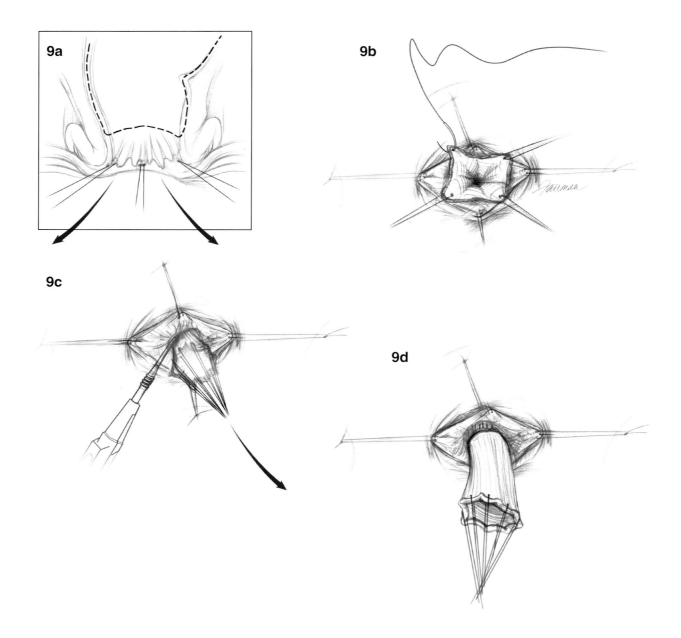

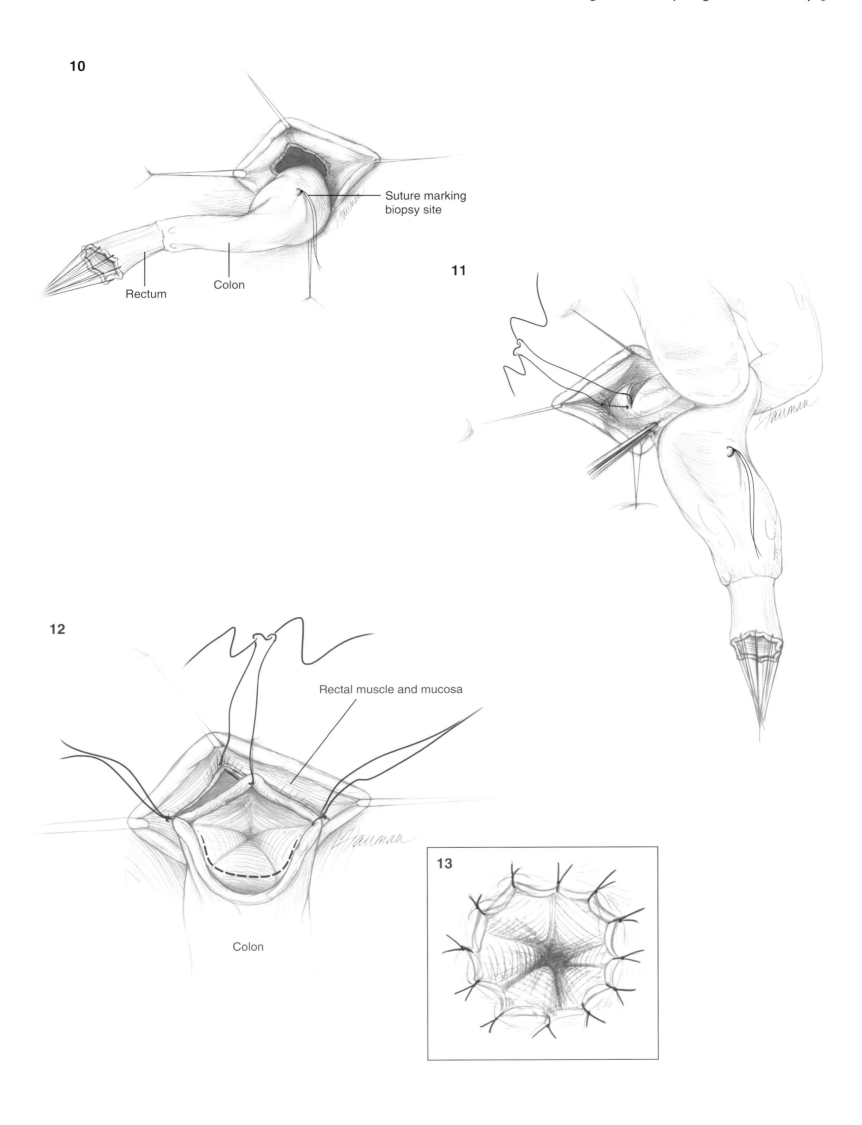

10

Suture marking
biopsy site

Rectum   Colon

11

12

Rectal muscle and mucosa

Colon

13

INDEX

Note: Page number followed by f indicate figure only.

INDEX

Note: Page number followed by f indicate figure only.

OPERATIONS